Rapid Response to Everyday Emergencies

➤ A NURSE'S GUIDE

LIPPINCOTT WILLIAMS & WILKINS
A **Wolters Kluwer** Company

Philadelphia • Baltimore • New York • London
Buenos Aires • Hong Kong • Sydney • Tokyo

STAFF

Executive Publisher
Judith A. Schilling McCann,
RN, MSN

Editorial Director
H. Nancy Holmes

Clinical Director
Joan M. Robinson, RN, MSN

Senior Art Director
Arlene Putterman

Editorial Project Manager
William Welsh

Clinical Project Manager
Mary Perrong, RN, CRNP, MSN,
APRN,BC

Editor
Elizabeth Jacqueline Mills

Clinical Editors
Karen A. Hamel, RN, BSN;
Tamara Kear, RN, MSN, CNN
Jana L. Sciarra, RN, CRNP, MSN

Copy Editors
Kimberly Bilotta (supervisor),
Amy Furman,
Kelly Pavlovsky,
Lisa Stockslager,
Pamela Wingrod

Designer
Jan Greenberg (project
manager)

Digital Composition Services
Diane Paluba (manager),
Joyce Rossi Biletz,
Donna S. Morris

Manufacturing
Patricia K. Dorshaw
(director), Beth J. Welsh

Editorial Assistants
Megan L. Aldinger,
Karen J. Kirk, Linda K. Ruhf

Indexer
Barbara Hodgson

RPDRSPONS — D N O S A J J M
07 06 05   10 9 8 7 6 5 4 3 2 1

**Library of Congress
Cataloging-in-Publication Data**
Rapid response to everyday emergencies: a nurse's guide.
     p. ; cm.
  Includes bibliographical references and index.
  1. Emergency nursing — Handbooks, manuals, etc. I. Lippincott Williams & Wilkins.
  [DNLM: 1. Nursing Care — methods — Handbooks. 2. Emergency Nursing — methods — Handbooks.   WY 49 R218 2006]
    RT120.E4R37 2006
    610.73'6 — dc22
ISBN 1-58255-430-7 (alk. paper)   2005002797

Rapid Response to *Everyday Emergencies*

➤ A NURSE'S GUIDE

Contents

Contributors and consultants

Haralee Abramo, RN, MSN
Director of Education
Los Robles Hospital and
  Medical Center
Thousand Oaks, Calif.

Karen Balich-Reitz, RN, MS
Quality Facilitator
MacNeal Hospital
Berwyn, Ill.

Anne L. Bateman, RN, EdD, APRN,BC, PMH
Assistant Professor, Nursing and
  Psychiatry
University of Massachusetts
Worcester

Laura M. Criddle, RN, MS, CEN, CCNS,
  CNRN
Doctoral Student
Oregon Health and Science
  University
Portland

Cynthia L. Dakin, RN, PhD
Assistant Professor
Northeastern University
Boston

Laura Favand, RN, BSN, MS
Chief Nurse Education and
  Training
Army Trauma Training Center
Ryder Trauma Center
Miami

Sharon Lee, RN, MS, BSN, FNP, CCRN
Family Nurse Practitioner,
  Emergency RN
Bryan LGH Medical Center
Lincoln, Nebr.

Elizabeth Molle, RN, MS
Nurse Educator
Middlesex Hospital
Middletown, Conn.

Ruthie Robinson, RN, MSN, CCRN, CEN, CNS
Director, Magnet Program and
  Clinical Research
Christus St. Elizabeth Hospital
Beaumont, Tex.

Belinda L. Spencer, RN, MSN, CCRN,
  APRN,BC
Chief Nurse
Army Trauma Training Center
Ryder Trauma Center
Miami

Warren Stewart, RN, BSN, CEN
Staff Nurse
Irwin Army Community Hospital
Ft. Riley, Kans.

Robin Walsh, RN, BSN, CEN
Clinical Nurse Supervisor
University Health Services at the
  University of Massachusetts
Amherst

Rita M. Wick, RN, BSN
Education Specialist
Berkshire Health Systems
Pittsfield, Mass.

Foreword

As a nursing student, I longed to work in an exciting, high-acuity practice setting. After graduation, as I began my career in the real world of professional nursing, I quickly learned that true emergencies can be terrifying events, especially to a novice. An interesting dichotomy emerged: Despite my initial desire to work in an action-packed setting, I suddenly wanted all of my patients to be absolutely stable. Each new crisis challenged my ability to respond competently and effectively cope with the aftermath of my actions. I would replay each scenario in my mind and wonder if I could have done anything differently.

It was a frustrating experience.

I eventually learned my lessons, but it wasn't easy. In those days, emergency care algorithms and protocols weren't widely available or even taught to most nurses. We were expected to adapt—and because of that, the stress and strain of learning how to rapidly respond weighed upon me heavily.

Luckily for you, *Rapid Response to Everyday Emergencies: A Nurse's Guide* is an all-new title specifically designed to demystify emergency situations by providing vital emergency-response information in a quick-scan format. This user-friendly handbook gives students and experienced nurses alike a practical need-to-know clinical reference that offers prioritized, highly bulleted guidance for instant crisis management.

The book's concise yet highly detailed structure is just one of many innovations that make it such a valuable reference. It begins with a chapter on emergency essentials, which includes an overview of how to conduct primary and secondary surveys—tools that, if used properly, rapidly identify life-threatening emergencies and enable you to prioritize your care. This chapter also discusses triage and basic life-support guidelines, which are two aspects of nursing care that every nurse should occasionally brush up on.

The rest of the book is broken down into chapters by either body system or trauma type, and the disorders in each chapter are listed in alphabetical order to facilitate its quick-access format. Forget about paging through this book to find what you need. *Rapid Response to Everyday Emergencies: A Nurse's Guide* allows you to locate information in a flash.

Once you're at the entry, the book speeds you along even faster. Crucial information pertinent to each emergency is presented up-front for easy access; pathophysiology and other background content follows. Just the right amount of supplemental information allows for a critique of the event and a discussion of clinical issues surrounding the emergency.

In addition to the core text, *Rapid Response to Everyday Emergencies: A Nurse's Guide* emphasizes key points in a variety of ways. Sidebars filled with insightful information abound, and eye-catching logos draw attention to some of the most important clinical points. *In Action* presents case studies of actual emergencies and provides in-depth analysis on how to best manage them. *Complications* highlights warning signs and symptoms to monitor for and the actions to take should they develop. *Alert* details crucial points in the management of crisis situations. The inclusion of appendices on emergency cardiac drugs and normal and abnormal serum drug levels enhance the book's overall utility.

In my experience, knowledge, focus, and anticipation are essential in emergency management. Knowledge involves recognition of the situation through assessment and critical thinking, as well as prioritizing actions. Focus is necessary to block out extraneous information and concentrate on critical aspects of care. Anticipation is vital to stay one step ahead, be prepared for complications that may arise, and to plan for ways to prevent the emergency altogether. *Rapid Response to Everyday Emergencies: A Nurse's Guide* illustrates this approach like no other book on the market. It's a part of my reference library, and I highly recommend that it become a part of yours.

Linda Laskowski-Jones, RN, MS, APRN,BC, CCRN, CEN
Director, Trauma, Emergency & Aeromedical Services
Christiana Care Health System – Christiana Hospital
Newark, Del.

1

Emergency essentials

What comes to mind when you hear the word emergency? Do you think of a motor vehicle accident, a drowning, or a patient with cardiac arrest coming through the doors of the emergency department (ED)? Or, do you visualize a postoperative patient experiencing respiratory distress or a patient falling while trying to walk to the bathroom? Emergencies occur everywhere. No matter what your area of expertise, you'll encounter emergencies in your nursing career. This chapter will give an overview of emergency situations and your role in responding to patients who need your help.

When a patient arrives in the ED by ambulance, it's important to get as much information as you can from the prehospital care providers. For instance, if the patient was involved in an accident, you'll want to know the following information:

➤ Mechanism of injury—How did the accident occur? What type of accident was it? If it was a motor vehicle accident, did the vehicle sustain exterior or interior damage? Was the patient restrained? Did the patient have to be extricated from the vehicle? Was he ambulatory at the scene? If the patient sustained a burn injury, was he found in an enclosed space? If the burn resulted from a fire, was the fire accompanied by an explosion?

➤ Injuries sustained—What injuries have the prehospital care providers identified or suspected? What are the patient's chief complaints?

➤ Vital signs—What vital signs have they obtained before arriving in the ED?

➤ Treatment—What treatment have they provided to the patient and how did he respond?

Prehospital care providers can give invaluable information to expedite diagnosis and treatment of the patient.

All patients with traumatic injuries should be assessed rapidly in a systematic method used consistently for all patients. The Emergency Nurses Association (ENA) has developed the Trauma Nursing Core Course to teach nurses such a method for assessing trauma patients. The ENA method uses primary and secondary surveys to rapidly identify life-threatening emergencies and prioritize care; these surveys are reviewed below.

➤ Primary survey

The primary survey begins with an assessment of airway, breathing, and circulation—the ABCs learned in nursing school. The ENA recommends additional assessment parameters—neurologic status, designated as disability (D), and exposure and environment, designated as (E). (See *Primary assessment of the trauma patient.*) The ABCDE primary survey consists of the following:

➤ *A:* Before you assess the airway of a trauma patient, immobilize the cervical spine by applying a cervical collar. Until proven otherwise, assume that the patient who has sustained a major trauma has a cervical spine injury. When continuing your assessment, note whether the patient can speak; if he can, he has a patent airway. Check for obstructions to the airway, such as the tongue (the most common obstruction), blood, loose teeth, or vomitus. Clear airway obstructions immediately, using the jaw thrust or chin lift technique to maintain cervical spine immobilization. You may need to use suction if blood or vomitus are present. Insert a nasopharyngeal or oropharyngeal airway if necessary—but remember that an oropharyngeal airway can only be used on an unconscious patient. An oropharyngeal airway stimulates the gag reflex in a conscious or semi-conscious patient. If a nasopharyngeal or oropharyngeal airway fails to provide a patent airway, the patient may require intubation.

➤ *B:* Assess the patient for spontaneous respirations, noting their rate, depth, and symmetry. Obtain oxygen saturation with pulse oximetry. Is he using accessory muscles to breathe? Do you hear breath sounds bilaterally? Do you detect tracheal deviation or jugular vein distention? Does the patient have an open chest wound? All major trauma patients require high-flow oxygen. If the patient doesn't have spontaneous respirations or if his breathing is ineffective, ventilate him by using a bag-valve-mask device until intubation can be achieved.

➤ *C:* Check for the presence of peripheral pulses. Determine the patient's blood pressure. What's his skin color—does he exhibit pallor, flushing, or some other discoloration? What's his skin temperature—is it warm, cool, or clammy to the touch? Is the patient diaphoretic? Is there obvious bleeding? All major trauma patients need at least two large-bore I.V. lines because they may require large amounts of fluids and blood. A fluid warmer should be used if possible. If the patient exhibits external bleeding, apply direct pressure over the site. If he has no pulse, initiate cardiopulmonary resuscitation immediately.

➤ *D:* Perform a neurologic assessment. Use the Glasgow Coma Scale to assess the patient's baseline mental status. You may also assess the patient using the mnemonic *AVPU,* in which A represents an alert and oriented patient, V indicates response to voice, P represents response to pain, and U indicates an unresponsive patient. Maintain cervical spine immobilization until X-rays confirm that there's no cervical injury. If the

➤ PRIMARY ASSESSMENT OF THE TRAUMA PATIENT

Parameter	Assessment	Interventions
A = Airway	➤ Airway patency	➤ Institute cervical spine immobilization until X-rays determine whether the patient has a cervical spine injury. ➤ Position the patient. ➤ To open the airway, make sure that the neck is midline and stabilized; next, perform the jaw-thrust maneuver.
B = Breathing	➤ Respirations (rate, depth, effort) ➤ Breath sounds ➤ Chest wall movement and chest injury ➤ Position of trachea (midline or deviation)	➤ Administer 100% oxygen with a bag-valve mask. ➤ Use airway adjuncts, such as an oropharyngeal or a nasopharyngeal airway, an endotracheal tube, an esophageal-tracheal combitube, or cricothyrotomy, as indicated. ➤ Suction the patient as needed. ➤ Remove foreign bodies that may obstruct breathing. ➤ Treat life-threatening conditions, such as pneumothorax or tension pneumothorax.
C = Circulation	➤ Pulse and blood pressure ➤ Bleeding or hemorrhage ➤ Capillary refill and color of skin and mucous membranes ➤ Cardiac rhythm	➤ Start cardiopulmonary resuscitation, medications, and defibrillation or synchronized cardioversion. ➤ Control hemorrhaging with direct pressure or pneumatic devices. ➤ Establish I.V. access and fluid therapy (isotonic fluids and blood). ➤ Treat life-threatening conditions such as cardiac tamponade.
D = Disability	➤ Neurologic assessment, including level of consciousness, pupils, and motor and sensory function	➤ Institute cervical spine immobilization until X-rays confirm the absence of cervical spine injury.
E = Exposure and environment	➤ Environmental exposure (extreme cold or heat) and injuries	➤ Examine the patient to determine the extent of injuries. ➤ Institute appropriate therapy determined by environmental exposure (warming therapy for hypothermia or cooling therapy for hyperthermia).

patient isn't alert and oriented, conduct further assessments during the secondary survey.

➤ *E:* Expose the patient to perform a thorough assessment. Remove all clothing to assess all of his injuries. Remember, if the patient has bullet holes or knife tears through his clothing, don't cut through these areas. Law enforcement will count on you to preserve evidence as necessary. Environmental control means keeping the patient warm. Remember, you have removed all of the patient's clothes. Cover him with warm blankets. You may need to use an overhead warmer, especially with an infant or a small child. Use fluid warmers when administering large amounts of I.V. fluids or blood. A cold patient has numerous problems with healing.

Remember that the primary ABCDE survey is a rapid assessment intended to identify life-threatening emergencies, which must be treated before the assessment continues.

➤ Secondary survey

After the primary survey is completed, perform a more detailed secondary survey, which includes a head-to-toe assessment. This part of the examination identifies all injuries sustained by the patient. At this time, a care plan is developed and diagnostic tests are ordered.

➤ Obtain a full set of vital signs initially including respirations, pulse, blood pressure, and temperature. If you suspect chest trauma, get blood pressures in both arms.

Next, perform the five interventions:

– Initiate cardiac monitoring.

– Obtain continuous pulse oximetry readings. Be aware, however, that readings may be inaccurate if the patient is cold or in hypovolemic shock.

– Insert a urinary catheter to monitor accurate intake and output measurements. Many urinary catheters also record core body temperatures. Don't insert a urinary catheter if there's blood at the urinary meatus.

– Insert a nasogastric (NG) tube for stomach decompression. Injuries, such as a facial fracture, contraindicate the use of an NG tube; if a facial fracture is suspected, insert the tube orally instead. Depending on your facility's policy and procedures, the physician may insert the NG tube when facial fracture is suspected.

– Obtain laboratory studies as ordered, such as type and crossmatching for blood; a complete blood count or hematocrit and hemoglobin level; toxicology and alcohol screens, if indicated; a pregnancy test, if necessary; and serum electrolyte levels.

➤ Facilitate the presence of the patient's family. Several organizations, including the ENA and the American Heart Association, endorse the practice of allowing the patient's family to be present during resuscitation.

> **MEMORY TIP: SAMPLE**

The acronym SAMPLE is a mnemonic that will help you remember the types of information you'll need to obtain for the patient's history.

Subjective: What does the patient say? How did the accident occur? Does he remember? What symptoms does he report?

Allergies: Does the patient have allergies and if so, to what is he allergic? Is he wearing a MedicAlert bracelet?

Medications: Does the patient take medications on a regular basis and if so, what medications? What medications has he taken in the past 24 hours?

Past medical history: Has the patient been treated for medical conditions and if so, what condition(s)? Has he had surgery and if so, what type of surgery?

Last meal eaten/Last tetanus shot/Last menstrual period: When was the last time the patient had anything to eat or drink? When did he have his most recent tetanus shot? (If unknown, administer one in the emergency department.) If the patient is a female of childbearing age, when was her last menstrual period? Could she be pregnant?

Events leading to injury: How did the accident occur? Inquire about precipitating factors, if any. For instance, the patient being seen for injuries sustained in a motor vehicle accident may have had the accident because he experienced a myocardial infarction while driving. Likewise, the patient who sustained a fall might have fallen because he tripped or became dizzy.

It's important, however, to assess the family's needs before offering permission to be present. Family members may need emotional and spiritual support from you or from a member of the clergy. If a family member wishes to be present during resuscitation, assign a medical professional to explain procedures as they're performed.

➤ Calm the patient's fears. During a tense trauma situation, the urgency of the assessment and treatment processes may cause you to overlook the patient's fears. Remember to talk to the patient and explain the examination and interventions being administered. An encouraging word and tone can go a long way to comfort and calm a frightened patient. Comfort measures also include the administration of pain medication and sedation as needed.

➤ Obtain the patient's history, remembering to obtain as much information as possible to determine the presence of coexisting conditions that could affect his care or factors that might have precipitated the trauma. (See *Memory tip: SAMPLE*.) Next, perform a head-to-toe assessment, starting at the patient's head and working your way down to his feet. Don't forget to check all posterior surfaces. Logroll the patient (with assistance, if necessary) to assess for injuries to the back. Address any life-threatening injuries immediately.

➤ *Triage*

Triage is a method of prioritizing patient care according to the type of illness or injury and the urgency of the patient's condition. It's used to ensure that each patient receives care appropriate to his need and in a timely manner.

Many people with nonurgent conditions come to the ED because it's their only source of medical care; this increase in nonurgent cases has necessitated a means of quickly identifying and treating those patients with more serious conditions. The triage nurse must be able to rapidly assess the nature and urgency of problems for many patients and prioritize their care based on that assessment.

The ENA has established guidelines for triage based on a five-tier system:

➤ Level I—resuscitation: This level includes patients who need immediate nursing and medical attention, such as those with cardiopulmonary arrest, major trauma, severe respiratory distress, and seizures.
➤ Level II—emergent: These patients need immediate nursing assessment and rapid treatment. Patients who may be assessed as level II include those with head injuries, chest pain, stroke, asthma, and sexual assault.
➤ Level III—urgent: These patients need quick attention, but can wait as long as 30 minutes for assessment and treatment. Such patients might report to the ED with signs of infection, mild respiratory distress, or moderate pain.
➤ Level IV—less urgent: Patients in this triage category can wait up to an hour for assessment and treatment; they might include those with an earache, chronic back pain, upper respiratory symptoms, and a mild headache.
➤ Level V—nonurgent: These patients can wait up to 2 hours (possibly longer) for assessment and treatment; those with sore throat, menstrual cramps, and other minor symptoms are typically assigned to level V.

If you can't decide which triage level is best for a patient, assign him the higher level.

Carefully document the patient's chief complaint and vital signs, your triage assessment, and the triage category to which you've assigned him. It's also important to document pertinent negatives. For example, if the patient is experiencing chest pain without cardiac symptoms, be sure to note "Patient complains of nonradiating left chest pain. Denies shortness of breath, diaphoresis, or nausea. Pain increases with movement and deep inspiration." Quote the patient when appropriate.

As you perform triage, tell the patients you interview that you are the triage nurse and that you'll be performing a screening assessment. Be attentive to what's occurring beyond your current assessment because it may be necessary to leave the patient if a patient with a more critical situation arrives in the ED. Maintain communication with patients waiting to be summoned to a treatment room because a patient's status may change—improving or worsening—during an extended period in the waiting room.

➤ *Emergencies throughout the hospital*

It's no surprise that emergencies aren't confined to the ED—they occur throughout the facility and you need to be prepared to respond regardless of the unit to which you're assigned.

Responding to an emergency situation always begins with the ABCDEs discussed earlier. Likewise, basic life support (BLS) is always performed the same way, whether it's done within or outside the ED. The American Heart Association BLS algorithm provides the following guidelines:

➤ Check responsiveness—call the patient and gently shake or tap him to see if there's a response.
➤ If no response, call for help.
➤ Open the airway—use the head tilt/chin lift method.
➤ Check breathing—look, listen, and feel for respirations.
➤ Breathe—if the patient isn't breathing, give two full breaths.
➤ Assess circulation—assess for signs of circulation for 10 seconds only.
➤ If circulation is present—continue rescue breathing and reassess circulation every minute.
➤ If circulation isn't present—begin chest compressions.

Patients experiencing cardiopulmonary arrest are managed with BLS as described above until advanced cardiac life support (ACLS) measures are available. ACLS involves advanced airway techniques (intubation), defibrillation, and emergency drug administration.

Falls are a commonly encountered emergency in most facilities. Again, assessing the ABCDEs is the first step in caring for the patient who has fallen. Follow the primary survey with the secondary survey. Assist the patient back to bed if possible. Document your findings in the medical record. Notify the primary care provider that the patient fell. Most facilities also require that you file an incident report when a patient falls. Reviewing the report, which documents the circumstances of the fall, may enable the staff to institute measures that will prevent or decrease the incidence of falls. Every patient should be assessed for fall risk upon admission and appropriate fall precautions instituted as needed.

Respiratory distress is another common emergency. Respiratory difficulties can be caused by many conditions, such as fluid overload, asthma, allergic reactions, and pulmonary embolus. In addition to the ABCDEs, it's important to provide verbal reassurance to the patient in respiratory distress to decrease his anxiety. Administer supplemental oxygen and, if not contraindicated, raise the head of the bed to ease respiratory effort. The patient may find it helpful to hang his legs off the side of the bed and lean on an overbed table. If he needs to assume this position, remain with him to prevent falls. Notify the primary care provider as soon as possible. Anticipate orders for a chest X-ray, arterial blood gas levels, an electrocardiogram, or a breathing treatment. The patient's history and reason for hospitalization can help you identify the reason for the respiratory distress.

An anaphylactic reaction is a severe allergic reaction that constitutes a life-threatening emergency situation; untreated anaphylaxis can lead to bronchoconstriction, circulatory collapse, and death. If the patient is receiving blood products, immediately discontinue them and replace with normal saline solution administered through new I.V. tubing. (Initiate an I.V. line if not already present.) Raise the head of the bed and apply high-flow oxygen. Notify the primary care provider immediately and have epinephrine available for administration. Other drugs that may be used to treat an anaphylactic reaction include antihistamines and corticosteroids. Discharge teaching for this patient will include wearing a MedicAlert bracelet and, possibly, carrying an epinephrine kit at all times.

➤ *Loss of consciousness*

A patient may experience loss of consciousness due to numerous conditions. His history and reason for hospitalization will provide clues to the etiology of the event, and the cause will guide the treatment. A few potential causes of loss of consciousness are listed below.
➤ Alcohol or drugs—Even the hospitalized patient may consume alcohol or drugs; he could have brought the substances into the facility himself or a visitor might have brought them. Do you smell alcohol on the patient's breath? Is there a history of alcohol consumption? Is there evidence of track marks? What's the patient's pupillary response? Is the breathing shallow? Does the patient respond to naloxone (Narcan)?
➤ Seizures—Is it possible that the patient has suffered a seizure? Is there a history of seizures? Has the patient experienced bladder or bowel incontinence?
➤ Metabolic disturbances—Does the patient have a history of liver or renal failure? Diabetes? Check the blood glucose level at the bedside. If the patient is hypoglycemic, does he respond to I.V. dextrose?
➤ Head trauma—Has the patient recently suffered head trauma? An elderly patient can experience a subdural hematoma days after a head injury.
➤ Stroke—If a stroke is suspected, a computed tomography scan of the brain will be needed.
➤ Infection—Has the patient exhibited signs or symptoms of meningitis or sepsis?

Remember that a loss of consciousness is scary for the patient. Not only may he require treatment for injuries resulting from the loss of consciousness, he may also require emotional support.

2

Cardiovascular emergencies

➤ *Acute peripheral arterial occlusion*

Peripheral arterial occlusion is an obstruction in a healthy artery or an
artery with progressive atherosclerosis caused by embolism, thrombosis,
or trauma. Arterial blood flow is occluded, and distal tissues become deprived of oxygen. Ischemia and infarction may follow.

Rapid assessment
Examine the affected limb for the five Ps — pain, pulselessness, paresthe-
sia, pallor, and paralysis:
➤ Pain — usually severe and sudden in an arm or leg (or in both legs in a
   patient with a saddle embolus)
➤ Pulselessness — diminished or absent arterial pulses when checked by
   Doppler and decreased or absent capillary refill
➤ Paresthesia — numbness, tingling, paresis, or a sensation of cold in the
   affected area
➤ Pallor — a line of color and temperature demarcation at the level of the
   obstruction
➤ Paralysis — some degree of limb paralysis.

 ALERT *Paralysis is a late sign of ischemia. Even after blood flow
is restored, a patient may have paralysis and neuropathy.*

   Ask the patient if he has a history of:
➤ intermittent claudication
➤ hypertension
➤ hyperlipidemia
➤ diabetes mellitus
➤ chronic arrhythmias such as atrial fibrillation
➤ drug use that may contribute to thrombus or embolus formation (such
   as hormonal contraceptives)
➤ smoking.

Immediate actions
If you suspect an acute arterial occlusion:
➤ Notify the physician.
➤ Place the patient on bed rest.

➤ Place the affected area in a dependent position to enhance blood flow.
➤ Give supplemental oxygen.
➤ Insert an I.V. catheter in an unaffected limb.
➤ Draw blood for diagnostic studies.
➤ Administer analgesics, such as morphine, possibly I.V. (to achieve adequate pain relief), heparin (to prevent further emboli formation), and thrombolytics (to dissolve a newly formed clot), as ordered.

Follow-up actions
➤ Perform frequent neurovascular checks.
➤ Mark the location on the patient's extremity where the pulses are palpable or audible to ensure consistent assessments.
➤ Document the status of each pulse immediately after each assessment, compare findings, and report changes immediately.
➤ Mark areas of discoloration or mottling on the patient's extremity and notify the physician of any area expansion.
➤ Watch for tissue swelling after successful thrombolytic therapy.
➤ Monitor prothrombin time, International Normalized Ratio, and partial thromboplastin time and other coagulation panels.
➤ Report values outside therapeutic levels.
➤ Watch for signs of bleeding.
➤ Prepare the patient for interventional radiology (angioplasty or stenting) or surgery (thrombectomy, arterial bypass, or amputation).
➤ Avoid clothing that restricts blood flow to the affected area.
➤ Prevent trauma to the affected area by using a soft-care mattress, cotton wraps or protectors for the heels, a foot cradle, and sheepskin.
➤ Avoid the use of heating pads or cold packs, to prevent burns.
➤ Perform teaching related to bleeding precautions and the effects of anticoagulants and thrombolytics.
➤ Provide a diet low in vitamin K (the antidote to warfarin).

Preventive steps
➤ Prophylactic anticoagulation is essential for patients at highest risk.
➤ Instruct patients that smoking cessation may prevent episodes of arterial occlusion.

Pathophysiology recap
➤ A clot in a peripheral artery hinders or stops blood flow to a specific area.
➤ The area is then deprived of oxygen and begins to experience cellular and tissue changes, which may progress to necrosis and, possibly, death.
➤ Risk factors include smoking, aging, intermittent claudication, diabetes mellitus, chronic arrhythmias, hypertension, hyperlipidemia, and using drugs that may contribute to thrombus or embolus formation such as hormonal contraceptives.

➤ *Air embolism*

An air embolism is a potentially lethal condition that occurs when air bubbles enter the circulatory system.

Rapid assessment
- ➤ Assess the rate, depth, pattern, and quality of respirations, noting dyspnea and tachypnea.
- ➤ Assess the patient's level of consciousness, noting confusion and lethargy.
- ➤ Obtain the patient's vital signs, including oxygen saturation.
- ➤ Ask about chest or joint pain.

Immediate actions
- ➤ Abort a central venous (CV) line insertion attempt, clamp the line, and leave it in place.
- ➤ Place the patient on his left side with his head down in Trendelenburg position.
- ➤ Provide 100% oxygen and prepare for endotracheal intubation and mechanical ventilation, if necessary.
- ➤ Notify the physician.
- ➤ During surgery, assist the surgeon to seal open blood vessels.
- ➤ Insert a peripheral I.V. line and administer I.V. fluids. (See *Managing air embolus,* pages 12 and 13.)

Follow-up actions
- ➤ Aspirate from the distal port of a CV catheter, if present, and attempt to remove air.
- ➤ Perform external cardiac compression in the case of cardiovascular collapse.
- ➤ Administer hyperbaric oxygen therapy.
- ➤ Prepare the patient for a transesophageal echocardiogram, Doppler ultrasound, and pulmonary artery catheter placement, as ordered.
- ➤ Administer beta-adrenergic blockers and, if seizures occur, anticonvulsants.

Preventive steps
- ➤ Eliminate air from the contents of a syringe before injecting its contents, and prime all I.V. fluid tubing.
- ➤ Place the patient in Trendelenburg position during CV line insertion.
- ➤ Use closed catheterization systems.
- ➤ Apply an occlusive dressing to the catheter site after CV catheter removal.

 ALERT *Air embolism may be delayed for 30 minutes or more after catheter removal. Monitor the patient for 1 hour after removal for signs and symptoms to be safe.*

IN ACTION

> MANAGING AIR EMBOLUS

You're helping Paul Stone, 55, to get out of bed and walk. He's taken only a few steps when he starts having difficulty breathing and complains of pain in his mid-chest and shoulder. He suddenly becomes very pale and says he feels nauseated and light-headed.

What's the situation?

Mr. Stone had a small bowel resection 2 days ago. This is his first attempt to walk postoperatively. He has a triple-lumen central vascular catheter inserted via the subclavian vein.

You call for assistance and help Mr. Stone back to bed. The dressing is still intact, but you notice a small amount of fluid on the floor. The junction of the catheter hub and tubing are outside the dressing, and you see that the tubing has pulled apart from one of the catheter hubs.

What's your assessment?

Based on Mr. Stone's signs and symptoms, you suspect an air embolus. The insertion site for his central vascular catheter is above the level of the heart, and Mr. Stone was standing when the tubing separated from the catheter hub. The venous pressure at the catheter tip is lower than the atmospheric pressure. When Mr. Stone took a breath, air was sucked into the right side of his heart through the open catheter lumen.

A large air bubble blocks blood flow from the right ventricle into the pulmonary artery. Blood continues to flow into the right side of the heart, causing it to pump harder. This increased workload and increased pressure of the right ventricle causes more air bubbles to break away from the air pocket and forces them into the pulmonary artery. This may result in decreased cardiac output, shock, and death.

What must you do immediately?

Close the open catheter lumen with the slide clamp on the catheter's extension leg or with another clamp such as a hemostat. If no other clamp is available, manually fold and pinch the tubing together.

Place Mr. Stone on his left side in the Trendelenburg position to move the air embolus away from the pulmonic valve.

Take his vital signs: heart rate, 140; respirations, 30; BP, 90/60 mm Hg. You listen to his chest and hear a continuous churning sound, a classic indication of an air embolus (although this sign isn't always present). His color is becoming cyanotic and he's still short of breath. You immediately administer 100% oxygen and page the surgeon stat. Oxygen causes the nitrogen in the air embolus to dissolve into the blood. The air bubble decreases in size as nitrogen moves into the blood. For very large air emboli, hyperbaric therapy may be needed to increase this process. Next, insert a peripheral I.V. line for emergency vascular access. Obtain specimens for arterial blood gas studies and prepare the patient for an electrocardiogram, which may show sinus tachycardia and nonspecific ST-segment and T-wave changes. Initially, a chest X-ray may be normal, but subsequent X-rays will probably

> **MANAGING AIR EMBOLUS** *(continued)*

show pulmonary edema, which can develop after an air embolus.

What should be done later?
If Mr. Stone continues to have symptoms for more than a few hours, other treatment may be necessary. The central vascular catheter may be used to aspirate the embolus, or the physician may insert a needle into the right ventricle percutaneously and aspirate the air embolus.

Because of your quick action with proper patient positioning and oxygen, Mr. Stone begins to stabilize within an hour after the catheter disconnection. Because air embolism is a significant risk for a patient with a central vascular catheter, always use tubing with a twist-lock connection and check all junctions frequently to make sure that they're secure, especially before the patient gets out of bed.

Hadaway, L.C. "Action Stat: Air embolus," *Nursing* 32(10):104, October 2002. Used with permission.

➤ In the operating room, surgical openings should be kept lower than the level of the heart.
➤ Tell scuba divers that they should obtain appropriate training.

Pathophysiology recap
➤ Air is introduced into the circulation.
➤ The air embolism obstructs blood flow through the vessels.
➤ The blood supply is diminished or cut off, and tissues are starved of oxygen, causing them to die.
➤ The effect of the air embolism depends on the part of the body to which the vessel supplies blood.
➤ Air emboli are most common:
  – during surgery (craniotomies, head and neck surgeries, vaginal deliveries, cesarean deliveries, spinal instrumentation procedures, and liver transplantations)
  – during CV line insertions
  – after accidental introduction of air into the circulation during I.V. therapy
  – during scuba diving
  – following penetrating wounds.

➤ *Angina*

Angina is severe pain in the chest that's typically described as "heaviness," "crushing," or "tightening." The pain may radiate to the arms or jaw. It occurs when oxygen demands of the heart exceed the oxygen supply to the heart muscle.

➤ UNDERSTANDING CHEST PAIN

Use this table to accurately assess chest pain.

Causes	Signs and symptoms
Angina pectoris	Aching, squeezing, pressure, heaviness, burning pain; usually subsides within 10 minutes
Acute myocardial infarction	Tightness or pressure; burning, aching pain, possibly accompanied by shortness of breath, diaphoresis, weakness, anxiety, or nausea; sudden onset; lasts 30 minutes to 2 hours
Pericarditis	Sharp and continuous; may be accompanied by friction rub; sudden onset
Dissecting aortic aneurysm	Excruciating, tearing pain; may be accompanied by blood pressure difference between right and left arm; sudden onset
Pulmonary embolus	Sudden, stabbing pain; may be accompanied by cyanosis, dyspnea, or cough with hemoptysis
Pneumothorax	Sudden and severe pain; sometimes accompanied by dyspnea, increased pulse rate, decreased breath sounds, or deviated trachea

Angina occurs in four major forms:
➤ *Stable.* The pain in this type of angina is predictable in frequency and duration; it can be relieved with nitrates and rest.
➤ *Unstable.* This pain is more intense and is easily induced. It lasts longer and occurs more frequently than stable angina. Unstable angina is also called pre-infarction angina and is classified as an acute coronary syndrome, along with a myocardial infarction (MI).
➤ *Prinzmetal's or variant angina.* The pain in Prinzmetal's angina results from unpredictable coronary artery spasm.
➤ *Microvascular.* This is an angina-like chest pain caused by impaired vasodilator reserve in a patient with normal coronary arteries.

 ALERT *In patients with coronary artery disease (CAD), angina of increasing frequency, severity, or duration (especially if not provoked by exertion, a heavy meal, or cold and wind) may signal an impending MI.*

Rapid assessment
➤ Assess the rate, depth, pattern, and quality of respirations.
➤ Assess the patient's level of consciousness.

Location	Precipitating factors	Alleviating factors
Substernal; may radiate to jaw, neck, arms, and back	Eating, physical effort, smoking, cold weather, stress, anger, hunger, lying down	Rest, nitroglycerin (*Note:* Unstable angina appears even at rest.)
Typically across chest, but may radiate to jaw, neck, arms, or back	Exertion, anxiety	Opioid analgesics such as morphine, nitroglycerin
Substernal; may radiate to neck or left arm	Deep breathing, supine position	Sitting up, leaning forward, anti-inflammatory drugs
Retrosternal, upper abdominal, or epigastric; may radiate to back, neck, or shoulders	Not applicable	Analgesics, surgery
Over lung area	Inspiration	Analgesics
Lateral thorax	Normal respiration	Analgesics, chest tube insertion

➤ Obtain the patient's vital signs and monitor blood pressure and heart rate.
➤ Ask the patient to describe the pain in detail, including its sensation, location, radiation, duration, and precipitating and alleviating factors. (See *Understanding chest pain.*)
➤ Assess for associated symptoms, such as dyspnea, tachycardia, palpitations, nausea, vomiting, fatigue, diaphoresis, pallor, weakness, syncope, or anxiety.

Immediate actions
➤ Provide supplemental oxygen and prepare the patient for intubation and mechanical ventilation, if necessary.
➤ Assist the patient to bed.
➤ Initiate continuous cardiac monitoring and obtain a 12-lead electrocardiogram and portable chest X-ray.
➤ Administer aspirin (to prevent platelet aggregation), nitrates (to vasodilate and to reduce pain), morphine (to reduce pain and provide sedation), and beta-adrenergic blockers (to reduce pain), as ordered.

Follow-up actions
➤ Monitor the patient's vital signs frequently.
➤ Ensure adequate rest.
➤ Obtain serum samples for creatine kinase, isoenzymes, and troponin, and coagulation studies.
➤ Prepare the patient for intra-aortic balloon pump insertion, angioplasty, coronary artery stenting, or coronary artery bypass grafting as his condition warrants.
➤ Administer daily aspirin and long-acting nitrates in the oral, patch, or paste form.

Preventive steps
➤ Instruct patients to practice heart-healthy living, with a heart-healthy diet, stress reduction, regular exercise and preventive care, maintaining a healthy weight, smoking cessation, and abstinence from alcohol.
➤ Instruct patients to avoid precipitating events, which vary on an individual basis, such as strenuous exercise or heavy lifting.

Pathophysiology recap
➤ Angina occurs when myocardial oxygen demands exceed the supply. This occurs when a thrombus progresses and occludes blood flow.
➤ Plaque in the coronary artery ruptures or erodes, resulting in platelet adhesions, fibrin clot formation, and activation of thrombin and subsequent occlusion of the coronary artery. Progressive obstruction of the coronary arteries leads to myocardial oxygen deprivation and tissue death.
➤ The most common cause of angina is CAD, which is usually a result of atherosclerosis. Risk factors for CAD include hyperlipidemia, hypertension, cigarette smoking, diabetes, heredity, obesity, sedentary lifestyle, stress, and personality factors. Males and those older than age 40 are also at increased risk for CAD.

➤ Cardiac arrest

Cardiac arrest is the absence of mechanical functioning of the heart muscle. The heart stops beating or beats abnormally and doesn't pump effectively. If blood circulation isn't restored within minutes, cardiac arrest can lead to the loss of arterial blood pressure, brain damage, and death.

Rapid assessment
➤ Assess the patient's level of consciousness.
➤ Assess for spontaneous respirations.
➤ Attempt to palpate a pulse.
➤ Attempt to obtain the patient's vital signs.
➤ Verify a "do-not-resuscitate" order in the patient's chart.

➤ DEFIBRILLATOR PADDLE PLACEMENT

Here's a guide to correct paddle placement for defibrillation.

Anterolateral placement

For anterolateral placement, place one paddle to the right of the upper sternum, just below the right clavicle, and the other over the fifth or sixth intercostal space at the left anterior axillary line.

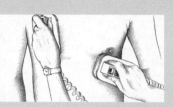

Anteroposterior placement

For anteroposterior placement, place the anterior paddle directly over the heart at the precordium, to the left of the lower sternal border. Place the flat posterior paddle under the patient's body beneath the heart and immediately below the scapulae (but not under the vertebral column).

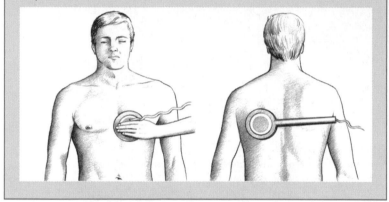

Immediate actions

➤ Notify the physician and resuscitation team.
➤ Initiate cardiopulmonary resuscitation.
➤ Monitor cardiac rhythm.
➤ Assist with endotracheal intubation and mechanical ventilation.
➤ Assist with defibrillation for ventricular fibrillation or pulseless ventricular tachycardia. (See *Defibrillator paddle placement.*)

 ALERT *Defibrillation should be performed for ventricular fibrillation or pulseless ventricular tachycardia within 2 to 3 minutes of the arrest for maximum effectiveness.*

➤ Perform interventions (such as temporary pacing) and administer medications according to advanced cardiac life support protocol until the patient recovers or is declared dead.
➤ Connect the patient to an oxygen saturation monitor and an automatic blood pressure cuff and perform a 12-lead electrocardiogram (ECG).

➤ IMPLANTABLE CARDIOVERTER-DEFIBRILLATOR REVIEW

An implantable cardioverter-defibrillator (ICD) has a programmable pulse generator and lead system that monitors the heart's activity, detects ventricular arrhythmias and other tachyarrhythmias, and responds with appropriate therapies. The range of therapies includes antitachycardia and antibradycardia pacing, cardioversion, and defibrillation. Newer defibrillators can also pace the atrium and ventricle.

Implantation of an ICD is similar to that of a permanent pacemaker. The cardiologist positions the lead (or leads) transvenously in the endocardium of the right ventricle (and the right atrium, if both chambers need pacing). The lead connects to a generator box implanted in the right or left upper chest near the clavicle.

Leadwire

Pulse generator

Follow-up actions
➤ Prepare the patient for hemodynamic monitoring (arterial line and pulmonary artery catheter insertion).
➤ Monitor the patient's cardiac rhythm and vital signs frequently.
➤ Provide emotional support to the patient's family and friends.
➤ Contact a chaplain or religious representative, if appropriate.
➤ Titrate medication administration rates to the desired effectiveness and parameters ordered by the physician and monitor the medication's effectiveness.

Preventive steps
➤ Instruct patients to practice heart-healthy living, with a heart-healthy diet, stress reduction, regular exercise and preventive care, maintaining a healthy weight, smoking cessation, and abstinence from alcohol.
➤ Patients with previous episodes of ventricular tachycardia or ventricular fibrillation should undergo electrophysiology studies and receive an implantable cardioverter-defibrillator. (See *Implantable cardioverter-defibrillator review.*)

Pathophysiology recap
➤ The heart's electrical signals are disrupted.

➤ The heart stops beating or the ventricles start to fibrillate.
➤ Blood isn't pumped to the brain or other vital organs.
➤ Circulatory and respiratory collapse occurs and, without prompt treatment, death ensues.

➤ *Cardiac arrhythmias*

Cardiac arrhythmias, also called *cardiac dysrhythmias,* are changes in the heart rate and rhythm caused by an abnormal electrical conduction or automaticity in the heart muscle. (See *Cardiac conduction system.*) Arrhythmias vary in severity from mild and asymptomatic with no treatment required to catastrophic ventricular fibrillation, which necessitates immediate resuscitation. (See *Dangerous cardiac arrhythmias,* pages 20 to 25.)

Rapid assessment
➤ Assess the rate, depth, pattern, and quality of respirations, noting dyspnea and tachypnea.
➤ Assess the patient for a decreased level of consciousness.

(Text continues on page 24.)

➤ CARDIAC CONDUCTION SYSTEM

Specialized fibers propagate electrical impulses throughout the heart's cells, causing the heart to contract. This illustration shows the elements of the cardiac conduction system.

Interatrial tract (Bachmann's bundle)
Sinoatrial node
Atrioventricular (AV) node
Right bundle branch
Internodal tracts
Bundle of His (AV bundle)
Left bundle branch
Purkinje fibers

➤ DANGEROUS CARDIAC ARRHYTHMIAS

Arrhythmia	Rapid assessment

ASYSTOLE

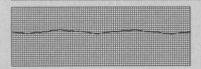

➤ Assess for unconsciousness.
➤ Assess for absence of spontaneous respirations.
➤ Palpate and confirm that the patient is pulseless.
➤ Attempt to obtain the patient's vital signs, noting lack of a blood pressure.

Assess electrocardiogram (ECG) strip for the following:
➤ no atrial or ventricular rhythm or rate
➤ P wave usually indiscernible; may be present but no impulse conduction
➤ PR interval not measurable
➤ QRS complex absent or occasional escape beats
➤ T wave absent
➤ a nearly flat line or, if a pacer is present, pacer spikes without a P wave or QRS complex in response.

PAROXYSMAL SUPRAVENTRICULAR TACHYCARDIA

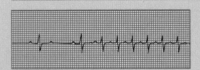

➤ Assess the patient's level of consciousness (LOC).
➤ Assess for dyspnea.
➤ Palpate for a rapid peripheral pulse and auscultate for a rapid apical pulse.
➤ Ask if the patient is having palpitations.
➤ Obtain the patient's vital signs, noting hypotension.
➤ Assess for syncope.

Assess the ECG strip for the following:
➤ regular atrial and ventricular rhythms
➤ regular atrial and ventricular rate 160 to 250 beats/minute
➤ P wave regular but aberrant; may be difficult to distinguish from the preceding T wave or not visible
➤ PR interval may not be measurable
➤ QRS complex normal or may be aberrantly conducted
➤ T wave usually indistinguishable
➤ abrupt start and stop to the rhythm alternating with baseline rhythm.

Immediate actions	Follow-up actions
➤ Start continuous cardiac monitoring, and verify rhythm in another lead. ➤ Check the chart for a "do-not-resuscitate" order. ➤ Perform cardiopulmonary resuscitation (CPR). ➤ Provide supplemental oxygen and intubate and mechanically ventilate the patient. ➤ Perform transcutaneous pacing. ➤ Identify and treat potentially reversible causes. Administer: ➤ atropine ➤ epinephrine.	➤ Monitor the patient's vital signs frequently. ➤ Prepare for possible arterial and pulmonary artery catheter insertion. ➤ Monitor arterial blood gas (ABG) results and treat abnormalities. ➤ Monitor serum electrolytes and treat abnormalities. ➤ Insert an indwelling urinary catheter. ➤ Monitor the patient's intake and output hourly. ➤ Provide emotional support to the patient's family.
➤ Assist the patient to bed. ➤ Provide supplemental oxygen. ➤ Ensure a patent I.V. line. If unstable: ➤ prepare for immediate synchronized cardioversion. If stable: ➤ assist with Valsalva's maneuver or carotid sinus massage (effective treatment for stable paroxysmal atrial tachycardia) ➤ if cardiac function is preserved, treatment priority: calcium channel blocker, beta-adrenergic blocker, digoxin, cardioversion; consider procainamide, amiodarone ➤ if ejection fraction is less than 40% or if the patient is in heart failure, treatment priority: digoxin, amiodarone, diltiazem.	➤ Monitor the patient's vital signs frequently. ➤ Monitor digoxin levels and withhold the next dose if toxicity is expected. ➤ Monitor ABG results and treat abnormalities. ➤ Monitor serum electrolytes and treat abnormalities. ➤ Prepare the patient for atrial overdrive pacing to suppress spontaneous depolarization of the ectopic pacemaker with a series of paced electrical impulses.

(continued)

➤ DANGEROUS CARDIAC ARRHYTHMIAS (continued)

Arrhythmia	Rapid assessment

SINUS BRADYCARDIA (SYMPTOMATIC)

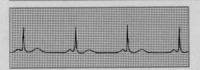

➤ Assess for altered mental status, dizziness, fainting, and blurred vision.
➤ Auscultate for crackles and dyspnea.
➤ Palpate for a peripheral pulse and auscultate for an apical pulse that's regular and less than 60 beats/minute.
➤ Auscultate for an S_3 heart sound.
➤ Ask the patient if he has chest pain.
➤ Obtain the patient's vital signs, noting hypotension.
➤ Assess for syncope. (Bradycardia-induced syncope is known as a *Stokes-Adams attack*.)
  Assess the ECG strip for the following:
➤ regular rhythm
➤ rate less than 60 beats/minute
➤ P wave normal and preceding QRS complex
➤ normal and constant PR interval
➤ normal QRS complex
➤ normal T wave
➤ QT normal or prolonged interval.

THIRD-DEGREE ATRIOVENTRICULAR BLOCK (COMPLETE HEART BLOCK)

➤ Assess the patient's LOC and mental status.
➤ Assess for dyspnea.
➤ Palpate for a slow peripheral pulse.
➤ Obtain the patient's vital signs, noting hypotension.
➤ Inspect for diaphoresis and pallor.
  Assess the ECG strip for the following:
➤ regular atrial rhythm
➤ regular ventricular rhythm and rate slower than atrial rate
➤ no relation between P waves and QRS complexes
➤ P wave may be buried in the QRS complex or T wave, or may occur without QRS complex
➤ PR interval not measurable, no constant interval
➤ normal or widened QRS complex
➤ usually normal T wave.

Immediate actions	Follow-up actions
➤ Provide supplemental oxygen. ➤ Ensure a patent I.V. line. ➤ Assist the patient to bed. ➤ Initiate continuous cardiac monitoring. ➤ Perform transcutaneous pacing and prepare for transvenous pacing if indicated. Administer: ➤ atropine (not effective in denervated transplanted hearts) ➤ catecholamine infusions: dopamine, epinephrine, or isoproterenol	➤ Monitor the patient's vital signs frequently. ➤ Monitor digoxin levels; withhold the next dose and notify the physician if toxicity is suspected. ➤ Monitor ABG results and treat abnormalities. ➤ Monitor serum electrolytes and treat abnormalities. ➤ Prepare the patient for permanent pacemaker insertion, if indicated.
➤ Provide supplemental oxygen. ➤ Ensure a patent I.V. line. ➤ Assist the patient to bed. ➤ Prepare for transcutaneous pacing. ➤ Maintain transcutaneous pacing until transvenous pacing is available. ➤ If unresponsive to transcutaneous pacing, transvenous pacing is delayed and signs and symptoms are severe – consider catecholamine infusion: dopamine, epinephrine, or isoproterenol.	➤ Monitor the patient's vital signs frequently. ➤ Monitor digoxin levels; withhold the next dose and notify the physician if toxicity is suspected. ➤ Withhold drugs that decrease the heart rate. ➤ Monitor ABG results and treat abnormalities. ➤ Monitor serum electrolytes and treat abnormalities. ➤ Prepare the patient for permanent pacemaker placement.

(continued)

> **DANGEROUS CARDIAC ARRHYTHMIAS** (continued)

Arrhythmia	Rapid assessment

VENTRICULAR FIBRILLATION

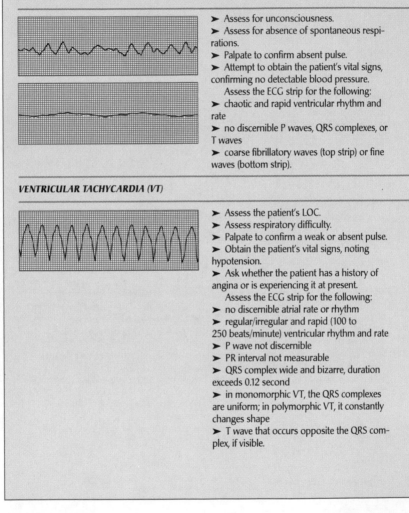

➤ Assess for unconsciousness.
➤ Assess for absence of spontaneous respirations.
➤ Palpate to confirm absent pulse.
➤ Attempt to obtain the patient's vital signs, confirming no detectable blood pressure.
  Assess the ECG strip for the following:
➤ chaotic and rapid ventricular rhythm and rate
➤ no discernible P waves, QRS complexes, or T waves
➤ coarse fibrillatory waves (top strip) or fine waves (bottom strip).

VENTRICULAR TACHYCARDIA (VT)

➤ Assess the patient's LOC.
➤ Assess respiratory difficulty.
➤ Palpate to confirm a weak or absent pulse.
➤ Obtain the patient's vital signs, noting hypotension.
➤ Ask whether the patient has a history of angina or is experiencing it at present.
  Assess the ECG strip for the following:
➤ no discernible atrial rate or rhythm
➤ regular/irregular and rapid (100 to 250 beats/minute) ventricular rhythm and rate
➤ P wave not discernible
➤ PR interval not measurable
➤ QRS complex wide and bizarre, duration exceeds 0.12 second
➤ in monomorphic VT, the QRS complexes are uniform; in polymorphic VT, it constantly changes shape
➤ T wave that occurs opposite the QRS complex, if visible.

➤ Palpate a radial pulse and auscultate the apical pulse and compare rate and strength.
➤ Obtain the patient's vital signs.
➤ Ask about pain or palpations and chest pain and have the patient describe how he's feeling.
➤ Monitor cardiac rhythm and obtain a 12-lead ECG to diagnose the specific arrhythmia.

Immediate actions	Follow-up actions
➤ Initiate CPR. ➤ Defibrillate the patient immediately up to three times with 200 joules, 200 to 300 joules, and then 360 joules or biphasic equivalent. ➤ Intubate and mechanically ventilate the patient. ➤ Ensure a patent I.V. line. Administer: ➤ epinephrine ➤ vasopressin ➤ antiarrhythmics (amiodarone, lidocaine, magnesium, or procainamide).	➤ Monitor the patient's vital signs frequently. ➤ Monitor ABG results and treat abnormalities. ➤ Monitor serum electrolytes and treat abnormalities. ➤ Prepare the patient for electrophysiology studies and possible implantable cardioverter-defibrillator placement.
➤ If the patient is unstable, perform immediate synchronized cardioversion. ➤ If the patient is stable, follow monomorphic or polymorphic algorithm. ➤ If the patient is pulseless, defibrillate immediately up to three times with 200 joules, 200 to 300 joules, and then 360 joules, or biphasic equivalent. ➤ Intubate and mechanically ventilate the patient, if indicated. ➤ Ensure a patent I.V. line. Administer: ➤ procainamide, sotalol, amiodarone, or lidocaine, if monomorphic VT ➤ beta-adrenergic blockers, lidocaine, amiodarone, procainamide, or sotalol, if polymorphic VT with normal baseline QT interval ➤ magnesium, isoproterenol, phenytoin or lidocaine, if polymorphic VT with long baseline QT interval (Also consider overdrive pacing.) ➤ epinephrine or vasopressin, or antiarrhythmics, if pulseless.	➤ Monitor the patient's vital signs frequently. ➤ Monitor ABG results and treat abnormalities. ➤ Monitor serum electrolytes and treat abnormalities. ➤ Prepare the patient for electrophysiology studies and implantable cardioverter-difibrillator placement.

Immediate actions
➤ Notify the physician.
➤ Provide supplemental oxygen.
➤ If the patient isn't breathing, begin rescue breathing and prepare the patient for endotracheal intubation and mechanical ventilation.

➤ If the patient is pulseless, administer cardiopulmonary resuscitation and perform defibrillation for pulseless ventricular tachycardia or ventricular fibrillation. (See *Monophasic and biphasic defibrillators.*)
➤ Use the advanced cardiac life support protocol to treat specific life-threatening arrhythmias.
➤ If asymptomatic, assist the patient back to bed.
➤ Administer medications to treat specific arrhythmias.
➤ Obtain a 12-lead ECG.

Follow-up actions
➤ Monitor the patient's cardiac rhythm.
➤ Monitor the patient's vital signs, including pulse oximetry and cardiac output, if available.
➤ Prepare the patient for transcutaneous or transvenous pacing, if appropriate. (See *Transcutaneous pacemaker,* page 28.)
➤ Attach the postoperative patient with pericardial pacing wires to an external pacing device with a charged battery and turn up the sensitivity.
➤ Pace the patient as ordered, and observe for capture and signs of improved cardiac output and palpate for a pulse.
➤ Prepare the patient with a permanent pacemaker for an interrogation.
➤ Report adverse drug effects immediately.
➤ Frequently monitor intake and output, serum electrolyte levels, and arterial blood gas values and detect and treat abnormalities.
➤ Prepare the patient for cardioversion, electrophysiology studies, an angiogram, internal cardiac defibrillator placement, pacemaker placement, or ablation, as indicated.

Preventive steps
➤ Maintain adequate oxygenation.
➤ Maintain normal fluid, acid-base, and electrolyte balance (especially potassium, magnesium, and calcium).
➤ Maintain normal drug levels.

 ALERT *If drug toxicity is suspected, withhold the next dose and notify the physician.*

Pathophysiology recap
Arrhythmias may result from enhanced automaticity, reentry, escape beats, or abnormal electrical conduction. Other causes include:
➤ congenital defects
➤ myocardial ischemia or infarction
➤ organic heart disease
➤ drug toxicity
➤ degeneration of the conductive tissue
➤ connective tissue disorders
➤ electrolyte imbalances
➤ cellular hypoxia

➤ MONOPHASIC AND BIPHASIC DEFIBRILLATORS

The two types of defibrillators – monophasic and biphasic – are discussed below.

Monophasic defibrillators

Monophasic defibrillators deliver a single current of electricity that travels in one direction between the two pads or paddles on the patient's chest. To be effective, a large amount of electrical current is required for monophasic defibrillation.

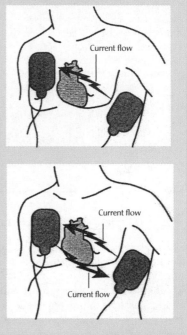

Biphasic defibrillators

Biphasic defibrillators have recently been introduced into hospitals. Pad or paddle placement is the same as with the monophasic defibrillator. The difference is that during biphasic defibrillation, the electrical current discharged from the pads or paddles travels in a positive direction for a specified duration and then reverses and flows in a negative direction for the remaining time of the electrical discharge.

Energy efficient

The biphasic defibrillator delivers two currents of electricity and lowers the defibrillation threshold of the heart muscle, making it possible to successfully defibrillate ventricular fibrillation (VF) with smaller amounts of energy.

Adjustable

The biphasic defibrillator can adjust for differences in impedance or resistance of the current through the chest. This reduces the number of shocks needed to terminate VF.

Reduced myocardial damage

Because the biphasic defibrillator requires lower energy levels and fewer shocks, damage to the myocardial muscle is reduced. Biphasic defibrillators used at the clinically appropriate energy level may be used for defibrillation and, in the synchronized mode, for synchronized cardioversion.

➤ hypertrophy of the heart muscle
➤ acid-base imbalance
➤ emotional stress.

➤ *TRANSCUTANEOUS PACEMAKER*

Transcutaneous pacing, also referred to as *external* or *noninvasive pacing*, delivers electrical impulses through externally applied cutaneous electrodes. The electrical impulses are conducted through an intact chest wall using skin electrodes placed in either anterior-posterior or sternal-apex positions. (Anterior-posterior placement is shown here.)

Transcutaneous pacing is the pacing method of choice in emergency situations because it's the least invasive technique and it can be instituted quickly.

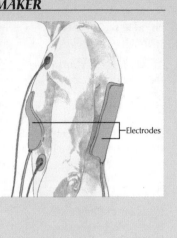
—Electrodes

➤ *Cardiac tamponade*

Cardiac tamponade is a rapid, unchecked rise in intrapericardial pressure that impairs diastolic filling and reduces cardiac output. The rise in pressure typically results from blood or fluid accumulation in the pericardial sac. If fluid accumulates rapidly, this condition requires emergency life-saving measures to prevent death. A slow accumulation and rise in pressure, as in pericardial effusion associated with malignant tumors, may not produce immediate symptoms because the fibrous wall of the pericardial sac can gradually stretch to accommodate as much as 1 to 2 L of fluid.

Rapid assessment

Monitor the patient for the classic signs of cardiac tamponade (Beck's triad):

➤ increased venous pressure (central venous pressure and pulmonary artery wedge pressure) and decreased cardiac output with jugular vein distention

➤ pulsus paradoxus (inspiratory drop in systemic blood pressure greater than 10 mm Hg)

➤ muffled heart sounds on auscultation.

 ALERT *A quiet heart with faint sounds typically accompanies only severe tamponade and occurs within minutes of the tamponade, as happens with cardiac rupture or trauma.*

Following your assessment for Beck's triad, you should:

➤ assess the rate, depth, pattern, and quality of respirations

➤ assess the patient for a decreased level of consciousness

➤ obtain the patient's vital signs, noting hypotension and decreased cardiac output, if available
➤ observe the electrocardiogram (ECG) tracing for arrhythmias.

Immediate actions
➤ Assist the patient to sit upright and lean forward.
➤ Administer oxygen therapy, and prepare the patient for endotracheal intubation and mechanical ventilation, if necessary.
➤ Prepare the patient for an echocardiogram to visualize the fluid collection.
➤ Prepare the patient for a pericardiocentesis or surgical creation of an opening to improve systemic arterial pressure and cardiac output. (See *Understanding pericardiocentesis,* pages 30 and 31.)
   If the patient is hypotensive:
➤ perform trial volume loading with crystalloids (such as I.V. normal saline solution) and colloids (such as albumin).
➤ administer inotropic drugs to improve myocardial contractility.

Follow-up actions
➤ Prepare the patient for a pulmonary artery catheter and arterial line insertion.
➤ Monitor the patient's vital signs frequently.
➤ Obtain a 12-lead ECG.
➤ Watch for complications of pericardiocentesis, such as ventricular fibrillation, vasovagal response, or coronary artery or cardiac chamber puncture.
➤ In traumatic injury, prepare the patient for a blood transfusion or a thoracotomy to drain reaccumulating fluid or to repair bleeding sites.
➤ In heparin-induced tamponade, administer the heparin antagonist protamine sulfate.
➤ In warfarin-induced tamponade, administer vitamin K.

 ALERT *Watch for a decrease in central venous pressure and a concomitant rise in blood pressure, which indicate relief of cardiac compression.*

➤ Infuse I.V. solutions to maintain blood pressure.
➤ Reassure the patient to reduce anxiety.

Preventive steps
➤ Instruct patients to practice heart-healthy living, with a heart-healthy diet, stress reduction, regular exercise and preventive care, maintaining a healthy weight, smoking cessation, and abstinence from alcohol.
➤ Instruct postoperative cardiac patients to maintain bed rest for 1 hour after pericardial pacing wires or pericardial sumps are discontinued.

➤ UNDERSTANDING PERICARDIOCENTESIS

Typically performed at the bedside in a critical care unit, pericardiocentesis involves the needle aspiration of excess fluid from the pericardial sac. It's the treatment of choice for life-threatening cardiac tamponade (except when fluid accumulates rapidly, in which case immediate surgery is usually preferred). Pericardiocentesis may also be used to aspirate fluid in subacute conditions, such as viral or bacterial infections and pericarditis. What's more, it provides a sample for laboratory analysis to confirm diagnosis and identify the cause of pericardial effusion.

Procedure

After starting continuous electrocardiogram (ECG) monitoring and administering a local anesthetic at the puncture site, the physician inserts the aspiration needle in one of three areas. He'll probably choose the xiphocostal approach, with needle insertion in the angle between the left costal margin and the xiphoid process, to avoid needle contact with the pleura and the coronary vessels, thus decreasing the risk of damage to these structures.

As an alternative, he may use the parasternal approach, inserting the needle into the fifth or sixth intercostal space next to the left side of the sternum, where the pericardium normally isn't covered by lung tissue; however, this method poses a risk of puncture of the left anterior descending coronary artery or the internal mammary artery.

He may opt for a third method, the apical approach, in which he inserts the needle at the cardiac apex; however, because this method poses the greatest risk of complications, such as pneumothorax, he'll need to proceed cautiously.

After inserting the needle tip, the physician slowly advances it into the pericardial sac to a depth of 1″ to 2″ (2.5 to 5 cm), or until he can aspirate fluid. He then clamps a hemostat to the needle at the chest wall to prevent needle movement.

The physician then slowly aspirates pericardial fluid. If he finds large amounts of fluid, he may place an indwelling catheter into the pericardial sac to allow continuous, slow drainage. After the physician has removed the fluid, he withdraws the needle and places a dressing over the puncture site.

Complications

Pericardiocentesis carries some risk of potentially fatal complications, such as inadvertent puncture of internal organs (particularly the heart, lung, stomach, or liver) or laceration of the myocardium or of a coronary artery. Therefore, keep emergency equipment readily available during the procedure.

Pathophysiology recap

➤ Fluid enters the pericardial space, resulting in a mechanical compression of the heart muscle.
➤ The range of motion and functioning of the heart is, therefore, limited.
➤ Cardiac output is decreased, resulting in poor tissue perfusion. (See *Understanding cardiac tamponade*, page 32.)

Nursing considerations

Before the procedure

➤ Help the patient comply by clearly explaining the procedure. Briefly discuss possible complications, such as arrhythmias and organ or artery puncture, but reassure him that such complications rarely occur. Tell him he'll have an I.V. line inserted to provide access for medications, if needed.

➤ Make sure that the patient (or a family member, if appropriate) has signed an informed consent form.

➤ Place the patient in a supine position in his bed, with his upper torso raised 60 degrees and his arms supported by pillows. Shave the needle insertion site on his chest if necessary, and clean the area with an antiseptic solution. Next, apply 12-lead ECG electrodes. If ordered, assist the physician in attaching the pericardial needle to the precordial lead (V) of the ECG and also to a three-way stopcock.

During the procedure

➤ Closely monitor the patient's blood pressure and hemodynamic parameters. Check the ECG pattern continuously for premature ventricular contractions and elevated ST segments, which may indicate that the needle has touched the ventricle; for elevated PR segments, which may indicate that the needle has touched the atrium; and for large, erratic QRS complexes, which may indicate that the needle has penetrated the heart. Also watch for signs of organ puncture, such as hypotension, decreased breath sounds, chest pain, dyspnea, hematoma, and tachycardia.

➤ Note and record the volume and character of aspirated fluid. Blood that has accumulated slowly in the patient's pericardial sac usually doesn't clot after it has been aspirated; blood from a sudden hemorrhage, however, will clot.

After the procedure

➤ Check the patient's vital signs at least hourly and maintain continuous ECG monitoring.

➤ Expect the patient's blood pressure to rise as the pressure from the fluid is relieved. Be alert for the development of recurring fluid collection; watch for decreased blood pressure, narrowing pulse pressure, increased central venous pressure, tachycardia, muffled heart sounds, tachypnea, pleural friction rub, jugular vein distention, anxiety, and chest pain. Notify the physician of these signs; he may need to repeat pericardiocentesis or surgically drain the pericardium in the operating room.

Potential causes of cardiac tamponade include:
➤ pericarditis
➤ heart surgery
➤ thoracic dissecting aortic aneurysm
➤ stab wounds to the heart
➤ lung cancer
➤ myocardial infarction.

➤ UNDERSTANDING CARDIAC TAMPONADE

The pericardial sac, which surrounds and protects the heart, is composed of several layers. The fibrous pericardium is the tough outermost membrane; the inner membrane, called the *serous membrane*, consists of the visceral and parietal layers. The visceral layer clings to the heart and is also known as the *epicardial layer*. The parietal layer lies between the visceral layer and the fibrous pericardium. The pericardial space — between the visceral and parietal layers — contains 10 to 30 ml of pericardial fluid. This fluid lubricates the layers and minimizes friction when the heart contracts.

In cardiac tamponade, blood or fluid fills the pericardial space, compressing the heart chambers, increasing intracardiac pressure, and obstructing venous return. As blood flow into the ventricles falls, so does cardiac output. Without prompt treatment, low cardiac output can cause death.

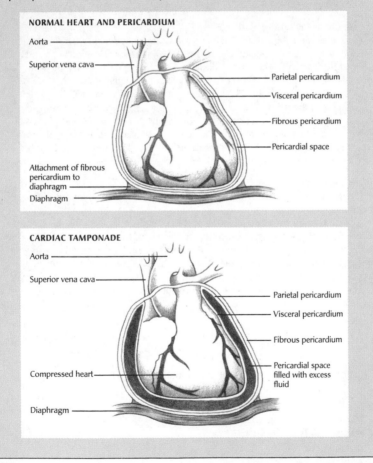

NORMAL HEART AND PERICARDIUM

Aorta
Superior vena cava
Parietal pericardium
Visceral pericardium
Fibrous pericardium
Pericardial space
Attachment of fibrous pericardium to diaphragm
Diaphragm

CARDIAC TAMPONADE

Aorta
Superior vena cava
Parietal pericardium
Visceral pericardium
Fibrous pericardium
Pericardial space filled with excess fluid
Compressed heart
Diaphragm

➤ *Dissecting aortic aneurysm*

A dissecting aortic aneurysm occurs with bleeding into and along the wall of the aorta. Blood enters the walls, separates the layers of the aorta, and creates a blood-filled cavity. It typically occurs in the ascending aorta or thoracic (chest) portion of the aorta, but can occur in the abdominal portion. An acute dissecting aneurysm is an emergency that requires surgical intervention.

Rapid assessment
➤ Assess the rate, depth, pattern, and quality of respirations.
➤ Assess the patient for an altered level of consciousness.
➤ Monitor the patient's vital signs.
➤ Assess cardiovascular status and monitor for weak or thready peripheral pulses, auscultate the apical pulse, and compare rate and strength.
➤ Auscultate for a "blowing" or "swishing" murmur over the aorta and for heart murmurs.
➤ Assess for pain, which is usually a sudden, excruciating pain in the chest or back that the patient may describe as a tearing sensation.

Immediate actions
➤ Initiate cardiac monitoring and perform a 12-lead electrocardiogram.
➤ Provide supplemental oxygen and assist with endotracheal intubation and mechanical ventilation, as necessary.
➤ Obtain a serum sample for hemoglobin level and hematocrit to evaluate blood loss.
➤ Administer I.V. fluids and blood products to increase intravascular volume and cardiac output.
➤ Give antihypertensives such as nitroprusside to decrease blood pressure and maintain systolic blood pressure at 90 to 100 mm Hg.
➤ Administer analgesics such as morphine to relieve pain.
➤ Give negative inotropic agents such as propranolol to reduce myocardial contractility and decrease cardiac workload.

Follow-up actions
➤ Monitor the patient's vital signs frequently.
➤ Watch for signs of shock and decreased tissue perfusion (hypotension, tachycardia, cyanosis, or a thready pulse).
➤ Prepare the patient for an echocardiogram, a chest X-ray, magnetic resonance imaging or computed tomography scan of the chest, or an angiogram.
➤ Obtain blood urea nitrogen, creatinine, and electrolyte levels to evaluate renal function.
➤ Prepare the patient for vascular surgery or aortic valve replacement if the aortic valve is compromised secondary to the dissection.

➤ **UNDERSTANDING DISSECTING AORTIC ANEURYSM**

In an abdominal aortic aneurysm, there's dilation of the aortic arterial wall. With dissection, there's bleeding into and along the wall of the aorta. As blood enters the walls, the layers of the aorta separate and a blood-filled cavity forms. Dissection typically occurs in the ascending aorta or thoracic (chest) portion of the aorta. See illustration below.

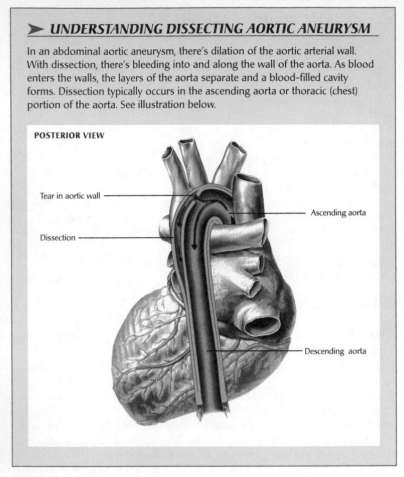

POSTERIOR VIEW

Tear in aortic wall

Dissection

Ascending aorta

Descending aorta

Preventive steps
➤ Obtain adequate treatment of the underlying condition, such as hypertension and Marfan syndrome.
➤ Strict blood pressure control, with medications and ultrasound monitoring every 3 to 4 months, should be performed for patients with chronic aneurysms.

Pathophysiology recap
➤ Blood enters in the intimal lining of the aorta, accumulates in between the layers of the aortic wall, and separates the vessel layers.
➤ As more blood enters the space, the aneurysm expands.

 ALERT *Rupture of a dissecting aortic aneurysm may be fatal in less than 1 hour. Prompt recognition and treatment is imperative.*

➤ Circulatory volume is lost to the aneurysm, cardiac output is decreased, and tissue perfusion is diminished. (See *Understanding dissecting aortic aneurysm*.)

➤ Risk factors include hypertension, atherosclerosis, degeneration of the medial layer of the vessel wall, congenital defects, and connective tissue disease such as Marfan syndrome.

➤ Endocarditis

Endocarditis is an infection or inflammation of the inner lining of the heart, the heart valves, or cardiac prostheses. If untreated, it's usually fatal. With proper treatment, however, about 70% of patients recover.

Rapid assessment
➤ Assess the rate, depth, pattern, and quality of respirations.
➤ Assess the patient's level of consciousness.
➤ Obtain the patient's vital signs, including temperature, noting a fever.
➤ Auscultate heart sounds for a loud, regurgitant murmur.
➤ Observe skin and mucous membranes for petechiae.
➤ Observe the electrocardiogram (ECG) tracing for arrhythmias.

Immediate actions
➤ Notify the physician.
➤ Provide supplemental oxygen.
➤ Draw blood for cultures.
➤ Obtain an allergy history.
➤ While awaiting results, or if blood cultures are negative, administer empiric antimicrobial therapy based on the likely infecting organism.
➤ Place the patient on bed rest.
➤ Administer an antipyretic.

Follow-up actions
➤ Monitor the patient's vital signs frequently.
➤ Obtain a 12-lead ECG.
➤ Observe for signs of heart failure (crackles, jugular vein distention, and dyspnea).
➤ Watch for signs of embolization (hematuria, pleuritic chest pain, left upper quadrant pain, or paresis).
➤ Monitor the white blood cell count and erythrocyte sedimentation rate, and obtain a blood sample to determine the rheumatoid factor status, which will be positive in rheumatic fever.
➤ Monitor blood urea nitrogen levels, creatinine clearance, and urine output to monitor for renal infarction.
➤ Begin antimicrobial therapy for 4 to 6 weeks.
➤ Prepare the patient for transesophageal echocardiography.

➤ **DEGENERATIVE CHANGES IN ENDOCARDITIS**

This illustration shows typical vegetations on the endocardium produced by fibrin and platelet deposits on infection sites.

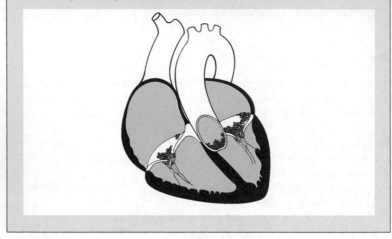

➤ Prepare the patient with severe valvular damage, especially aortic or mitral insufficiency, or an infected prosthetic valve for corrective surgery.

Preventive steps
➤ At-risk patients with a murmur or valvular disease should take prophylactic antibiotics when undergoing dental or surgical procedures or invasive testing.
➤ Instruct patients to practice good hygiene, including thorough hand washing.
➤ Instruct patients to thoroughly wash and cook food.

Pathophysiology recap
➤ An infection occurs in the endocardium, heart valves, or cardiac prosthesis.
➤ The most common causative organisms are bacterial: the group A nonhemolytic streptococci and enterococci.
➤ The causative agent can also be viral, fungal, or rickettsial.
➤ Fibrin and platelets aggregate on valve tissue and engulf circulating infectious organisms. This causes friable cardiac vegetation that may embolize to the spleen, kidneys, central nervous system, and lungs. (See *Degenerative changes in endocarditis.*)

➤ Heart failure

Heart failure occurs when the heart can't pump enough blood to meet the body's metabolic needs. It results in intravascular and interstitial volume overload and poor tissue perfusion. The symptoms of heart failure restrict the ability to perform activities of daily living for many patients.

Rapid assessment
➤ Assess the rate, depth, pattern, and quality of respirations, noting dyspnea, tachypnea, orthopnea, and labored breathing.
➤ Auscultate breath sounds for crackles and diminished breath sounds.
➤ Palpate for a weak peripheral pulse.
➤ Obtain the patient's vital signs, noting decreased oxygen saturation and increased central venous pressure and pulmonary artery wedge pressure, if available.
➤ Observe for peripheral edema.

Immediate actions
➤ Provide supplemental oxygen and prepare the patient for endotracheal intubation and mechanical ventilation, if necessary.
➤ Assist the patient into bed.
➤ Place the patient in Fowler's position.
➤ Administer as ordered:
  – angiotensin-converting enzyme inhibitors for the patient with left ventricle dysfunction—to reduce preload and afterload
  – digoxin—to increase myocardial contractility, improve cardiac output, reduce ventricular volume, and decrease ventricular stretch
  – diuretics—to reduce fluid volume overload and venous return
  – beta-adrenergic blockers in the patient with New York Heart Association class II or III heart failure caused by left ventricular systolic dysfunction—to prevent remodeling
  – inotropic therapy with dobutamine or milrinone—for acute treatment of heart failure exacerbation
  – electrolyte supplementation (especially potassium) after the administration of diuretics—to prevent imbalances such as hypokalemia and the arrhythmias that they may cause.

Follow-up actions
➤ Initiate cardiac monitoring.
➤ Prepare the patient for arterial line and pulmonary artery catheter insertion.
➤ Elevate the lower extremities to promote venous drainage.
➤ Apply antiembolism stockings and assist with range-of-motion exercises.
➤ Monitor for calf pain and tenderness to detect for thrombus formation due to poor venous return and venous stasis.

➤ Monitor the patient for signs of complications such as pulmonary edema. (See *Pulmonary edema.*)
➤ Ensure adequate rest.
➤ Obtain a baseline weight.
➤ Insert an indwelling urinary catheter.
➤ Monitor intake and output every hour.
➤ Limit oral fluid intake and dietary sodium.
➤ Monitor serum electrolyte and digoxin levels.
➤ Monitor for signs of digoxin toxicity.

 ALERT *Signs of digoxin toxicity include anorexia, vomiting, confusion, a slow or an irregular pulse rate, seeing a yellow halo around objects and, in elderly patients, flulike symptoms.*

➤ Coronary artery bypass surgery or angioplasty may be necessary in patients with heart failure due to coronary artery disease.
➤ Other invasive procedures include use of a mechanical ventricular assist device, an implantable cardioverter-defibrillator, or a biventricular pacemaker.
➤ Heart transplantation may be required for patients receiving aggressive medical treatment but still experiencing limitations or repeated hospitalizations.

Preventive steps
➤ Initiate lifestyle modifications, including regular exercise, weight loss, smoking cessation, stress reduction, and reduced sodium, alcohol, and fat intake.
➤ Instruct patients to practice compliance with and timely administration of maintenance doses of diuretics and cardiac medications.

Pathophysiology recap
➤ The heart is subjected to acute or chronic stress.
➤ Adequate tissue oxygenation is preserved by compensatory mechanisms by the tissues and organs, which respond to the change in cardiac pumping.
➤ Heart failure occurs when these compensatory mechanisms can't preserve oxygenation of tissues and organs. (See *Heart failure: How it happens,* page 40.)
➤ Heart failure may be either left-sided or right-sided.
➤ Left-sided heart failure results from impaired ejection of blood from the left ventricle.
➤ Right-sided heart failure results from impaired ejection of blood from the right ventricle.
➤ Right-sided heart failure can occur independently of left-sided heart failure, but it's typically a result of it.

COMPLICATIONS

➤ *PULMONARY EDEMA*

Pulmonary edema is a life-threatening disorder that results in accumulation of fluid in the extravascular spaces of the lung. It usually occurs as a complication of left-sided heart failure or other cardiac disorders. It may result from fluid overload and noncardiac conditions, such as impaired pulmonary lymphatic drainage and Hodgkin's disease. Rapid fluid accumulation can result in death.

Signs and symptoms
➤ Crackles or wheezing
➤ Decreased level of consciousness
➤ Diastolic S_3 gallop
➤ Dyspnea on exertion, paroxysmal nocturnal dyspnea, or orthopnea
➤ Hypotension
➤ Jugular vein distention
➤ Labored and rapid breathing
➤ Persistent cough producing pink, frothy sputum
➤ Restlessness and anxiety
➤ Sweaty, cold, and clammy skin
➤ Tachycardia
➤ Weak, thready pulse

Treatment
➤ Administer oxygen to enhance gas exchange and improve oxygenation.
➤ Prepare the patient for endotracheal intubation and mechanical ventilation, if necessary.
➤ Administer:
  – diuretics, such as furosemide and bumetanide, to increase urination and help mobilize extravascular fluid
  – morphine, to reduce anxiety and dyspnea and to dilate systemic venous bed (thus promoting blood flow from the pulmonary circulation to the periphery)
  – positive inotropic agents, such as digoxin and inamrinone, to enhance contractility
  – vasopressors, such as dobutamine, to enhance contractility and promote vasoconstriction in peripheral vessels
  – antiarrhythmics for arrhythmias related to decreased cardiac output
  – vasodilators, such as nitroprusside, to decrease preload, afterload, and peripheral vascular resistance.

Nursing considerations
➤ Give prescribed drugs and oxygen.
➤ Place the patient in high Fowler's position.
➤ Restrict fluids and sodium intake.
➤ Promote rest and relaxation.
➤ Provide emotional support.

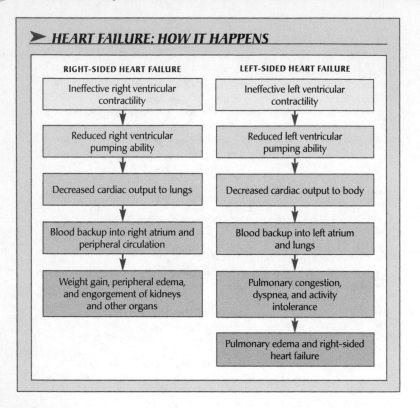

➤ *HEART FAILURE: HOW IT HAPPENS*

RIGHT-SIDED HEART FAILURE	LEFT-SIDED HEART FAILURE
Ineffective right ventricular contractility	Ineffective left ventricular contractility
Reduced right ventricular pumping ability	Reduced left ventricular pumping ability
Decreased cardiac output to lungs	Decreased cardiac output to body
Blood backup into right atrium and peripheral circulation	Blood backup into left atrium and lungs
Weight gain, peripheral edema, and engorgement of kidneys and other organs	Pulmonary congestion, dyspnea, and activity intolerance
	Pulmonary edema and right-sided heart failure

➤ *Hypertensive crisis*

Hypertensive crisis refers to the abrupt, acute, and marked increase in blood pressure from the patient's baseline that ultimately leads to acute and rapidly progressing end-organ damage (See *What happens in hypertensive crisis.*) Typically, the diastolic blood pressure is greater than 120 mm Hg.

Rapid assessment
➤ Assess the patient's level of consciousness, noting irritability and confusion.
➤ Obtain the patient's vital signs, noting a diastolic pressure of greater than 120 mm Hg several times at an interval of at least 2 minutes.

Immediate actions
➤ Administer supplemental oxygen.
➤ Initiate cardiac monitoring and perform a 12-lead electrocardiogram.
➤ Prepare the patient for arterial catheter insertion.

➤ WHAT HAPPENS IN HYPERTENSIVE CRISIS

Hypertensive crisis is a severe rise in arterial blood pressure caused by a disturbance in one or more of the regulating mechanisms. If left untreated, hypertensive crisis may result in renal, cardiac, or cerebral complications and, possibly, death.

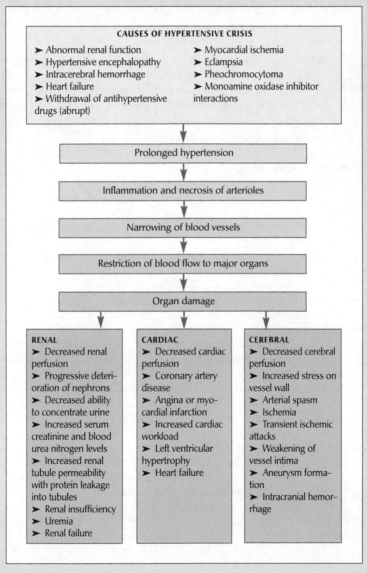

CAUSES OF HYPERTENSIVE CRISIS

➤ Abnormal renal function
➤ Hypertensive encephalopathy
➤ Intracerebral hemorrhage
➤ Heart failure
➤ Withdrawal of antihypertensive drugs (abrupt)

➤ Myocardial ischemia
➤ Eclampsia
➤ Pheochromocytoma
➤ Monoamine oxidase inhibitor interactions

↓

Prolonged hypertension

↓

Inflammation and necrosis of arterioles

↓

Narrowing of blood vessels

↓

Restriction of blood flow to major organs

↓

Organ damage

↓

RENAL
➤ Decreased renal perfusion
➤ Progressive deterioration of nephrons
➤ Decreased ability to concentrate urine
➤ Increased serum creatinine and blood urea nitrogen levels
➤ Increased renal tubule permeability with protein leakage into tubules
➤ Renal insufficiency
➤ Uremia
➤ Renal failure

CARDIAC
➤ Decreased cardiac perfusion
➤ Coronary artery disease
➤ Angina or myocardial infarction
➤ Increased cardiac workload
➤ Left ventricular hypertrophy
➤ Heart failure

CEREBRAL
➤ Decreased cerebral perfusion
➤ Increased stress on vessel wall
➤ Arterial spasm
➤ Ischemia
➤ Transient ischemic attacks
➤ Weakening of vessel intima
➤ Aneurysm formation
➤ Intracranial hemorrhage

➤ Administer I.V. antihypertensive therapy, such as sodium nitroprusside, labetalol, nitroglycerin, and hydralazine.

 ALERT *Remember that nitroprusside is metabolized to thiocyanate, which is excreted by the kidneys. Be alert for signs and symptoms of thiocyanate toxicity (fatigue, nausea, tinnitus, blurred vision, and delirium). If signs are present, send a serum thiocyanate level; if it's greater than 10 mg/dl, notify the physician.*

➤ Titrate I.V. antihypertensive medications according to the desired response and parameters set by the physician.

 ALERT *Care must be taken not to reduce the patient's blood pressure too rapidly because the patient's autoregulatory control is impaired. The current recommendation is to reduce blood pressure by no more than 25% of the mean arterial pressure over the first 2 hours. Further reductions should occur over the next few days.*

➤ Administer analgesics for headache or pain.

Follow-up actions
➤ Monitor the patient's vital signs frequently.
➤ Watch for signs of heart failure (crackles, dyspnea, and jugular vein distention).
➤ Monitor intake and output, noting a positive balance and a urine output of less than 30 ml/hr.
➤ Monitor blood urea nitrogen and serum creatinine levels to assess renal perfusion.
➤ Assess vision for blurriness and diplopia.
➤ Keep the environment quiet and use low lighting.

Preventive steps
➤ Instruct patients to practice heart-healthy living, with a heart-healthy diet, stress reduction, regular exercise and preventive care, maintaining a healthy weight, smoking cessation, and abstinence from alcohol.
➤ Obtain adequate management of primary hypertension.
➤ Obtain adequate management of conditions that cause secondary hypertension, such as pheochromocytoma or Cushing's syndrome.

Pathophysiology recap
➤ Prolonged hypertension leads to inflammation and necrosis of arterioles, narrowing of blood vessels, restriction of blood flow to major organs, and organ damage (especially renal, cardiac, and cerebral). If untreated, prolonged hypertension may result in death.
➤ Hypertensive crisis is most common in patients with a known history of preexisting, untreated, or uncontrolled hypertension.

➤ *Myocardial contusion*

A myocardial contusion is a bruising of the heart muscle caused by blunt trauma to the chest. The heart muscle usually returns to normal functioning without permanent damage.

Rapid assessment
➤ Assess the rate, depth, pattern, and quality of respirations.
➤ Assess the patient's level of consciousness.
➤ Obtain the patient's vital signs, including oxygen saturation.
➤ Auscultate heart sounds for murmurs.
➤ Auscultate lung sounds for crackles.
➤ Inspect and treat the injured area.
➤ Ask the patient about a constant angina-like substernal chest pain and other associated symptoms.

Immediate actions
➤ Provide supplemental oxygen as needed.
➤ Initiate cardiac monitoring and observe for arrhythmias.
➤ Place the patient on bed rest in semi-Fowler's position to ease breathing.
➤ Administer antiarrhythmics, analgesics, anticoagulants (in severely decreased cardiac output, to prevent thrombus formation), and cardiac glycosides (to increase contractility).

Follow-up actions
➤ Prepare the patient for central venous (CV) line or pulmonary artery catheter insertion.
➤ Monitor the patient's vital signs, including CV pressure and pulmonary artery wedge pressure, frequently.
➤ Obtain a 12-lead electrocardiogram.
➤ Monitor for signs of complications, such as cardiogenic shock and cardiac tamponade.
➤ Obtain blood samples for aspartate aminotransferase, alanine aminotransferase, lactate dehydrogenase, creatine kinase (CK), and CK-MB.
➤ Prepare the patient for echocardiography, computed tomography scan, and nuclear heart and lung scans.
➤ Prepare the patient for a temporary pacemaker, if necessary.

Preventive steps
➤ Instruct patients to wear seat belts and, if possible, purchase an automobile with air bags.

Pathophysiology recap

➤ Blunt chest trauma can result in a myocardial contusion when the force of the impact compresses the heart between the sternum and the spinal column, leading to bruising of the myocardium.

➤ This causes capillary hemorrhage, varying in size from petechiae to hemorrhage of the full thickness of the myocardium.

➤ If myocardial function is seriously compromised, myocardial contusion can become life-threatening.

➤ It commonly affects the right ventricle because of this chamber's location.

➤ Myocardial contusion is typically caused by:
   – a motor vehicle accident that forces the chest wall against the steering wheel
   – a fall (typically from higher than 20 feet) or other direct blow that results in sternal or anterior thoracic compression
   – cardiopulmonary resuscitation.

➤ *Myocardial infarction*

A myocardial infarction (MI) occurs when diminished blood flow reduces the amount of oxygen that reaches the heart, resulting in irreversible damage and death of the heart muscle. An MI is categorized as an acute coronary syndrome, along with unstable angina. The degree of coronary occlusion determines whether acute coronary syndrome is unstable angina, a non-Q-wave MI, or a Q-wave MI. An MI is also commonly called a *heart attack*.

Rapid assessment

➤ Assess the rate, depth, pattern, and quality of respirations, noting dyspnea, tachypnea, and shallow respirations.

➤ Assess the patient for a decreased level of consciousness.

➤ Auscultate heart sounds for gallops and murmurs and lung sounds for crackles.

➤ Obtain the patient's vital signs, including oxygen saturation.

➤ Observe electrocardiogram (ECG) tracing.

➤ Ask the patient to describe his chest pain and associated symptoms, if any.

 ALERT *The cardinal symptom of an MI is persistent, intense substernal pain that may radiate to the left arm, jaw, neck, or shoulder blades. This pain is unrelieved by rest or nitroglycerin, and may last several hours. Some patients with an MI, such as elderly patients and those with diabetes, may not experience pain at all. Other pa-*

tients experience only mild pain; for example, female patients who experience atypical chest pain with an MI may present with complaints of indigestion and fatigue.*

Immediate actions
➤ Notify the physician.
➤ Provide supplemental oxygen therapy and prepare the patient for endotracheal intubation and mechanical ventilation, if necessary.
➤ Assist the patient back to bed.
➤ Initiate cardiac monitoring.
➤ Obtain a 12-lead ECG.
➤ Emergency drugs such as epinephrine, a defibrillator, and a transcutaneous pacemaker should be readily available.
➤ Administer as ordered:
  – aspirin—to prevent platelet aggregation
  – nitroglycerin—to relieve chest pain and promote vasodilatation
  – I.V. morphine—to reduce pain and provide sedation
  – thrombolytic therapy—to restore vessel patency and minimize necrosis (Therapy should be started within 12 hours of the onset of symptoms unless contraindicated.)
  – antiarrhythmics—to treat cardiac arrhythmias
  – angiotensin-converting enzyme inhibitors—to prevent heart failure, usually started after thrombolytic therapy is complete and blood pressure is stable
  – beta-adrenergic blockers—to reduce the heart's workload.

Follow-up actions
➤ Monitor the patient's vital signs and oxygen saturation frequently.
➤ Prepare the patient for pulmonary artery catheterization.
➤ Follow thrombolytic therapy with a continuous I.V. heparin infusion.
➤ Monitor creatine kinase (CK), CK-MB, and troponin levels, which rise 6 to 8 hours after the onset of ischemia, for a 72-hour period.
➤ Prepare the patient for pacemaker insertion or cardioversion, if necessary.
➤ Prepare the patient for an echocardiogram and scans using I.V. technetium-99.
➤ Prepare the patient for a primary percutaneous transluminal coronary angioplasty as an alternative to thrombolytic therapy. (See *Understanding angioplasty,* page 46.)
➤ Prepare the patient for coronary artery bypass graft surgery, if necessary.
➤ Insert an indwelling urinary catheter.
➤ Monitor intake and output hourly, and report a urine output of less than 30 ml/hour to the physician.

➤ UNDERSTANDING ANGIOPLASTY

Percutaneous transluminal coronary angioplasty is used to open an occluded coronary artery without opening the chest.

First, the physician threads the catheter to the insertion site (visualized by angiography). Next, he inserts a double-lumen balloon catheter through the guide catheter and directs the balloon through the occlusion.

When the balloon is within the occlusion, it's inflated, resulting in arterial stretching and plaque fracture. Multiple inflations–deflations may be necessary to successfully clear the occluded artery.

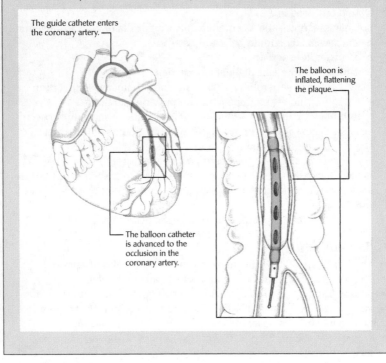

The guide catheter enters the coronary artery.

The balloon is inflated, flattening the plaque.

The balloon catheter is advanced to the occlusion in the coronary artery.

➤ Obtain a baseline weight.
➤ Apply antiembolism stockings.
➤ Provide a calm, quiet environment.
➤ Provide emotional support.
➤ Watch for signs and symptoms of post-MI complication, such as cardiogenic shock, thromboembolism, papillary muscle dysfunction or rupture, rupture of the ventricular septum, rupture of the myocardium, and ventricular aneurysm. (See *Ventricular aneurysm.*)

COMPLICATIONS

➤ *VENTRICULAR ANEURYSM*

Typically occurring in the left ventricle, a ventricular aneurysm produces ventricular wall dysfunction. This complication may develop within 4 to 6 weeks after a myocardial infarction (MI). It occurs when the MI destroys a large muscular section of the left ventricle. The ventricular wall remodels and gradually thins in the area of the infarction. Under intracardiac pressure, this layer stretches and forms a separate noncontractile sac (aneurysm).

Signs and symptoms
➤ Arrhythmias such as premature ventricular contractions
➤ Crackles and rhonchi
➤ Double, diffuse, or displaced apical impulse
➤ Edema
➤ Gallop rhythm
➤ Irregular peripheral pulse rhythm
➤ Jugular vein distention, if heart failure is present
➤ Pulsus alternans
➤ Visible or palpable systolic precordial bulge

Treatment
➤ Depends on the size of the aneurysm and the presence of complications
➤ May require only routine medical examination to follow the patient's condition
➤ May require aggressive measures, such as cardioversion, defibrillation, and endotracheal intubation
➤ No activity restrictions, unless surgical interventions are needed
➤ Medications may include antiarrhythmics, cardiac glycosides, diuretics, analgesics, antihypertensives, nitrates, and anticoagulants
➤ Surgical interventions may include embolectomy or aneurysmectomy with myocardial revascularization
➤ Weight reduction, if appropriate
➤ Low-fat diet

Nursing considerations
➤ Monitor the patient's vital signs and hemodynamic status.
➤ Assess heart and lung sounds.
➤ Monitor cardiac rhythm, especially for ventricular arrhythmias.
➤ Assess the patient's fluid balance status.
➤ Prepare the patient for surgery, if indicated.
➤ Be alert for sudden changes in sensorium that may indicate cerebral embolization and for signs that suggest renal failure or an MI.
➤ Provide psychological support for the patient and his family.

➤ *UNDERSTANDING THROMBUS FORMATION*

A thrombus is a blood clot in a blood vessel or a blood clot in the heart.

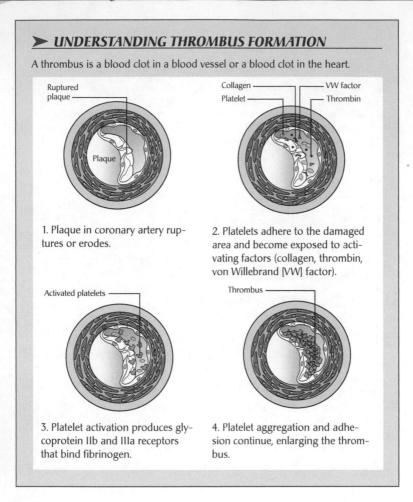

1. Plaque in coronary artery ruptures or erodes.

2. Platelets adhere to the damaged area and become exposed to activating factors (collagen, thrombin, von Willebrand [VW] factor).

3. Platelet activation produces glycoprotein IIb and IIIa receptors that bind fibrinogen.

4. Platelet aggregation and adhesion continue, enlarging the thrombus.

Preventive steps
➤ Instruct patients to practice heart-healthy living, with a heart-healthy diet, stress reduction, regular exercise and preventive care, maintaining a healthy weight, smoking cessation, and abstinence from alcohol and illegal drugs, especially cocaine.
➤ A daily aspirin regimen is indicated for individuals with coronary artery disease or history of an MI.

Pathophysiology recap
➤ An MI begins with rupture or erosion of plaque, which results in platelet adhesions, fibrin clot formation, and activation of thrombin. (See *Understanding thrombus formation*.)

➤ A clot or thrombus in the artery disrupts blood flow and oxygen delivery to the heart muscle, leading to tissue death.
➤ The area of damaged heart muscle loses its ability to contract, forcing the rest of the heart muscle to compensate.

➤ *Myocarditis*

Typically uncomplicated and self-limiting, myocarditis is an inflammation of the heart's muscular tissue. Occasionally, it may become serious and, if untreated or untreatable, scarring and permanent heart muscle damage occur.

Rapid assessment
➤ Assess for a history of a viral illness.
➤ Assess the patient's respiratory status, noting shortness of breath and an inability to lie flat.
➤ Assess the patient for fatigue, restlessness, or confusion.
➤ Auscultate heart sounds, noting abnormal heart beats.
➤ Obtain the patient's vital signs, noting decreased oxygen saturation and increased temperature.
➤ Assess for peripheral edema.
➤ Observe for other signs of infection, such as fever, rash, red throat, itchy eyes, and swollen joints.
➤ Ask the patient whether he's experiencing chest pain and if so, to describe it.

Immediate actions
➤ Provide supplemental oxygen.
➤ Initiate continuous cardiac monitoring.
➤ Obtain blood for culture and antibody titers.
➤ Administer as ordered:
  – nonsteroidal anti-inflammatory agents—to reduce inflammation and pain
  – antibiotics—to treat bacterial infection
  – diuretics—to decrease preload and edema
  – inotropic drugs—to increase contractility
  – antiarrhythmics—to treat arrhythmias if necessary

 ALERT *Use caution when administering antiarrhythmics because they can depress myocardial contractility.*

  – anticoagulation therapy—to prevent emboli
  – corticosteroids and immunosuppressants—to reduce the inflammatory response (This treatment is controversial and limited to life-threatening complications.)

– cardiac glycosides—to increase contractility.

 ALERT *Cardiac glycosides should be administered cautiously because some patients with myocarditis may show a paradoxical sensitivity to even small doses.*

Follow-up actions
➤ Monitor the patient's vital signs frequently.
➤ Prepare the patient for diagnostic tests, including a 12-lead electrocardiogram, chest X-ray, echocardiogram and, rarely, a heart muscle biopsy.
➤ Prepare the patient for pacemaker insertion, if necessary.
➤ Monitor the patient for signs of heart failure.
➤ Monitor for elevated white blood cell count, erythrocyte sedimentation rate, creatine kinase (CK), CK-MB, aspartate aminotransferase, and lactate dehydrogenase levels.
➤ Institute a sodium restriction to reduce fluid retention.
➤ Maintain modified bed rest.

Preventive steps
➤ Instruct patients to obtain prompt treatment of causative disorders.
➤ Instruct patients to practice good hygiene, including thorough hand washing.
➤ Instruct patients to thoroughly wash and cook food.

Pathophysiology recap
➤ In myocarditis, the heart muscle becomes inflamed by a viral, bacterial, helminthic, or parasitic infection, a hypersensitive immune reaction, radiation therapy, or chemical poisons.
➤ The heart muscle weakens, which produces symptoms of heart failure.
➤ Sometimes only a small portion of the heart is involved, but serious cases may involve the entire heart, possibly resulting in sudden death.
➤ More commonly, the heart tries to heal the damaged or dead muscle itself and forms scar tissue. This scar tissue doesn't contract or help the heart to pump.

➤ Pacemaker malfunction

A pacemaker malfunction occurs when a temporary or permanent pacemaker fails to produce an adequate electrical stimulation to cause the heart muscle to contract or when the heart muscle fails to respond to the electrical stimulus generated by the artificial pacemaker.

Rapid assessment
➤ Assess the rate, depth, pattern, and quality of respirations.
➤ Assess the patient for an altered level of consciousness.
➤ Auscultate for an apical pulse and palpate for a carotid or radial pulse and compare the rate and rhythm.
➤ Obtain the patient's vital signs.
➤ Observe the electrocardiogram (ECG) tracing in the paced mode and determine the nature of the malfunction.

Immediate actions
➤ Provide supplemental oxygen and prepare the patient for endotracheal intubation and mechanical ventilation, if necessary.
➤ If a temporary pacemaker is being used, troubleshoot by changing the battery lead wires and pacemaker box, ensuring that all connections are intact, and turning the sensitivity up. (See *Temporary pacemaker malfunctions,* pages 52 and 53.)
➤ Observe for appropriately located pacemaker spikes with the appropriate ECG tracing after the spike.
➤ Palpate for a correlating pulse.
➤ Initiate cardiopulmonary resuscitation according to the advanced cardiac life support protocol, if a pulse is absent.
➤ Initiate external transcutaneous pacing as necessary.

Follow-up actions
➤ Monitor the patient's vital signs and cardiac output frequently.
➤ Obtain a 12-lead ECG.
➤ Prepare the patient with a permanent pacemaker for pacemaker interrogation, reprogramming, battery change, placement, or replacement.

Preventive steps
➤ Instruct patients to schedule and obtain regular pacemaker interrogations and battery changes.
➤ Instruct patients to carefully manage temporary pacing equipment.

Pathophysiology recap
➤ Pacemaker malfunctions are generally traced back to mechanical failure, battery failure, or problems at the electrode-to-myocardium communication site. The pacemaker fails to produce an adequate electrical stimulation to cause the heart muscle to contract, or the heart muscle fails to respond to the electrical stimulus generated by the artificial pacemaker.

➤ TEMPORARY PACEMAKER MALFUNCTIONS

Occasionally, a temporary pacemaker may fail to function correctly. When this occurs, you need to take immediate action to correct the problem. See below for steps to take when your patient's pacemaker fails to pace, capture, or sense intrinsic beats.

Failure to pace
The ECG shows no pacemaker activity when activity should be present.

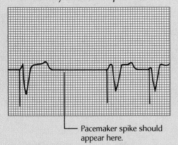

Pacemaker spike should appear here.

Nursing interventions
➤ Check connections to the cable and the position of the pacing electrode in the patient (by X-ray).
➤ If the pulse generator is on but indicators aren't flashing, change the battery. If that doesn't help, change the pulse generator.
➤ Adjust the sensitivity setting.

Failure to capture
The ECG shows pacemaker spikes but the heart isn't responding.

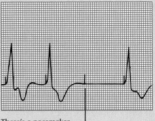

There's a pacemaker spike but no response from the heart.

Nursing interventions
➤ If the patient's condition has changed, notify the physician and ask for new settings.
➤ If the pacemaker settings are altered, return them to their correct positions.
➤ If the heart isn't responding, check all connections; increase milliamperes slowly (according to facility policy or the physician's order); turn the patient on his left side, then on his right; and schedule an anteroposterior or lateral chest X-ray to determine the position of the electrode.

➤ *Papillary muscle rupture*

Papillary muscle rupture is an acute and progressive condition caused by trauma or a myocardial infarction (MI). It typically affects the posterior papillary muscle of the heart and contributes to 5% of deaths after an MI.

Rapid assessment
➤ Observe the pattern, rate, depth, and quality of respirations.
➤ Assess the patient for an altered level of consciousness.

Failure to sense intrinsic beats (undersensing)

The ECG shows pacemaker spikes anywhere in the cycle (the pacemaker fires, but at the wrong times or for the wrong reasons).

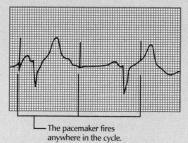

The pacemaker fires anywhere in the cycle.

Nursing interventions

➤ If the pacemaker is undersensing, turn the sensitivity control completely to the right.
➤ If the pacemaker isn't functioning correctly, change the battery or pulse generator.
➤ Remove items in the room that may cause electromechanical interference (such as razors, radios, and cautery

devices). Check ground wires on the bed and other equipment for damage. Unplug each piece and see if the interference stops. When you locate the cause, ask a staff engineer to check it.
➤ If the pacemaker is still firing on the T wave, notify the physician and turn off the pacemaker. Have atropine available in case the heart rate drops. Call a code and institute cardiopulmonary resuscitation if needed.

➤ Obtain the patient's vital signs and hemodynamic parameters, noting increased central venous pressure (CVP) and pulmonary artery wedge pressure (PAWP), and decreased cardiac output, if available.
➤ Auscultate heart sounds for a new pansystolic murmur and apical thrill.

Immediate actions

➤ Provide supplemental oxygen and assist with endotracheal intubation and mechanical ventilation, if necessary.
➤ Prepare the patient for arterial line and pulmonary artery catheter insertion.

➤ Monitor for and treat signs and symptoms of heart failure.
➤ Prepare the patient for intra-aortic balloon pump therapy.
➤ Administer vasodilators (nitroprusside), calcium channel blockers, diuretics, digoxin, inotropic agents, and afterload-reducing agents.

Follow-up actions
➤ Monitor the patient's vital signs and hemodynamic parameters, including CVP, PAWP, and cardiac output, frequently.
➤ Obtain a 12-lead electrocardiogram.
➤ Insert an indwelling urinary catheter.
➤ Monitor intake and output.
➤ Provide a calm, quiet environment.
➤ Prepare the patient for diagnostic studies, including an echocardiogram, a chest X-ray, and an angiogram.
➤ Prepare the patient for mitral valve replacement or coronary artery bypass graft surgery.

Preventive steps
➤ Instruct patients to practice heart-healthy living, with a heart-healthy diet, stress reduction, regular exercise and preventive care, maintaining a healthy weight, smoking cessation, and abstinence from alcohol and illegal drugs, especially cocaine.
➤ The use of fibrinolytic agents to prevent papillary muscle rupture is under investigation.

Pathophysiology recap
➤ The papillary muscles are a column of myocardium projecting into the cavity of the left ventricle.
➤ They are continuous with the wall of the ventricle at the base and attached to the chordae tendineae of the mitral valve at the apex.
➤ There are anterior and posterior papillary muscles connected to the anterior and posterior mitral valve leaflets, respectively.
➤ Contraction of the papillary muscles helps maintain systolic closure of the valve.
➤ When the papillary muscle ruptures due to trauma or ischemia, life-threatening mitral regurgitation occurs.

➤ Pericarditis

Pericarditis is an inflammation of the pericardium—the fibroserous sac that envelops, supports, and protects the heart. It occurs in acute and chronic forms. Acute pericarditis can be fibrinous or effusive, with purulent, serous, or hemorrhagic exudates. Chronic constrictive pericarditis is characterized by dense fibrous pericardial thickening.

Rapid assessment

➤ Assess for a history of a bacterial, fungal, or viral illness (infectious pericarditis).
➤ Assess the patient's respiratory status.
➤ Assess the patient's level of consciousness.
➤ Obtain the patient's vital signs, including temperature, noting a fever.
➤ Auscultate the heart, noting muffled and distant sounds and a pericardial friction rub.
➤ Palpate the chest, noting a diminished or absent apical pulse.
➤ Ask the patient to describe the pain he's experiencing, which is typically a tight chest pain or pleuritic pain that increases with deep inspiration and decreases when the patient sits up and leans forward.
➤ Ask the patient or check the chart for allergies and a recent history of chest trauma, myocardial infarction (MI), or bacterial infection.

Immediate actions

➤ Provide supplemental oxygen as needed based on oxygen saturation.
➤ Institute cardiac monitoring and monitor for cardiac arrhythmias and ST- and T-wave changes.
➤ Maintain bed rest as long as the fever and pain persist to help reduce metabolic needs.
➤ Place the patient in an upright position to relieve dyspnea and chest pain.
➤ Obtain blood for culture and antistreptolysin-O titers.
➤ Administer analgesics to relieve pain and nonsteroidal anti-inflammatory drugs (NSAIDs) to reduce inflammation. If the patient doesn't respond to NSAIDs, give corticosteroids as ordered.

 ALERT *Corticosteroids must be used cautiously because the disorder may recur when the drug therapy stops.*

➤ Initiate antibiotic, antifungal, or antiviral therapy if an infectious cause is suspected.

Follow-up actions

➤ Monitor the patient's vital signs and hemodynamic parameters including pulmonary artery pressure measurements, if available.

 ALERT *Keep in mind that central venous pressure, pulmonary artery pressure, and pulmonary artery wedge pressure will be elevated with pericarditis. Be alert for decreases in cardiac output, which suggest increasing effusion.*

➤ Monitor cardiac rhythm and obtain a 12-lead electrocardiogram, as ordered.
➤ Watch for and report signs and symptoms of pericardial tamponade.
➤ Place a pericardiocentesis set at the bedside and prepare the patient for pericardiocentesis, as necessary.

➤ Prepare the patient for an echocardiogram and a chest X-ray.
➤ Monitor for an increased erythrocyte sedimentation rate and white blood cell count.
➤ If pericarditis is chronic or constrictive, prepare the patient for a partial or total pericardectomy.
➤ Provide emotional support.

Preventive steps
➤ Instruct patients to practice good hygiene, including thorough hand washing.
➤ Instruct patients to thoroughly wash and cook food.
➤ Instruct patients to practice heart-healthy living, with a heart-healthy diet, stress reduction, regular exercise and preventive care, maintaining a healthy weight, smoking cessation, and abstinence from alcohol and illegal drugs.

Pathophysiology recap
➤ Pericardial tissue is damaged by a bacterial, fungal, or viral infection; neoplasms; high-dose radiation; uremia; a hypersensitivity or autoimmune disease, such as rheumatic fever; previous cardiac injury, such as an MI, trauma, or surgery; drugs; or idiopathic factors.
➤ Chemical mediators of inflammation (prostaglandins, histamines, bradykinins, and serotonin) are released into the surrounding tissue, initiating an inflammatory response.
➤ Friction occurs as the inflamed pericardial layers rub against each other.
➤ Histamines and other chemical mediators cause vessels to dilate and increase permeability.
➤ Vessel walls leak fluid and protein into the tissues, causing extracellular edema.
➤ Macrophages, neutrophils, and monocytes invade the area and create an exudate composed of necrotic tissue and cells.
➤ The contents of the cavity autolyze and are reabsorbed into normal tissue.

➤ Shock, cardiogenic

Cardiogenic shock is sometimes called *pump failure*. It's a condition of diminished cardiac output that severely impairs tissue perfusion. It reflects severe left-sided heart failure and occurs as a serious complication in nearly 15% of all patients hospitalized with an acute myocardial infarction (MI). Cardiogenic shock typically affects patients whose area of infarction exceeds 40% of muscle mass; in such patients, mortality may exceed 85%.

ALERT *Cardiogenic shock is the most lethal form of shock. Most patients die within 24 hours of its onset. The prognosis for those who survive is poor.*

Rapid assessment
➤ Assess the rate, depth, pattern, and quality of respirations, noting tachypnea and shallow respirations.
➤ Assess the patient's level of consciousness, noting restlessness and confusion.
➤ Assess for signs of poor tissue perfusion such as cold, pale, clammy skin.
➤ Palpate peripheral pulses, noting thready and weak pulses.
➤ Obtain the patient's vital signs, noting a drop in the systolic blood pressure.
➤ Obtain hemodynamic parameters, including central venous pressure and pulmonary artery wedge pressure; note decreased cardiac output, if available.
➤ Observe the electrocardiogram tracing for arrhythmias.

Immediate actions
➤ Provide supplemental oxygen and prepare the patient for endotracheal intubation and mechanical ventilation, if necessary.
➤ Initiate and maintain at least two I.V. lines with large-gauge needles for fluid and drug administration.
➤ Administer as ordered:
  – I.V. fluids (normal saline or lactated Ringer's solution)
  – colloids
  – blood products
  – vasopressors (dopamine)—to increase cardiac output, blood pressure, and renal blood flow
  – inotropic agents (dobutamine)—to increase myocardial contractility and increase cardiac output
  – a potent vasoconstrictor (norepinephrine)—to increase blood pressure
  – vasodilators (nitroglycerin or nitroprusside) with a vasopressor—to further improve cardiac output by decreasing afterload and preload
  – diuretics—to reduce preload in the setting of fluid volume overload
  – antiarrhythmics—to treat arrhythmias if necessary
  – thrombolytic therapy—to restore coronary artery blood flow if shock is due to an MI.

Follow-up actions
➤ Monitor the patient's vital signs frequently.
➤ Monitor arterial blood gas values, complete blood count, and electrolyte levels and treat abnormalities.
➤ Insert an indwelling urinary catheter.
➤ Monitor intake and output hourly.

➤ **CARDIOGENIC SHOCK: HOW IT HAPPENS**

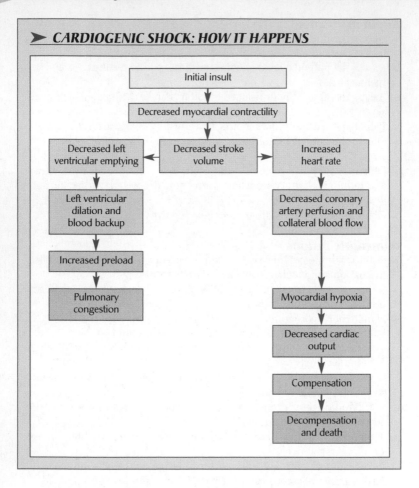

➤ Prepare the patient for an intra-aortic balloon pump (IABP) mechanical-assist device that attempts to improve coronary artery perfusion and decrease cardiac workload.
➤ If drug therapy and the IABP fail, prepare the patient for a ventricular assist device (VAD) to be inserted.
➤ If a VAD fails, prepare the patient for cardiac transplantation.
➤ Prepare the patient for coronary artery revascularization to restore coronary artery blood flow if shock is due to an MI.
➤ Prepare the patient for surgery if shock is due to papillary muscle rupture or a ventricular septal defect.

Preventive steps
➤ Reinforce to patients that prevention requires timely, thorough, and aggressive identification and treatment of causative disorders.

Pathophysiology recap
➤ Cardiogenic shock can result from any condition that causes significant left ventricular dysfunction with reduced cardiac output, such as an MI (most common), myocardial ischemia, papillary muscle dysfunction, and end-stage cardiomyopathy. (See *Cardiogenic shock: How it happens*.)

➤ Shock, hypovolemic

Hypovolemic shock most commonly results from acute blood loss, about 20% of total volume, GI bleeding, internal or external hemorrhage, or any condition that reduces circulating intravascular volume or other body fluids. Without sufficient blood or fluid replacement, it may lead to irreversible damage to organs and systems.

Rapid assessment
➤ Assess the rate, depth, pattern, and quality of respirations.
➤ Assess the patient's level of consciousness.
➤ Obtain the patient's vital signs, noting a mean arterial pressure less than 60 mm Hg, a narrowing pulse pressure, and a decreased central venous pressure.
➤ Test for orthostatic blood pressure readings.
➤ Palpate peripheral pulses, noting rapid, thready, and weak pulses.
➤ Observe for pallor and cold, clammy skin.

Immediate actions
➤ Place the patient in semi-Fowler's position.
➤ Provide supplemental oxygen and assist with intubation and mechanical ventilation, if necessary.
➤ Initiate cardiopulmonary resuscitation, if necessary.
➤ Institute cardiac monitoring.
➤ Obtain a serum sample for hematocrit.
➤ Restore circulating volume by administering, as ordered:
  − I.V. fluid, such as normal saline solution—to restore filling pressures
  − colloids, such as albumin or other plasma expanders—to increase volume until blood is available

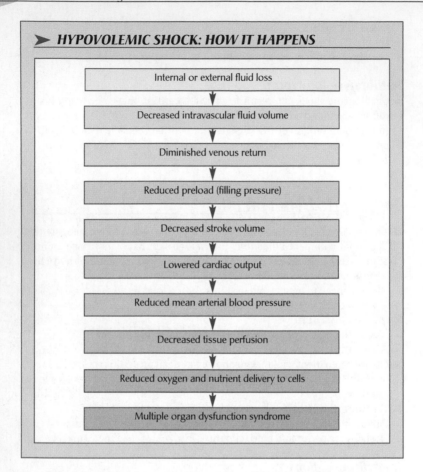

➤ HYPOVOLEMIC SHOCK: HOW IT HAPPENS

Internal or external fluid loss
↓
Decreased intravascular fluid volume
↓
Diminished venous return
↓
Reduced preload (filling pressure)
↓
Decreased stroke volume
↓
Lowered cardiac output
↓
Reduced mean arterial blood pressure
↓
Decreased tissue perfusion
↓
Reduced oxygen and nutrient delivery to cells
↓
Multiple organ dysfunction syndrome

– blood products—to restore blood loss and improve blood oxygen-carrying capacity
– vasopressors, such as dopamine and norepinephrine—to improve perfusion and maintain blood pressure.

Follow-up actions
➤ Monitor the patient's vital signs frequently.
➤ Monitor arterial blood gas values.
➤ Check skin color and the capillary refill time and report a refill greater than 2 seconds.
➤ Prepare the patient for arterial line and pulmonary artery catheter insertion.
➤ Insert an indwelling urinary catheter.

➤ Monitor intake and output hourly.
➤ Insert a nasogastric (NG) tube if bleeding from the GI tract is suspected.
➤ Maintain NG tube patency and check stools, emesis, and gastric drainage for occult blood.
➤ Watch for signs of impeding coagulopathy.
➤ Draw coagulation studies to monitor for disseminated intravascular coagulation.
➤ Monitor serum potassium, sodium, lactate dehydrogenase, creatinine, and blood urea nitrogen levels.
➤ Provide emotional support.
➤ Keep the patient's room quiet and comfortable.
➤ Prepare the patient for surgery to correct the cause if necessary.

Preventive steps
➤ Recognize patients with conditions that reduce blood volume as at-risk patients.
➤ Estimate fluid loss and replace as necessary to prevent hypovolemic shock.

Pathophysiology recap
➤ Hypovolemic shock stems from reduced intravascular blood volume, which leads to decreased cardiac output and inadequate tissue perfusion.
➤ The subsequent tissue anoxia prompts a shift in cellular metabolism from aerobic to anaerobic pathways.
➤ This results in an accumulation of lactic acid, which produces metabolic acidosis.
➤ Multisystem organ failure occurs. (See *Hypovolemic shock: How it happens.*)

➤ Shock, septic

Septic shock is characterized by low systemic vascular resistance and elevated cardiac output. It's thought to occur in response to an infection that releases microbes or one of the immune mediators.

Rapid assessment
In the hyperdynamic phase, assess for:
➤ increased cardiac output
➤ peripheral vasodilatation
➤ decreased systemic vascular resistance
➤ pink, flushed, warm, and dry skin
➤ altered level of consciousness (LOC)

➤ rapid and shallow respirations
➤ low urine output
➤ rapid, full, bounding pulses
➤ normal or high blood pressure.
   In the hypodynamic phase, assess for:
➤ decreased cardiac output
➤ peripheral vasoconstriction
➤ increased systemic vascular resistance
➤ inadequate tissue perfusion
➤ pale, cyanotic, cold, and clammy skin
➤ mottled peripheral areas
➤ decreased LOC, up to and including obtundation and coma
➤ rapid and shallow respirations
➤ low urine output
➤ irregular, thready, or absent pulse
➤ hypotension
➤ crackles or rhonchi
➤ decreased pulmonary artery wedge pressure and increased cardiac output.

Immediate interventions
➤ Administer supplemental oxygen and assist with endotracheal intubation and mechanical ventilation, if necessary.
➤ Place the patient in semi-Fowler's position.
➤ Initiate cardiac monitoring.
➤ Administer as ordered:
   – antipyretics—to reduce fever
   – antibiotics—to eradicate the causative organism
   – I.V. fluids, such as normal saline solution, colloids, or blood products—to maintain intravascular volume
   – vasopressors, such as dopamine and norepinephrine—to improve perfusion and maintain blood pressure
   – monoclonal antibodies, tumor necrosis factor, endotoxin, and interleukin 1—to counteract septic shock mediators (investigational).

Follow-up interventions
➤ Obtain blood samples for culture prior to starting antibiotic therapy, if possible.
➤ Remove, send for culture, and re-insert, if necessary, any possible infectious sources (arterial and I.V. lines, urinary catheters).
➤ Prepare the patient for pulmonary artery catheter insertion.
➤ Monitor the patient's vital signs, including temperature and cardiac output, and calculate systemic vascular resistance frequently.

➤ Obtain an arterial blood gas analysis.
➤ Prepare the patient for a computed tomography scan and chest X-ray to reveal the infective source.
➤ Insert an indwelling urinary catheter.
➤ Monitor intake and output hourly.
➤ Monitor complete blood count, blood urea nitrogen and creatinine levels, prothrombin time, partial thromboplastin time, International Normalized Ratio, and blood glucose levels.
➤ Provide a calm, relaxing environment.
➤ Prepare the patient for surgery to repair or eliminate the infectious source.
➤ Discontinue or decrease the dosage of immunosuppressive drugs.
➤ Institute infection control precautions and use aseptic technique for all invasive procedures.

Preventive steps
➤ Practice good hygiene, including thorough hand washing, especially if the patient is immunosuppressed.
➤ Practice sterile technique and infection control precautions.

Pathophysiology recap
➤ An organism gains entry into the body through an alteration in the body's normal defenses or through artificial devices that penetrate the body, such as I.V., intra-arterial, and urinary catheters or knife or bullet wounds.
➤ An immune response is triggered when the bacteria release endotoxins.
➤ Macrophages secrete tumor necrosis factor (TNF) and interleukins, which in turn increase the release of platelet-activating factor (PAF), prostaglandins, leukotrienes, thromboxane A2, kinins, and complement.
➤ Vasodilation and vasoconstriction, increased capillary permeability, reduced systemic vascular resistance, microemboli, and an elevated cardiac output occur.
➤ To this point, the patient is in the hyperdynamic phase of shock. After this point, he's in the hypodynamic phase.
➤ Endotoxins also stimulate the release of histamine, further increasing capillary permeability.
➤ Myocardial depressant factor, TNF, PAF, and other factors depress myocardial function.
➤ Cardiac output falls, resulting in multisystem organ failure. (See *Septic shock: How it happens,* page 64.)

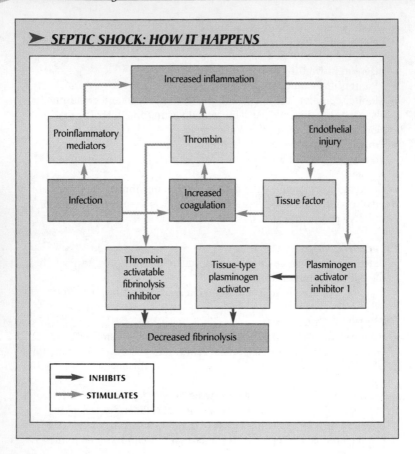

➤ SEPTIC SHOCK: HOW IT HAPPENS

➤ *Thrombophlebitis*

Thrombophlebitis is an acute condition characterized by inflammation and thrombus formation. It may occur in deep (intermuscular or intramuscular) or superficial (subcutaneous) veins. Deep vein thrombophlebitis affects small veins, such as the soleal venous sinuses, or large veins, such as the vena cava and the femoral, iliac, and subclavian veins, causing venous insufficiency.

Rapid assessment
➤ Palpate pulses.
➤ Obtain the patient's vital signs, including temperature, noting a fever.
➤ Assess the color, temperature, sensation, and movement of the affected extremity.

While keeping in mind that some patients are asymptomatic, if you suspect deep vein thrombophlebitis, assess for:
➤ severe pain
➤ fever
➤ chills
➤ malaise
➤ possibly, swelling and cyanosis of the affected arm or leg
➤ positive Homans' sign (pain on dorsiflexion of the foot).
If you suspect superficial thrombophlebitis, assess for:
➤ heat
➤ pain
➤ swelling
➤ rubor
➤ tenderness
➤ induration along the length of the affected vein.

Immediate actions
➤ Maintain bed rest.
➤ Elevate the affected arm or leg.
➤ Apply warm, moist soaks to the affected area.
➤ Administer analgesics, anti-inflammatory drugs (for superficial thrombophlebitis), heparin or low-molecular-weight heparin, and thrombolytics (for acute, extensive, deep vein thrombosis).

Follow-up actions
➤ If you suspect deep vein thrombophlebitis, prepare the patient for duplex Doppler ultrasonography, impedance plethysmography, plethysmography, and phlebography.
➤ If deep vein thrombophlebitis causes complete venous occlusion, prepare the patient for ligation, vein plication, or clipping.
➤ Prepare the patient for embolectomy and insertion of a vena caval umbrella or filter.
➤ Measure and record the circumference of the affected arm or leg daily on a consistent, marked area, and compare this measurement to the other arm or leg.
➤ Watch for signs of pulmonary emboli.
➤ After the acute episode of deep vein thrombophlebitis subsides, apply antiembolism stockings and tell the patient that he may resume his normal activity.
➤ Administer warfarin.
➤ Perform close monitoring of anticoagulant therapy using partial thromboplastin time for heparin and prothrombin time and International Normalized Ratio for warfarin.
➤ Watch for signs and symptoms of bleeding.

Preventive steps

➤ After some types of surgery, especially major abdominal or pelvic operations, prophylactic doses of anticoagulants may reduce the risk of deep vein thrombophlebitis and pulmonary embolism.

➤ To prevent thrombophlebitis in high-risk patients, perform range-of-motion exercises while the patient is on bed rest, use intermittent pneumatic calf massage during lengthy surgical or diagnostic procedures, apply antiembolism stockings postoperatively, and encourage early ambulation.

Pathophysiology recap

➤ A thrombus occurs when an alteration in the epithelial lining causes platelet aggregation and consequent fibrin entrapment of red and white blood cells and additional platelets.

➤ Thrombus formation is more rapid in areas where blood flow is slower because of greater contact between platelet and thrombin accumulation.

➤ The rapidly expanding thrombus initiates a chemical inflammatory process in the vessel epithelium, which leads to fibrosis.

➤ The enlarging clot may occlude the vessel lumen partially or totally, or it may detach and embolize to lodge elsewhere in the systemic circulation.

➤ Deep vein thrombophlebitis may be idiopathic, but it typically results from endothelial damage, accelerated blood clotting, and reduced blood flow.

➤ Predisposing factors for deep vein thrombophlebitis are prolonged bed rest, trauma, surgery, childbirth, and the use of hormonal contraceptives.

➤ It's typically progressive, leading to pulmonary embolism, a potentially lethal complication.

➤ Causes of superficial thrombophlebitis include trauma, infection, I.V. drug abuse, and chemical irritation due to extensive use of the I.V. route for medications and diagnostic tests.

➤ It's usually self-limiting and seldom leads to pulmonary embolism.

3
Respiratory emergencies

➤ *Acute respiratory distress syndrome*

In acute respiratory distress syndrome (ARDS), inflammation of the lungs and accumulation of fluid in the alveoli leads to low blood oxygen levels. ARDS is a life-threatening condition, with mortality of 20% to 30%.

Rapid assessment
➤ Assess for dyspnea, tachypnea, accessory muscle use, and other signs of respiratory distress.
➤ Auscultate for crackles or diminished or absent breath sounds.
➤ Observe for a dry cough or a cough that produces frothy sputum.
➤ Assess the patient for a decreased level of consciousness.
➤ Obtain the patient's vital signs, noting fever, increased pulse and respiratory rate, and decreased oxygen saturation. (See *A closer look at pulse oximetry,* page 68.)
➤ Observe the electrocardiogram (ECG) tracing for arrhythmias.

Immediate actions
➤ Administer humidified oxygen and if hypoxemia doesn't resolve immediately, prepare the patient for endotracheal (ET) intubation and mechanical ventilation with positive end expiratory pressure to help improve oxygenation.
➤ Initiate ECG and oxygen saturation monitoring.
➤ Obtain an arterial blood gas (ABG) analysis.
➤ Additional medications are generally required to minimize restlessness and allow ventilation when ET intubation and mechanical ventilation are instituted. Administer sedatives, opioids, and neuromuscular blocking agents, as ordered.

 ALERT *Hypoxemia despite increased supplemental oxygen is the hallmark of ARDS.*

Follow-up actions
➤ Monitor the patient's vital signs frequently.
➤ Prepare the patient for arterial line and pulmonary artery catheter placement.

➤ *A CLOSER LOOK AT PULSE OXIMETRY*

Used to monitor arterial oxygen saturation, pulse oximetry may be intermittent or continuous. Normal oxygen saturation levels are 95% to 100% for adults. Lower levels may indicate hypoxemia and warrant intervention.

Interfering factors

Certain factors can interfere with the accuracy of oximetry readings. For example, an elevated bilirubin level may falsely lower oxygen saturation readings, whereas elevated carboxyhemoglobin or methemoglobin levels can falsely elevate oxygen saturation readings.

Some intravascular substances, such as lipid emulsions and dyes, can also prevent accurate readings. Other interfering factors include excessive light (such as from phototherapy or direct sunlight), excessive patient movement, excessive ear pigment, hypothermia, hypotension, and vasoconstriction.

Some acrylic nails and certain colors of nail polish (blue, green, black, and brown-red) may also interfere with readings.

➤ Place the patient in the prone position to increase oxygenation. (See *Prone positioning.*)
➤ Prepare the patient for a chest X-ray.
➤ Monitor ABG values and mixed venous blood gas values.
➤ Maintain the ET tube and mechanical ventilator. (See *Securing an ET tube*, pages 70 and 71.)
➤ Perform chest physiotherapy and tracheal suctioning, as needed.
➤ Obtain and send a sputum sample for culture.
➤ Obtain and send blood samples for culture, toxicology, and serum amylase level.
➤ Insert an indwelling urinary catheter.
➤ Monitor intake and output every hour.
➤ Maintain fluid restriction.
➤ Monitor for complications, such as arrhythmias, disseminated intravascular coagulation, GI bleeding, infection, malnutrition, paralytic ileus, pneumothorax, pulmonary fibrosis, renal failure, thrombocytopenia, and tracheal stenosis.
➤ Provide emotional support.
➤ Provide a calm, quiet environment.
➤ Administer as ordered:
 – sedatives and analgesics at routine intervals if the patient on mechanical ventilation is receiving neuromuscular blocking agents
 – sodium bicarbonate—to reverse metabolic acidosis based on ABG results
 – I.V. fluids—to maintain blood pressure by treating hypovolemia
 – vasopressors, such as dopamine and norepinephrine—to maintain blood pressure
 – antimicrobial drugs if necessary—to treat infection

➤ PRONE POSITIONING

Prone positioning (also known as *proning*) is a therapeutic maneuver to improve oxygenation and pulmonary function in the patient with acute lung injury or acute respiratory distress syndrome (ARDS). It involves physically turning the patient face down, which shifts blood flow to regions of the lung that are better ventilated.

The criteria for prone positioning commonly include:
➤ acute onset of acute respiratory failure
➤ hypoxemia, specifically a partial pressure of arterial oxygen/fraction of inspired oxygen (PaO_2/FIO_2) ratio of 300 or less for acute lung injury or a PaO_2/FIO_2 ratio of 200 or less for ARDS
➤ radiologic evidence of diffuse bilateral pulmonary infiltrates.

With the right equipment, prone positioning may aid diaphragm movement by allowing the abdomen to expand more fully. It's usually used for 6 or more hours per day, for up to 10 days, until the patient's need for a high concentration of inspired oxygen resolves.

Equipment innovations
Equipment, such as a lightweight, cushioned frame that straps to the front of the patient before turning, minimizes the risks associated with moving the patient and keeps him prone for several hours at a time.

Indications for prone positioning
Good candidates for prone positioning include mechanically ventilated patients with ARDS who require high concentrations of inspired oxygen. In patients who respond, prone positioning may correct severe hypoxemia. It may also facilitate maintenance of adequate oxygenation (PaO_2 greater than 60%) in patients with acute lung injury while decreasing the risk of ventilator-induced lung injury. The effect of prone positioning on survival rates hasn't been established.

Contraindications for prone positioning
Patients whose heads can't be supported in a face-down position and those who can't tolerate a head–down position are poor candidates for prone positioning. Relative contraindications include increased intracranial pressure, spinal instability, unstable bone fractures, multiple trauma, left-sided heart failure (nonpulmonary respiratory failure), shock, abdominal compartment syndrome, abdominal surgery, extreme obesity (weight greater than 300 lb [136.1 kg]), and pregnancy. Hemodynamically unstable patients (systolic blood pressure less than 90 mm Hg) who don't show improvement with aggressive fluid resuscitation and vasopressors should be thoroughly evaluated before being placed in the prone position.

– diuretics—to reduce interstitial and pulmonary edema
– electrolyte supplementation—to correct sodium or potassium imbalance.

➤ SECURING AN ET TUBE

Before securing an endotracheal (ET) tube in place, make sure the patient's face is clean, dry, and free from beard stubble. If possible, suction his mouth and dry the tube just before securing. Also, check the reference mark on the tube to ensure correct placement. After securing, always check for bilateral breath sounds to make sure that the tube hasn't been displaced by manipulation. Confirm tube placement with the 5-point auscultation technique (listen over the left and right anterior chest, left and right midaxillary chest, and over the stomach) and with an end-tidal carbon dioxide detector.

Remember these warning signs of ET tube displacement:
➤ The tube appears much longer than it should and isn't positioned at the original reference mark.
➤ The low pressure ventilator alarm sounds.
➤ The patient shows signs and symptoms of hypoxemia: tachypnea, tachycardia, diaphoresis, agitation, and arrhythmias such as bradycardia.

If the ET tube is displaced, remove the tube and ventilate the patient with 100% oxygen with a bag-valve mask; notify the physician that the patient needs to be reintubated.

To secure the ET tube, use one of the methods described here. The American Heart Association recommends using a commercial tracheal tube holder rather than using the adhesive tape method. Alternatively, the tube may be taped in place to prevent dislodgment.

Method 1

An ET tube holder, which may be made of hard plastic or other material, is a convenient way to secure an ET tube. Tube holders are available in adult and pediatric sizes, and some models include an attached bite block.

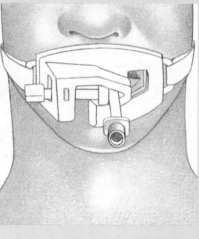

The strap is placed around the patient's neck and secured around the tube with Velcro fasteners (as shown at right). The style and manner of use vary by manufacturer, so check the instructions enclosed with the tube holder you're using for correct placement and care.

Preventive steps

➤ Instruct patients that smoking cessation is essential for the prevention of ARDS.
➤ Help patients identify and avoid allergens that may cause anaphylaxis.
➤ Instruct patients to utilize appropriate safety equipment to avoid exposure to noxious gases.

Method 2

Cut one piece of 1″ cloth adhesive tape long enough to wrap around the patient's head and overlap in front. Then cut an 8″ (20.3-cm) piece of tape and center it on the longer piece, with the sticky sides together. Next, cut a 5″ (12.7-cm) slit in each end of the longer tape (as shown top right).

Apply a skin adhesive product to the patient's cheeks and under his nose and lower lip.

Place the top half of one end of the tape under the patient's nose and wrap the lower half around the ET tube. Place the lower half of the other end of the tape along his lower lip, and wrap the top half around the tube (as shown bottom right).

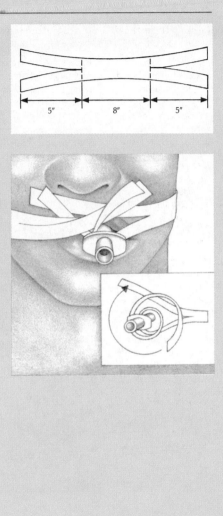

Pathophysiology recap

➤ ARDS results from the loss of integrity of the alveolar-capillary membrane.

➤ The membrane alteration results in increased permeability to plasma.

➤ Fluid enters the alveolar space, disrupting the function of pulmonary surfactant.

➤ UNDERSTANDING ARDS

These diagrams show the process and progression of acute respiratory distress syndrome (ARDS).

In phase 1, injury reduces normal blood flow to the lungs. Platelets aggregate and release histamine (H), serotonin (S), and bradykinin (B).

In phase 2, the released substances inflame and damage the alveolar capillary membrane, increasing capillary permeability. Fluids then shift into the interstitial space.

In phase 3, capillary permeability increases and proteins and fluids leak out, increasing interstitial osmotic pressure and causing pulmonary edema.

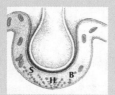 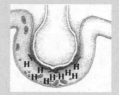

In phase 4, decreased blood flow and fluids in the alveoli damage surfactant and impair the cell's ability to produce more. The alveoli then collapse, impairing gas exchange.

In phase 5, oxygenation is impaired, but carbon dioxide (CO_2) easily crosses the alveolar capillary membrane and is expired. Blood oxygen O_2 and CO_2 levels are low.

In phase 6, pulmonary edema worsens and inflammation leads to fibrosis. Gas exchange is further impeded.

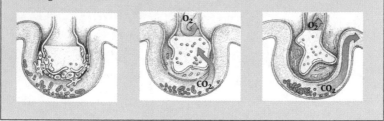

➤ Microatelectasis occurs and gas exchange is impaired.
➤ Pulmonary perfusion is altered, causing ventilation-perfusion mismatch with shunting of blood through unventilated alveoli.
➤ Common causes include indirect or direct lung trauma, anaphylaxis, aspiration of gastric contents, diffuse pneumonia, drug overdose, idiosyncratic drug reaction, near drowning, inhalation of noxious gases, or septic shock. (See *Understanding ARDS*.)

➤ *Acute respiratory failure*

Acute respiratory failure occurs when the lungs can't expand adequately to oxygenate the blood or eliminate carbon dioxide. In patients with normal lung tissue, respiratory failure is indicated by a partial pressure of arterial carbon dioxide ($Paco_2$) above 50 mm Hg and a partial pressure of arterial oxygen (Pao_2) below 50 mm Hg.

Rapid assessment

➤ Assess the rate, depth, pattern, and quality of breathing, noting nasal flaring, accessory muscle use, and tachypnea.
➤ Assess the patient for agitation, anxiety, or a decreased level of consciousness.
➤ Obtain the patient's vital signs, noting decreased oxygen saturation.
➤ Auscultate for diminished breath sounds, wheezes, crackles, and rhonchi.

 ALERT *If you auscultate crackles, pulmonary edema is the suspected cause of respiratory failure.*

➤ Percuss for hyperresonance in patients with chronic obstructive pulmonary disease (COPD) and a flat or dull sound in patients with atelectasis or pneumonia.
➤ Observe for ashen, cool, clammy skin and cyanotic mucous membranes.

Immediate actions

➤ Provide supplemental oxygen and prepare the patient for endotracheal intubation and mechanical ventilation, if necessary.
➤ Place the patient in semi-Fowler's position.
➤ Assist the patient to perform pursed-lip breathing to prevent alveolar collapse.
➤ Obtain an arterial blood gas (ABG) analysis.
➤ Prepare the patient for pulmonary artery catheter insertion.
➤ Administer as ordered:
 – reversal agents such as naloxone—to treat overdose
 – antibiotics—to combat infection
 – corticosteroids—to reduce inflammation
 – positive inotropic agents—to increase cardiac output
 – vasopressors—to maintain blood pressure
 – diuretics—to reduce fluid overload and edema.

Follow-up actions

➤ Monitor the patient's vital signs, pulse oximetry, and respiratory status frequently.
➤ Monitor ABG values and serum electrolytes, and treat abnormalities.
➤ Perform a 12-lead electrocardiogram.
➤ Monitor for an increased white blood cell count.
➤ Perform chest physiotherapy.

➤ Perform tracheal suctioning and send sputum and blood for culture and Gram stain.
➤ Prepare the patient for a chest X-ray.
➤ Provide a calm, relaxing environment.

Preventive steps
➤ Obtain adequate and aggressive management of causative disorders.
➤ Perform careful administration of opioids, sedatives, and tranquilizers.
➤ Practice aggressive pulmonary toileting.

Pathophysiology recap
➤ A decrease in respiratory effort or airway obstruction leads to alveolar hypoventilation.
➤ Blood that passes through the lungs isn't oxygenated and $PaCO_2$ levels rise, PaO_2 levels decrease, pH decreases, and respiratory acidosis develops.
➤ The other organs attempt to compensate.
➤ Tissue hypoxemia causes tissues to resort to anaerobic metabolism, causing lactic acid buildup and metabolic acidosis.
➤ Metabolic and respiratory acidosis increase the acidity of the blood, which interferes with body systems.
➤ Causes of acute respiratory failure include COPD, pneumonia, bronchospasm, ventilatory failure, pneumothorax, atelectasis, cor pulmonale, pulmonary edema, pulmonary emboli, central nervous system (CNS) disease, and CNS depression due to head trauma or misuse of opioids, sedatives, or tranquilizers.

➤ Airway obstruction

An airway obstruction is a partial or complete blockage of the upper airway structures that lead to the lungs. If not recognized early, it progresses to respiratory arrest. Obstruction of the airway is considered life-threatening.

Rapid assessment
➤ Assess the patient's respiratory status for spontaneous respirations, an effective cough reflex, use of accessory muscles, and presence of breath sounds.
➤ Assess level of consciousness.
➤ Assess for the cause of the obstruction.
    If you note these signs, suspect a partial obstruction:
➤ diaphoresis
➤ tachycardia
➤ restlessness and anxiety
➤ forceful coughs with frequent wheezing between coughs (partial obstruction with good air exchange)

➤ **MEMORY TIP: THE 5 Cs OF COMPLETE AIRWAY OBSTRUCTION**

For an easy way to remember key symptoms of complete airway obstruction, just think of the 5 Cs:

> **C**hoking event
>
> **C**essation of coughing and inability to speak
>
> **C**onsciousness level change
>
> **C**yanosis
>
> **C**ardiac arrest.

➤ weak ineffective cough and wheezing, whistling, or high-pitched noise (stridor) on inhalation (partial obstruction with poor air exchange).

If you note these signs, suspect a complete airway obstruction:
➤ cessation of coughing and the inability to make a sound
➤ gasping for air, paradoxical chest movement, and the absence of breath sounds
➤ restlessness, agitation, panic, or increasing anxiety
➤ hypoxemia and hypercapnia
➤ a change in the level of consciousness or unconsciousness
➤ cyanosis, pallor, or increased respiratory difficulty
➤ cardiac arrest. (See *Memory tip: The 5 Cs of complete airway obstruction.*)

Immediate actions
➤ Treat a partial airway obstruction with poor air exchange as a complete airway obstruction.
➤ If the patient is conscious, perform abdominal thrusts to relieve the obstruction.
➤ If the obstruction isn't relieved and the patient becomes unconscious, place him in the supine position, call for help, perform a series of abdominal thrusts to remove the foreign object, and follow American Heart Association guidelines for airway obstruction.
➤ Open the airway by using the head-tilt, chin-lift maneuver or the jaw-thrust maneuver. (See *Opening an airway,* page 76.)

 ALERT *Ensure that cervical spine injury has been ruled out by history, assessment, or X-ray before performing the head-tilt, chin-lift maneuver.*

➤ If the obstruction isn't relieved, prepare the patient for cricothyroidotomy, tracheotomy, laryngoscopy, endotracheal intubation, or bronchoscopy, to determine the cause of the obstruction, attempt to relieve it, and allow for oxygenation.

➤ *OPENING AN AIRWAY*

To open the airway, use the head-tilt, chin-lift maneuver or the jaw-thrust maneuver, as appropriate. Both methods are described here.

Head-tilt, chin-lift maneuver

In many cases of airway obstruction, the muscles controlling the patient's tongue have relaxed, causing the tongue to obstruct the airway. If the patient doesn't appear to have a neck injury, use the head-tilt, chin-lift maneuver to open his airway. Use these steps to carry out this maneuver:

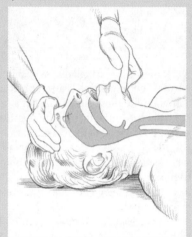

➤ Place your hand closest to the patient's head on his forehead.
➤ Apply firm pressure – firm enough to tilt the patient's head back.
➤ Place the fingertips of your other hand under the bony portion of the patient's lower jaw, near the chin.
➤ Lift the patient's chin. Be sure to keep his mouth partially open (as shown at right). Avoid placing your fingertips on the soft tissue under the patient's chin because this may inadvertently obstruct the airway you're trying to open.
    Note: The head-tilt, chin-lift maneuver shouldn't be used unless it's known that the patient doesn't have a cervical spine injury.

Using the jaw-thrust maneuver

If you suspect a neck injury, use the jaw-thrust maneuver to open the patient's airway. Use these steps to carry out this maneuver:

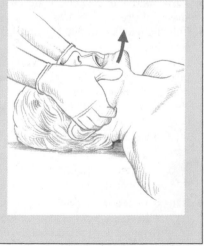

➤ Kneel at the patient's head with your elbows on the ground.
➤ Rest your thumbs on the patient's lower jaw near the corners of his mouth, pointing your thumbs toward his feet.
➤ Place your fingertips around the lower jaw.
➤ To open the airway, lift the lower jaw with your fingertips (as shown at right).

➤ If the object is removed and ventilation is successful, but the patient has no pulse, begin cardiopulmonary resuscitation.

Follow-up actions
➤ Monitor the patient's respiratory status and vital signs, including oxygen saturation, frequently.
➤ When an obstruction is related to the tongue or an accumulation of tenacious secretions, insert an oral airway.
➤ Prepare the patient for a chest X-ray.
➤ Provide emotional support.

Preventive steps
➤ Prompt detection and intervention is necessary to prevent a partial airway obstruction from progressing to a complete airway obstruction.
➤ Assess the swallowing ability and gag reflex of patients who are at risk and keep the head of bed elevated 30 degrees or higher.
➤ Make sure that diet orders agree with the patient's swallowing abilities.
➤ Arrange a swallow evaluation and exercises for patients who are at risk.
➤ Be sure that the patient knows to keep foreign objects, such as pen caps and coins, out of the oral cavity.

Pathophysiology recap
➤ Airway obstruction is an interruption in the flow of air through the nose, mouth, pharynx, or larynx.
➤ Oxygen can't flow to the lungs, gas exchange is impaired or prevented, and hypoxia occurs.
    A patient's airway can become obstructed or compromised by:
➤ the tongue (most common)
➤ vomitus
➤ food
➤ edema (of the tongue, the larynx, and smoke inhalation edema)
➤ aspiration of a foreign object
➤ teeth
➤ saliva or tenacious secretions
➤ decreased muscle tone when a person is unconscious or unresponsive
➤ peritonsillar or pharyngeal abscesses
➤ tumors of the head or neck
➤ cerebral disorders (stroke)
➤ trauma of the face, trachea, or larynx
➤ burns to the head, face, or neck
➤ viral and bacterial infections (such as croup or epiglottiditis)
➤ anaphylaxis.

➤ *Anaphylactic shock*

Anaphylactic shock is a dramatic, widespread, acute atopic reaction marked by the sudden onset of rapidly progressive urticaria and respiratory distress. A severe anaphylactic reaction may precipitate vascular collapse, leading to systemic shock and, sometimes, death.

Rapid assessment
➤ Assess the patient for exposure to a possible allergen at any time within the 24 hours preceding the onset of the reaction.
➤ Assess the patient's respiratory status, noting shortness of breath, sneezing, nasal pruritus, and signs and symptoms of laryngeal edema.
➤ Assess the patient's level of consciousness and neurologic status.
➤ Assess for other primary signs, such as diaphoresis, urticaria, and angioedema.
➤ Obtain the patient's vital signs, including oxygen saturation, noting hypotension and decreased saturation.

Immediate actions
➤ Provide supplemental oxygen and prepare the patient for endotracheal intubation or tracheostomy and mechanical ventilation, if necessary.
➤ Immediately inject epinephrine 1:1,000 aqueous solution, and repeat every 5 to 20 minutes, as needed.
➤ If the patient is conscious and normotensive, give epinephrine I.M. or subcutaneously.
➤ For severe reactions in which the patient has lost consciousness and is hypotensive, give I.V. epinephrine.
➤ If the patient is experiencing cardiac arrest, begin cardiopulmonary resuscitation. If the patient has a latex allergy, be sure to perform emergency interventions using latex-free equipment. (See *Managing a latex allergy reaction.*)

Follow-up actions
➤ Monitor the patient's vital signs closely.
➤ Watch for signs of shock.
➤ Insert an indwelling urinary catheter.
➤ Monitor intake and output every hour.
➤ Show the patient how to use an anaphylaxis kit and assist him in obtaining a medical identification naming his allergies. (See *How to use an anaphylaxis kit,* page 80.)
➤ Administer as ordered:
  – volume expanders (plasma, a plasma expander, saline solution, or albumin), as needed—to increase intravascular volume and blood pressure

> **MANAGING A LATEX ALLERGY REACTION**

If you determine that your patient is having an allergic reaction to latex, act immediately. Make sure that you perform emergency interventions using latex-free equipment. If the latex product that caused the reaction is known, remove it and perform the following measures:
➤ If the allergic reaction develops during medication administration or a procedure, stop it immediately.
➤ Assess airway, breathing, and circulation.
➤ Administer 100% oxygen and monitor oxygen saturation.
➤ Start an I.V. line with lactated Ringer's or normal saline solution.
➤ Administer epinephrine according to the patient's symptoms.
➤ Administer famotidine by the I.V. route, as ordered.
➤ If bronchospasm is evident, treat it with nebulized albuterol.
➤ Secondary treatment for a latex allergy reaction is aimed at treating the swelling and tissue reaction to the latex as well as breaking the chain of events associated with the allergic reaction. It includes I.V. administration of diphenhydramine or methylprednisolone.
➤ Document the event and the exact cause (if known). If latex particles have entered the I.V. line, insert a new I.V. line with a new catheter, new tubing, and new infusion attachments as soon as possible.

– I.V. vasopressors, such as norepinephrine and dopamine—to increase blood pressure
– corticosteroids—to decrease inflammation
– I.V. diphenhydramine—to decrease the histamine response
– I.V. aminophylline—to bronchodilate and improve oxygenation.

 ALERT *Aminophylline should be administered over 10 to 20 minutes when treating bronchospasm. Rapid infusion may cause or aggravate severe hypotension.*

Preventive steps
➤ Instruct patients to avoid exposure to known allergens.
➤ If a patient must receive a drug to which he's allergic, gradually increase doses of the antigen or administer corticosteroids in advance.
➤ A patient with a history of allergies should receive a drug with a high anaphylactic potential only after cautious pretesting for sensitivity.

Pathophysiology recap
Previous sensitization or exposure to the specific antigen results in the production of specific immunoglobulin E antibodies by plasma cells and helper T cells. (See *Understanding anaphylaxis*, page 81.)

(Text continues on page 82.)

➤ HOW TO USE AN ANAPHYLAXIS KIT

If the physician has prescribed an anaphylaxis kit for the patient to use in an emergency, explain that the kit contains everything he needs to treat an allergic reaction:
➤ prefilled syringe containing two doses of epinephrine
➤ alcohol swabs
➤ antihistamine tablets.
   Instruct the patient to notify the physician immediately if anaphylaxis occurs (or to ask someone else to call) and to use the anaphylaxis kit as outlined here.

Getting ready
➤ Take the prefilled syringe from the kit and remove the needle cap. Hold the syringe with the needle pointing up. Expel air from the syringe by pushing in the plunger until it stops.
➤ Next, clean about 4″ (10 cm) of the skin on your arm or thigh with an alcohol swab. (If you're right-handed, clean your left arm or thigh; if you're left-handed, clean your right arm or thigh.)

Injecting the epinephrine
➤ Rotate the plunger one-quarter turn to the right so that it's aligned with the slot. Insert the entire needle — like a dart — into the skin.
➤ Push down on the plunger until it stops. It will inject 0.3 ml of the drug. Withdraw the needle. (_Note:_ This dose is for a patient older than age 12. The dose and administration for an infant and for a child age 12 and younger must be directed by a physician.)

Taking the antihistamine tablets
➤ Chew and swallow the antihistamine tablets. (A child age 12 and younger should follow the directions supplied by the physician or provided in the kit.)

Following up
➤ Apply ice packs — if available — to the sting site. Avoid exertion, keep warm, and see a physician or go to an emergency facility immediately.
➤ _Important:_ If you don't notice an improvement within 10 minutes, give yourself a second injection by following the directions in the kit. If the syringe has a preset second dose, don't depress the plunger until you're ready to give the second injection. Proceed as before, following the injection instructions.

Special instructions
➤ Keep the kit handy for emergency treatment at all times.
➤ Ask the pharmacist for storage guidelines.
➤ Periodically check the epinephrine in the preloaded syringe. A pinkish brown solution must be replaced.
➤ Note the kit's expiration date and replace the kit before that date.

➤ UNDERSTANDING ANAPHYLAXIS

1. Response to antigen
Immunoglobulin (Ig) M and IgG recognize and bind to an antigen.

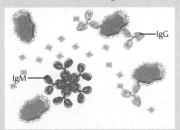

COMPLEMENT CASCADE, ◆

2. Release of chemical mediators
Activated IgE on basophils promotes the release of mediators: histamine, serotonin, and leukotrienes.

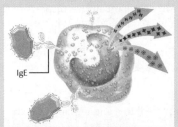

**HISTAMINE, H; LEUKOTRIENES, ✳;
SEROTONIN, ◆**

3. Intensified response
Mast cells release more histamine and eosinophil chemotactic factor of anaphylaxis (ECF-A), which create venule-weakening lesions.

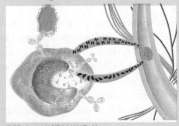

ECF-A ◖; HISTAMINE, H

4. Respiratory distress
In the lungs, histamine causes endothelial cell destruction and fluid leakage into alveoli.

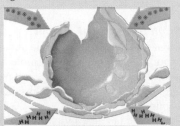

HISTAMINE, H; LEUKOTRIENES, ✳

5. Deterioration
Meanwhile, mediators increase vascular permeability, causing fluid leak from the vessels.

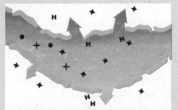

**BRADYKININ, ●; HISTAMINE, H;
PROSTAGLANDINS, +; SEROTONIN, ◆**

6. Failure of compensatory mechanisms
Endothelial cell damage causes basophils and mast cells to release heparin and mediator-neutralizing substances. However, anaphylaxis is now irreversible.

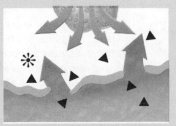

HEPARIN, ▲; LEUKOTRIENES, ✳

➤ *Bronchospasm*

Bronchospasm is a sudden tightening of the muscles that support the bronchiole tubes that causes the tubes to constrict and narrow, thereby obstructing the normal flow of air into the lungs. If bronchospasm isn't promptly diagnosed and treated, air exchange is hindered as air is trapped in the alveolar sacs of the lungs.

Rapid assessment

➤ Measure the respiratory rate and observe the depth and pattern of respirations, noting dyspnea, prolonged expiration, accessory muscle use, nasal flaring, and other signs of respiratory distress.
➤ Auscultate the lungs for wheezing, rhonchi, and diminished breath sounds.
➤ Obtain the patient's vital signs, noting decreased oxygen saturation.
➤ Assess the patient for an altered level of consciousness.
➤ Palpate for a rapid pulse.
➤ Assess the skin and mucous membranes for cyanosis.

Immediate actions

➤ Provide supplemental oxygen, perform rescue breathing, or prepare the patient for endotracheal intubation and mechanical ventilation, as necessary.
➤ Obtain an arterial blood gas sample for analysis. (See *Obtaining a sample for ABG analysis.*)
➤ Initiate continuous electrocardiogram (ECG) monitoring.
➤ Administer as ordered:
  – bronchodilators—to dilate the bronchial tree and enhance gas exchange
  – epinephrine—to treat an allergic reaction
  – corticosteroids—to decrease the inflammatory response
  – nebulizer therapies—to dilate the bronchial tree, enhance expectoration, and improve gas exchange.

Follow-up actions

➤ Monitor the patient's respiratory status, including breath sounds and oxygen saturation.

 ALERT *Be prepared to take immediate action if a patient stops wheezing, but continues to show signs of respiratory distress. The abrupt cessation of wheezing may result from severe bronchial constriction that narrows the airways during inhalation and exhalation. So little air passes through the narrowed airways that no sound is made. This lack of sound is a sign of imminent respiratory collapse. If not already intubated, the patient needs endotracheal intubation and mechanical ventilation.*

> ➤ **OBTAINING A SAMPLE FOR ABG ANALYSIS**

Follow these steps to obtain a sample for arterial blood gas (ABG) analysis:
➤ After performing Allen's test, perform a cutaneous arterial puncture (or, if an arterial line is in place, draw blood from the arterial line).
➤ Use a heparinized blood gas syringe to draw the sample.
➤ Eliminate all air from the sample, place it on ice immediately, and transport it for analysis.
➤ Apply pressure to the puncture site for 3 to 5 minutes. If the patient is receiving anticoagulants or has a coagulopathy, hold the puncture site longer than 5 minutes if necessary.
➤ Tape a gauze pad firmly over the puncture site. If the puncture site is on the arm, don't tape the entire circumference because this may restrict circulation.

➤ Monitor the patient's vital signs and ECG for arrhythmias due to hypoxia and bronchodilator administration.
➤ Prepare the patient for pulmonary function tests, a chest X-ray, and an ECG.

Preventive steps
➤ Facilitate identification and avoidance of the cause of bronchospasm.
➤ Initiate strict management of conditions that place the patient at risk for bronchospasm.

Pathophysiology recap
➤ The muscles surrounding the bronchial tubes tighten, which narrows air passages and interrupts the flow of air into and out of the lungs.
➤ Asthma is the most common cause of bronchospasm; however, chronic obstructive pulmonary disease and hypersensitivity reaction to an allergen also cause this condition. Other causes include exercise (during or within minutes of stopping); airway irritation due to suctioning, airway insertion, or the presence of an endotracheal tube; and induction, administration, or recovery process from anesthesia.

➤ Croup

Croup is a severe inflammation and obstruction of the upper airway. It affects more males than females and usually occurs in children ages 3 months to 5 years during the winter.

Rapid assessment
➤ Assess for dyspnea, tachypnea, accessory muscle use, nasal flaring, and other signs of respiratory distress.

➤ Assess the patient for a decreased level of consciousness.
➤ Obtain the patient's vital signs, noting decreased oxygen saturation.
➤ Auscultate for rhonchi, wheezing, and diminished breath sounds.
➤ Listen to the patient to detect audible wheezing and difficulty speaking.

Immediate actions
➤ Provide supplemental oxygen.
➤ Place the child in an upright or Fowler's position.
➤ Administer as ordered:
  – antipyretics — to reduce fever
  – antibiotics — to treat the causative organism
  – racemic epinephrine — to dilate the bronchial tree and decrease respiratory distress
  – corticosteroids — to reduce inflammation
  – analgesics — to reduce the pain.

Follow-up actions
➤ Provide cool humidification during sleep.
➤ If the patient's fever is greater than 102° F (38.9° C), administer sponge baths and provide a hypothermia blanket to reduce the temperature.
➤ Isolate patients suspected to have respiratory syncytial virus (RSV) and parainfluenza infections and practice careful infection control measures.
➤ Prepare the patient for throat culture, a chest X-ray, and laryngoscopy.
➤ Provide adequate rest and emotional support.

Preventive steps
➤ Instruct patients to practice good hygiene, including thorough hand washing.
➤ Instruct patients to avoid close contact with people who are known to have a respiratory infection.
➤ Provide vaccinations for diphtheria, *Haemophilus influenzae,* and measles.

Pathophysiology recap
➤ Croup usually results from a viral infection.
➤ Parainfluenza viruses cause two-thirds of such infections; adenoviruses, RSV, influenza and measles viruses, and bacterial (pertussis, diphtheria, and mycoplasma) infections account for the rest.
➤ Inflammatory swelling and spasms constrict the larynx and reduce air flow.
➤ The inflammatory changes almost completely obstruct the larynx (which includes the epiglottis) and significantly narrow the trachea.

➤ Flail chest

Flail chest can occur in multiple rib fractures, rib and sternum fractures, or thoracic surgery. A segment of the chest wall becomes unstable, disconnects from the thoracic cage, and demonstrates paradoxical respiration. Flail chest is considered a life-threatening injury.

Rapid assessment

➤ Observe for paradoxyical respirations—the injured area moves in the opposite direction of the rest of the chest.

➤ Observe the patient's respiratory pattern, rate, and depth, comparing both sides and noting dyspnea and tachypnea.

➤ Auscultate lung sounds for absent breath sounds on the affected side.

➤ Assess the patient for a decreased level of consciousness.

➤ Obtain the patient's vital signs, noting decreased oxygen saturation.

➤ Auscultate heart rate and rhythm.

Immediate actions

➤ Place the patient in semi-Fowler's position.

➤ Provide supplemental oxygen at a high flow rate under positive pressure and assist with endotracheal intubation and mechanical ventilation, if necessary.

➤ Support the flail segment by firmly wrapping the chest, using a sandbag or I.V. bag, or by lying the patient down on the affected side in bed.

➤ Administer analgesics.

➤ Obtain an arterial blood gas analysis.

Follow-up actions

➤ Perform tracheal suctioning.

➤ Watch for signs of tension pneumothorax or hemothorax.

➤ Administer I.V. lactated Ringer's or normal saline solution.

➤ Prepare the patient for surgical stabilization of the flail segment, if necessary.

Preventive steps

➤ Instruct patients to wear seat belts and, if possible, purchase an automobile with air bags.

Pathophysiology recap

➤ Multiple rib fractures cause the chest wall to become unstable.

➤ When the patient takes a breath, the negative pressure "sucks in" the unstable segment. This isn't harmful unless increased ventilatory pressures are necessary, as with airway obstruction or underlying pulmonary contusion.

➤ The paradoxical rib motion becomes more severe, making respiration inefficient as the patient's pulmonary condition worsens.

➤ **Hemothorax**

Hemothorax occurs when blood enters the pleural cavity, between the parietal and visceral pleura.

Rapid assessment
➤ Assess the rate, depth, pattern, and quality of respirations and compare both sides.
➤ Assess for tachypnea and dyspnea.
➤ Assess the patient for a decreased level of consciousness.
➤ Obtain the patient's vital signs, noting hypotension and decreased oxygen saturation.
➤ Auscultate for absent breath sounds on the affected side.
➤ Percuss the lung fields for tympany.

Immediate actions
➤ Provide supplemental oxygen and prepare the patient for endotracheal intubation and mechanical ventilation, if necessary.
➤ Prepare the patient for thoracentesis and chest tube insertion.
➤ Connect the chest tube to suction as ordered.
➤ Administer as ordered:
   – I.V. fluids and supplemental blood products—to increase intravascular volume, blood pressure, and hematocrit
   – opioids—to treat pain and provide sedation during thoracentesis or chest tube insertion.

Follow-up actions
➤ Continue to monitor the patient's vital signs and oxygen saturation.
➤ Prepare the patient for a chest X-ray.
➤ Observe the content of the chest tube drainage container every hour for the amount and quality of drainage. Notify the physician if the amount of drainage is greater than 200 ml in one hour.
➤ Watch for hypotension and other signs and symptoms of shock.
➤ Prepare the patient for thoracotomy if necessary.

Preventive steps
➤ Instruct patients to wear seat belts and, if possible, purchase an automobile with air bags.

Pathophysiology recap
➤ Accumulation of blood occurs in the pleural space. Depending on the cause of hemothorax and the amount of blood present in the pleural cavity, it may be associated with lung collapse and mediastinal shift.
➤ Pneumothorax (air in the pleural cavity) commonly occurs with hemothorax.

➤ Causes include blunt or penetrating chest trauma, pneumonia, tuberculosis, tumors, a dissecting thoracic aneuryom, and anticoagulant therapy.

➤ Pneumonia

Pneumonia is an infection of the lung parenchyma. It's a common illness that can range from mild to severe and can cause death. The severity of the infection depends on the causative organism and the patient's age and general health.

Rapid assessment
➤ Observe the rate, depth, pattern, and quality of respirations, noting dyspnea, tachypnea, and shallow respirations.
➤ Assess the patient for a decreased level of consciousness.
➤ Obtain the patient's vital signs, noting decreased oxygen saturation and increased temperature.
➤ Auscultate for rhonchi, crackles, or diminished breath sounds.
➤ Percuss the lung fields.
➤ Monitor the patient's cough and the secretions produced.
➤ Test for vocal fremitus.

Immediate actions
➤ Provide supplemental, humidified oxygen and prepare the patient for endotracheal intubation and mechanical ventilation, if necessary.
➤ Obtain an arterial blood gas (ABG) analysis.
➤ Administer broad-spectrum antimicrobial therapy.

Follow-up actions
➤ Monitor the patient's vital signs, including temperature and oxygen saturation, frequently.
➤ Maintain bed rest.
➤ Perform chest physiotherapy and tracheal suctioning, as needed.
➤ Obtain a sputum sample for culture.
➤ Monitor intake and output.
➤ Monitor ABG levels and the white blood cell count.
➤ Prepare the patient for a chest X-ray or bronchoscopy.
➤ Practice infection control measures.
➤ Provide fever reducing measures.
➤ Provide a calm, quiet environment.
➤ Administer as ordered:
  – antimicrobial therapy—to treat the specific causative agent
  – bronchodilators—to increase gas exchange in the alveoli
  – antitussives—to control coughing
  – antipyretics—to reduce fever
  – analgesics—to control pain

> ## ➤ PNEUMONIA IN OLDER ADULTS

Older adults are at greater risk for developing pneumonia because weakened chest musculature — a normal occurrence in aging — reduces their ability to clear secretions. Those in long-term care facilities are especially susceptible.

Bacterial pneumonia is the most common type of pneumonia found in older adults; viral pneumonia is the second most common type. Aspiration pneumonia results from impaired swallowing and a diminished gag reflex due to stroke or prolonged illness.

An older adult with pneumonia may present with fatigue, a slight cough, and a rapid respiratory rate. Pleuritic pain and fever may also be present. However, remember that the absence of fever doesn't mean an absence of infection in an older adult, who may develop a subnormal body temperature in response to infection.

    − I.V. fluids — to increase intravascular volume and help decrease tenacious secretions
    − corticosteroids — to decrease inflammation.

Preventive steps
➤ Instruct patients to avoid pulmonary irritants, such as dust, environmental pollutants, and smoking.

Pathophysiology recap
➤ Pneumonia is most common in debilitated individuals and older adults. (See *Pneumonia in older adults.*)

Bacterial pneumonia
➤ An infection triggers alveolar inflammation and edema, capillary engorgement, and stasis.
➤ The alveolar capillary membrane loses integrity, blood and exudates fill the alveoli, and atelectasis occurs.

Viral pneumonia
➤ The infection causes interstitial inflammation and desquamation of the bronchiolar epithelial cells.
➤ The process spreads to the alveoli, which fill with fluid and blood.

Aspiration pneumonia
➤ Inflammatory changes are triggered by the aspiration of gastric juices.
➤ Surfactant is inactivated, leading to alveolar collapse.
➤ Gastric juices, which are acidic, damage the lung tissue and alveoli, and solid contents contained in gastric juices may lodge in the airway and reduce the flow of air.

➤ *Pneumothorax, spontaneous*

Spontaneous pneumothorax occurs when air or gas enters the pleural space, causing the lung to collapse. It occurs without a traumatic injury to the chest or lung.

Rapid assessment

- ➤ Assess the rate, depth, pattern, and quality of respirations and chest wall movement.
- ➤ Obtain the patient's vital signs, including oxygen saturation.
- ➤ Auscultate for breath sounds bilaterally, noting absent sounds on the affected side.
- ➤ Assess the patient for a decreased level of consciousness.
- ➤ Observe cough.
- ➤ Assess for chest pain or tightness.

Immediate actions

- ➤ Provide supplemental oxygen and prepare the patient for endotracheal intubation and mechanical ventilation, if necessary.
- ➤ Obtain an arterial blood gas analysis.
- ➤ Prepare the patient for a chest tube insertion.

Follow-up actions

- ➤ Maintain the chest tube to suction and observe the color and consistency of the drainage.
- ➤ Monitor the patient's vital signs, including oxygen saturation.
- ➤ Administer analgesics.
- ➤ Prepare the patient for a chest X-ray.
- ➤ Prepare the patient for surgery if necessary.

Preventive steps

- ➤ Initiate management of pulmonary disorders that increase the risk of spontaneous pneumothorax.
- ➤ To prevent recurrence, tell the patient to avoid high altitudes, scuba diving, and flying in unpressurized aircraft.
- ➤ Instruct patients that smoking cessation reduces risk of pneumothorax.

Pathophysiology recap

Primary spontaneous pneumothorax

- ➤ Primary spontaneous pneumothorax occurs in a patient with no previously diagnosed lung disorder.
- ➤ It's generally caused by the rupture of an air- or fluid-filled sac in the lung called a bleb or bullae.

Secondary spontaneous pneumothorax

- ➤ Secondary spontaneous pneumothorax occurs in a patient with previously diagnosed lung disease.

➤ It usually occurs in patients with chronic obstructive pulmonary disease.
➤ Other causes include pneumonia, asthma, cystic fibrosis, lung cancer, tuberculosis, and interstitial lung disease.

➤ *Pneumothorax, tension*

Tension pneumothorax is a collapsed lung resulting from trapped air in the pleural space. The air enters the space during inspiration but doesn't exit during expiration. Tension pneumothorax can lead to hypotension, shock, and death. (See *Understanding tension pneumothorax*.)

Rapid assessment
➤ Assess the rate, depth, pattern, and quality of respirations and chest wall movement.
➤ Assess the patient for restlessness or change in level of consciousness.
➤ Obtain the patient's vital signs, noting decreased oxygen saturation and hypotension.
➤ Auscultate for breath sounds bilaterally, noting absent sounds on the affected side.
➤ Auscultate for distant heart sounds.
➤ Palpate for subcutaneous emphysema.
➤ Observe for mediastinal shift toward the unaffected side and jugular vein distention.
➤ Observe cough.
➤ Assess for chest pain or tightness.

Immediate actions
➤ Provide supplemental oxygen and prepare the patient for endotracheal intubation and mechanical ventilation, if necessary.
➤ Obtain an arterial blood gas analysis.
➤ Prepare the patient for a chest tube insertion.
➤ Connect the chest tube to suction, as ordered.

Follow-up actions
➤ Maintain the chest tube to suction and observe the color and consistency of drainage.
➤ Monitor the patient's vital signs, including oxygen saturation.
➤ Administer analgesics.
➤ Prepare the patient for a chest X-ray.
➤ Prepare the patient for surgery, if necessary.

Preventive steps
➤ Instruct patients to avoid chest trauma if possible.

➤ UNDERSTANDING TENSION PNEUMOTHORAX

In tension pneumothorax, air accumulates intrapleurally and can't escape. As intrapleural pressure increases, the lung on the affected side collapses.

On inspiration, the mediastinum shifts toward the unaffected lung, impairing ventilation.

On expiration, the mediastinal shift distorts the vena cava and reduces venous return.

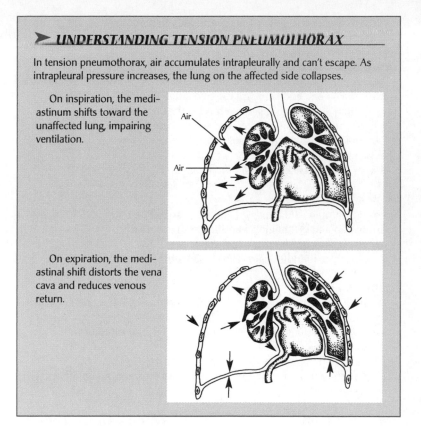

Pathophysiology recap

➤ Air enters the pleural space though an opening during inspiration and doesn't exit during expiration.
➤ The trapped air accumulates and causes pressure to build up in the chest.
➤ The increase in pressure causes the lung to collapse on that side.
➤ The pressure may also cause structures in the chest to be moved out of their normal anatomical position toward the other side of the chest. This shift can cause the other lung to be compromised and may inhibit blood return to the heart.

➤ *Pneumothorax, traumatic*

Traumatic pneumothorax is caused by a chest injury that causes air to collect between the lung and the inner chest wall, causing the lung to collapse. *Open pneumothorax* involves the introduction of atmospheric air via an opening in the pleural cavity. *Closed pneumothorax* is due to the introduction of atmospheric air from within the lung itself.

Rapid assessment
➤ Assess the rate, depth, pattern, and quality of respirations and chest wall movement, and compare the two sides.
➤ Auscultate for absent breath sounds on the affected side.
➤ Assess the patient for an altered level of consciousness.
➤ Obtain the patient's vital signs, noting decreased oxygen saturation and hypotension.
➤ Assess pain and ask the patient to describe it.

Immediate actions
➤ Provide supplemental oxygen and prepare the patient for endotracheal intubation and mechanical ventilation, if necessary.
➤ Obtain an arterial blood gas analysis.
➤ Prepare the patient for chest tube insertion.

Follow-up actions
➤ Maintain the chest tube to suction and observe the color and consistency of drainage.
➤ Monitor the patient's vital signs, including oxygen saturation.
➤ Administer analgesics.
➤ Prepare the patient for a chest X-ray.
➤ Prepare the patient for surgery (for open or recurrent pneumothorax), if necessary.

Preventive steps
➤ Instruct patients to wear seat belts and, if possible, purchase an automobile with airbags.
➤ Teach patients general safety practices that can help prevent injury such as the use of safety equipment while playing sports.

Pathophysiology recap
➤ Traumatic pneumothorax is commonly the result of a blunt or penetrating chest injury, such as an injury sustained in a motor vehicle accident or a gunshot wound to the chest.
➤ Traumatic pneumothorax can also occur as a complication of medical procedures, including bronchial biopsy, pleural biopsy, thoracentesis, and central venous catheter insertion.
➤ Traumatic pneumothorax usually occurs with hemothorax.

Open pneumothorax
➤ Open pneumothorax is also called a *sucking chest wound* or *communicating pneumothorax.*
➤ Atmospheric air (positive pressure) flows directly into the pleural cavity (negative pressure).

➤ The air pressure in the pleural cavity becomes positive, and the lung collapses, resulting in decreased total lung capacity, vital capacity, and lung compliance as well as a ventilation-perfusion mismatch.

Closed pneumothorax
➤ Air enters the pleural space from within the lung.
➤ Pleural pressure increases.
➤ The lung can't expand during normal inspiration.

➤ Pulmonary edema

Fluid accumulation in the extravascular spaces of the lung, called *pulmonary edema,* frequently occurs as a complication of left-sided heart failure or other cardiac disorders. Pulmonary edema may be chronic or may develop suddenly and rapidly; the acute form may cause death. Reexpansion pulmonary edema is a rare noncardiac form of pulmonary edema that may occur as a complication of therapeutic procedures such as thoracentesis.

Rapid assessment
➤ Assess the rate, depth, pattern, and quality of respirations, noting dyspnea on exertion, chronic dyspnea, paroxysmal nocturnal dyspnea, or orthopnea and labored breathing.
➤ Assess the patient for an altered level of consciousness.
➤ Obtain the patient's vital signs and hemodynamic parameters, noting decreased oxygen saturation, increased central venous pressure and pulmonary artery wedge pressure, decreased cardiac output, and hypotension.
➤ Auscultate for crackles, wheezing, and diminished breath sounds.
➤ Auscultate the heart for an S_3 gallop.
➤ Observe the patient cough and check for pink, frothy sputum.
➤ Inspect for jugular vein distention.

Immediate actions
➤ Provide supplemental oxygen and prepare the patient for endotracheal intubation and mechanical ventilation, if necessary.
➤ Place the patient in high Fowler's position.
➤ Obtain an arterial blood gas analysis.
➤ Administer as ordered:
 – diuretics, such as furosemide and bumetanide—to increase urination, which helps mobilize extravascular fluid
 – positive inotropic agents, such as digoxin or inamrinone—to enhance contractility in myocardial dysfunction
 – vasopressors, if necessary—to enhance contractility and promote vasoconstriction in peripheral vessels
 – antiarrhythmics, if necessary—to treat arrhythmias related to decreased cardiac output

IN ACTION

➤ *MANAGING REEXPANSION PULMONARY EDEMA*

Responding to the call bell, you find Jackie Smith, 43, awake and alert but coughing and markedly dyspneic and tachypneic at rest. The head of the bed is elevated 90 degrees, and she denies chest pain. You take her vital signs: BP, 105/60 mm Hg; apical heart rate, 120 and regular; respirations, 28 and labored; and oxygen saturation (SpO_2), 92%. You auscultate inspiratory crackles over her right hemithorax.

What's the situation?
Ms. Smith, who has a history of cancer of the right breast, was admitted to your unit a few hours ago because of a nonproductive cough and progressive dyspnea over the past 2 weeks. Her admission chest X-ray showed a large right pleural effusion. About an hour ago, her physician performed a diagnostic and therapeutic thoracentesis and removed about 2,500 ml of blood-tinged pleural fluid. Ms. Smith's dyspnea resolved, and a repeat chest X-ray showed reexpansion of the right lung.

What's your assessment?
Although you consider that Ms. Smith has a pneumothorax, a possible complication of thoracentesis, the crackles you identified on physical assessment don't fit; you would expect decreased or absent breath sounds instead. The more likely explanation for your patient's sudden change in clinical status is reexpansion pulmonary edema.

This type of pulmonary edema is a relatively rare complication that can follow expansion of a pneumothorax or too-rapid removal of a large pleural effusion, as in Ms. Smith's case. The onset is typically abrupt, occurring within the first hour of lung reexpansion, but it can also develop up to 24 hours later. Usually only the reexpanded lung is involved, but sometimes the contralateral lung is affected as well.

Some patients may be asymptomatic with evidence of pulmonary edema apparent only on X-ray; others may develop hypoxemia and hypotension that can progress to respiratory failure and cardiac arrest. Common signs and symptoms

– arterial vasodilators such as nitroprusside—to decrease peripheral vascular resistance, preload and afterload
– morphine—to reduce anxiety and dyspnea and to dilate systemic venous bed, thereby promoting blood flow from the pulmonary circulation to the periphery. (See *Managing reexpansion pulmonary edema*.)

Follow-up actions
➤ Monitor the patient's vital signs frequently.
➤ Prepare the patient for central venous or pulmonary artery catheter insertion.
➤ Obtain an electrocardiogram.
➤ Insert an indwelling urinary catheter.

include dyspnea, tachypnea, tachycardia, a cough, and unilateral crackles. Some patients develop cyanosis, chest pain, hypotension, diaphoresis, and pink, frothy sputum or frank hemoptysis.

What must you do immediately?

Stay with Ms. Smith and ask a colleague to notify her physician. Provide emotional support, administer oxygen at 4 L/minute by nasal cannula, ensure that she has patent I.V. access, and continue to monitor her vital signs, including SpO_2. Obtain a stat 12-lead electrocardiogram (ECG) and chest X-ray.

The ECG is normal except for sinus tachycardia, with no evidence of ischemia. The X-ray shows no pneumothorax or reaccumulation of the effusion, but a unilateral alveolar filling pattern involving the entire right lung is visible.

You administer 40 mg of furosemide I.V., as ordered, and continue to monitor the patient's clinical status carefully. Although reexpansion pulmonary edema resolves spontaneously in many cases, other cases require endotracheal intubation and mechanical ventilation.

What should be done later?

Following diuresis, Ms. Smith's pulmonary status improves dramatically. Her respirations are now 18 and unlabored, her SpO_2 is 98% on room air, her heart rate is 94 and regular, and lungs are clear. Ms. Smith remains stable and is discharged home in a few days.

Because the most common cause of massive pleural effusion is malignancy, especially of the lung and breast, Ms. Smith's pleural fluid analysis results will be used to help guide further treatment. Malignant pleural effusion tends to be recurrent, so teach her signs and symptoms to look for and make sure that she knows when to notify her physician.

Hayes, D.D. "Action Stat: Reexpansion pulmonary edema," *Nursing* 33(12):96, December 2003. Used with permission.

➤ Monitor intake and output.
➤ Restrict fluids and sodium intake.
➤ Monitor serum electrolyte levels and treat abnormalities.
➤ Prepare the patient for a chest X-ray and an echocardiogram.

Preventive steps

➤ Initiate management of the conditions that can cause pulmonary edema.
➤ Provide a low-salt diet and fluid restriction for patients known to be at risk.

Pathophysiology recap

➤ In pulmonary edema, blood isn't adequately pumped out of the heart, which causes pressure to build up in the veins of the lungs.

➤ Fluid is forced into the alveoli, which hinders normal oxygen exchange, causing shortness of breath and hypoxia.
➤ Causes include myocardial infarction, mitral or aortic valve disorders, infection, hypervolemia, and inhalation of heat or poison gas. Heart diseases that cause weakening or stiffening of the muscle of the heart (such as cardiomyopathy) may also result in pulmonary edema. Pulmonary disorders, such as pneumonia and pulmonary veno-occlusive disease, may also cause pulmonary edema.

➤ Pulmonary embolism

A pulmonary embolism is an obstruction of the pulmonary arterial bed. It occurs when a mass—such as a dislodged thrombus—lodges in a pulmonary artery branch, partially or completely obstructing the artery, which causes ventilation-perfusion mismatch, hypoxemia, and intrapulmonary shunting.

Rapid assessment
➤ Assess for dyspnea and pleuritic or anginal pain.
➤ Assess the patient for a decreased level of consciousness.
➤ Palpate a pulse.
➤ Obtain the patient's vital signs, noting a low-grade fever, tachycardia, and hypotension.
➤ Observe the patient's cough, noting blood-tinged sputum.
➤ Auscultate heart sounds for a S_3 and S_4 gallop.
➤ Auscultate lung sounds for crackles and a pleural friction rub.
➤ Assess the extremities for the location of the original area of thrombosis.
➤ Ask the patient whether he's experiencing pain and if so, to describe it.

Immediate actions
➤ Provide supplemental oxygen and prepare the patient for endotracheal intubation and mechanical ventilation, if necessary.
➤ Initiate cardiac monitoring.
➤ Obtain an arterial blood gas analysis.
➤ Administer as ordered:
 – heparin—to inhibit new thrombus formation
 – fibrinolytic therapy—to enhance fibrinolysis of pulmonary emboli and remaining thrombi

 ALERT *Always be sure to have the antidotes for agents readily available. These include protamine sulfate for heparin, vitamin K for warfarin, and epsilon-aminocaproic acid for thrombolytics.*

 – vasopressors, if necessary—to treat hypotension
 – antibiotic therapy (for septic embolus)—to treat the causative bacteria.

Follow-up actions
➤ Monitor the patient's vital signs, including oxygen saturation, frequently.
➤ Prepare the patient for pulmonary artery catheter insertion.
➤ Obtain a 12-lead electrocardiogram.
➤ Prepare the patient for a ventilation-perfusion scan, pulmonary angiography, a chest X-ray, and magnetic resonance imaging of the chest.
➤ Monitor partial thromboplastin time while giving heparin.
➤ Administer warfarin, as ordered, and monitor prothrombin time and International Normalized Ratio.
➤ Watch for signs of bleeding and institute bleeding precautions.
➤ Prepare the patient for a vena cava ligation, plication, or insertion of a device (umbrella filter) to filter blood returning to the heart and lungs, if necessary.
➤ Prepare the patient for surgical embolectomy if necessary.
➤ Provide gentle range-of-motion exercises.

 ALERT *Never vigorously massage the patient's legs; doing so could dislodge thrombi.*

Preventive steps
➤ Patients at risk for pulmonary embolism may require low-molecular-weight heparin to prevent postoperative venous thromboembolism.
➤ Implement sequential compression devices or antiembolism stockings immediately after surgical procedures, such as large abdominal surgeries, that place the patient at high risk.
➤ Encourage early postoperative ambulation.

Pathophysiology recap
➤ In most patients, pulmonary embolism results from a dislodged thrombus that originates in the leg veins or, less commonly, the pelvic, renal, and hepatic veins, the right side of the heart, or the upper extremities.
➤ Thrombus formation is the result of vascular wall damage, venous stasis, or hypercoagulability of the blood.
➤ Trauma, clot dissolution, sudden muscle spasm, intravascular pressure changes, or a change in peripheral blood flow can cause the thrombus to loosen or fragment.
➤ The thrombus, now called an embolus, floats to the heart's right side and enters the lung through the pulmonary artery where it will dissolve, continue to fragment, or grow.
➤ The embolus prevents the alveoli from producing enough surfactant to maintain alveolar integrity.
➤ The alveoli collapse and atelectasis develops.
➤ There are many risk factors for pulmonary embolism. (See *Risk factors for pulmonary embolism,* page 98.)

➤ RISK FACTORS FOR PULMONARY EMBOLISM

Many disorders and treatments heighten the risk of pulmonary embolism. Surgery and prolonged bed rest, for example, can promote venous stasis, thereby increasing the risk. Other risk factors appear below.

Predisposing disorders
- ➤ Autoimmune hemolytic anemia
- ➤ Cardiac disorders
- ➤ Diabetes mellitus
- ➤ History of thromboembolism, thrombophlebitis, or vascular insufficiency
- ➤ Infection
- ➤ Long bone fracture
- ➤ Lung disorders, especially chronic disorders
- ➤ Manipulation or disconnection of central lines
- ➤ Osteomyelitis
- ➤ Polycythemia
- ➤ Sickle cell disease

Venous stasis
- ➤ Age older than 40
- ➤ Burns
- ➤ Obesity
- ➤ Orthopedic casts
- ➤ Prolonged bed rest or immobilization
- ➤ Recent childbirth

Venous injury
- ➤ I.V. drug abuse
- ➤ I.V. therapy
- ➤ Leg or pelvic fractures or injuries
- ➤ Surgery, particularly of the legs, pelvis, abdomen, or thorax

Increased blood coagulability
- ➤ Cancer
- ➤ Use of high-estrogen hormonal contraceptive agents

➤ Respiratory acidosis

Respiratory acidosis is an acid-base disturbance characterized by reduced alveolar ventilation, as shown by hypercapnia (partial pressure of arterial carbon dioxide [$Paco_2$] above 45 mm Hg). It can be acute or chronic, and the prognosis varies according to the severity of the underlying disturbance and the patient's general clinical condition.

Rapid assessment
➤ Assess the rate, depth, pattern, and quality of respirations, noting dyspnea and shallow respirations.

➤ *ABG RESULTS IN RESPIRATORY ACIDOSIS*

This chart shows typical arterial blood gas (ABG) findings in uncompensated and compensated respiratory acidosis.

	Uncompensated	Compensated
pH	< 7.35	Normal
Paco$_2$ (mm Hg)	> 45	> 45
HCO$_3^-$ (mEq/L)	Normal	> 26

➤ Assess the patient for apprehension, confusion, or other changes in level of consciousness.
➤ Obtain the patient's vital signs, noting increased pulse and respiratory rate and possible decrease in oxygen saturation.
➤ Auscultate for diminished or absent breath sounds.
➤ Assess for decreased deep tendon reflexes.
➤ Observe for tremors and warm, flushed skin.
➤ Assess for nausea and vomiting.
➤ Obtain an arterial blood gas (ABG) analysis. (See *ABG results in respiratory acidosis*.)

Immediate actions
➤ Provide supplemental oxygen and prepare the patient for endotracheal intubation and mechanical ventilation, if necessary.
➤ Administer:
  – bronchodilators—to open the alveoli and enhance gas exchange
  – antibiotics—to prevent pulmonary infection or treat the causative organism
  – sodium bicarbonate—to increase serum pH and treat acidosis

ALERT *Dangerously low blood pH (less than 7.15) can produce profound central nervous system (CNS) and cardiovascular deterioration; careful administration of I.V. sodium bicarbonate may be required.*

  – I.V. fluid, such as normal saline solution with sodium bicarbonate—to increase intravascular volume, blood pressure, and serum pH.

Follow-up actions
➤ Monitor the patient's vital signs, including oxygen saturation, frequently.

ALERT *Be aware that pulse oximetry, used to monitor oxygen saturation, won't reveal increasing carbon dioxide levels.*

➤ Treat the underlying cause.
➤ Monitor ABG values and serum electrolyte levels, and treat abnormalities.
➤ Perform tracheal suctioning, as needed.
➤ Administer vigorous chest physiotherapy.
➤ Encourage turning, coughing, and deep breathing.
➤ Monitor intake and output.
➤ Prepare the patient for dialysis, charcoal, or bronchoscopy, if necessary.

Preventive steps
➤ Instruct patients that smoking cessation is essential in preventing recurrence of respiratory acidosis.
➤ Monitor dose and levels of CNS depressant drugs.

Pathophysiology recap
➤ Depressed ventilation causes carbon dioxide retention and an increase in hydrogen ion concentration, resulting in respiratory acidosis.

➤ Respiratory alkalosis

Respiratory alkalosis is an acid-base disturbance characterized by a decrease in the partial pressure of arterial carbon dioxide ($PaCO_2$) to less than 35 mm Hg. It may be acute, resulting from a sudden increase in ventilation; or chronic, which may be difficult to identify because of renal compensation.

Rapid assessment
➤ Assess the rate, depth, pattern, and quality of spontaneous respirations, noting dyspnea, tachypnea, and deep breathing.
➤ Assess for anxiety, restlessness, or changes in level of consciousness.
➤ Obtain the patient's vital signs, including oxygen saturation.
➤ Obtain an arterial blood gas (ABG) analysis. (See *ABG results in respiratory alkalosis.*)
➤ Assess for increased deep tendon reflexes and check the muscles for twitching, spasms, and strength.
➤ Assess for paresthesia and tetany.
➤ Assess the patient's pain level.

Immediate actions
➤ Provide supplemental oxygen and prepare the patient for endotracheal intubation and mechanical ventilation, if necessary.
➤ Assist the patient to breathe into a paper bag, if indicated.
➤ Institute safety measures and seizure precautions.
➤ Administer as ordered:
  – diamox—to promote bicarbonate excretion through the kidneys
  – analgesics—to relieve the pain that may be causing the condition.

> **ABG RESULTS IN RESPIRATORY ALKALOSIS**

This chart shows typical arterial blood gas (ABG) findings in uncompensated and compensated respiratory alkalosis.

	Uncompensated	Compensated
pH	> 7.45	Normal
Paco$_2$ (mm Hg)	< 35	< 35
HCO$_3^-$ (mEq/L)	Normal	< 22

Follow-up actions
> Monitor the patient's vital signs, including oxygen saturation.
> Treat the underlying cause.
> Send blood samples for toxicology screening, especially salicylate poisoning.
> Monitor ABG values and serum electrolyte levels.
> Provide adequate rest periods.

Preventive steps
> Instruct patients that smoking cessation helps prevent the recurrence of respiratory alkalosis.
> Instruct patients to take aspirin in recommended doses.
> Adequately control pain with analgesics and guided imagery.

Pathophysiology recap
> Alveolar hyperventilation and hypocapnia result in respiratory alkalosis.
> Uncomplicated respiratory alkalosis leads to a decrease in hydrogen ion concentrations, which results in an elevated blood pH.
> Hypercapnia occurs when the elimination of carbon dioxide by the lungs exceeds carbon dioxide production at the cellular level.

> Respiratory arrest

Respiratory arrest, the prolonged absence of spontaneous breathing, usually coincides with cardiac arrest. It's the third of three stages of respiratory compromise: respiratory distress, respiratory failure, and respiratory arrest.

Rapid assessment
> Assess the patient's level of consciousness, noting depressed sensorium, agitation, or unconsciousness.
> Assess for a patent airway.

➤ Assess for absence of spontaneous respirations, a rise or fall of the chest, air movement from the mouth or nose, and gasping for air, stridor, and an irregular respiratory pattern.
➤ Palpate for a peripheral pulse.
➤ Auscultate for diminished or absent breath sounds.
➤ Obtain the patient's vital signs, noting decreased oxygen saturation, tachycardia, and hypertension.
➤ Assess for cyanosis and mottling.

Immediate actions
➤ Determine the patient's responsiveness and call for help.
➤ Attempt to open the airway.
➤ If the airway is obstructed, relieve the obstruction through a series of subdiaphragmatic, abdominal thrusts in a child or adult, or five back blows followed by five chest thrusts in an infant.
➤ If a cervical spine injury is suspected, use the modified jaw-thrust technique to open the airway.
➤ If the obstruction is cleared, assess the patient's respiratory status and perform rescue breathing if necessary.
➤ If the airway is patent, check the pulse; if no pulse, then implement cardiopulmonary resuscitation.
➤ Provide supplemental oxygen and prepare the patient for endotracheal intubation or tracheostomy and mechanical ventilation.
➤ Initiate cardiac monitoring.

Follow-up actions
➤ Monitor the patient's vital signs frequently.
➤ Monitor arterial blood gas values and serum electrolytes, and treat abnormalities promptly.
➤ Prepare the patient for a chest X-ray and bronchoscopy or laryngoscopy.
➤ Provide emotional support to the patient and his family.

Preventive steps
➤ Initiate thorough and aggressive treatment of causative conditions.
➤ Institute safety measures to prevent aspiration of foreign objects.

Pathophysiology recap
➤ Secondary respiratory arrest results from insufficient circulation.
➤ Complete respiratory arrest is the absence of spontaneous ventilatory movement with cyanosis; it may develop quickly in a conscious victim because of a foreign body obstruction.
➤ If the respiratory arrest is prolonged, cardiac arrest will follow because of impairment of cardiac oxygenation and function related to hypoxemia.
➤ Respiratory arrest is the leading cause of cardiac arrest in infants and children; in adults, cardiac arrest usually leads to respiratory arrest.

➤ Effective pulmonary gas exchange involves several functions, including a clear airway, normal lungs and chest wall, and adequate pulmonary circulation.
➤ A compromise of any of these anatomic structures or functions can affect respiration.

Primary respiratory arrest
➤ Primary respiratory arrest results from airway obstruction, decreased respiratory drive, or respiratory muscle weakness.
➤ While airway obstruction can be partial or complete, the most common cause in an unconscious victim is upper airway obstruction due to tongue displacement into the oropharynx secondary to a loss of muscle tone.
   Other potential causes of upper airway obstruction include:
➤ accumulation of blood, mucus, or vomitus
➤ foreign body aspiration
➤ spasms or edema of the larynx
➤ edema of the pharynx
➤ inflammation of the upper airway
➤ neoplasm
➤ trauma.
   Causes of lower airway obstruction include:
➤ aspiration of gastric contents
➤ severe bronchospasm
➤ conditions that fill the alveoli of the lungs with fluid such as pulmonary hemorrhage.

➤ Respiratory depression

Respiratory depression implies inadequate ventilation. It's a condition of slow, weak respirations, usually less than 12 per minute, that don't ventilate or perfuse the lungs. If respiratory depression isn't corrected, it leads to acidemia.

Rapid assessment
➤ Assess for a patent airway.
➤ Assess the rate, depth, pattern, and quality of respirations, noting a rate of less than 12 breaths/minute, dyspnea, stridor, and air hunger.
➤ Assess for hypoventilation with an overdose of sedatives or opioids.
➤ Assess for other signs of overdose, such as diaphoresis, dilated or constricted pupils, coma, tremors, seizure activity, or neurologic posturing.
➤ Auscultate the lungs for crackles and rhonchi.
➤ Assess for restlessness or agitation, a depressed level of consciousness, or unresponsiveness.
➤ Palpate for a pulse.

➤ Obtain the patient's vital signs, noting tachycardia and decreased oxygen saturation.
➤ Inspect the skin and mucous membranes for cyanosis or pallor.

Immediate actions
➤ Place the patient in semi-Fowler's position.
➤ Provide supplemental oxygen and prepare the patient for endotracheal intubation or tracheostomy and mechanical ventilation.
➤ Perform rescue breathing and cardiopulmonary resuscitation, if necessary.
➤ Initiate continuous cardiac monitoring.
➤ Administer the appropriate sedative or opioid antagonist, if necessary. (See *Common antidotes.*)
➤ Obtain an arterial blood gas (ABG) analysis.
➤ Obtain an electrocardiogram.
➤ Obtain blood samples for toxicology.
➤ Administer I.V. fluids to increase intravascular volume and blood pressure, flumazenil to reverse effects of benzodiazepines, nalaxone to reverse effects of opiods, or antiarrhythmics to treat arrhythmias caused by hypoxia.

 ALERT *When administering flumazenil and naloxone, watch for signs of withdrawal. Flumazenil may precipitate seizures, especially in patients who have ingested tricyclic antidepressants or have been on long-term sedation with benzodiazepines.*

Follow-up actions
➤ Monitor the patient's vital signs frequently.
➤ Prepare the patient for arterial and pulmonary artery catheter insertion.
➤ Monitor ABG results.
➤ Perform tracheal suctioning and chest physiotherapy, as needed.
➤ Insert an indwelling urinary catheter.
➤ Monitor intake and output hourly.
➤ Prepare the patient for a chest X-ray and pulmonary function tests.
➤ Provide a calm, quiet environment.

Preventive steps
➤ Initiate thorough and aggressive management of causative disorders.

Pathophysiology recap
➤ Respiratory depression is a serious complication and commonly occurs in patients sedated with anesthesia or medications such as opioids.
➤ The respiratory rate may decrease gradually or abruptly cease.
➤ Any change from respiratory function reflected in previous assessments and data must be considered as potential respiratory depression.
➤ If uncorrected, progressive carbon dioxide retention and hypoxemia can result in systemic acidemia.

➤ COMMON ANTIDOTES

This chart lists drugs or toxins commonly involved in respiratory depression and their antidotes.

Drug or toxin	Antidote
Acetaminophen	Acetylcysteine (Mucomyst, Acetadote)
Anticholinergics, tricyclic antidepressants	Physostigmine (Antilirium)
Benzodiazepines	Flumazenil (Romazicon)
Calcium channel blockers	Calcium chloride
Cyanide	Amyl nitrate, sodium nitrate, and sodium thiosulfate; methylene blue
Digoxin, cardiac glycosides	Digoxin immune fab (Digibind)
Ethylene glycol or methanol	Fomepizole (Antizol)
Heparin	Protamine sulfate
Insulin	Glucagon
Iron	Deferoxamine (Desferal)
Lead	Edetate calcium disodium (Calcium Disodium Versenate)
Opioids	Naloxone (Narcan), nalmefene (Revex), naltrexone (Depade, ReVia)
Organophosphates, anticholinesterases	Atropine, pralidoxime (Protopam)

➤ It may be caused by an impairment at various levels of the respiratory system, including the central nervous system, the upper and lower airways, and alveolar spaces or chest wall as well as the impairment of normal mechanisms of ventilation or the blood and circulatory system.

➤ *Respiratory syncytial virus*

Respiratory syncytial virus (RSV) is the leading cause of lower respiratory tract infection in infants and young children and upper respiratory infections in adults. It's the suspected cause of fatal respiratory disease in infants. RSV can cause serious illness in adults who are immunocompromised, elderly people living in institutions, and patients with underlying cardiopulmonary disease.

Rapid assessment
> Assess the rate, depth, pattern, and quality of respirations, noting dyspnea, tachypnea, nasal flaring, and retraction.
> Assess for malaise and a decreased level of consciousness.
> Auscultate lung sounds for wheezing, rhonchi, and crackles.
> Obtain the patient's vital signs, noting decreased oxygen saturation and increased temperature.
> Observe for nasal congestion and nasal and pharyngeal inflammation.
> Inspect for otitis media.
> Inspect for cyanosis.

Immediate actions
> Place the patient in semi-Fowler's position.
> Provide supplemental oxygen and prepare the patient for endotracheal intubation or tracheostomy and mechanical ventilation, if necessary.
> Institute contact isolation precautions.
> Administer as ordered:
  - ribavirin in aerosol form
  - I.V. fluids such as normal saline solution.

Follow-up actions
> Monitor the patient's vital signs, including oxygen saturation, frequently.
> Monitor arterial blood gas values.
> Obtain cultures of nasal and pharyngeal secretions and serum RSV antibody titers.
> Perform percussion, drainage, and suction when necessary.
> Use a croup tent, as needed.
> Monitor intake and output.
> Prepare the patient for a chest X-ray.
> Provide adequate nutrition and avoidance of overhydration.
> Provide frequent rest periods.

Preventive steps
> Instruct patients to practice good hygiene, including frequent, thorough hand washing, especially around infants and toddlers.
> Instruct patients to avoid contact with infants and children and people with a cold or fever.
> When possible, try to keep young children away from infants to prevent the spread of RSV.
> Instruct patients to not smoke around infants.
> Instruct parents to avoid taking premature and low-birth-weight infants into crowds.

➤ A monthly palivizumab (Synagis) injection is recommended for infants younger than age 2 who are at high risk.

Pathophysiology recap
➤ Infection is caused by RSV, a subgroup of myxoviruses resembling paramyxovirus.
➤ The virus is transmitted from person to person by respiratory secretions.
➤ The virus attaches to cells, eventually resulting in necrosis of the bronchiolar epithelium; in severe infection, peribronchiolar infiltration of lymphocytes and mononuclear cells occurs.
➤ Intra-alveolar thickening and filling of the alveolar spaces with fluid results.
➤ Narrowing of the airway passages on expiration prevents air from leaving the lungs, causing progressive overinflation.

➤ Status asthmaticus

Status asthmaticus is a life-threatening situation resulting from an acute asthma attack. If untreated or if the patient doesn't respond to treatment with pharmacotherapy after 24 hours, status asthmaticus is diagnosed.

Rapid assessment
➤ Assess for recent exposure to an allergen.
➤ Observe the rate, depth, pattern, and quality of respirations, noting dyspnea, tachypnea, and accessory muscle use.
➤ Auscultate the lungs for wheezing and diminished breath sounds.
➤ Assess for lethargy, confusion, and fatigue.
➤ Obtain the patient's vital signs, noting an increased heart rate and decreased oxygen saturation.
➤ Monitor for pulsus paradoxus.
➤ Observe the patient's cough and the secretions produced.
➤ Percuss for hyperresonance over the chest wall.
➤ Test for vocal fremitus.
➤ Obtain an arterial blood gas (ABG) analysis.

Immediate actions
➤ Remove precipitating factors, if identifiable.
➤ Provide humidified supplemental oxygen and prepare the patient for endotracheal intubation and mechanical ventilation, if necessary.

 ALERT *Remember that oxygen can be toxic and directly injure the lung if given too long or at excessive concentrations. Therefore, use the lowest fraction of inspired oxygen necessary to maintain adequate oxygenation for the shortest time possible.*

➤ Institute continuous electrocardiogram monitoring.
➤ Administer as ordered:

– bronchodilators—to dilate the bronchial tree and enhance gas exchange
– epinephrine—to treat an allergic reaction
– corticosteroids—to decrease inflammation
– nebulizer therapies (anticholinergic agents)—to dilate the bronchial tree
– I.V. fluids such as normal saline solution—to increase intravascular volume and thin tenacious secretions.

Follow-up actions
➤ Monitor the patient's vital signs frequently.
➤ Monitor ABG values.
➤ Monitor intake and output.
➤ Perform chest physiotherapy; encourage coughing and deep breathing.

 ALERT *During the acute phase of status asthmaticus, chest physiotherapy is contraindicated because of the patient's respiratory distress as well as the hyperreactiveness of the airways.*

➤ Assist with relaxation techniques.
➤ Provide a calm, quiet environment.

Preventive steps
➤ Instruct patients to avoid precipitating factors such as environmental irritants or allergens.
➤ Initiate desensitization to specific antigens to decrease the severity of asthma attacks with future exposure.

Pathophysiology recap
➤ Immunoglobulin (Ig) E antibodies attached to histamine-containing mast cells and receptors on cell membranes initiate intrinsic asthma attacks.
➤ Antigen exposure occurs and the IgE antibody combines with the antigen.
➤ On subsequent antigen exposure, mast cells degranulate and release mediators.
➤ Mast cells in the lung are stimulated to release histamine and the slow-reacting substance of anaphylaxis.
➤ Histamine attaches to receptor sites in the larger bronchi, where it causes swelling in smooth muscle and inflammation, irritation, and swelling in mucous membranes. This causes dyspnea, prolonged expiration, and an increased respiratory rate. (See *Understanding asthma*.)
➤ Leukotrienes attach to receptor sites in the smaller bronchi and cause local swelling of smooth muscle and prostaglandins to travel to the lungs via the bloodstream.
➤ Prostaglandins enhance the effect of histamine, causing an audible wheeze and cough.
➤ Histamine stimulates mucus secretion by the mucous membranes, narrowing the bronchial lumen further.

➤ UNDERSTANDING ASTHMA

In asthma, hyperresponsiveness of the airways and bronchospasms occur. These illustrations show how an asthma attack progresses.

➤ Histamine (H) attaches to receptor sites in larger bronchi, causing swelling of the smooth muscles.

➤ Leukotrienes (L) attach to receptor sites in the smaller bronchi and cause swelling of smooth muscle. Leukotrienes also cause prostaglandins to travel through the bloodstream to the lungs, where they enhance histamine's effects.

➤ Histamine stimulates the mucous membranes to secrete excessive mucus, further narrowing the bronchial lumen. On inhalation, the narrowed bronchial lumen can still expand slightly; on exhalation, however, the increased intrathoracic pressure closes the bronchial lumen completely.

➤ Mucus fills lung bases, inhibiting alveolar ventilation. Blood is shunted to alveoli in other parts of the lungs, but it still can't compensate for diminished ventilation.

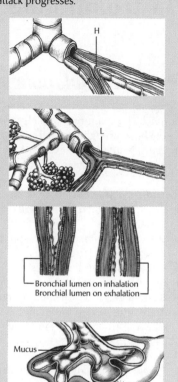

Bronchial lumen on inhalation
Bronchial lumen on exhalation

Mucus

➤ Goblet cells secrete viscous mucus, resulting in coughing, wheezing, and respiratory distress.

➤ On inhalation, the narrowed bronchial lumen can still expand slightly, allowing air to reach the alveoli.

➤ On exhalation, increased intrathoracic pressure closes the bronchial lumen completely.

➤ When status asthmaticus develops, hypoxemia worsens and the expiratory rate and volume decrease even further.

➤ Gas exchange is impeded, airway resistance is increased, hypoxia increases, the patient tires and hypoventilates, and partial pressure of arterial carbon dioxide ($Paco_2$) levels rise.

➤ Respiratory acidosis develops.

➤ The situation becomes life-threatening when no air is audible on auscultation (a silent chest) and $Paco_2$ rises to over 70 mm Hg.

4

Gastrointestinal emergencies

➤ *Abdominal trauma, blunt*

Nonpenetrating injuries to the abdomen are known as *blunt abdominal trauma*. These injuries typically result from motor vehicle accidents, sports injuries, fights, or falls. The prognosis for patients with this type of injury depends on the extent of the injury and on the organs damaged, but it's generally improved by prompt diagnosis and surgical repair.

Rapid assessment
➤ Obtain the patient's vital signs, noting tachycardia and hypotension, if present.
➤ Observe for spontaneous respirations.
➤ Auscultate breath sounds.
➤ Palpate for peripheral pulses.
➤ Auscultate heart sounds and apical rate.
➤ Auscultate for bowel sounds or abdominal bruits.
➤ Assess the patient for tenderness, abdominal splinting or rigidity, nausea, vomiting, pallor, and cyanosis. Pain may be severe and may radiate beyond the abdomen; for example, the patient may report pain in the shoulders.
➤ Assess for signs of injury, such as bruises, abrasions, contusions, and distention.

 ALERT *Be alert for signs and symptoms of massive blood loss: hypotension; cyanosis; anxiety; oliguria; confusion; restlessness; pale, cool, clammy skin; and a rapid, weak, thready pulse. If you detect these signs, prepare the patient for I.V. fluid and blood product administration to replace intravascular volume and treat blood loss.*

Immediate actions
➤ To maintain airway and breathing, intubate the patient and provide mechanical ventilation as necessary; otherwise, provide supplemental oxygen.
➤ Keep the patient's cervical spine immobilized unless injury to this area has been ruled out.
➤ Using large-bore needles, start two I.V. lines for monitoring and rapid infusion of normal saline or lactated Ringer's solution (or blood transfusions if the patient's condition is hemodynamically unstable).

➤ Draw blood for complete blood count, type and cross match, and serum electrolytes while inserting the large-bore I.V. catheter.
➤ Insert a nasogastric tube and, if necessary, an indwelling urinary catheter.
➤ Assist the physician with a diagnostic peritoneal lavage if indicated.
➤ Give an analgesic for pain, as indicated.
➤ Treat injuries as needed.

Follow-up actions
➤ Monitor the patient's vital signs.
➤ Monitor intake and output hourly.
➤ Monitor stomach aspirate and urine for blood.
➤ Prepare the patient for a central venous or pulmonary artery catheter and arterial line insertion, as needed.
➤ Monitor arterial blood gas values.
➤ Monitor hemoglobin and hematocrit levels and administer blood products as ordered.
➤ Monitor serum electrolytes and treat abnormalities.
➤ Provide care to injuries as ordered.
➤ Monitor the patient for signs and symptoms of infection, especially peritonitis.
➤ Prepare the patient for surgery, if necessary, making sure that he or a responsible family member has signed an informed consent form.

 ALERT *An informed consent form is necessary unless surgery must be performed immediately to save the patient's life. The patient may not sign the form if under the influence of opioid analgesics or other agents.*

➤ If the injury was caused by a motor vehicle accident, find out whether the police were notified and, if not, notify them.

Preventive steps
➤ Encourage the patient to wear a seat belt while driving or riding as a passenger in a motor vehicle.
➤ Advise the patient to use ladders safely and according to manufacturers' recommendations to avoid the risk of falls.

Pathophysiology recap
➤ Blunt abdominal injuries usually result from motor vehicle accidents, fights, falls from heights, and sports accidents.
➤ Generally, damage to a solid abdominal organ (liver, spleen, pancreas, or kidney) causes hemorrhage, whereas damage to a hollow organ (stomach, intestine, gallbladder, or bladder) causes rupture and release of the affected organ's contents (including bacteria) into the abdomen, which, in turn, produces inflammation.
➤ Because a blunt abdominal injury may damage major blood vessels as well as internal organs, the most immediate life-threatening conse-

➤ EFFECTS OF BLUNT ABDOMINAL TRAUMA

When a blunt object strikes a person's abdomen, it increases intra-abdominal pressure. Depending on the force of the blow, the trauma can lacerate the liver and spleen, rupture the stomach, bruise the duodenum, and damage the kidneys.

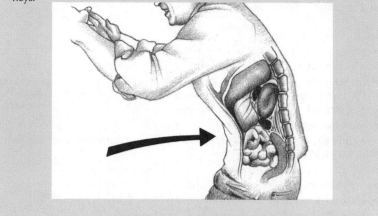

quences are hemorrhage and hypovolemic shock; later threats include infection. (See *Effects of blunt abdominal trauma.*)

➤ *Appendicitis*

The most common abdominal surgical disease, appendicitis is an inflammation of the vermiform appendix due to an obstruction. Since the advent of antibiotics, the incidence and mortality from appendicitis have declined; however, if untreated, gangrene and perforation will develop within 36 hours.

Rapid assessment

- ➤ Obtain vital signs, noting hypotension, tachycardia, and increased temperature.
- ➤ Assess for a history of generalized or localized colicky periumbilical or epigastric pain, followed by anorexia, nausea, and episodes of vomiting.
- ➤ Assess the patient for pain localized in the right lower quadrant of the abdomen (McBurney's point).
- ➤ Assess for abdominal "boardlike" rigidity, retractive respirations, increasing abdominal tenderness, increasingly severe abdominal spasms, constipation (diarrhea is also possible) and, almost invariably, rebound tenderness.

ALERT *Sudden cessation of abdominal pain indicates a perforation or infarction of the appendix.*

Immediate actions
➤ Withhold oral solids and liquids.
➤ Administer I.V. fluids to prevent dehydration.

ALERT *Never apply heat to the right lower quadrant of the patient's abdomen or administer a cathartic or an enema; these actions may cause the appendix to rupture.*

➤ Obtain a serum sample for a complete blood count, noting increased white blood cells.
➤ Prepare the patient for surgery. Appendectomy is the only effective treatment.
➤ With appendicitis complicated by peritonitis, insert a nasogastric tube to decompress the stomach and reduce nausea and vomiting. (See *Inserting a nasogastric tube,* page 114.)
➤ To minimize pain, place the patient in Fowler's position.
➤ Administer I.V. antibiotics as ordered.

Follow-up actions
➤ Monitor the patient's postoperative vital signs and pain level.
➤ Administer pain medications as ordered.
➤ Monitor intake and output hourly.
➤ Administer a systemic antibiotic to reduce postoperative wound infection.
➤ Teach and assist the patient to cough, breathe deeply, and turn frequently to prevent pulmonary complications.
➤ Assess and document bowel sounds, passing of flatus, and bowel movements. In a patient whose nausea and abdominal rigidity have subsided, these signs indicate that he may resume oral fluids; advance diet as tolerated.
➤ Help the patient ambulate as soon as possible after surgery (within 24 hours).
➤ Monitor the patient for postoperative complications. The complaint that "something gave way" may indicate that wound dehiscence has occurred. Continuing pain and fever may signal an abscess. If an abscess or peritonitis develops, incision and drainage may be necessary. Monitor wound drainage.

Preventive steps
➤ Appendicitis can't be prevented; it typically develops suddenly, with no apparent direct cause.
➤ Patients with severe abdominal pain or right lower quadrant pain should seek medical attention immediately to prevent rupture of an inflamed appendix.

➤ *INSERTING A NASOGASTRIC TUBE*

Usually inserted to decompress the stomach, a nasogastric (NG) tube can also prevent vomiting after major surgery. Inserting an NG tube requires close observation of the patient and verification of proper placement. Follow these steps to insert an NG tube and confirm its proper placement.

For insertion:
➤ Explain the procedure to the patient, and gather and prepare all necessary equipment.
➤ Help the patient into high Fowler's position unless contraindicated, and help her keep her neck in a neutral position.
➤ To determine how long the NG tube must be to reach the stomach, hold the end of the tube at the tip of the patient's nose. Extend the tube to the patient's earlobe and then down to the xiphoid process (as shown to the right).

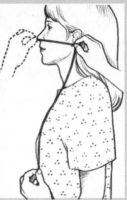

➤ Mark this distance on the tubing with tape. (Average measurements for an adult range from 22" to 26" [56 to 66 cm].)
➤ Lubricate the first 3" (7.6 cm) of the tube with a water-soluble gel.
➤ Instruct the patient to hold her head straight and upright. Grasp the tube with the end point-ing downward, curve it if necessary, and care-fully insert it into the more patent nostril.
➤ Aim the tube downward and toward the ear closer to the chosen nostril. Advance it slowly.
➤ Unless contraindicated, offer the patient a cup or glass of water with a straw. Direct her to sip and swallow as you slowly advance the tube. (If you aren't using water, ask the patient to swallow.)
➤ As you carefully advance the tube and the patient swallows, watch for signs of respiratory distress, which may mean the tube is in the bronchus and must be removed immediately. Evaluate the patient and, if appropriate, reattempt the procedure.
➤ Stop advancing the tube when the tape mark reaches the patient's nostril.
➤ Secure the NG tube to the patient's nose with hypoallergenic tape or other designated tube holder.
For confirmation of proper placement:
➤ Attach a catheter-tip or bulb syringe to the NG tube and try to aspirate stomach contents. If you don't obtain stomach contents, position the patient on her left side to move the contents into the stomach's greater curvature and aspirate again.
➤ If you still can't aspirate stomach contents, advance the tube 1" to 2" (2.5 to 5 cm) and try to aspirate stomach contents again. Examine the aspirate and place a small amount on the pH test strip. Probability of a gastric placement is increased if the aspirate has a typical gastric fluid appearance (grassy green, clear and colorless with mucus threads, or brown) and the pH is ≤ 5.
➤ If these tests don't confirm proper tube placement, you'll need X-ray confir-mation.

Pathophysiology recap
➤ Appendicitis probably results from an obstruction of the intestinal lumen caused by a fecal mass, stricture, barium ingestion, or viral infection.
➤ This obstruction triggers an inflammatory process that can lead to infection, thrombosis, necrosis, and perforation.
➤ If the appendix ruptures or perforates, the infected contents spill into the abdominal cavity, causing peritonitis, the most common and most perilous complication of appendicitis.

➤ Bowel infarction

Bowel infarction is a result of decreased blood flow to the major mesenteric vessels. It leads to vasoconstriction and vasospasm of the bowel and contracted bowel with mucosal ulceration.

Rapid assessment
➤ Obtain vital signs, noting tachycardia and hypotension.
➤ Assess for abdominal pain and abdominal distention with tenderness and guarding.
➤ Auscultate for absent or hypoactive bowel sounds.
➤ Ask about vomiting, bloody diarrhea, and weight loss.
➤ Barium studies, angiography, and a computed tomography scan may reveal the area or location of infarction.
➤ Assess skin temperature and capillary refill.

Immediate actions
➤ Initiate and maintain nothing-by-mouth status.
➤ Assess depth, pattern, and rate of respirations, and prepare the patient for endotracheal intubation and mechanical ventilation, if necessary.
➤ Obtain a serum sample for arterial blood gas analysis, lactic acid, electrolytes, complete blood count, prothrombin time, International Normalized Ratio, and partial thromboplastin time.
➤ Obtain a baseline abdominal girth and weight.
➤ Monitor skin temperature and capillary refill.
➤ Insert large bore I.V. lines and administer I.V. fluid replacement, as ordered.
➤ Administer vasoactive agents, such as dopamine, as ordered.
➤ Initiate the administration of anticoagulants, such as heparin, as ordered.

Follow-up actions
➤ Monitor vital signs frequently.
➤ Prepare the patient for barium studies, angiography, and a computed tomography scan to reveal the area or location of infarction.

➤ Prepare the patient for a sigmoidoscopy to confirm the diagnosis of ischemic bowel.
➤ Prepare the patient for surgical repair, as indicated.
➤ Administer analgesics to control pain and antibiotics to prevent infection, as ordered.
➤ Monitor intake and output hourly.
➤ Observe electrolytes and glucose levels for imbalances and treat as ordered.
➤ Provide nutritional support, as ordered.
➤ Watch for signs and symptoms of thromboemboli.
➤ Monitor prothrombin time, International Normalized Ratio, and partial thromboplastin time for patients taking anticoagulants. Notify the physician of your findings so that he can titrate the doses accordingly.
➤ Monitor patients taking anticoagulants for signs and symptoms of bleeding.

Preventive steps
➤ Advise the patient with endocarditis or atrial fibrillation who takes Coumadin to follow up with his physician for blood work to ensure his dose is appropriate.
➤ Advise the patient taking medications to lower cholesterol to follow up with his physician for blood monitoring and medication dosage changes.

Pathophysiology recap
➤ Decreased blood flow to the mesenteric vessels leads to spasms.
➤ When the spasms subside, the muscles of the bowel are fatigued and can't receive essential oxygen and nutrients.
➤ The bowel becomes edematous and cyanotic and necrosis can occur.
➤ As pressure in the bowel lumens increases, perforation can occur, leading to peritonitis or abscess formation.
➤ Bowel infarction can be caused by thrombosis after a myocardial infarction, cholesterol plaques in the aorta that become dislodged, arteriosclerosis, cirrhosis of the liver, hypercoagulation (as seen in polycythemia or after splenectomy), or reduced perfusion from heart failure or shock. In patients with endocarditis or atrial fibrillation, emboli may cause bowel infarction.

➤ Esophageal varices rupture

Esophageal varices are dilated, tortuous veins in the submucosa of the lower esophagus resulting from portal hypertension. Rupture of these vessels can cause sudden and massive bleeding. If the patient experiences a major loss of blood volume (approximately 40%), death can occur within 30 minutes.

Rapid assessment

➤ Assess the patient's level of consciousness (LOC).

 ALERT *Be sure to establish a baseline for the patient's LOC. If he has underlying hepatic disease, his LOC may be altered due to hepatic encephalopathy, making it difficult to determine whether changes are due to hypovolemia alone. Correlate changes in the LOC with additional findings, such as prolonged capillary refill; decreased distal pulses; cool, pale extremities; and hemodynamic parameters to evaluate for continued hypovolemia.*

➤ Observe the rate, depth, and pattern of the patient's respirations, and auscultate breath sounds.
➤ Assess the patient's vital signs, noting tachycardia, tachypnea, decreased oxygen saturation, and hypotension.
➤ Auscultate the patient's apical rate and palpate for peripheral pulses.
➤ Observe visible blood loss and approximate the amount.
➤ Assess the patient's skin color and capillary refill.

Immediate actions

➤ Perform cardiopulmonary resuscitation as necessary.
➤ Provide supplemental oxygen and prepare the patient for endotracheal intubation and mechanical ventilation as necessary.
➤ Suction the patient orally to help clear his airway.
➤ Place the patient in semi-Fowler's position to maximize chest expansion and prevent aspiration.
➤ Administer I.V. fluid replacement and blood component therapy, as ordered.
➤ Obtain a serum sample for complete blood count, serum electrolytes, prothrombin time, International Normalized Ratio, partial thromboplastin time, arterial blood gas analysis, and type and screen.
➤ Assist with central venous line or pulmonary artery catheter insertion.
➤ Administer, as ordered:
  – I.V. vasopressin therapy — to stop bleeding temporarily
  – beta-adrenergic blockers — to decrease portal venous pressure
  – somatostatin therapy — to decrease splanchnic blood flow, as ordered.

 ALERT *Nitroglycerin may need to be administered along with vasopressin to provide cardiac protection from vasoconstriction.*

➤ Insert an indwelling urinary catheter.
➤ Institute continuous cardiac monitoring to evaluate for arrhythmias.
➤ Begin lactulose therapy to promote elimination of old blood from the GI tract, which combats excessive production and accumulation of ammonia.
➤ Assist the physician to perform nasogastric (NG) intubation with gastric lavage using room temperature normal saline solution. (See *Gastric lavage*, page 118.)

➤ *GASTRIC LAVAGE*

For patients with gastric or esophageal bleeding, gastric lavage may be used to stop bleeding. It may also be used after poisoning or drug overdose to flush out the stomach and remove ingested substances.

Normal saline solution is usually used for lavage to prevent rapid electrolyte loss.

Types of gastric tubes

When irrigating the stomach of a patient with profuse gastric bleeding, a wide-bore gastric tube usually is best. Typically inserted orally, these tubes remain in place only long enough to complete the lavage and evacuate stomach contents.

Ewald tube

In an emergency, using a single-lumen tube with several openings at the distal end, such as an Ewald tube, allows you to siphon large amounts of gastric contents quickly.

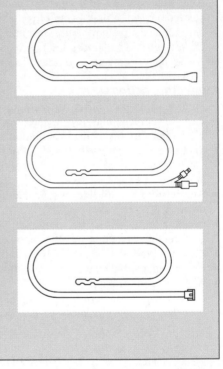

Levacuator tube

A Levacuator tube has two lumens. Use the larger lumen for evacuating gastric contents and the smaller lumen for instilling an irrigant.

Edlich tube

An Edlich tube is a single-lumen tube with four openings near the closed distal tip. A funnel or syringe may be connected at the proximal end. Like the Ewald tube, the Edlich tube lets you siphon large quantities of gastric contents quickly.

 ALERT *Don't attempt NG intubation in a patient with known esophageal varices without a physician present. Intubation can cause further rupture.*

Follow-up actions

➤ Institute safety measures to protect the patient from self-harm.
➤ Monitor the patient's vital signs closely.
➤ Administer medications, as ordered.

> **TREATMENT MODALITIES FOR RUPTURED ESOPHAGEAL VARICES**

If medical management doesn't resolve ruptured esophageal varices, the physician may decide that the patient requires one of the following procedures to treat this condition:
> sclerotherapy via endoscopy, to cause fibrosis and obliteration of the varices
> endoscopic banding, to ligate the varices
> balloon tamponade, to help control hemorrhage by applying pressure to the bleeding site
> portosystemic shunts when bleeding can't be controlled by endoscopic or pharmacologic methods or balloon tamponade
> percutaneous transhepatic embolization, to block the collateral vessels of the stomach that supply blood to the varices
> transjugular intrahepatic portosystemic shunts, to decrease portal hypertension.

In general, the patient's condition determines the treatment of choice. For example, if the patient is having massive bleeding along with respiratory complications, the physician may choose to perform balloon tamponade, stabilize the patient, and then have him undergo sclerotherapy or banding. A patient who has already undergone sclerotherapy and continues to have variceal rupture and bleeding may require a transjugular intrahepatic portosystemic shunt.

> Monitor the patient's hemoglobin level and hematocrit at least every 4 hours until stable.
> Monitor intake and output hourly.
> Watch for signs and symptoms of fluid overload (crackles, jugular vein distention) with blood product administration.

 ALERT *Increases in central venous pressure, pulmonary artery pressure, and pulmonary artery wedge pressure indicate fluid overload.*

> As necessary, prepare the patient for shunting procedure or surgery. (See *Treatment modalities for ruptured esophageal varices.*)
> Assist with sclerotherapy or banding as necessary, monitoring the patient's respiratory status closely for complications.
> If the patient requires balloon tamponade with a Blakemore tube, assist with insertion. Maintain balloon pressure as ordered, usually between 20 and 45 mm Hg, and deflate the balloon at ordered intervals.

 ALERT *After an esophageal balloon has been inserted, stay alert for respiratory complications because the inflated balloon can partially or totally obstruct the airway. Suction oral secretions from above the inflated balloon using a proximal tube or additional lumen of the tube, and ensure that this tube or lumen is labeled for suction purposes only. Assess breath sounds at least every hour, and keep scissors at the bedside (to cut all lumens) in case total airway occlusion oc-*

COMPLICATIONS

➤ *ACUTE UPPER GI BLEED*

Upper GI bleeding occurs above the ligament of Treitz (where the duodenum meets the jejunum), and includes bleeding in the esophagus, stomach, and duodenum. Upper GI bleeding may result from ruptured esophageal varices, peptic ulcer disease, Mallory-Weiss syndrome, or erosive gastritis. It accounts for significant morbidity and mortality.

Signs and symptoms
➤ Bright red blood in nasogastric tube drainage or vomitus (hematemesis)
➤ Drainage or vomitus that looks like coffee grounds (if blood has been exposed to gastric acid after spending time in the stomach)
➤ Melena (black, tarry, sticky stools)
➤ Other signs and symptoms, according to amount of blood lost:
  – 500 to 750 ml (10% to 15% of total blood volume) – asymptomatic
  – 750 to 1,200 ml (15% to 25% of total blood volume) – anxiety, restlessness, tachycardia, tachypnea, hypotension; however, normal urine output
  – 1,200 to 1,500 ml (25% to 35% of total blood volume) – anxiety, restlessness, agitation, tachycardia, tachypnea, orthostatic hypotension, decreased urine output
  – 1,500 to 2,000 ml (35% to 50% of total blood volume) – anxiety, agitation, confusion; tachycardia; tachypnea; hypotension, with systolic blood pressure less than 60 mm Hg; oliguria; diaphoresis; cool, clammy skin; pallor
The patient's condition will continue to deteriorate if bleeding isn't controlled.

Treatment
Treatment focuses on stopping the bleeding and providing fluid resuscitation while maintaining the patient's vital functions. Treatment may include fluid volume replacement, respiratory support as indicated, gastric intubation with gastric lavage and gastric pH monitoring, and endoscopic or surgical repair of bleeding sites. Pharmacologic therapy may include histamine-2 receptor antagonists and other agents.

Nursing considerations
➤ Ensure a patent airway and assess breathing and circulation.
➤ Assess the patient for the extent of blood loss and begin fluid resuscitation, as ordered.
➤ Obtain a type and crossmatch for blood component therapy.
➤ Administer supplemental oxygen and monitor pulse oximetry and arterial blood gas levels for signs of hypoxemia.
➤ Monitor for signs of hypovolemic shock.
➤ Assist with insertion of a central venous or pulmonary artery catheter to evaluate the patient's hemodynamic status.
➤ When available, begin blood component therapy, as ordered.
➤ Assess the patient's level of consciousness every 30 minutes until his condition stabilizes.

curs. Ensure that the tube and all connections are secure and taped, with firm traction applied to the tube. Check traction and balloon pressure at least every 2 hours.

➤ Provide emotional support and reassurance appropriately if massive GI bleeding occurs, which is always a frightening experience.
➤ Keep the patient as quiet and comfortable as possible to minimize oxygen demands, but remember that tolerance of sedatives and tranquilizers may be decreased because of liver damage.
➤ Clean the patient's mouth, which may be dry and flecked with dried blood.
➤ The patient may need evaluation for possible liver transplantation.

Preventive steps
➤ Treating the underlying cause of liver disease, or treating existing esophageal varices with medications such as beta-adrenergic blockers or endoscopic banding, may prevent bleeding episodes.

Pathophysiology recap
➤ Portal hypertension (elevated blood pressure in the portal vein) occurs, producing splenomegaly with thrombocytopenia, dilated collateral veins (such as esophageal varices), and ascites.
➤ Esophageal varices may rupture because of mechanical irritation, such as from coarse or unchewed food; straining on defecation; or vigorous coughing. (See *Acute upper GI bleed.*)

➤ Intestinal obstruction

Intestinal obstruction is a partial or complete blockage of the lumen in the small or large bowel. A complete obstruction in any part of the bowel, if untreated, can cause death within hours from shock and vascular collapse.

Rapid assessment
➤ Determine the patient's level of consciousness.
➤ Obtain the patient's vital signs, noting hypotension, tachycardia, and increased temperature.
➤ Assess rate, depth, and pattern of spontaneous respirations.
➤ Assess the patient's muscle strength and deep tendon reflexes.
   To detect small-bowel obstruction:
➤ Assess for colicky pain, nausea, vomiting, and constipation.
➤ Auscultate for high-pitched, loud, musical, or tinkling bowel sounds, borborygmi, and rushes (occasionally loud enough to be heard without a stethoscope).
➤ Palpate for abdominal tenderness with moderate distention. Rebound tenderness may occur when the obstruction has caused strangulation with ischemia.

➤ Assess for vomiting of fecal contents, which indicates complete obstruction.

To detect large-bowel obstruction:

➤ Assess for constipation, colicky abdominal pain (which eventually becomes continuous), nausea (usually without vomiting at first), and abdominal distention; later, the patient may vomit fecal contents.

Immediate actions

➤ Provide supplemental oxygen as necessary.
➤ Perform nasogastric intubation as necessary.
➤ Initiate blood replacement and I.V. fluid administration.
➤ Obtain an arterial blood gas sample to help confirm metabolic alkalosis or acidosis.
➤ Insert an indwelling urinary catheter.
➤ Obtain serum samples for complete blood count, electrolytes, and lactic acid.
➤ Administer analgesics, sedatives, and antibiotics, as ordered.
➤ Observe for and report signs of perforation.

Follow-up actions

➤ Monitor vital signs frequently.
➤ Prepare the patient for abdominal X-rays to confirm the diagnosis, showing the presence and location of intestinal gas or fluid.
➤ Monitor for signs and symptoms of shock and infection.
➤ Observe for signs of dehydration (thick, swollen tongue; dry, cracked lips; and dry oral mucous membranes).
➤ Record the amount and color of drainage from the nasogastric tube. Irrigate the tube with normal saline solution to maintain patency, as ordered.
➤ Keep the patient in semi-Fowler's position as much as possible to promote pulmonary ventilation and ease respiratory distress from abdominal distention.
➤ Encourage ambulation and activity to help promote the return of peristalsis.
➤ Auscultate for bowel sounds, and observe the patient for signs of returning peristalsis (passage of flatus and mucus through the rectum).
➤ Advance the patient's diet as tolerated and ordered.
➤ Obtain a consultation from a nutritionist and provide nutritional support, including total parenteral nutrition, if necessary.
➤ Prepare the patient and his family for the possibility of surgery and provide emotional support and positive reinforcement afterward.
➤ Arrange for an enterostomal therapist to visit and teach the patient who has had an ostomy.

Preventive steps

➤ Recommend a high-fiber diet, increased fluid intake, and regular exercise to maintain normal bowel function.

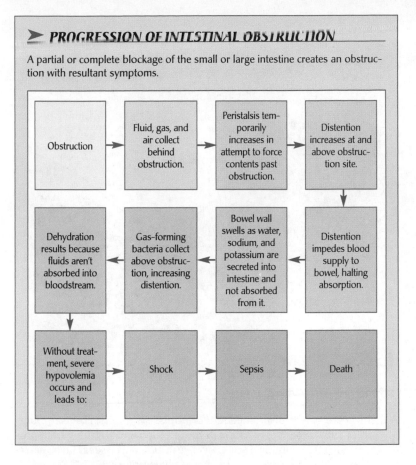

> ➤ PROGRESSION OF INTESTINAL OBSTRUCTION

A partial or complete blockage of the small or large intestine creates an obstruction with resultant symptoms.

➤ Teach the patient the signs and symptoms of bowel obstruction and advise him that early detection is critical to prevent such severe complications as perforation and bowel ischemia.

Pathophysiology recap

➤ Intestinal obstructions are most likely to occur from adhesions caused by previous abdominal surgery, an external hernia, volvulus, Crohn's disease, radiation enteritis, an intestinal wall hematoma (after trauma or anticoagulant therapy), or a neoplasm.

➤ When intestinal obstruction occurs, fluid, air, and gas collect near the site. (See *Progression of intestinal obstruction.*)

➤ Intestinal obstruction may be simple, in which blockage prevents intestinal contents from passing with no other complications; strangulated, in which the blood supply to part or all of the obstructed section is cut off and the lumen is blocked; or close-looped, in which both ends of a bowel section are occluded, isolating it from the rest of the intestine.

➤ **VIEWING A MALLORY-WEISS TEAR**

A Mallory-Weiss tear is usually singular and longitudinal; these tears result from prolonged or forceful vomiting. About 60% of Mallory-Weiss tears involve the cardia; 15%, the terminal esophagus; and 25%, the region across the esophagogastric junction.

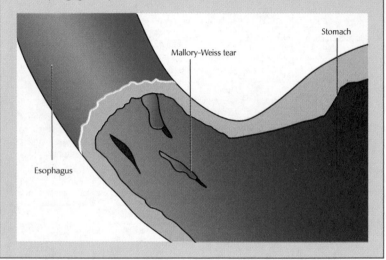

➤ Mallory-Weiss tear

A Mallory-Weiss tear (also called *Mallory-Weiss syndrome*) is a tear in the mucosa or submucosa of the cardia or lower esophagus resulting from prolonged or forceful vomiting. (See *Viewing a Mallory-Weiss tear.*) It's characterized by mild to massive, usually painless bleeding.

Rapid assessment
➤ Obtain the patient's vital signs, noting hypotension and tachycardia.
➤ Observe the rate, depth, and pattern of respirations.
➤ Assess the patient's swallowing ability.
➤ Ask about recent forceful vomiting, followed by vomiting of bright red blood (which may be mild to massive).
➤ Ask about accompanying epigastric or back pain.
➤ Determine if the patient passed large amounts of blood rectally a few hours to several days after normal vomiting.

Immediate actions
➤ Initiate and maintain nothing-by-mouth status.
➤ Provide supplemental oxygen, if necessary.

➤ Place the patient in semi-Fowler's position to prevent aspiration.
➤ Provide support for the patient, particularly if bleeding has frightened him.
➤ Keep the patient warm.
➤ Limit the patient's activity to prevent further bleeding.
➤ Obtain serum samples for the hemoglobin level and hematocrit.
➤ Insert a large-bore (14G to 18G) I.V. line and start a temporary infusion of normal saline solution, as ordered, in case a transfusion is necessary.
➤ Obtain blood for coagulation studies (prothrombin time, partial thromboplastin time, and platelet count) and typing and crossmatching. Keep units of matched blood on hand and transfuse blood if ordered.

Follow-up actions
➤ Prepare the patient for fiber-optic endoscopy to confirm the presence of Mallory-Weiss tears.
➤ Avoid giving the patient medications that may cause nausea or vomiting.
➤ If severe bleeding continues, be prepared to assist with such procedures as angiography with infusion of a vasoconstrictor, endoscopy with electrocoagulation, transcatheter embolization or thrombus formation with an autologous blood clot or other hemostatic material, or surgery to suture each laceration (reserved for massive recurrent or uncontrollable bleeding).
➤ Monitor intake and output.
➤ Prepare the patient and his family for surgery, if necessary.
➤ Obtain a consultation from a nutritionist and provide nutritional support, if necessary.
➤ Prepare the patient for a swallow study, if necessary.

Preventive steps
➤ Counsel the patient to avoid alcohol, aspirin, and other substances that irritate the GI tract.
➤ Encourage the patient with alcoholism to join a support group, such as Alcoholics Anonymous, or refer him for counseling.
➤ Encourage the patient with bulimia to seek medical treatment.

Pathophysiology recap
➤ Forceful or prolonged vomiting may cause Mallory-Weiss tears.
➤ These tears in the gastric mucosa probably occur when the upper esophageal sphincter fails to relax during vomiting; lack of sphincter coordination may occur following excessive intake of alcohol.
➤ Other factors or conditions that can increase intra-abdominal pressure and predispose a person to esophageal tearing include coughing, straining during bowel movements, trauma, seizures, childbirth, hiatal hernia, esophagitis, gastritis, and atrophic gastric mucosa.

➤ RANSON'S CRITERIA

The severity of acute pancreatitis is determined by the existence of certain characteristics. The more criteria met by the patient, the more severe the episode of pancreatitis and, therefore, the greater the risk of mortality.

On admission
Admission criteria include:
➤ patient older than age 55
➤ white blood cell count greater than 16,000/µl
➤ serum glucose greater than 200 mg/dl
➤ lactate dehydrogenase greater than 350 U/L
➤ aspartate aminotransferase greater than 250 U/L.

After admission
During the first 48 hours after admission, criteria include:
➤ 10% decrease in hematocrit
➤ blood urea nitrogen level increase greater than 5 mg/dl
➤ serum calcium less than 8 mg/dl
➤ base deficit greater than 4 mEq/L
➤ partial pressure of arterial oxygen less than 60 mm Hg
➤ estimated fluid sequestration greater than 6 L.

Mortality is less than 1% among patients who meet fewer than three of the criteria. When three to four of the criteria are met, it increases to 15% to 20%; with five or six criteria, mortality is 40%.

➤ Pancreatitis, acute

Pancreatitis, inflammation of the pancreas, occurs in acute and chronic forms and may be due to edema, necrosis, or hemorrhage. In males, this disease is commonly associated with alcoholism, abdominal trauma, or penetrating peptic ulcers; in females, with biliary tract disease. Drugs, such as glucocorticoids, sulfonamides, thiazides, procainamide, tetracycline, and nonsteroidal anti-inflammatory drugs, can also induce the disorder. The severity of pancreatitis and the risk of mortality are predicted by using Ranson's criteria. (See *Ranson's criteria*.)

Rapid assessment
➤ Assess the patient's level of consciousness.
➤ Observe the pattern, rate, and depth of respirations, and auscultate breath sounds, noting diminished sounds on the left and crackles.
➤ Obtain vital signs, noting hypotension, tachycardia, tachypnea, increased temperature, and decreased oxygen saturation.
➤ Ask about intense epigastric pain centered close to the umbilicus and radiating to the back, which is typically aggravated by eating fatty foods, consuming alcohol, and lying in a recumbent position.

➤ Ask about persistent nausea, vomiting, diminished bowel activity, and restlessness.
➤ Auscultate bowel sounds and assess for abdominal distention and ascites.
➤ Observe for mottled skin, jaundice, icteric sclera, Cullen's sign (bluish periumbilical discoloration), and Turner's sign (bluish flank discoloration).

Immediate actions
➤ Initiate and maintain nothing-by-mouth status.
➤ Place the patient in a comfortable position that maximizes air exchange, such as semi-Fowler's or high Fowler's.
➤ Provide supplemental oxygen and prepare for endotracheal intubation and mechanical ventilation or thoracentesis, if necessary.
➤ Assist with a central venous or pulmonary artery catheter and arterial line insertion.
➤ Obtain serum samples for complete blood count and serum electrolyte, amylase, lipase, and arterial blood gas levels.

> **ALERT** *Stay especially alert for signs and symptoms of hypokalemia (hypotension, muscle weakness, apathy, confusion, and cardiac arrhythmias), hypomagnesemia (hypotension, tachycardia, confusion, tremors, twitching, tetany, and hallucinations), and hypocalcemia (positive Chvostek's and Trousseau's signs, seizures, and prolonged QT interval on the electrocardiogram). Have emergency equipment readily available.*

➤ Insert an indwelling urinary catheter.
➤ Insert a nasogastric tube and connect to low intermittent suction, as ordered.
➤ Measure the patient's abdominal girth.
➤ Administer, as ordered:
  – I.V. fluids, such as normal saline solution or lactated Ringer's solution — to increase intravascular volume
  – diuretics — to treat crackles
  – vasoconstrictors — to increase blood pressure
  – antibiotics — to treat bacterial infection
  – analgesics — to relieve pain
  – antacids — to neutralize gastric secretions
  – histamine-2 receptor antagonists — to decrease hydrochloric acid production
  – anticholinergics — to reduce vagal stimulation and inhibit pancreatic enzyme secretion.

Follow-up actions
➤ Monitor the patient's vital signs closely.
➤ Check nasogastric (NG) tube placement every 4 hours and irrigate with normal saline solution for patency.

➤ Monitor NG tube drainage, vomitus, and stool for blood.
➤ Monitor serum electrolyte levels and treat abnormalities.
➤ Allow for periods of rest and activity.
➤ Monitor serum peak and trough levels of antibiotics, as appropriate.
➤ Administer parenteral nutrition, as ordered.
➤ Monitor blood glucose levels and administer insulin, as ordered.
➤ Monitor intake and output and obtain daily weights.
➤ When bowel sounds become active, anticipate switching to enteral or oral feedings and advance diet as tolerated or ordered.
➤ Perform range-of-motion exercises to maintain joint mobility.
➤ Perform meticulous skin care.
➤ Provide emotional support to the patient.
➤ Prepare the patient for surgery, as needed.

Preventive steps
➤ Advise the patient to avoid factors that precipitate acute pancreatitis, especially alcohol.
➤ Explain that observing proper safety precautions can prevent abdominal trauma, which may result in acute pancreatitis.

Pathophysiology recap
➤ Acute pancreatitis occurs in two forms: edematous (interstitial) pancreatitis, which causes fluid accumulation and swelling; and necrotizing pancreatitis, which causes cell death and tissue damage.
➤ The inflammation that occurs in both types is caused by premature activation of enzymes, which leads to tissue damage.
➤ If pancreatitis damages the islets of Langerhans, diabetes mellitus may result.
➤ Sudden severe pancreatitis causes massive hemorrhage and total destruction of the pancreas, manifested as diabetic acidosis, shock, or coma.

➤ Peptic ulcer, perforated

Peptic ulcers are circumscribed lesions that extend through the muscularis mucosa layer of the gastric or duodenal lining. Perforation occurs when the peptic ulcer erodes the lining of the stomach or duodenum to a point where the gut becomes connected to the peritoneal cavity. (See *What happens when peptic ulcers perforate.*)

Rapid assessment
➤ Assess the patient's level of consciousness.
➤ Obtain the patient's vital signs, noting hypotension, tachycardia, and increased temperature.

➤ *WHAT HAPPENS WHEN PEPTIC ULCERS PERFORATE*

When a peptic ulcer erodes completely through the gastric or duodenal lining, contents – such as undigested food – leak into the normally sterile peritoneal cavity (as shown below), resulting in peritonitis and increased risk of infection, hemorrhage, and abscess formation.

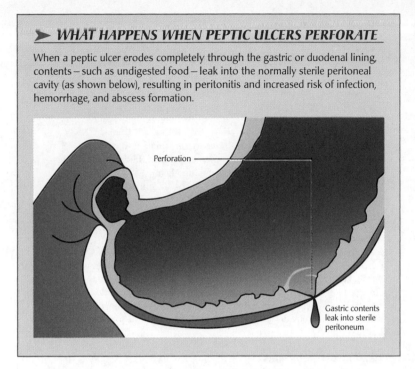

Perforation

Gastric contents leak into sterile peritoneum

➤ Ask about a sudden onset of constant, radiating abdominal pain and tenderness, dyspepsia, anorexia, nausea, vomiting, and bloody or coffee-grounds emesis
➤ Observe for signs of peritonitis, including a rigid boardlike abdomen.
➤ Auscultate for bowel sounds, noting if they are absent.
➤ Observe the patient's skin color and capillary refill.

ALERT *Remember that 10% of patients with perforated ulcers have no previous signs or symptoms of peptic ulcer disease.*

Immediate actions
➤ Provide supplemental oxygen, as needed.
➤ Withhold oral fluids and solids.
➤ Administer I.V. fluids and electrolytes and pain medication, as ordered.
➤ Insert a nasogastric (NG) tube for gastric suction and decompression.
➤ Insert an indwelling urinary catheter.
➤ Obtain serum samples for complete blood count, serum electrolyte, prothrombin time, International Normalized Ratio, partial thromboplastin time, and arterial blood gas analysis.
➤ Assist with a central venous or pulmonary artery catheter and arterial line insertion.

COMPLICATIONS

➤ *DUMPING SYNDROME*

In dumping syndrome (also known as *rapid gastric emptying*), undigested food passes too rapidly from the stomach into the jejunum (lower end of the small intestine). It occurs as a result of certain types of gastric surgery.

Signs and symptoms
➤ Early signs and symptoms (which may occur from a few minutes to 45 minutes after a meal) occur as a result of increased blood flow to the intestines and include weakness, sweating, dizziness, and fainting.
➤ Late signs and symptoms (which typically occur 3 hours or more after a meal) result from increased insulin release that causes hypoglycemia and include sweating, anxiety, shakiness, hypotension, and headache.

Treatment
Most patients recover from dumping syndrome within 16 months after the procedure. Treatment is mainly symptomatic and involves changes in eating habits. Lying down and resting may help early signs and symptoms to pass. Eating candy or drinking sweet liquid, such as juice, which help to raise blood sugar, should help relieve late signs and symptoms. Increasing intake of soluble fiber (found in fresh fruits and vegetables) may also help to relieve rapid gastric emptying.

Nursing considerations
➤ Advise the patient to eat four to six small, high-protein, low-carbohydrate meals throughout the day.
➤ Instruct the patient to drink liquids between meals rather than with them.
➤ Tell the patient to notify his physician if he experiences signs of GI bleeding, such as vomiting blood; passing dark, tarry stools; or having bright red bleeding with bowel movements.

➤ Administer histamine-2 receptor antagonists or proton pump inhibitors as ordered to inhibit acid production.
➤ Give antibiotics in combination with proton pump inhibitors as ordered to treat *H. pylori*.

Follow-up actions
➤ Monitor the patient's vital signs closely.
➤ Monitor intake and output.
➤ Monitor hemoglobin level and hematocrit at least every 4 hours, and transfuse as ordered.
➤ Prepare the patient for an upper GI series to confirm the presence and location of the ulcers.
➤ Prepare the patient for surgery, as needed.
➤ Monitor the patient for preoperative complications, such as peritonitis, hemorrhage, and shock; also monitor him for postoperative complica-

tions, such as hemorrhage; shock; iron, folate, or vitamin B_{12} deficiency anemia (from malabsorption or continued blood loss); and dumping syndrome. (See *Dumping syndrome.*)

Preventive steps

➤ Advise patients at risk for ulcer formation, such as the elderly and those with peptic ulcer disease, to avoid the use of nonsteroidal anti-inflammatory drugs (NSAIDs). If NSAIDs must be used, recommend the use of a proton-pump inhibitor to lessen gastric irritation.
➤ Counsel the patient to avoid stressful situations, excessive intake of coffee, and ingestion of alcoholic beverages during exacerbations of peptic ulcer disease.
➤ Encourage the patient who smokes to enroll in a smoking-cessation program.

Pathophysiology recap

➤ With peptic ulcer perforation, gastric and duodenal contents leak into the normally sterile peritoneum.
➤ Peritonitis follows, increasing the risk of infection and abscess formation.

➤ Peritonitis

Peritonitis is an acute or chronic inflammation of the peritoneum, the membrane that lines the abdominal cavity and covers the visceral organs. Inflammation may extend throughout the peritoneum or may be localized as an abscess. Mortality is 10%, with death usually resulting from bowel obstruction; mortality was much higher before the introduction of antibiotics.

Rapid assessment

➤ Assess the patient's vital signs, noting hypotension, tachycardia, and temperature of 103° F (39.4° C) or higher.
➤ Observe the patient for signs and symptoms of dehydration, including oliguria, thirst, pinched skin, and a dry, swollen tongue.
➤ Obtain the patient's history, including reports of sudden, severe, and diffuse abdominal pain that's intensified and localized to the area of the underlying disorder.
➤ Ask the patient about nausea and vomiting.
➤ Assess for abdominal rigidity, which along with nausea and vomiting, may indicate paralytic ileus. (See *Paralytic ileus,* page 132.)
➤ Observe the patient for weakness, pallor, excessive sweating, and cold skin, which are caused by an excessive loss of fluid, electrolytes, and protein into the abdominal cavity.

COMPLICATIONS

➤ *PARALYTIC ILEUS*

Paralytic ileus is a physiologic form of intestinal obstruction that usually develops in the small bowel after abdominal surgery. It causes decreased or absent intestinal motility that usually disappears spontaneously after 2 to 3 days.

This condition can develop as a response to trauma, toxemia, or peritonitis or as a result of electrolyte deficiencies (especially hypokalemia) and the use of certain drugs, such as ganglionic blocking agents and anticholinergics. It can also result from vascular causes, such as thrombosis or embolism. Excessive air swallowing may contribute to it, but paralytic ileus brought on by this factor alone seldom lasts for more than 24 hours.

Signs and symptoms
➤ Severe, continuous abdominal discomfort with nausea and vomiting
➤ Abdominal distention
➤ Absent or diminished bowel sounds
➤ Constipation
➤ Flatus and small, liquid stools

Treatment
Paralytic ileus lasting longer than 48 hours requires intubation for decompression and nasogastric suctioning. Isotonic fluids should be administered to restore intravascular volume and correct electrolyte disorders.

When paralytic ileus results from surgical manipulation of the bowel, treatment may also include administration of a prokinetic drug, such as metoclopramide or erythromycin.

Nursing considerations
➤ Warn those receiving cholinergic agents to expect certain paradoxical adverse effects, such as intestinal cramps and diarrhea.
➤ Assess frequently for returning bowel sounds.

Immediate actions
➤ Place the patient in semi-Fowler's position to help him deep-breathe with less pain to prevent pulmonary complications and help localize purulent exudate in the lower abdomen or pelvis.
➤ Withhold oral fluids and solids to decrease peristalsis and prevent perforation; administer I.V. parenteral fluids and electrolytes, as ordered.
➤ Administer I.V. antibiotics, as ordered.
➤ Insert a nasogastric (NG) tube to decompress the bowel; be prepared to insert a rectal tube to facilitate the passage of flatus.
➤ Administer analgesics, as ordered.
➤ Assist with central venous or pulmonary artery catheter and arterial line insertion.
➤ Obtain serum samples for complete blood count, serum electrolytes, and arterial blood gas analysis.

➤ Administer I.V. fluids, such as normal saline solution or lactated Ringer's solution, to increase intravascular volume.

Follow-up actions

➤ Monitor vital signs closely.
➤ Prepare the patient for abdominal X-ray, computed tomography scan, or ultrasound to confirm the diagnosis.
➤ Counteract mouth and nose dryness due to fever and NG intubation with regular cleaning and lubrication.
➤ Prepare the patient for surgery, if ordered.

After surgery to evacuate the peritoneum:
➤ Maintain parenteral fluid and electrolyte administration, as ordered.
➤ Accurately record fluid intake and output, including NG tube and drain output.
➤ Place the patient in Fowler's position to promote drainage (through drainage tube) by gravity.
➤ Move the patient carefully because the slightest movement will intensify the pain.
➤ Keep the side rails up and implement other safety measures if fever and pain disorient the patient.
➤ Encourage and assist ambulation, as ordered, usually on the first postoperative day.
➤ Watch for signs of dehiscence (the patient may complain that "something gave way") and abscess formation (continued abdominal tenderness and fever).
➤ Frequently assess for peristaltic activity by listening for bowel sounds and checking for gas, bowel movements, and a soft abdomen.
➤ Gradually decrease parenteral fluids and increase oral fluids.

Preventive steps

➤ Early treatment of GI inflammatory conditions and preoperative and postoperative antibiotic therapy help prevent peritonitis.

Pathophysiology recap

➤ Although the GI tract normally contains bacteria, the peritoneum is sterile.
➤ When bacteria invade the peritoneum due to inflammation and perforation of the GI tract, peritonitis results.
➤ Bacterial invasion of the peritoneum typically results from appendicitis, diverticulitis, peptic ulcer, ulcerative colitis, volvulus, strangulated obstruction, abdominal neoplasm, or a stab wound.
➤ Peritonitis may also occur following chemical inflammation, as in the rupture of a fallopian or ovarian tube or the bladder, perforation of a gastric ulcer, or released pancreatic enzymes.
➤ In chemical and bacterial inflammation, accumulated fluids containing protein and electrolytes make the transparent peritoneum opaque, red, inflamed, and edematous.

➤ *Pseudomembranous enterocolitis*

Marked by severe diarrhea, pseudomembranous enterocolitis is an acute inflammation and necrosis of the small and large intestines, which usually affects the mucosa but may extend into the submucosa and, rarely, other layers. This rare condition typically results in death within 1 to 7 days because of severe dehydration and toxicity, peritonitis, or perforation.

Rapid assessment
➤ Obtain the patient's vital signs, noting hypotension, tachycardia, and increased temperature.
➤ Ask about an onset of copious watery or bloody diarrhea, abdominal pain, and fever, followed by profuse watery diarrhea (with up to 30 stools per day) and abdominal pain.
➤ Auscultate bowel sounds, noting hyperactive sounds.
➤ Assess for abdominal distention and bloating.
➤ Assess for signs and symptoms of dehydration, such as dry muscle membranes, poor skin turgor, and oligura.

Immediate actions
➤ If your patient has *Clostridium difficile,* place him on isolation precautions according to your facility's policy.
➤ Determine whether the patient is receiving broad-spectrum antibiotic therapy; if he is, discontinue this therapy immediately.
➤ Obtain a stool culture to identify *C. difficile* before administering metronidazole or vancomycin.
➤ Initiate I.V. fluids to treat or prevent dehydration.
➤ Obtain a serum sample for complete blood count and electrolytes.
➤ Make sure that the patient has a safe path to the bathroom and that assistive devices are in reach.
➤ Administer vasopressors, such as dopamine, if needed to maintain blood pressure after fluid replacement has been given.
➤ Insert an indwelling urinary catheter, if necessary.

Follow-up actions
➤ Monitor vital signs frequently.
➤ Monitor intake and output hourly.
➤ Monitor for signs and symptoms of dehydration, peritonitis, and perforation.
➤ Check serum electrolytes daily and monitor for signs of hypokalemia, especially malaise, and a weak, rapid, irregular pulse.
➤ Provide electrolyte supplementation as necessary.
➤ Provide meticulous skin care.

 ALERT *Excessive diarrhea may cause skin excoriation and breakdown. To decrease excoriation and facilitate drainage measurement, insert a rectal tube or large indwelling catheter*

(inserted but not inflated) into the rectum and attach it to a drainage bag to gravity, as ordered.
➤ Prepare the patient for a rectal biopsy through sigmoidoscopy to confirm the diagnosis.
➤ Test follow-up stool cultures for *C. difficile* after treatment.

Preventive steps
➤ Advise the patient who developed the disorder because of broad-spectrum antibiotic therapy to avoid these agents.
➤ Teach the patient the signs and symptoms of pseudomembranous enterocolitis and caution him to report symptoms of recurrence immediately.

Pathophysiology recap
➤ Necrotic mucosa is replaced by a pseudomembrane filled with staphylococci, leukocytes, mucus, fibrin, and inflammatory cells.
➤ Although the exact cause of pseudomembranous enterocolitis is unknown, some researchers believe that *C. difficile* plays a role in its development.
➤ Pseudomembranous enterocolitis has occurred postoperatively in debilitated patients who undergo abdominal surgery and in patients treated with broad-spectrum antibiotics.

➤ *Wound dehiscence and evisceration*

Wound dehiscence occurs when the edges of a surgical wound fail to join or separate even after they appear to be healing normally. It may lead to evisceration, in which a portion of the viscera—usually a bowel loop—protrudes through the incision.

Rapid assessment
➤ Obtain the patient's vital signs, noting hypotension and tachycardia.
➤ Ask about a "popping sensation" after retching, coughing, or straining.
➤ Observe for a serosanguineous exudate from the wound, an indication of wound dehiscence; or the presence of visible coils of intestine, an indication of evisceration. (See *Recognizing dehiscence and evisceration,* page 136.)

Immediate actions
➤ Initiate and maintain nothing-by-mouth status because the patient may need to return to the operating room.
➤ Keep the patient in bed and stay with him while someone else notifies the physician.
➤ Using sterile technique, cover the extruding wound contents with warm, sterile normal saline soaks.

➤ RECOGNIZING DEHISCENCE AND EVISCERATION

In wound dehiscence, the layers of the surgical wound separate. In evisceration, the viscera (in this case, a loop of bowel) protrude through the surgical incision.

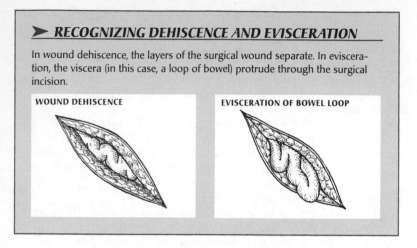

WOUND DEHISCENCE

EVISCERATION OF BOWEL LOOP

➤ Maintain the patient on absolute bed rest in low Fowler's position (elevated no more than 20 degrees) with his knees flexed to prevent injury and reduce stress on an abdominal incision.
➤ Provide reassurance and support to ease the patient's anxiety.
➤ Administer I.V. fluids to replace fluid losses from the wound as ordered.
➤ Administer analgesics as necessary.

Follow-up actions
➤ Monitor the patient's vital signs closely.
➤ Moisten the dressings every hour by withdrawing saline solution from the container through the syringe and gently squirting the solution onto the dressings.

 ALERT *When moistening the dressings, inspect the color of the viscera. If it appears dusky or black, notify the physician immediately. With its blood supply interrupted, a protruding organ may become ischemic and necrotic.*

➤ Withhold oral fluids and solids and prepare the patient for surgery.

Preventive steps
➤ Teach the patient to support the incision with a pillow or cushion before changing position, coughing, or sneezing.
➤ Advise patients who will be undergoing surgery that a healthy diet will help prevent wound dehiscence and evisceration.

Pathophysiology recap
➤ Dehiscence occurs when collagen fibers in the healing wound aren't mature enough to hold an incision closed without sutures.
➤ As a result, separation of the skin and tissue layers in the wound occurs, usually 3 to 11 days after surgery or development of the wound.

5
Neurologic emergencies

➤ Brain abscess

Also known as an *intracranial abscess,* a brain abscess is a free or encapsulated collection of pus usually found in the temporal lobe, cerebellum, or frontal lobes. It can vary in size and may occur singly or in multiple locations.

Rapid assessment
➤ Obtain the patient's vital signs, noting hypotension, tachycardia, and increased temperature.
➤ Assess for increased intracranial pressure (ICP) as well as constant intractable headache worsened by straining, nausea, and vomiting.
➤ Obtain the patient's history, paying special attention to recent infection—especially of the middle ear, mastoid, nasal sinuses, heart, or lungs—or congenital heart disease.
➤ Assess for ocular disturbances, such as nystagmus, decreased vision, and unequal pupil size.
➤ Observe the patient for signs of infection, such as fever, pallor, chills, and malaise. (If the abscess is encapsulated, these symptoms may not develop.)
➤ Assess the patient's level of consciousness (LOC), which will vary from drowsiness to deep stupor according to the abscess size and location.
   Assess for the following findings; again, they will vary with the abscess site:
➤ temporal lobe abscess —auditory-receptive dysphasia, central facial weakness, and hemiparesis
➤ cerebellar abscess —dizziness, coarse nystagmus, gaze weakness on the lesion side, tremor, and ataxia
➤ frontal lobe abscess —expressive dysphasia, hemiparesis with unilateral motor seizure, drowsiness, inattention, and mental function impairment.

Immediate actions
➤ Maintain the patient on bed rest with the head of the bed elevated less than 30 degrees.
➤ Administer supplemental oxygen and provide mechanical ventilation as needed.

➤ Maintain seizure and safety precautions.
➤ Assist with ICP monitoring, if necessary.
➤ Insert an indwelling urinary catheter.
➤ Obtain serum samples for electrolytes and white blood cells.
➤ Provide a calm, quiet environment to prevent increased ICP.
➤ Administer, as ordered:
  – antibiotics — to combat the underlying infection
  – anticonvulsants — to help prevent seizures
  – I.V. fluids with osmotic diuretics and glucocorticoids — to decrease ICP and cerebral edema
  – stool softeners — to prevent straining, which increases ICP.

Follow-up actions
➤ Monitor the patient's vital signs frequently.
➤ Monitor intake and output hourly because fluid overload can contribute to cerebral edema.
➤ Frequently assess the patient's neurologic status, especially LOC, speech, and sensorimotor and cranial nerve functions. Watch for signs of increased ICP (decreased LOC, vomiting, abnormal pupil response, and depressed respirations), which may lead to cerebral herniation with such signs as fixed and dilated pupils, widened pulse pressure, bradycardia or tachycardia, and absent respirations.
➤ Prepare the patient for surgery, if necessary.
➤ Explain the surgical procedure to the patient and his family and make sure that the patient or a legal guardian has signed an informed consent form.
➤ Maintain a calm, quiet environment; schedule activities; and limit tracheal suctioning, if appropriate, to prevent increases in ICP.
➤ Obtain a consultation from a physical and occupational therapist, as ordered.
➤ Provide passive range-of-motion exercises to all extremities.
  Postoperatively:
➤ Continue frequent neurologic assessments. Monitor the patient's vital signs and intake and output.
➤ Watch for signs of meningitis (nuchal rigidity, headaches, chills, and sweats), an ever-present threat.
➤ Be sure to change a damp dressing often, using sterile technique and noting the amount of drainage. Never allow bandages to remain damp. To promote drainage and prevent reaccumulation of purulent material in the abscess, position the patient on the operative side. Measure drainage from surgical drains as instructed by the surgeon.
➤ If the patient remains stuporous or comatose for an extended period, give meticulous skin care to prevent pressure ulcers and position him in Fowler's or low Fowler's position to preserve function and prevent contractures.

➤ If the patient requires isolation because of postoperative drainage, make sure that he and his family understand the reasons for this precaution.
➤ Assist the patient to ambulate as soon as possible to prevent immobility and encourage independence.

Preventive steps
➤ As ordered, give prophylactic antibiotics to patients who have experienced open skull fractures or penetrating head wounds.
➤ Stress the need for treatment of otitis media, mastoiditis, dental abscess, and other infections.

Pathophysiology recap
➤ Brain abscess usually begins with localized inflammatory necrosis and edema, septic thrombosis of vessels, and suppurative encephalitis.
➤ This is followed by thick encapsulation of accumulated pus and adjacent meningeal infiltration by neutrophils, lymphocytes, and plasma cells. Increasing pressure in the brain results in more damage.
➤ Brain abscess is usually secondary to some other infection, especially otitis media, sinusitis, dental abscess, mastoiditis, and human immunodeficiency virus infection. Other causes include subdural empyema; bacterial endocarditis; bacteremia; pulmonary or pleural infection; pelvic, abdominal, and skin infections; and cranial trauma, such as a penetrating head wound or open skull fracture.
➤ Brain abscess occurs in about 2% of children with congenital heart disease, possibly because the hypoxic brain is a good culture medium for bacteria.
➤ Untreated brain abscess is usually fatal; even with treatment, the prognosis is only fair, and about 30% of patients develop focal seizures.

➤ Cerebral aneurysm and subarachnoid hemorrhage

A cerebral aneurysm is a localized dilation of a cerebral artery that most commonly results from a congenital weakness in the arterial wall. Cerebral aneurysms may arise at an arterial junction in the circle of Willis, the circular anastomosis forming the major cerebral arteries at the base of the brain. (See *Common sites of cerebral aneurysm,* page 140.)

Cerebral aneurysms can rupture and cause bleeding into the subarachnoid space (subarachnoid hemorrhage).

Rapid assessment
➤ Obtain the patient's vital signs, noting hypotension, bradycardia, tachycardia, tachypnea, bradypnea, and decreased oxygen saturation.
➤ Obtain the patient's history, if possible, paying particular attention to reports of a sudden severe headache, nausea, and vomiting.

> **COMMON SITES OF CEREBRAL ANEURYSM**

Cerebral aneurysms usually arise at the arterial bifurcation in the circle of Willis and its branches. The illustration below shows the most common sites around this circle.

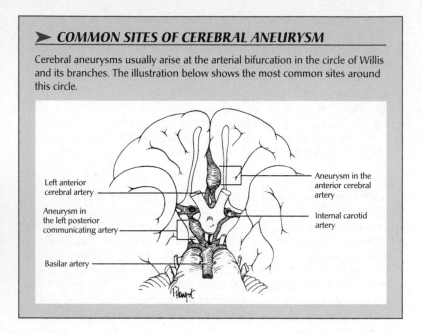

Left anterior cerebral artery

Aneurysm in the left posterior communicating artery

Basilar artery

Aneurysm in the anterior cerebral artery

Internal carotid artery

➤ Ask about symptoms that occurred during the preceding several days, such as headache, nuchal rigidity, stiff back and legs, and intermittent nausea—these premonitory symptoms may indicate rupture of a cerebral aneurysm.

➤ Assess the patient for an altered level of consciousness (LOC), which varies depending on the severity and location of bleeding.

➤ Examine the patient for nuchal rigidity, back and leg pain, fever, restlessness, irritability, occasional seizures, and blurred vision; these indicate meningeal irritation due to bleeding.

➤ Assess for hemiparesis, hemisensory defects, dysphagia, and visual defects. (See *Hunt-Hess classifications for subarachnoid hemorrhage.*)

➤ Observe for diplopia, ptosis, dilated pupils, and an inability to rotate the eye, findings caused by compression of the oculomotor nerve, which may indicate that the aneurysm is located near the internal carotid artery.

Immediate actions

➤ Impose aneurysm precautions to minimize the risk of rebleeding before repair and to avoid increased ICP: facilitate bed rest in a quiet, darkened room (keep the head of the bed flat or under 30 degrees, as ordered); limit visitations; and restrict physical activity. Advise the patient to avoid straining with bowel movements. Explain the purpose of these restrictive measures.

> ## HUNT-HESS CLASSIFICATIONS
> ## FOR SUBARACHNOID HEMORRHAGE
>
> The severity of symptoms accompanying subarachnoid hemorrhage varies from patient to patient, depending on the site and the amount of bleeding. The Hunt-Hess classification identifies five grades that differentiate subarachnoid hemorrhage from a ruptured cerebral aneurysm:
>
> ➤ Grade I (minimal bleeding): The patient is alert and oriented, without symptoms.
>
> ➤ Grade II (mild bleeding): The patient is alert and oriented, with a mild to severe headache and nuchal rigidity.
>
> ➤ Grade III (moderate bleeding): The patient is lethargic and confused or drowsy, with nuchal rigidity and, possibly, a mild focal deficit such as hemiparesis.
>
> ➤ Grade IV (severe bleeding): The patient is stuporous, with nuchal rigidity and, possibly, mild to severe focal deficits, hemiplegia, early decerebrate rigidity, and vegetative disturbances.
>
> ➤ Grade V (moribund; commonly fatal): If the rupture is nonfatal, the patient is in a deep coma, with severe neurologic deficits, such as decerebrate rigidity and a moribund appearance.

➤ Initiate and maintain seizure and safety precautions.

➤ Maintain a patent airway and provide supplementary oxygen.

➤ Assist with the insertion of an intracranial pressure monitoring catheter.

➤ Give I.V. fluids (colloids and crystalloids), as ordered, and monitor I.V. infusions to avoid increased ICP.

➤ Obtain a serum sample for arterial blood gas analysis. Prepare the patient for diagnostic testing, such as computed tomography.

➤ Administer, as ordered:
 – vasoconstrictors — to keep blood pressure within parameters set by the physician (usually 20 mm Hg above normal)
 – corticosteroids — to decrease edema
 – phenobarbital or another sedative — to promote sedation, help decrease ICP, and prevent seizures
 – nimodipine to prevent and treat vasospasm
 – stool softeners or mild laxatives — to prevent straining, which increases ICP
 – histamine-2 receptor blocker — to prevent GI irritation from stress and corticosteroid administration.

Follow-up actions
Perform the following actions whether or not the patient will undergo surgical repair, focusing on ensuring comfort, preventing increased ICP, and minimizing the risk of other complications.

➤ Monitor the patient's vital signs frequently; immediately report significant changes, especially a rise or significant decrease in systolic pressure.

➤ Monitor the patient's LOC frequently and report changes.

➤ Turn the patient often. Encourage occasional deep breathing and leg movement. Warn the patient to avoid all unnecessary physical activity. Assist with active range-of-motion (ROM) exercises; if the patient is paralyzed, perform regular passive ROM exercises.

➤ Watch for these danger signals, which may indicate an enlarging aneurysm, rebleeding, intracranial clot, increased ICP, vasospasm, or other complication: decreased LOC, a unilateral enlarged pupil, the onset or worsening of hemiparesis or motor deficit, increased blood pressure, slowed pulse, worsening of headache or the sudden onset of a headache, renewed or worsened nuchal rigidity, and renewed or persistent vomiting. (See *Increased intracranial pressure*.)

➤ If the patient has facial weakness, assess the gag reflex and assist him during meals, placing food in the unaffected side of his mouth.

➤ If the patient can't swallow, insert a nasogastric tube, as ordered, and give all tube feedings slowly.

➤ If the patient can eat, provide a high-fiber diet to prevent straining at stool, which can increase ICP.

➤ If the patient is receiving steroids, monitor for GI bleeding and check the stool for occult blood.

➤ With facial nerve palsy, administer artificial tears or ointment to the affected eye, and tape the eye shut at night to prevent corneal damage.

➤ To minimize stress, encourage relaxation techniques. Avoid using restraints because these can cause agitation and raise ICP.

➤ Prevent deep vein thrombosis by applying antiembolism stockings or sequential compression sleeves.

➤ If the patient can't speak, establish a simple means of communication or use cards or a notepad. Encourage family interaction but don't allow overstimulation.

➤ Provide emotional support, and include the patient's family in his care as much as possible. Encourage family members to adopt a realistic attitude, but don't discourage hope.

➤ Prepare the patient for a cerebral angiogram, computed tomography scan, or magnetic resonance imaging of the head to visualize the aneurysm.

➤ Before discharge, make a referral to a visiting nurse or a rehabilitation center when necessary, and teach the patient and family how to recognize signs of rebleeding.

If surgery is scheduled:

➤ Prepare the patient for surgery.

➤ Explain the procedure to the patient and his family. Traditional surgical repair involves clipping, ligating, or wrapping the aneurysm with mus-

COMPLICATIONS

➤ *INCREASED INTRACRANIAL PRESSURE*

The pressure exerted within the intact skull by the intracranial volume – about 10% blood, 10% cerebrospinal fluid (CSF), and 80% brain tissue – is called *intracranial pressure* (ICP). When an injury to the brain causes blood, CSF, and brain tissue to expand within the limited space of the rigid skull, increased ICP occurs.

Increased ICP can result from many conditions that cause injury to the brain. Such conditions include trauma (contusion, laceration, and intracranial hemorrhage), cerebral edema (stroke, infection, hypoxia, and postsurgical complications), hydrocephalus, or the development of a space-occupying lesion (tumor, abscess, and aneurysm).

Signs and symptoms

Early signs of increased ICP include:

➤ altered level of consciousness – subtle loss of orientation, restlessness and anxiety, irritability, sudden quietness (less talkative or interactive), or requiring increased stimulation to obtain a response from the patient

➤ pupillary changes – pupil changes on the side of the lesion, unilateral hippus (one pupil constricts, then dilates), sluggish reaction of both pupils, or unequal pupils.

The patient may experience sudden muscle weakness with motor changes on the side opposite the lesion. He may display a positive pronator drift (with palms up, one hand pronates). Intermittent increases in blood pressure may also occur.

Late signs include fixed and dilated pupils, accompanied by profound weakness, increased systolic blood pressure, profound bradycardia, and abnormal respirations. The patient will be unarousable.

Treatment

Management of increased ICP may involve the administration of medications. Osmotic diuretic agents, such as mannitol, reduce cerebral edema by temporarily shrinking intracranial contents. Corticosteroids lower elevated ICP by reducing sodium and water concentration in the brain; however, their use is controversial. A barbiturate-induced coma depresses the reticular activating system and reduces the brain's metabolic demand; the reduced demand for oxygen and energy lessens cerebral blood flow, thereby lowering ICP.

Withdrawal of CSF through an intracranial drainage system reduces CSF volume, thereby reducing ICP. Although less commonly used, surgical removal of a skull-bone flap provides room for the swollen brain to expand. Hematoma evacuation may be performed.

Nursing considerations

➤ Assess the patient's clinical status and take routine and neurologic vital signs every hour or as ordered.

(continued)

> ➤ *INCREASED INTRACRANIAL PRESSURE (continued)*

➤ Calculate cerebral perfusion pressure hourly or, if possible, monitor cerebral blood flow.
➤ Administer medications, as ordered.
➤ Restrict fluid intake, usually to 1,200 to 1,500 ml/day, to help prevent developing or worsening cerebral edema.
➤ Reduce fever by administering acetaminophen, as ordered, and providing cooling measures because fever raises brain metabolism (which increases cerebral blood flow, resulting in increased ICP).

cle. Newer interventional radiology techniques utilize endovascular coil placement and balloon-assisted coiling.
➤ Make sure that the patient or a legal guardian has signed an informed consent form.

Preventive steps
➤ Advise the patient to avoid coffee and other stimulants and aspirin to reduce the risk of aneurysm rupture.
➤ Advise the patient to monitor his blood pressure daily and to follow-up with his physician to make sure it's within the physician's parameters.
➤ Counsel the patient who smokes to enter a smoking-cessation program to reduce the risk of aneurysm formation.

Pathophysiology recap
➤ Cerebral aneurysm may result from a congenital defect, a degenerative process, or a combination of both.
➤ Blood flow exerts pressure against a congenitally weakened arterial wall, stretching it like an overblown balloon and making it likely to rupture.
➤ After such rupture, blood spills into the space normally occupied by cerebrospinal fluid, known as a subarachnoid hemorrhage.
➤ Blood may also spill into the brain tissue, which can result in potentially fatal increased ICP.

➤ Cerebral contusion

A cerebral contusion is bruising of the brain tissue caused by a severe blow to the head. This injury disrupts normal nerve functions in the bruised area and may cause loss of consciousness, hemorrhage, edema, and even death.

Rapid assessment

➤ Assess the patient's level of consciousness (LOC), noting a loss of consciousness and its duration or, if the patient is conscious, noting whether he's drowsy, confused, disoriented, agitated, or even violent.
➤ Assess the patient's rate, depth, and pattern of respirations.
➤ Assess the patient's vital signs, noting labored respirations.
➤ Examine the patient for scalp wounds.
➤ Observe for hemiparesis or unilateral numbness, decorticate or decerebrate posturing, and unequal pupillary response.
➤ Assess for aphasia.
➤ Test the patient's motor responses and deep tendon reflexes.

 ALERT *A lucid period followed by rapid deterioration suggests epidural hematoma.*

Immediate actions

➤ Initiate and maintain bed rest with the head of the bed elevated less than 30 degrees to prevent increased intracranial pressure. (Elevate the head after spinal injury is ruled out.)
➤ Institute and maintain seizure and other safety precautions.
➤ Obtain a serum sample for arterial blood gas analysis.
➤ Provide supplemental oxygen and prepare for endotracheal (ET) intubation or tracheotomy if facial trauma precludes oral ET intubation.
➤ Assist with the insertion of an intracranial pressure monitoring (ICP) device, if necessary.
➤ Start I.V. fluids with lactated Ringer's or normal saline solution.
➤ Administer mannitol to reduce cerebral edema, as ordered.
➤ Obtain a serum sample for typing and crossmatching, complete blood count, and arterial blood gas analysis.
➤ Insert an indwelling urinary catheter.
➤ If the patient is unconscious, insert an oral or nasogastric tube to prevent aspiration.
➤ Carefully observe the patient for cerebrospinal fluid (CSF) leakage from the nostrils and ear canals.
➤ If CSF leakage develops, raise the head of the bed 30 degrees.

 ALERT *If CSF leaks from the ear, position the patient so that the ear drains naturally. If you detect CSF leakage from the nose, place a gauze pad under the patient's nostrils. Be sure to tell him not to blow his nose but to wipe it instead. Don't pack the ear or nose.*

➤ Treat injuries as necessary.

 ALERT *Abnormal respirations and decreased LOC may indicate a breakdown in the brain's respiratory center and a possible impending tentorial herniation — a neurologic emergency.*

Follow-up actions
➤ Monitor the patient's vital signs, including ICP and LOC, frequently.
➤ Prepare the patient for a diagnostic computed tomography scan or magnetic resonance imaging of the head, if scheduled.
➤ Monitor intake and output.
➤ If spinal injury is ruled out, keep the head of the bed at 30 degrees. Enforce bed rest.
➤ Clean and dress any superficial scalp wounds. (If the skin has been broken, tetanus prophylaxis may be necessary.)
➤ Provide a calm, quiet environment and schedule daily activities to ensure the patient doesn't receive excess stimulation, which can increase ICP.
➤ Prepare the patient for a craniotomy, if scheduled.
➤ Explain the procedure to the patient and his family and make sure that the patient or a legal guardian has signed an informed consent form.

Preventive steps
➤ Strongly encourage the patient to use safety precautions to prevent any type of head injury, including seat belts, age-appropriate car and booster seats for infants and children, helmets for bicycle or motorcycle riding, and hard hats in designated construction areas.

Pathophysiology recap
➤ Cerebral contusion results from acceleration-deceleration or coup-contrecoup injuries. Such injuries can occur directly beneath the site of impact when the brain rebounds against the skull from the force of a blow, when the force of the blow drives the brain against the opposite side of the skull, or when the head is hurled forward and stopped abruptly.
➤ When these injuries occur, the brain continues moving and slaps against the skull (acceleration), and then rebounds (deceleration).
➤ These injuries can also cause the brain to strike against bony prominences inside the skull, causing intracranial hemorrhage or hematoma that may result in tentorial herniation.

➤ Concussion

Also called a *closed head injury,* a concussion results from a sharp blow to the head that results in an alteration in mental status. A patient may experience a concussion due to a fall, a motor vehicle accident, a sports-related accident, or child or elder abuse. Recovery is usually complete within 24 to 48 hours; however, repeated injuries have a cumulative effect on the brain.

Rapid assessment

➤ Assess the patient's level of consciousness (LOC).
➤ Obtain the patient's vital signs.
➤ Obtain a thorough history, including the event that caused the injury; if the patient can't supply this information (for example, if he can't remember how he sustained the injury), interview his family, eyewitnesses, or emergency personnel.
➤ Ask whether the patient lost consciousness or vomited or whether he's experiencing dizziness, nausea, or severe headache.
➤ Ask the patient's family members or eyewitnesses whether the patient seemed to experience personality changes, such as irritability, lethargy, or other behavior that's out of character.
➤ Examine the patient for additional injuries. Palpate the skull for tenderness or hematomas.

 ALERT *Examine children, infants, and elderly patients for other signs of abuse; report them, if found.*

➤ Determine whether the patient is experiencing anterograde amnesia (he can't recall the events that immediately preceded the injury) and retrograde amnesia (he can't recall the events that immediately followed the injury); the presence of anterograde amnesia and the duration of retrograde amnesia may correlate with the severity of the injury.

 ALERT *If the patient has an altered LOC or if a neurologic examination reveals abnormalities, the injury may be more severe than a concussion. The patient should undergo a computed tomography scan, and a neurosurgeon should be consulted immediately.*

➤ Assess the patient's pupillary reaction to light and the size, shape, and equality of the pupils.

Immediate actions

➤ Initiate and maintain bed rest with the head of the bed at 30 degrees.
➤ Initiate and maintain seizure precautions.
➤ Provide a calm, quiet environment.
➤ Explain to the patient that he will have to undergo at least 4 hours of observation before discharge.
➤ Provide nonopioid medication, such as Tylenol, for pain or headache. (Opioids may alter the patient's neurologic examination.)

Follow-up actions

➤ Monitor the patient's vital signs and LOC frequently, reporting changes to the physician.
➤ Prepare the patient for a computed tomography scan of the head, if necessary.
➤ Perform a neurologic examination at least every hour, and report changes to the physician.

➤ If the patient has a normal CT scan and is stable after 4 hours of observation, prepare him for discharge.

➤ Explain postconcussion syndrome—characterized by headache, dizziness, vertigo, anxiety, and fatigue—to the patient and his family and inform them that it may persist for several weeks after the injury.

Preventive steps

➤ Strongly encourage the patient to use safety precautions to prevent head injury, including seat belts, age-appropriate car and booster seats for infants and children, helmets for bicycle or motorcycle riding, and hard hats in designated construction areas.

Pathophysiology recap

➤ A sudden, forceful blow to the head causes the brain to strike the skull, causing temporary neural dysfunction.

➤ Dystonic reaction

A dystonic reaction is marked by slow, involuntary movements of large-muscle groups in the limbs, trunk, and neck, usually a result of an extra-pyramidal reaction to a drug. These reactions may cause the patient severe anxiety and distress as well as discomfort, but they are rarely life threatening.

Rapid assessment

➤ Obtain the patient's vital signs.

➤ Obtain the patient's history, including the prescription drug regimen.

➤ Ask the patient about situations that aggravate the condition (for example, walking and emotional stress) and measures that bring relief (such as sleep).

➤ Ask the patient about pain and the duration of each occurrence.

➤ Assess for flexion of the foot, hyperextension of the legs, extension and pronation of the arms, arching of the back, and abnormal postures of the head and neck, including grimacing, oculogyric crisis (deviation of the eye), protrusion of the tongue, trismus, and extension and rotation of the neck (spasmodic torticollis).

➤ Assess the patient's muscle strength, deep tendon reflexes, and gait.

Immediate actions

➤ Implement measures to ensure the patient's physical safety, such as raising and padding his bed rails.

➤ Ensure a clear and safe pathway to the bathroom and doorway. The patient may require assistance with ambulation initially.

➤ Administer I.V. anticholinergic agents (or benzodiazepines, if the patient doesn't respond to anticholinergics). Rapid relief of symptoms should occur after administration of an anticholinergic drug.

➤ Provide emotional support.
➤ Instruct the patient in the use of assistive devices, if necessary.

Follow-up actions
➤ Monitor the patient's vital signs.
➤ Monitor the patient's ability to perform activities of daily living.
➤ Administer pain medication, as ordered.
➤ Provide emotional support and encouragement.
➤ Encourage patients taking medications that cause dystonic reactions not to discontinue them abruptly without consulting a physician.
➤ Continue oral anticholinergic drug treatment for 48 to 72 hours to prevent recurrence.

Preventive steps
➤ Administer an anticholinergic agent to prevent recurrence in the patient who's receiving neuroleptic drug therapy.
➤ The physician may need to switch the patient to a neuroleptic drug less likely to produce a dystonic reaction.

Pathophysiology recap
➤ Dystonic reactions, which are unpredictable, appear to result from a disturbance of the dopaminergic-cholinergic balance in the basal ganglia.
➤ Dystonic reactions are typically induced by certain medications, including neuroleptics (antipsychotics), antiemetics, and antidepressants, although they may be hereditary or idiopathic in some patients.

➤ Encephalitis

A severe inflammation of the brain, encephalitis is usually caused by a mosquito-borne (or, in some areas, tick-borne) virus. Other modes of transmission include ingestion of infected goat's milk and accidental injection or inhalation of the virus. Eastern equine encephalitis (a mosquito-borne viral form) may produce permanent neurologic damage and commonly causes death.

Rapid assessment
➤ Obtain the patient's vital signs, noting increased temperature.
➤ Determine the patient's level of consciousness, perform a neurologic examination, and test his cognitive abilities. (See *Performing a rapid neurologic examination, page 150.*)

 ALERT *The assessment should focus on early changes in intracranial dynamics. Continued swelling may result in cranial nerve compression, causing changes in pupillary reaction to light, ptosis, eyelid droop, and an eye rotating outward.*

> **PERFORMING A RAPID NEUROLOGIC EXAMINATION**

To assess neurologic function in the patient with encephalitis, include the following:
➤ *Orientation* – the patient's knowledge of where he is, and the year, season, date, day, and month
➤ *Registration and recall* – the patient's ability to recall three objects that you name
➤ *Attention and calculation* – the patient's ability to focus on what you're saying
➤ *Language* –the patient's ability to name objects, repeat words clearly, read, and follow a written command
➤ *Focus on recall of recent event* – the patient's ability to recall your name, what he had for breakfast, and who came to visit.
  As you elicit answers, be particularly concerned about the restless patient and about the patient who requires more stimulation to provide the same responses to the above questions.

➤ Ask about a sudden onset of headache and vomiting that may have progressed to signs and symptoms of meningeal irritation (stiff neck and back) and neuronal damage (drowsiness, coma, paralysis, seizures, ataxia, tremors, nausea, vomiting, and organic psychoses).
➤ Ask about taste and smell disturbances, which are signs of herpes encephalitis.

Immediate actions
➤ Initiate and maintain bed rest, safety, and seizure precautions.
➤ Provide a calm, quiet environment.
➤ Assist the physician in obtaining cerebrospinal fluid (CSF) and blood samples to detect the presence of the virus. (This will confirm the diagnosis.)
➤ Monitor for signs of progression of a herniation pattern (abnormal posturing movements to noxious stimuli, such as decerebration, decortication, and flaccidity).
➤ Administer, as ordered:
  – acyclovir — to treat herpes encephalitis
  – I.V. anticonvulsants — to treat and prevent seizures
  – glucocorticoids — to reduce cerebral inflammation and edema
  – sedatives — to help decrease intracranial pressure (ICP)
  – acetaminophen — to relieve headache and reduce fever
  – antibiotics — to treat associated infections such as pneumonia
  – mild laxatives or stool softeners — to prevent straining and increased ICP
  – I.V. fluids — to prevent dehydration.

ALERT *Give acyclovir by slow I.V. infusion only. The patient must be well hydrated and the infusion must be given over 1 hour to avoid kidney damage. Watch for adverse effects, such as nausea, diarrhea, pruritus, and rash. Check the infusion site often to avoid infiltration and phlebitis.*

 ALERT *Be careful not to cause fluid overload, which can increase cerebral edema.*

Follow-up actions

➤ Monitor the patient's vital signs, LOC, neurologic status, and cognitive abilities frequently.
➤ Position the patient carefully to prevent joint stiffness and neck pain. Turn him regularly and provide range-of-motion exercises.
➤ Maintain adequate nutrition with small, frequent meals or supplementation with gastric tube or parenteral feedings.
➤ Monitor intake and output.
➤ Provide good mouth care.
➤ Maintain a quiet environment. Darkening the room may decrease photophobia and headache.
➤ Provide emotional support and reassurance.
➤ Attempt to frequently reorient the patient who is delirious or confused. Providing a calendar or clock in the patient's room may be helpful.
➤ Reassure the patient and his family that behavior changes caused by encephalitis usually disappear. If a neurologic deficit is severe and appears permanent, refer the patient to a rehabilitation program as soon as the acute phase has passed.

Preventive steps

➤ Advise the patient to obtain immunizations, especially against measles, mumps, and rubella.
➤ Teach the patient to prevent mosquito bites by using insect repellents containing DEET, wearing protective clothing (such as long-sleeved shirts and pants) while outdoors (especially at dawn and dusk), and eliminating areas of standing water, which can serve as mosquito breeding sites.

Pathophysiology recap

➤ In encephalitis, intense lymphocytic infiltration of brain tissues and the leptomeninges causes cerebral edema, degeneration of the brain's ganglion cells, and diffuse nerve cell destruction.
➤ Encephalitis generally results from infection with arboviruses specific to rural areas. However, in urban areas, it's typically caused by enteroviruses (coxsackievirus, poliovirus, and echovirus).
➤ Other causes include herpesvirus, mumps virus, human immunodeficiency virus, adenoviruses, and demyelinating diseases after measles, varicella, rubella, or vaccination.

➤ Epidural hematoma

An epidural hematoma is a traumatic accumulation of blood between the inner wall of the skull and the outer membrane that covers the brain (the dura mater). This type of injury occurs more commonly in young people because the dura mater isn't as firmly attached to the skull wall as it is in older people. If untreated, epidural hematoma may result in permanent brain damage or death.

Rapid assessment

➤ Assess the patient for an altered level of consciousness (LOC) and alternating periods of loss of consciousness and alertness with progression to neurologic deterioration and unconsciousness.

➤ Perform a neurologic evaluation, noting contralateral motor deficits, ipsilateral pupillary dilation, and presence of seizures (due to increased intracranial pressure [ICP]).

➤ Assess the patient's rate, depth, and pattern of respirations, and auscultate the lungs.

➤ Obtain the patient's vital signs, noting hypotension and tachycardia.

 ALERT *Bilateral pupillary dilation, bilateral decerebrate response, increased systemic blood pressure, and decreased pulse are indications of progressive neurologic degeneration due to uncontrolled bleeding. If bleeding isn't halted, profound coma, with irregular respiratory patterns, will occur.*

Immediate actions

➤ Initiate and maintain bed rest with the head of the bed at 30 degrees; also follow safety and seizure precautions.

➤ Provide supplemental oxygen, and assist with endotracheal intubation or tracheotomy, as necessary (for a patient with a Glasgow coma scale score of 8 or less and unable to protect his airway).

 ALERT *Abnormal respirations associated with decreased LOC may indicate a breakdown in the brain's respiratory center and an impending tentorial herniation—a neurologic emergency.*

➤ Provide a calm, quiet environment.

➤ Obtain blood samples for complete blood count, prothrombin time, International Normalized Ratio, and arterial blood gas analysis.

➤ Discontinue anticoagulants, and check with the physician about further treatment orders.

➤ Clean and dress any superficial scalp wounds using strict sterile technique. (If the skin has been broken, the patient may need tetanus prophylaxis.) Assist with suturing if needed. Carefully cover scalp wounds with a sterile dressing; control bleeding as necessary.

➤ Obtain a computed tomography scan or magnetic resonance imaging to identify abnormal masses or structural shifts within the cranium.

➤ Consult the neurosurgeon and prepare the patient for surgery to evacuate the hematoma.
➤ Administer, as ordered:
  – anticonvulsants — to control or prevent seizure activity
  – hyperosmotic diuretics — to reduce cerebral edema
  – antipyretics — to reduce temperature
  – mannitol or furosemide — to decrease ICP.

Follow-up actions
➤ Continue to assess the patient's vital signs and neurologic status, including LOC and pupil size, every 15 minutes. If the patient's condition
worsens or fluctuates, notify the physician.
➤ Assist with the insertion of an intracranial pressure monitoring device,
if necessary, and calculate cerebral perfusion pressure.
➤ Carefully observe the patient for cerebrospinal fluid (CSF) leakage from
the nose or ears. Check the bed sheets for a blood-tinged spot surrounded by a lighter ring (halo sign). Elevate the head of the bed 30 degrees.
(Anything that produces jugular compression can lead to increased ICP.)
Be sure to keep his head properly aligned.
➤ Position the patient so that secretions drain properly. If you detect CSF
leakage from the nose, place a gauze pad under the nostrils. If CSF leaks
from the ear, position the patient so his ear drains naturally — don't
pack the ear or nose. If the patient requires suctioning, suction him
through the mouth, not the nose, to avoid introducing bacteria into the
CSF.
➤ If the patient is unconscious, insert a orogastric tube to prevent aspiration.
➤ Monitor intake and output frequently to help maintain a normovolemic
state.
➤ Monitor wounds for signs and symptoms of infection.

Preventive steps
➤ Although an epidural hematoma isn't preventable after a head injury
has occurred, the patient can minimize the risk of head injury by wearing a seatbelt, a helmet when bicycling or motorcycle riding, and other
protective equipment while playing sports or during work or recreational activities.

Pathophysiology recap
➤ Epidural hematomas result from direct trauma, most commonly a skull
fracture, which causes a laceration of the blood vessel (typically the
middle meningeal artery), producing hemorrhage into the epidural
space.
➤ The collection of blood that forms, or hematoma, rapidly increases the
ICP as it exerts pressure directly on the brain. This may result in additional brain injury.

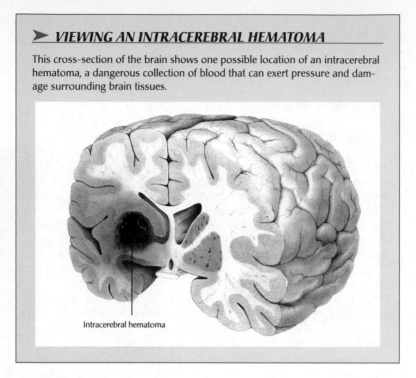

➤ VIEWING AN INTRACEREBRAL HEMATOMA

This cross-section of the brain shows one possible location of an intracerebral hematoma, a dangerous collection of blood that can exert pressure and damage surrounding brain tissues.

Intracerebral hematoma

➤ *Intracerebral hematoma*

An intracerebral hematoma is a traumatic or spontaneous disruption of cerebral blood vessels in the brain parenchyma resulting in neurologic deficits, which vary depending on the site and amount of bleeding. Hematoma collection may be isolated to one area of a cerebral hemisphere, or it may occur in other brain structures, such as the thalamus, basal ganglia, pons, or cerebellum. (See *Viewing an intracerebral hematoma.*)

Rapid assessment
➤ Obtain the patient's vital signs.
➤ Evaluate the patient's neurologic status, noting alterations in the level of consciousness (LOC), vision changes, dysphasia (difficulty speaking), dysphagia (difficulty swallowing), loss of balance or coordination, and seizure activity.
➤ Test for motor deficits and decorticate or decerebrate responses. (See *Comparing decerebrate and decorticate postures.*)
➤ Ask about headache, nausea, and vomiting.
➤ Assess the patient's rate, pattern, and depth of respirations, and auscultate the lung fields.

COMPARING DECEREBRATE AND DECORTICATE POSTURES

Decerebrate (extension) posture results from damage to the upper brain stem. In this posture, the arms are adducted and extended, with the wrists pronated and the fingers flexed. The legs are stiffly extended, with plantar flexion of the feet.

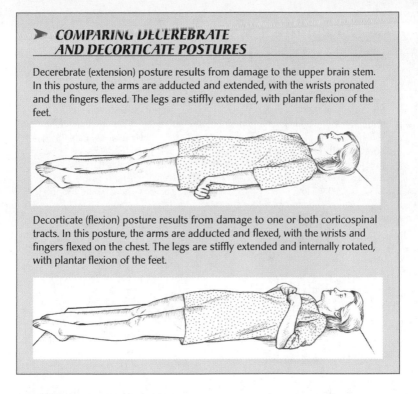

Decorticate (flexion) posture results from damage to one or both corticospinal tracts. In this posture, the arms are adducted and flexed, with the wrists and fingers flexed on the chest. The legs are stiffly extended and internally rotated, with plantar flexion of the feet.

 ALERT *Abnormal respirations may indicate a breakdown in the brain's respiratory center and an impending tentorial herniation — a neurologic emergency.*

Immediate actions
- Assess for additional injuries.
- Initiate and maintain bed rest with the head of the bed at 30 degrees; also initiate and maintain seizure and safety precautions.
- Provide supplemental oxygen, and prepare for endotracheal intubation and mechanical ventilation, as necessary.
- Assist with the insertion of an intracranial pressure monitoring device, if necessary, and calculate cerebral perfusion pressure.
- Provide a calm, quiet environment.
- Monitor the patient's vital signs continuously and assess for additional injuries.
- Clean and dress superficial scalp wounds using strict sterile technique. (If the skin has been broken, the patient may need tetanus prophylaxis.) Assist with suturing, if needed. Carefully cover scalp wounds with a sterile dressing; control bleeding, as necessary.
- Administer, as ordered:

➤ *CRANIOTOMY: A WINDOW TO THE BRAIN*

To perform a craniotomy, the surgeon incises the skin, clamps the aponeurotic layer, and retracts the skin flap. He then incises and retracts the muscle layer and scrapes periosteum off the skull.

Next, using an air-driven or electric drill, he drills a series of burr holes in the corners of the skull incision. During drilling, warm saline solution is dripped into the burr holes and the holes are suctioned to remove bone dust. When drilling is complete, the surgeon uses a dural elevator to separate the dura from the bone around the margin of each burr hole. He then saws between the burr holes to create a bone flap. He either leaves this flap attached to the muscle and retracts it or detaches the flap completely and removes it. In either case, the flap is wrapped to keep it moist and protected. Finally, the surgeon incises and retracts the dura, exposing the brain.

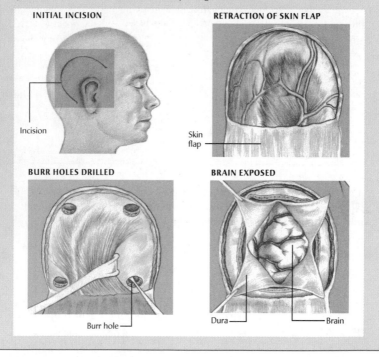

INITIAL INCISION

Incision

RETRACTION OF SKIN FLAP

Skin flap

BURR HOLES DRILLED

Burr hole

BRAIN EXPOSED

Dura — Brain

– corticosteroids or osmotic diuretics — to reduce the risk of increased intracranial pressure (ICP)
– anticonvulsants — to control or prevent seizure activity
– analgesics — to control pain
– blood products and I.V. fluids — to replace blood volume lost during hemorrhage
– antipyretics — to treat fever.

Follow-up actions

➤ Continue to check the patient's vital signs and neurologic status, including LOC and pupil size, every 15 minutes. If the patient's condition worsens or fluctuates, consult the physician.

➤ Prepare the patient for a diagnostic computed tomography scan or magnetic resonance imaging of the head.

➤ Carefully observe the patient for cerebrospinal fluid (CSF) leakage. Check the bed sheets for a blood-tinged spot surrounded by a lighter ring (halo sign). Elevate the head of the bed 30 degrees. (Anything that produces jugular compression can lead to increased ICP). Be sure to keep his head properly aligned.

➤ Position the patient so that secretions drain properly. If you detect CSF leakage from the nose, place a gauze pad under the nostrils. If CSF leaks from the ear, position the patient so his ear drains naturally—don't pack the ear or nose. If the patient requires suctioning, suction him through the mouth, not the nose, to avoid introducing bacteria into the CSF.

➤ If the patient is unconscious, insert an oragastric tube to prevent aspiration.

➤ Monitor intake and output frequently to help maintain a normovolemic state.

➤ Cluster nursing activities to provide for rest periods, thus reducing the risk of sustained increases in ICP.

➤ Monitor wounds for signs and symptoms of infection.

➤ Prepare the patient for craniotomy, as indicated. (See *Craniotomy: A window to the brain.*)

Preventive steps

➤ Initiate treatment of hypertension to reduce the patient's risk of developing intracerebral hematoma.

Pathophysiology recap

➤ Traumatic hemorrhage results from shear forces caused by brain movement; blood vessel laceration and hemorrhage into the cerebral tissue result. This bleeding irritates the tissues, causing cerebral edema.

➤ The pressure exerted on the brain from the cerebral edema and the presence of the hematoma can rapidly damage the tissues.

➤ Frontal and temporal lobes of the brain are common sites for intracerebral hematoma. Trauma is associated with few intracerebral hematomas; most are the result of hypertension.

➤ *Meningitis*

In meningitis, the brain and the spinal cord meninges become inflamed, usually as a result of a viral or, less commonly, bacterial infection. Such inflammation may involve all three meningeal membranes—the dura mater, the arachnoid, and the pia mater. The prognosis is good and complications are rare if the disease is recognized early and the infecting organism responds to antibiotics; however, mortality in untreated meningitis is 70% to 100%.

Rapid assessment

➤ Obtain the patient's vital signs, noting hypotension, tachycardia, decreased oxygen saturation, and increased temperature.
➤ Ask about chills, malaise, headache, vomiting, and papilledema.
➤ Assess the rate, depth, and pattern of respirations, and auscultate breath sounds.
➤ Perform a neurologic assessment, noting the patient's level of consciousness (LOC).

 ALERT *Stay especially alert for a temperature increase up to 102° F (38.9° C), a deteriorating LOC, onset of seizures, and altered respirations, all of which may signal an impending crisis.*

➤ Assess for irritability, nuchal rigidity, positive Brudzinski's and Kernig's signs, exaggerated and symmetrical deep tendon reflexes, and opisthotonos (a spasm in which the back and extremities arch backward so that the body rests on the head and heels). (See *Assessing Brudzinski's and Kernig's signs.*)
➤ Assess for photophobia, diplopia, and other visual problems.
➤ Observe the electrocardiogram for sinus arrhythmias.

ALERT *An infant may not show clinical signs of infection. Assess for fretful demeanor, refusal to eat, and profuse vomiting. Dehydration due to vomiting prevents the characteristic bulging fontanel that indicates increased intracranial pressure (ICP). As the illness progresses, you may observe twitching, seizures (in 30% of infants), or coma.*

Immediate actions

➤ Initiate and maintain bed rest with the head of the bed at 30 degrees. Also initiate and maintain seizure and safety precautions.
➤ Provide supplemental oxygen and prepare for endotracheal intubation and mechanical ventilation, if necessary.
➤ Provide a calm, quiet environment.
➤ Assist the physician in performing a lumbar puncture and obtaining a cerebrospinal fluid (CSF) culture and sensitivity tests to identify the infecting organism (viruses aren't detected by these tests).
➤ Insert an indwelling urinary catheter, if necessary.
➤ Place the patient on isolation precautions, as determined by facility policy.
➤ Obtain serum samples for complete blood count.
➤ Administer, as ordered:
  – I.V. antibiotics — to treat the infection
  – mannitol — to decrease cerebral edema
  – anticonvulsants or sedatives — to reduce restlessness

➤ ASSESSING BRUDZINSKI'S AND KERNIG'S SIGNS

When positive, Brudzinski's sign and Kernig's signs indicate meningeal irritation. Follow these guidelines to test for the two signs.

Brudzinski's sign
With the patient in the supine position, place your hand under his neck and flex it forward, chin to chest. This test is positive if he flexes his ankles, knees, and hips bilaterally. In addition, the patient typically complains of pain when the neck is flexed.

BRUDZINSKI'S SIGN

Pain

Kernig's sign
With the patient in the supine position, flex his hip and knee to form a 90-degree angle. Next, attempt to extend this leg. If he exhibits pain, resistance to extension, and spasm, the test is positive.

KERNIG'S SIGN

Pain

– acetaminophen — to relieve headache and fever
– stool softeners or mild laxatives — to prevent straining and increased ICP.

Follow-up actions
➤ Monitor the patient's vital signs frequently.
➤ Assess the patient's neurologic function frequently. Observe his LOC and check for signs of increased ICP (agitation, restlessness, confusion, vomiting, seizures, and a change in motor function and vital signs). Also, watch for signs of cranial nerve involvement (ptosis, strabismus, and diplopia).
➤ Position the patient carefully to prevent joint stiffness and neck pain.
➤ Turn the patient often, according to a planned positioning schedule.
➤ Assist with range-of-motion exercises.
➤ Monitor nutritional intake and obtain a consult from a nutritionist to determine the need for supplements or nasogastric tube or parenteral feedings.
➤ Provide reassurance and support.
➤ Reassure the family that the delirium and behavior changes caused by meningitis usually disappear.
➤ If a severe neurologic deficit appears permanent, refer the patient to a rehabilitation program as soon as the acute phase of this illness has passed.

➤ Monitor the patient for adverse effects of I.V. antibiotics and other medications.

Preventive steps
➤ Teach patients with chronic sinusitis or other chronic infections the importance of proper medical treatment.
➤ Follow strict sterile technique when treating patients with head wounds or skull fractures.

Pathophysiology recap
➤ The microorganism typically enters the central nervous system by one of four routes: the blood (most common); a direct opening between CSF and the environment as a result of trauma; along the cranial and peripheral nerves; and through the mouth or nose.
➤ Microorganisms can be transmitted to an infant via the umbilical cord and bloodstream.
➤ Meningitis commonly begins as an inflammation of the pia-arachnoid, which may progress to congestion of adjacent tissues and destruction of some nerve cells.
➤ Meningitis is almost always a complication of another bacterial infection—bacteremia (especially from pneumonia, empyema, osteomyelitis, or endocarditis), sinusitis, otitis media, encephalitis, myelitis, or brain abscess— usually caused by *Neisseria meningitidis, Haemophilus influenzae* (in children and young adults), or *Streptococcus pneumoniae* (in adults).
➤ Meningitis may also follow a skull fracture, a penetrating head wound, lumbar puncture, or ventricular shunting procedures.

➤ Neurogenic shock

In neurogenic shock, a temporary loss of autonomic function below the level of a spinal cord injury produces cardiovascular changes. Neurogenic shock is a type of distributive shock in which vasodilation causes a state of hypovolemia. It occurs most commonly at the level of T6 or above.

Rapid assessment
➤ Assess the patient's level of consciousness.
➤ Assess the rate, depth, and pattern of respirations, and auscultate breath sounds.
➤ Palpate for peripheral pulses, and auscultate the apical heart rate.
➤ Assess the patient's vital signs, noting hypotension and bradycardia.
➤ Observe the patient for warm, dry skin below the level of the injury.

Immediate actions
➤ Place the patient on bed rest with the head of the bed elevated 30 degrees to help increased blood pressure and blood flow to the brain.

➤ Obtain a blood sample for arterial blood gas analysis.
➤ Provide supplemental oxygen and prepare the patient for endotracheal intubation and mechanical ventilation, as necessary.
➤ Initiate cardiac and hemodynamic monitoring.
➤ Insert an indwelling urinary catheter.
➤ Treat hypothermia with a warming blanket.
➤ Administer, as ordered:
  – I.V. fluids, such as normal saline solution or lactated Ringer's solution — to increase intravascular volume and blood pressure
  – vasopressors — to increase blood pressure
  – blood products — to increase intravascular volume
  – an osmotic diuretic, such as mannitol, if urine output is decreased — to increase renal blood flow
  – atropine or transcutaneous pacing — to treat symptomatic bradycardia.

Follow-up actions
➤ Monitor the patient's vital signs frequently.
➤ Prepare the patient for diagnostic tests to determine the cause of the disorder.
➤ Assess skin color and temperature.
➤ Monitor intake and output, and watch for signs of dehydration and fluid overload.
➤ Provide meticulous skin care, and reposition the patient frequently to prevent skin breakdown.
➤ Monitor complete blood count and serum electrolyte values; treat abnormalities, as ordered.
➤ Apply antiembolism stockings to prevent deep venous thrombosis.
➤ Explain all procedures and their purposes to the patient. Provide emotional support to the patient and his family.
➤ Facilitate the patient's transfer to a spinal cord injury center

Preventive steps
➤ Neurogenic shock can't be prevented.

Pathophysiology recap
➤ Neurogenic shock is an abnormal vasomotor response that occurs secondary to the disruption of sympathetic impulses from the brain stem to the thoracolumbar area.
➤ It may result from spinal cord injury, spinal anesthesia, vasomotor center depression, medications, or hypoglycemia.
➤ A loss of sympathetic vasoconstrictor tone in the vascular smooth muscle and reduced autonomic function lead to widespread arterial and venous vasodilation.
➤ Venous return is reduced as blood pools in the venous system, leading to a drop in cardiac output and hypotension.
➤ Hypotension typically resolves within 48 to 72 hours.

➤ *Neuroleptic malignant syndrome*

Neuroleptic malignant syndrome is a rare, life-threatening neurologic disorder caused by an adverse reaction to neuroleptic or antipsychotic drugs. If untreated, stupor, coma, and death may occur.

Rapid assessment
- ➤ Perform a neurologic assessment, noting alterations in mental status, involuntary movements, and confusion.
- ➤ Obtain the patient's vital signs, noting labile blood pressure and increased temperature.
- ➤ Observe rate, depth, and pattern of respirations, and auscultate lung sounds, noting pulmonary congestion.
- ➤ Observe for dysarthria and muscle rigidity.
- ➤ Assess for dysphagia and excessive saliva secretion.
- ➤ Observe for pallor and excessive sweating.

Immediate actions
- ➤ Initiate the patient on bed rest; institute safety precautions.
- ➤ Provide supplemental oxygen, and prepare for endotracheal intubation and mechanical ventilation, if necessary.
- ➤ Initiate hypothermia therapy, if necessary.
- ➤ Institute aspiration precautions.
- ➤ Discontinue the offending neuroleptic agent immediately.
- ➤ Administer, as ordered:
  - vasopressors or vasodilators — to increase or decrease blood pressure, respectively
  - I.V. fluids — to increase intravascular volume and blood pressure
  - diuretics — to treat pulmonary congestion
  - nonopioid analgesics — to decrease pain without altering the neurologic examination.

Follow-up actions
- ➤ Monitor the patient's vital signs and neurologic status closely. Report changes to the physician.
- ➤ Monitor intake and output.
- ➤ Provide meticulous skin and mouth care.
- ➤ Observe for psychotic behavior while the patient is off antipsychotic medications. Ensure a safe environment for the patient and others.
- ➤ Assist with activities of daily living, as necessary.
- ➤ Provide range-of-motion exercises.
- ➤ Provide emotional support to the patient and his family.
- ➤ Prepare the patient for electroconvulsive therapy, if necessary.

Preventive steps
- ➤ Make sure that the patient's chart includes a notation about not prescribing the offending neuroleptic drug.

COMPLICATIONS

➤ *RHABDOMYOLYSIS*

In rhabdomyolysis, toxins released by deteriorating muscle cells cause kidney damage and, in some cases, acute renal failure. Rhabdomyolysis may result from neuroleptic malignant syndrome, blunt trauma, extensive burn injury, prolonged immobilization, drug therapy, exposure to toxins, or viral, bacterial, or fungal infection.

Signs and symptoms
➤ Dark urine
➤ Fever
➤ Malaise
➤ Muscle pain (especially in the thighs, calves, or lower back)
➤ Myalgia
➤ Nausea and vomiting
➤ Tenderness
➤ Weakness

Treatment
Early, aggressive hydration may prevent complications from rhabdomyolysis by rapidly eliminating myoglobin from the kidneys. I.V. hydration and diuretics promote diuresis. Bicarbonate may be administered to prevent myoglobin from breaking down into toxic compounds in the kidney. Dialysis, renal replacement therapy and, in severe cases, kidney transplantation may be necessary.

Nursing considerations
➤ Monitor intake and output, vital signs, electrolyte levels, daily weight, and laboratory results (especially blood urea nitrogen, creatine kinase, and creatinine levels).
➤ Watch for signs of renal failure (such as decreasing urine output and increasing urine specific gravity).
➤ To prevent rhabdomyolysis, ensure adequate hydration and monitor the patient for adverse reactions to prescribed drugs.

➤ Ask the patient about a history of neuroleptic malignant syndrome before administering a drug known to cause it.

Pathophysiology recap
➤ In most cases, neuroleptic malignant syndrome occurs within 2 weeks of starting neuroleptic drug therapy, but signs and symptoms may develop at any time during the treatment period.
➤ The drugs implicated in causing neuroleptic malignant syndrome all have dopamine D2-receptor antagonist properties, which decrease dopamine activity in the central nervous system.
➤ This decrease in dopamine activity is what causes the characteristic signs and symptoms as well as rhabdomyolysis. (See *Rhabdomyolysis*.)

> ## **TYPES OF SKULL FRACTURES**
>
> Skull fractures are linear, comminuted, or depressed.
> ➤ A linear fracture is a common hairline break, without displacement of structures.
> ➤ A comminuted fracture splinters or crushes the bone into several fragments.
> ➤ A depressed fracture pushes the bone toward the brain.
>   In children, the skull's thinness and elasticity allow a depression to occur without a fracture. However, a linear fracture that crosses a suture line increases the possibility of epidural hematoma.

➤ *Skull fracture*

A skull fracture may be simple (closed) or compound (open) and may or may not displace bone fragments. (See *Types of skull fractures.*) Because possible damage to the brain is the first concern rather than the fracture itself, a skull fracture is considered a neurosurgical condition.

   Skull fractures are also classified according to location, such as sphenoidal fracture, temporal fracture, or basilar fracture. A sphenoidal fracture may damage the optic nerve, causing blindness. A temporal fracture may cause unilateral deafness or facial paralysis. A basilar fracture commonly produces hemorrhage from the nose, pharynx, or ears; blood under the periorbital skin (periorbital ecchymoses, or *raccoon eyes*) and under the conjunctiva; and Battle's sign (supramastoid ecchymosis), sometimes with bleeding behind the eardrum. This type of fracture may also cause cerebrospinal fluid (CSF)—even brain tissue—to leak from the nose or ears. (See *Recognizing periorbital ecchymoses.*)

 ALERT *A basilar skull fracture is at the base of the skull and involves the cribriform plate and frontal sinuses. Because of the danger of grave cranial complications and meningitis, basilar fractures are usually far more serious than vault fractures.*

Rapid assessment
➤ Assess the rate, depth, and pattern of respirations, and auscultate breath sounds.
➤ Assess the patient's vital signs, noting hypotension, tachycardia, and changes in his respiratory pattern.
➤ Determine the cause of the trauma.
➤ Ask the patient if he has had a persistent, localized headache.
➤ Observe for scalp wounds, such as abrasions, contusions, lacerations, or avulsions, noting profuse bleeding, which can be heavy enough to induce hypovolemic shock.
➤ Ask the patient if he lost consciousness at the time of injury or if he vomited shortly after sustaining it.

➤ **RECOGNIZING PERIORBITAL ECCHYMOSES**

It's usually easy to differentiate bilateral periorbital ecchymoses *(raccoon eyes)* associated with basilar skull fracture from a black eye that occurs with facial trauma. Raccoon eyes (shown here) are always bilateral. They develop 2 to 3 days after a closed-head injury that results in basilar skull fracture. In contrast, periorbital ecchymosis that occurs with facial trauma is frequently unilateral, although both eyes can be affected. It usually develops within hours after injury.

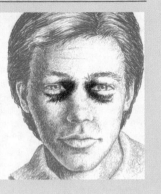

➤ Perform a neurologic assessment, noting mental status changes, disorientation, altered level of consciousness (LOC), decreased or abnormal pupillary response, and altered motor function and deep tendon reflexes.

 ALERT *Observe for CSF draining from the patient's nose or ears, which may indicate a dural injury. Leaking CSF may mix with blood making it difficult to identify. Place a small amount of drainage from the nose or ear on a gauze pad; if CSF is present, it will form a yellowish ring ("halo sign"). The fluid will test positive for glucose. Instruct the patient not to blow his nose but to wipe it instead. If CSF leaks from the ear, position the patient so the ear drains naturally; don't pack the ear or nose.*

 ALERT *Jagged bone fragments that pierce the dura mater or the cerebral cortex may cause subdural, epidural, or intracerebral hemorrhage or hematoma, resulting in hemiparesis, unequal pupils, dizziness, seizures, projectile vomiting, decreased pulse and respiratory rates, and progressive unresponsiveness.*

Immediate actions

➤ Initiate and maintain bed rest with the head of the bed at 30 degrees. Also institute seizure, safety, and aspiration precautions.
➤ Provide supplemental oxygen, and prepare for endotracheal intubation and mechanical ventilation, if necessary.
➤ Insert a large-bore I.V. catheter, and obtain serum samples for complete blood count, prothrombin time, International Normalized Ratio, partial thromboplastin time, type and crossmatch, serum electrolytes, and arterial blood gas analysis.
➤ Gently clean and cover scalp wounds carefully with a sterile dressing; control bleeding and assist with suturing, as necessary.

➤ TREATMENT OF SKULL FRACTURES

Treatment modalities for skull fractures vary according to the type and severity of the fracture.

Linear fractures

Although occasionally even a simple linear skull fracture can tear an underlying blood vessel or cause cerebrospinal fluid (CSF) leakage, linear fractures generally require only mild supportive treatment, including mild analgesics, such as acetaminophen, and cleaning, debridement, and repair of any wounds.

If the patient with a skull fracture hasn't lost consciousness, he should be observed in the emergency department for at least 4 hours. After this observation period, if his vital signs are stable, the CT scan is normal, and the neurosurgeon concurs, the patient can be discharged. At this time, the patient should be given an instruction sheet to follow for 24 to 48 hours of observation at home.

Vault and basilar fractures

More severe vault fractures, especially depressed fractures, usually require a craniotomy to elevate or remove fragments that have been driven into the brain and to extract foreign bodies and necrotic tissue, thereby reducing the risk of infection and further brain damage. Other treatments for severe vault fractures include antibiotic therapy and, in profound hemorrhage, blood transfusions.

Treatment for basilar fractures may include prophylactic antibiotics to prevent the onset of meningitis from CSF leaks as well as close observation for secondary hematomas and hemorrhages.

➤ Assist the physician to insert an intracranial pressure monitoring device.
➤ Insert an indwelling urinary catheter.
➤ Provide emotional support.
➤ Keep in mind that individual treatment will be based on the type and severity of the fracture. (See *Treatment of skull fractures.*)
➤ Prepare the patient for a computed tomography (CT) scan to determine the location of the fracture, and obtain a CT scan and magnetic resonance imaging to assess for brain damage.
➤ Administer, as ordered:
— I.V. fluids — to increase intravascular volume
— blood products — to increase intravascular volume and replace losses
– mannitol — to decrease ICP, if necessary
– antibiotics — to prevent a CSF or wound infection
– tetanus toxoid — as prophylaxis
– nonopioid analgesics — to control pain.

 ALERT *Don't administer hypotonic fluids, such as dextrose 5% in water, because they can cause cerebral edema.*

ALERT *Don't administer opioid analgesics or sedatives—they may depress respirations, increase carbon dioxide levels, lead to increased intracranial pressure, and mask changes in the patient's neurologic status. Give acetaminophen or another mild analgesic for pain. If the patient requires a gastric tube, choose an orogastric tube if you suspect a basilar skull fracture.*

Follow-up actions

➤ Monitor the patient's vital signs, LOC, and neurological status frequently, and report any changes.

➤ If the patient's nose is draining CSF, wipe it, being careful to not let him blow it. If an ear is draining, cover it lightly with sterile gauze — don't pack it.

➤ Perform tracheal suctioning through the mouth, not the nose, to prevent the introduction of bacteria if a CSF leak is present.

➤ Monitor for signs and symptoms of infection.

➤ Monitor intake and output hourly.

➤ Assist the patient with activities of daily living, as necessary. Obtain a consultation with a physical or occupational therapist as ordered.

➤ Monitor the patient's nutritional status, and obtain a consultation with a nutritionist to determine the need for supplemental nutrition.

➤ Perform wound care as ordered, and teach the patient and his family how to care for the wound.

➤ Remind the patient to return to the facility immediately if his LOC decreases, if his headache persists after several doses of mild analgesics, if he vomits more than once, or if weakness develops in his arms or legs.

➤ Prepare the patient for surgery, if necessary, explaining that you will need to shave the patient's head to provide a clean area for surgery.

➤ After surgery, monitor the patient's vital signs and neurologic status frequently, watching for changes in the LOC. Because skull fractures and brain injuries heal slowly, don't expect dramatic postoperative improvement.

Preventive steps

➤ Advise the patient to minimize risk of head injury by wearing a seatbelt, a helmet when bicycling or motorcycle riding, and other protective equipment while playing sports or during work or recreational activities.

Pathophysiology recap

➤ Like concussions and cerebral contusions or lacerations, skull fractures invariably result from a traumatic blow to the head. Motor vehicle accidents, bad falls, and severe beatings (especially in children) top the list of causes.

➤ Spinal cord injury

Usually the result of trauma to the head or neck, spinal cord injuries (SCIs)—other than spinal cord damage — include fractures, contusions, and compressions of the vertebral column. The danger from such injuries lies in associated damage to the spinal cord.

Rapid assessment

➤ Assess the rate, pattern, and depth of respirations, and auscultate lung sounds, noting crackles, rhonchi, or absent breath sounds indicating ineffective airway clearance.

➤ Perform a neurologic assessment, noting the patient's level of consciousness (LOC) and diminished motor and sensory function.

➤ Obtain vital signs, noting decreased oxygen saturation.

➤ Observe the patient's electrocardiogram for changes.

➤ Obtain the patient's history, including incidence of trauma, neoplastic lesions, endocrine disorders, or infections that could produce a spinal abscess.

➤ Inquire about muscle spasms and back or neck pain that worsens with movement.

➤ Observe surface wounds for signs of infection.

➤ Note point tenderness (indicates cervical fracture), pain that radiates to other body areas (indicates dorsal and lumbar fractures), or other symptoms that indicate the area of injury.

➤ Ask the patient to report other signs and symptoms because they will be based on the type and severity of injury. (See *Types of spinal cord injury,* pages 170 and 171.)

Immediate actions

➤ Provide supplemental oxygen and prepare for endotracheal intubation and mechanical ventilation, if necessary.

 ALERT *If the patient isn't intubated when admitted to the emergency department, hemorrhage and edema at the injury site can predispose him to increasing cord damage that ultimately leads to a higher level of dysfunction and altered respiratory function, necessitating mechanical ventilation.*

➤ Stabilize the patient's spine. (See *Managing spinal cord injury,* pages 172 and 173.)

 ALERT *If a cervical spine injury hasn't been ruled out, don't hyperextend the patient's neck for intubation. Perform nasal intubation or orotracheal intubation with the cervical spine immobilized manually.*

➤ Initiate continuous cardiac monitoring.

➤ Assist with a central venous or pulmonary artery catheter and arterial line insertion, if necessary.

➤ Obtain blood samples for arterial blood gas analysis and serum electrolytes.
➤ Insert a nasogastric tube and attach it to low intermittent suction for gastric decompression.

 ALERT *Paralytic ileus is a common problem for patients with SCI, usually occurring within the first 72 hours after the injury.*

➤ Insert an indwelling urinary catheter.
➤ Assist with measures to help the patient maintain body temperature because his abilities to conserve (vasoconstrict) and lose (vasodilate) heat are lost.
➤ Prepare the patient for surgical stabilization, if indicated.
➤ Apply antiembolism stockings to prevent deep venous thrombosis.
➤ Obtain spinal and chest X-rays as ordered.
➤ Obtain myelography, magnetic resonance imaging (MRI), or a computed tomography (CT) scan to locate the fracture and site of compression. CT scans or MRI also reveal spinal cord edema and may reveal a spinal mass.
➤ Administer vasopressors, as ordered, to increase blood pressure.

 ALERT *Hypotension occurs in the patient with an SCI because of a loss of vascular motor control below the level of the injury, causing vasodilation and a relative hypovolemia.*

Follow-up actions
➤ Monitor the patient's vital signs, LOC, neurologic status, and respiratory status frequently.

 ALERT *Assess the patient frequently for signs and symptoms of autonomic dysreflexia, a complication of SCI that requires immediate attention. (See* Autonomic dysreflexia, *page 174.)*

➤ Perform tracheal suctioning, as needed.
➤ Monitor intake and output, and institute a bladder and bowel training program, including intermittent catheterization and bowel retraining, as appropriate.
➤ Institute measures to prevent skin breakdown from immobilization including turning (as appropriate), repositioning, padding, and care of any devices, such as a halo jacket (for example, pin-site care) or traction.
➤ Monitor insertion sites for signs of infection.
➤ Encourage mobility as appropriate within the restrictions of the patient's condition and injury, including assistance with range-of-motion (ROM) exercises.

 ALERT *Stay alert for orthostatic hypotension, which may occur in a patient with an SCI to the cervical or high thoracic area. This sudden drop in blood pressure could lead to cerebral hypoxia and loss of consciousness. To prevent orthostatic hypotension, change the patient's position slowly and perform ROM exercises every 2 hours.*

➤ TYPES OF SPINAL CORD INJURY

Injury to the spinal cord is classified as complete or incomplete. An incomplete spinal injury may be anterior cord syndrome, central cord syndrome, or Brown-Séquard's syndrome, depending on the area of the cord affected. This chart highlights the characteristic signs and symptoms of each.

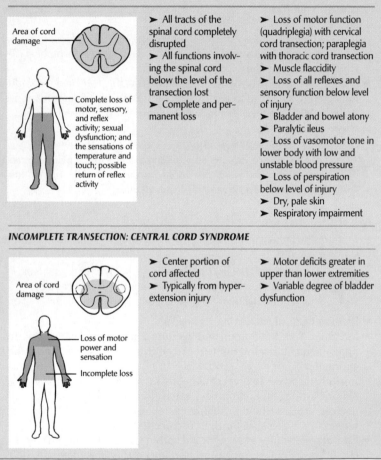

Type	Description	Signs and symptoms
COMPLETE TRANSECTION		
Area of cord damage Complete loss of motor, sensory, and reflex activity; sexual dysfunction; and the sensations of temperature and touch; possible return of reflex activity	➤ All tracts of the spinal cord completely disrupted ➤ All functions involving the spinal cord below the level of the transection lost ➤ Complete and permanent loss	➤ Loss of motor function (quadriplegia) with cervical cord transection; paraplegia with thoracic cord transection ➤ Muscle flaccidity ➤ Loss of all reflexes and sensory function below level of injury ➤ Bladder and bowel atony ➤ Paralytic ileus ➤ Loss of vasomotor tone in lower body with low and unstable blood pressure ➤ Loss of perspiration below level of injury ➤ Dry, pale skin ➤ Respiratory impairment
INCOMPLETE TRANSECTION: CENTRAL CORD SYNDROME		
Area of cord damage Loss of motor power and sensation Incomplete loss	➤ Center portion of cord affected ➤ Typically from hyperextension injury	➤ Motor deficits greater in upper than lower extremities ➤ Variable degree of bladder dysfunction

➤ Begin rehabilitation as soon as possible. Keep in mind that the patient with an SCI may need extensive rehabilitation depending on the level of injury and prognosis for recovery. If he requires ventilatory dependency, placement in an extended care facility may be necessary.

➤ Provide emotional support to the patient and his family; allow the patient to verbalize his concerns.

Type	Description	Signs and symptoms
INCOMPLETE TRANSECTION: ANTERIOR CORD SYNDROME		

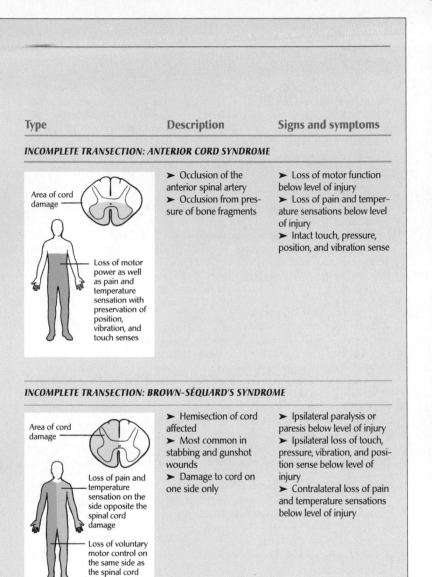

INCOMPLETE TRANSECTION: ANTERIOR CORD SYNDROME

Area of cord damage

Loss of motor power as well as pain and temperature sensation with preservation of position, vibration, and touch senses

➤ Occlusion of the anterior spinal artery
➤ Occlusion from pressure of bone fragments

➤ Loss of motor function below level of injury
➤ Loss of pain and temperature sensations below level of injury
➤ Intact touch, pressure, position, and vibration sense

INCOMPLETE TRANSECTION: BROWN-SÉQUARD'S SYNDROME

Area of cord damage

Loss of pain and temperature sensation on the side opposite the spinal cord damage

Loss of voluntary motor control on the same side as the spinal cord damage

➤ Hemisection of cord affected
➤ Most common in stabbing and gunshot wounds
➤ Damage to cord on one side only

➤ Ipsilateral paralysis or paresis below level of injury
➤ Ipsilateral loss of touch, pressure, vibration, and position sense below level of injury
➤ Contralateral loss of pain and temperature sensations below level of injury

Preventive steps
➤ Instruct patients to always wear a seat belt while driving or riding in a motor vehicle, and use age-appropriate car seats and booster seats for infants and children.

IN ACTION

➤ *MANAGING SPINAL CORD INJURY*

Jim Morris, 22, arrives in your emergency department by ambulance following a mountain-biking accident. He's alert and oriented, but anxious and tearful. He says he hasn't been able to move or feel his arms or legs since the accident occurred 3 hours ago. The paramedics have taken cervical spine precautions and tell you that Mr. Morris has no other apparent injuries.

You take his vital signs: blood pressure, 80/43 mm Hg; heart rate, 61; respirations, 22; and oxygen saturation, 95% on room air.

What's the situation?

Mr. Morris went over his handlebars when he hit a rock. He has no other medical problems.

His airway is patent and he's breathing well. When you assess him, he has no movement or sensation in response to tactile stimulation in either leg or his trunk. He can shrug both shoulders and can slightly raise his arms off the bed away from his body. He has a minimal ability to bend his elbows, but no ability to straighten the bent elbow or to grasp your hands. He does feel a pins-and-needles sensation in his thumbs.

What's your assessment?

Based on the absence of movement and sensation in his arms and legs, you suspect that Mr. Morris has sustained a traumatic neurologic injury at the C5-C6 level.

Traumatic swelling of the spinal cord can compromise function at one or two levels above and below the level of the injury. This could be disastrous in Mr. Morris's case because breathing is controlled at the C4 level. Also, he's showing signs of spinal shock, including hypotension and bradycardia from the loss of sympathetic tone. Hypotension may lead to ischemia, which could further injure the spinal cord. However, because this is neurologic, not hypovolemic shock, beware of trying to raise his blood pressure by giving fluids. More volume probably won't help and could lead to pulmonary edema or worsen an associated head injury.

What must you do immediately?

After assessing Mr. Morris's airway, breathing, and circulation, place him on 2 L/minute of oxygen via nasal cannula, continuous pulse oximetry, and cardiac

➤ Encourage patients to keep firearms and ammunition locked away in a cabinet or safe.

➤ Advise patients to install handrails on all stairways, use safety gates at the top and bottom of stairways when young children are in the home, and use a step stool with handles or a grab bar to reach high or hard-to-reach objects to prevent falls around the home.

➤ Encourage patients to play sports safely. Tell them to always wear required protective gear, and avoid head-first moves (such as sliding head-first into a base).

monitoring. Check his vital signs every 15 minutes. Have intubation equipment ready.

Establish two I.V. lines. Replace fluids only as necessary to replace losses. As ordered, administer dopamine or another vasopressor to support Mr. Morris's blood pressure. Have atropine at the bedside in case he develops symptomatic bradycardia.

Because Mr. Morris's injury occurred less than 8 hours ago, prepare to administer methylprednisolone (30 mg/kg initial I.V. bolus over 15 minutes) to reduce edema. Wait 45 minutes, then start a continuous infusion of 5.4 mg/kg/hour that will run for 23 hours, as prescribed. (Depending on the patient's response, the methylprednisolone infusion may run for a total of 48 hours.) Insert an indwelling urinary catheter to prevent bladder distention from urine retention and to monitor intake and output.

Keep the patient immobilized and prepare him for a lateral cervical spine X-ray and a computed tomography (CT) scan of the cervical spine. Perform serial neurologic assessments frequently (at least every hour for the first 24 hours) so that you don't miss a significant change in his condition.

What should be done later?

Mr. Morris's condition remains unchanged. The CT scan results demonstrate an unstable C6 fracture and subluxation of bilateral facets at C5-C6. The neurosurgeon may attempt closed reduction or, more likely, perform surgery to repair the damage. Mr. Morris will be admitted to the intensive care unit where he'll be closely monitored for complications, such as deep vein thrombosis, pulmonary embolism, and pneumonia.

Mr. Morris may need a nasogastric tube with intermittent suction to prevent vomiting and aspiration and to monitor for GI bleeding (an adverse effect of methylprednisolone therapy). Administer anxiolytics, as needed. Arrange for referrals to social services and counseling to help him and his family deal with the life-changing effects of spinal cord injury.

Hedger, A. "Action Stat: Spinal Cord Injury," *Nursing* 32(12):96, December 2002. Used with permission.

➤ Tell patients not to dive into water where there may be rocks or the depth of the water is unknown.

Pathophysiology recap

➤ An SCI causes scarring and meningeal thickening, leaving nerves in the area of the injury blocked or tangled.

➤ Mechanisms involved with spinal cord trauma include:
  – hyperextension from acceleration-deceleration forces and sudden reduction in the anteroposterior diameter of the spinal cord

COMPLICATIONS

➤ *AUTONOMIC DYSREFLEXIA*

Also known as *autonomic hyperreflexia,* autonomic dysreflexia is a serious medical condition that occurs after the resolution of spinal shock. Dysreflexia is caused by noxious stimuli, most commonly a distended bladder or skin lesion.

Signs and symptoms
➤ Sudden, severe elevation in blood pressure

Above level of injury
➤ Cutaneous vasodilation
➤ Sweating
➤ Throbbing headache

Below level of injury
➤ Chills
➤ Pallor
➤ Piloerection
➤ Vasoconstriction

Treatment
Treatment focuses on eliminating the stimulus; rapid identification and removal may eliminate the need for pharmacologic control of headache and hypertension.

Nursing considerations
➤ Immediately elevate the head of the bed if autonomic dysreflexia is suspected, and monitor blood pressure and heart rate every 3 to 5 minutes.
➤ Determine and treat the underlying stimulus for the event, such as a blocked catheter, fecal impaction, or urinary tract infection.
➤ Administer antihypertensive agents, as ordered.

– hyperflexion from sudden and excessive force, propelling the neck forward or causing an exaggerated movement to one side
– vertical compression from force applied from the top of the cranium along the vertical axis through the vertebra
– rotational forces from twisting, which adds shearing force.
➤ Most serious SCIs result from motor vehicle accidents, falls, diving into shallow water, and gunshot wounds; less serious injuries result from lifting heavy objects and minor falls.

➤ *Status epilepticus*

Status epilepticus is a continuous or recurrent seizure state lasting at least 10 minutes; it occurs in all seizure types. The most life-threatening example is generalized tonic-clonic status epilepticus, a continuous generalized tonic clonic seizure. With status epilepticus, the patient doesn't return to full consciousness before another seizure occurs.

Rapid assessment
➤ Determine the patient's level of consciousness and neurologic status.
➤ Assess the rate, pattern, and depth of respirations.
➤ If possible, obtain the patient's history, including diagnosis of epilepsy. History may also reveal inconsistent use of anticonvulsant medications, alcohol abuse, recent head injury, infection, or headaches.
➤ The physical examination typically reveals ongoing seizure activity of either a partial or generalized type. (See *Types of seizures,* pages 176 and 177.)

Immediate actions
➤ Institute and maintain seizure and safety precautions.
➤ Provide supplemental oxygen and prepare the patient for endotracheal intubation and mechanical ventilation, if possible.
➤ Use an oral airway to maintain airway patency; however, don't force it into the patient's mouth because this may cause further injury when the jaw becomes rigid.
➤ Institute continuous cardiac monitoring to evaluate for arrhythmias.
➤ Obtain blood samples for serum electrolytes and arterial blood gas analysis.
➤ Monitor blood glucose levels for hypoglycemia (a possible cause or effect of the patient's continued seizures).
➤ Administer, as ordered, I.V. anticonvulsant agents (fast-acting first, following by long-acting agents), I.V. dextrose 50% in water if the patient is hypoglycemic, and I.V. magnesium if the patient has hypomagnesemia.

Follow-up actions
➤ Monitor the patient's vital signs every 2 to 5 minutes.
➤ Monitor the patient's neurologic status at least every 5 to 10 minutes until stable.
➤ Monitor the patient's response to anticonvulsant agents. Explain that anticonvulsants are tapered gradually to determine if seizure activity has abated. If seizures continue, prepare for general anesthesia with pentobarbital, propofol, or midazolam.
➤ Assist the patient in obtaining a medical alert bracelet if he doesn't have one.
➤ Teach the patient's family what to do when the patient has a seizure in order to keep him safe.
➤ Provide emotional support.
➤ If alcohol withdrawal is determined to be the underlying cause, administer I.V. thiamine to prevent Wernicke's encephalopathy.

➤ TYPES OF SEIZURES

The various types of seizures – partial, generalized, status epilepticus, and unclassified – have distinct signs and symptoms.

Partial seizures

Arising from a localized area of the brain, partial seizures cause focal symptoms. These seizures are classified by their effect on consciousness and whether they spread throughout the motor pathway, causing a generalized seizure.

➤ A simple partial seizure begins locally and generally doesn't cause an alteration in consciousness. It may present with sensory symptoms (lights flashing, smells, and auditory hallucinations), autonomic symptoms (sweating, flushing, and pupil dilation), and psychic symptoms (dream states, anger, and fear). The seizure lasts for a few seconds and occurs without preceding or provoking events. This type can be motor or sensory.

➤ A complex partial seizure alters consciousness. Amnesia for events that occur during and immediately after the seizure is a differentiating characteristic. During the seizure, the patient may follow simple commands. This seizure usually lasts for 1 to 3 minutes.

Generalized seizures

As the term suggests, generalized seizures cause a generalized electrical abnormality within the brain. They can be convulsive or nonconvulsive and include several types:

➤ Absence seizures occur most commonly in children, although they may affect adults. They usually begin with a brief change in the level of consciousness, indicated by blinking or rolling eyes, a blank stare, and slight mouth movements. The patient retains his posture and continues preseizure activity without difficulty. Typically, each seizure lasts from 1 to 10 seconds. If not properly treated, seizures can recur as often as 100 times per day. An absence seizure is a nonconvulsive seizure, but it may progress to a generalized tonic–clonic seizure.

Preventive steps

➤ Teach the patient with a seizure disorder about his medications and the need for compliance with the dosage and schedule. Caution the patient to monitor the amount of medication remaining so that he doesn't run out of it.

➤ Explain the importance of having anticonvulsant blood levels checked at regular intervals even if the seizures are under control.

➤ Teach the patient measures to help him control and decrease the occurrence of seizures. These may include taking medication on time, eating balanced meals to avoid hypoglycemia, avoiding trigger factors (flashing lights, loud noises or music, video games, television), limiting alcohol intake or eliminating it altogether, treating illnesses early, and decreasing stress.

➤ Myoclonic seizures are brief, involuntary muscular jerks of the body or extremities, commonly occurring in the early morning.

➤ Clonic seizures are characterized by bilateral rhythmic movements.

➤ Tonic seizures are characterized by a sudden stiffening of muscle tone, usually of the arms, but possibly including the legs.

➤ Generalized tonic-clonic seizures typically begin with a loud cry, precipitated by air rushing from the lungs through the vocal cords. The patient then loses consciousness and falls to the ground. The body stiffens (tonic phase) and then alternates between episodes of muscle spasm and relaxation (clonic phase). Tongue biting, incontinence, labored breathing, apnea, and subsequent cyanosis may occur. The seizure stops in 2 to 5 minutes, when abnormal electrical conduction ceases. When the patient regains consciousness, he's confused and may have difficulty talking. If he can talk, he may complain of drowsiness, fatigue, headache, muscle soreness, and arm or leg weakness. He may fall into a deep sleep after the seizure.

➤ Atonic seizures are characterized by a general loss of postural tone and a temporary loss of consciousness. They occur in young children and are sometimes called *drop attacks* because they cause the child to fall.

Status epilepticus

Status epilepticus is a continuous seizure state that can occur in all seizure types. The most life-threatening example is generalized tonic-clonic status epilepticus, a continuous generalized tonic-clonic seizure. Status epilepticus is accompanied by respiratory distress leading to hypoxia or anoxia. It can result from abrupt withdrawal of anticonvulsant medications, hypoxic encephalopathy, acute head trauma, metabolic encephalopathy, or septicemia secondary to encephalitis or meningitis.

Unclassified seizures

This category is reserved for seizures that don't fit the characteristics of partial or generalized seizures or status epilepticus. Included as unclassified are events that lack the data to make a more definitive diagnosis.

Pathophysiology recap

➤ Status epilepticus results when inhibitory neurons can't slow and stop the firing excitatory neurons that occur during seizure activity.

➤ The result is ongoing, repetitive seizures; without treatment, the resulting hypoxia and anoxia are fatal.

➤ Most commonly, status epilepticus results from noncompliance with anticonvulsant mediation therapy or decreased serum drug levels secondary to alcohol abuse or infection.

➤ Stroke

A stroke, also known as a *cerebrovascular accident*, is a sudden impairment of cerebral circulation in one or more of the blood vessels supplying

➤ ASSESSMENT FINDINGS IN STROKE

A stroke can leave one patient with mild hand weakness and another with complete unilateral paralysis. In both patients, the functional loss reflects damage to the brain area normally perfused by the occluded or ruptured artery. In general, assessment findings associated with a stroke may include:
➤ altered level of consciousness (LOC)
➤ anxiety
➤ headache
➤ numbness on one side
➤ speech difficulties
➤ unilateral limb weakness
➤ vertigo
➤ vision disturbances (diplopia, hemianopsia, and ptosis).
    Typical assessment findings based on the artery affected are highlighted in the chart below.

Affected artery	Assessment findings
Middle cerebral artery	➤ Aphasia ➤ Dysphasia ➤ Hemiparesis of affected side (more severe in face and arm than in leg) ➤ Visual field deficits
Carotid artery	➤ Altered LOC ➤ Aphasia ➤ Bruits ➤ Headaches ➤ Numbness ➤ Paralysis ➤ Ptosis ➤ Sensory changes ➤ Vision disturbances on affected side ➤ Weakness
Vertebrobasilary artery	➤ Amnesia ➤ Ataxia ➤ Diplopia ➤ Dysphagia ➤ Numbness around lips and mouth ➤ Nystagmus ➤ Poor coordination ➤ Slurred speech ➤ Visual field deficits ➤ Vertigo ➤ Weakness on affected side

➤ **ASSESSMENT FINDINGS IN STROKE** *(continued)*

Affected artery	Assessment findings
Anterior cerebral artery	➤ Confusion ➤ Impaired motor and sensory functions ➤ Incontinence ➤ Loss of coordination ➤ Numbness, especially in leg on affected side ➤ Personality changes ➤ Weakness
Posterior cerebral artery	➤ Coma ➤ Cortical blindness ➤ Dyslexia ➤ Perseveration (abnormally persistent replies to questions) ➤ Sensory impairment ➤ Visual field deficits (homonymous hemianopsia)

the brain. A stroke interrupts or diminishes oxygen supply and commonly causes serious damage or necrosis to brain tissues. The sooner circulation returns to normal after stroke, the better chances are for a complete recovery. However, about half of those who survive a stroke remain permanently disabled and experience a recurrence within weeks, months, or years.

Signs and symptoms of a stroke will vary among individuals, depending on the artery affected (and, consequently, the portion of the brain it supplies), the severity of damage, and the extent of collateral circulation that develops to help the brain compensate for decreased blood supply. (See *Assessment findings in stroke.*)

Rapid assessment
➤ Call your facility's stroke team, if available, which should be comprised of specially trained nurses who respond to potential stroke patients.
➤ Evaluate the patient and complete a neurologic assessment using an assessment tool such as the N.I.H. Stroke Scale. (See *Using the N.I.H. Stroke Scale,* pages 180 and 181.)
➤ Assess the patient using a stroke assessment tool such as the Cincinnati prehospital stroke scale (See *Cincinnati prehospital stroke scale,* page 182.)
➤ Observe the rate, pattern, and depth of respirations.
➤ Observe the patient's vital signs, noting hypertension, hypotension, tachycardia, or bradycardia.

➤ USING THE N.I.H. STROKE SCALE

Category	Description	Score	Baseline Date/time	Date/Time
1a. Level of consciousness (LOC)	Alert	0	2/15/05	
	Drowsy	1	1100	
	Stuporous	2	1	
	Coma	3		
1b. LOC questions (Month, age)	Answers both correctly	0		
	Answers one correctly	1	0	
	Incorrect	2		
1c. LOC commands (Open/close eyes, make fist, let go)	Obeys both correctly	0		
	Obeys one correctly	1	1	
	Incorrect	2		
2. Best gaze (Eyes open – patient follows examiner's finger or face)	Normal	0	0	
	Partial gaze palsy	1		
	Forced deviation	2		
3. Visual (Introduce visual stimulus/threat to patient's visual field quadrants)	No visual loss	0		
	Partial hemianopsia	1	1	
	Complete hemianopsia	2		
	Bilateral hemianopsia	3		
4. Facial palsy (Show teeth, raise eyebrows, and squeeze eyes shut)	Normal	0		
	Minor	1	2	
	Partial	2		
	Complete	3		
5a. Motor arm – left (Elevate extremity to 90 degrees and score drift/movement)	No drift	0		
	Drift	1		
	Can't resist gravity	2	4	
	No effort against gravity	3		
	No movement	4		
	Amputation, joint fusion (explain)	9		
5b. Motor arm – right (Elevate extremity to 90 degrees and score drift/movement)	No drift	0		
	Drift	1		
	Can't resist gravity	2	0	
	No effort against gravity	3		
	No movement	4		
	Amputation, joint fusion (explain)	9		
6a. Motor leg – left (Elevate extremity to 30 degrees and score drift/movement)	No drift	0		
	Drift	1		
	Can't resist gravity	2	4	
	No effort against gravity	3		
	No movement	4		
	Amputation, joint fusion (explain)	9		

> **USING THE N.I.H. STROKE SCALE** *(continued)*

Category	Description	Score	Baseline Date/time	Date/Time
6b. Motor leg – right (Elevate extremity to 30 degrees and score drift/movement)	No drift Drift Can't resist gravity No effort against gravity No movement Amputation, joint fusion (explain)	 0 1 2 3 4 9	 0	
7. Limb ataxia (Finger-nose, heel down shin)	Absent Present in one limb Present in two limbs	0 1 2		
8. Sensory (Pinprick to face, arm, trunk, and leg – compare side to side)	Normal Partial loss Severe loss	0 1 2	R L 0 2	R L
9. Best language (Name items; describe a picture and read sentences)	No aphasia Mild to moderate aphasia Severe aphasia Mute	0 1 2 3	 1	
10. Dysarthria (Evaluate speech clarity by patient repeating listed words)	Normal articulation Mild to moderate dysarthria Near to unintelligible or worse Intubated or other physical barrier	0 1 2 9	 1	
11. Extinction and inattention (Use information from previous testing to identify neglect or double simultaneous stimuli testing)	No neglect Partial neglect Complete neglect	0 1 2	 0	
		Total	17	

➤ Observe and assess for right-sided signs and symptoms that indicate a stroke in the left hemisphere and for left-sided signs and symptoms that indicate a stroke in the right hemisphere.

➤ Assess cranial nerve function, keeping in mind that a stroke that causes cranial nerve damage produces signs of cranial nerve dysfunction on the same side as the hemorrhage or infarct.

➤ Ask about and assess for a sudden onset of hemiparesis or hemiplegia or a gradual onset of dizziness, mental disturbances, or seizures.

➤ *CINCINNATI PREHOSPITAL STROKE SCALE*

If any one of the three signs described here is abnormal, the probability of a stroke is 72%.

Facial droop

Tell the patient to show his teeth or smile. If he hasn't had a stroke, both sides of his face will move equally. If he has had a stroke, one side of his face won't move as well as the other side.

NORMAL

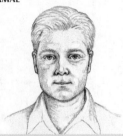

STROKE PATIENT WITH FACIAL DROOP ON RIGHT SIDE OF FACE

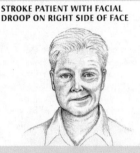

Arm drift

Tell the patient to close her eyes and hold both arms straight out in front of her for 20 seconds. If she hasn't had a stroke, her arms won't move or, if they do move, they'll move the same amount. Other findings, such as pronator grip, may be helpful.

If the patient has had a stroke, one arm won't move or one arm will drift down compared with the other arm.

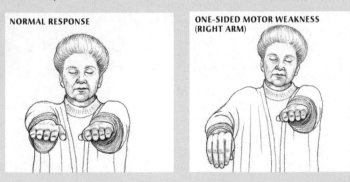

NORMAL RESPONSE

ONE-SIDED MOTOR WEAKNESS (RIGHT ARM)

Abnormal speech

Have the patient say, "You can't teach an old dog new tricks." If he hasn't had a stroke, he'll use correct words and his speech won't be slurred. If he has had a stroke, his words will be slurred, he may use the wrong words, or he may be unable to speak at all.

Adapted with permission from Kothan, R., et al. "Early Stroke Recognition: Developing an Out-of-Hospital NIH Stroke Scale," *Academy of Emergency Medicine* 4(10):986-90, October 1997.

➤ Ask about a loss of consciousness.
➤ Listen for aphasia or dysphasia and assess dysphagia.
➤ Assess the patient's motor function and deep tendon reflexes.

Immediate actions

➤ Initiate and maintain the patient on bed rest with the head of the bed at 30 degrees. Also institute seizure and safety precautions.
➤ Provide supplemental oxygen and prepare for endotracheal intubation and mechanical ventilation, if necessary.
➤ Initiate the algorithm for treating a suspected stroke. (See *Suspected stroke treatment algorithm,* pages 184 and 185.)
➤ Obtain a blood sample for prothrombin time (PT), International Normalized Ratio (INR), partial thromboplastin time (PTT), complete blood count, serum electrolytes, and arterial blood gas analysis.
➤ Assist the physician to insert an intracranial pressure monitoring device, if necessary.
➤ Prepare the patient for a computed tomography scan, magnetic resonance imaging, cerebral angiography, or digital subtraction angiography, as ordered.
➤ Administer, as ordered:
  – I.V. fluids — making sure to avoid overhydration, which may increase intracranial pressure (ICP)
  – thrombolytic therapy — making sure to institute bleeding precautions and assess the patient for signs and symptoms of bleeding every 15 to 30 minutes
  – fibrinolytic therapy — for the patient who has had an ischemic stroke, within 60 minutes of the patient's arrival in the emergency department (see *Indications for fibrinolytic therapy,* page 186)
  – anticoagulants, such as heparin — if the patient exhibits signs of stroke progression, unstable signs of stroke (such as a transient ischemic attack [TIA]), or evidence of embolic stroke
  – anticonvulsants — to prevent or treat seizures
  – stool softeners or mild laxatives — to prevent straining and increased ICP
  – steroids — to decrease inflammation
  – histamine-2 receptor blockers — to prevent GI damage from stress or steroids.

Follow-up actions

➤ Monitor the patient's vital signs, LOC, and neurologic status frequently, and report changes.
➤ Monitor PT, INR, PTT in patients taking anticoagulants or thrombolytics and anticonvulsants, if necessary.
➤ Apply antiembolism stockings or intermittent sequential compression devices.

(Text continues on page 186.)

➤ SUSPECTED STROKE TREATMENT ALGORITHM

This algorithm is used for suspected stroke. The patient's survival depends on prompt recognition of symptoms and treatment.

Detection, Dispatch, Delivery to Door

Immediate general assessment: first 10 minutes after arrival
➤ Assess airway, breathing, and circulation and vital signs.
➤ Provide oxygen by nasal cannula.
➤ Obtain I.V. access; obtain blood samples (complete blood count, electrolyte levels, coagulation studies).
➤ Check blood glucose levels; treat if indicated.
➤ Obtain 12-lead electrocardiogram; check for arrhythmias.
➤ Perform general neurologic screening assessment.
➤ Alert stroke team, neurologist, radiologist, computed tomography (CT) technician.

Immediate neurologic assessment: first 25 minutes after arrival
➤ Review patient history.
➤ Establish onset (< 3 hours required for fibrinolytics).
➤ Perform physical examination.
➤ Perform neurologic examination: Determine level of consciousness (Glasgow Coma Scale) and level of stroke severity (NIH Stroke Scale or Hunt and Hess Scale).
➤ Order urgent noncontrast CT scan (door-to-CT scan performed: goal < 25 minutes from arrival).
➤ Read CT scan (door-to-CT scan read: goal < 45 minutes from arrival).
➤ Perform lateral cervical spine X-ray (if patient is comatose or has a history of trauma).

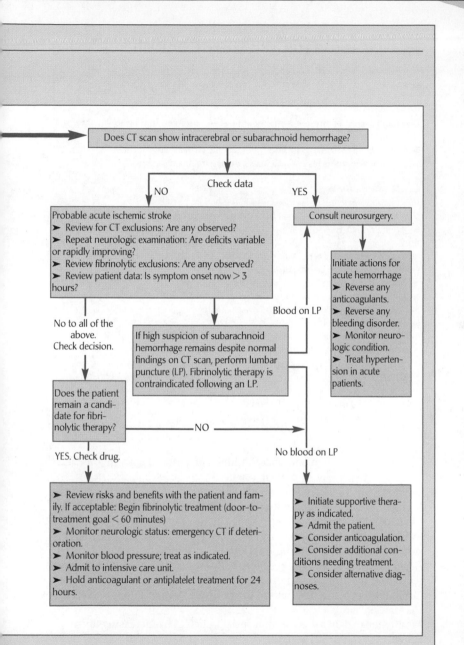

Does CT scan show intracerebral or subarachnoid hemorrhage?

Check data

NO   YES

Probable acute ischemic stroke
➤ Review for CT exclusions: Are any observed?
➤ Repeat neurologic examination: Are deficits variable or rapidly improving?
➤ Review fibrinolytic exclusions: Are any observed?
➤ Review patient data: Is symptom onset now > 3 hours?

Consult neurosurgery.

Initiate actions for acute hemorrhage
➤ Reverse any anticoagulants.
➤ Reverse any bleeding disorder.
➤ Monitor neurologic condition.
➤ Treat hypertension in acute patients.

No to all of the above.
Check decision.

Blood on LP

If high suspicion of subarachnoid hemorrhage remains despite normal findings on CT scan, perform lumbar puncture (LP). Fibrinolytic therapy is contraindicated following an LP.

Does the patient remain a candidate for fibrinolytic therapy?

NO

No blood on LP

YES. Check drug.

➤ Review risks and benefits with the patient and family. If acceptable: Begin fibrinolytic treatment (door-to-treatment goal < 60 minutes)
➤ Monitor neurologic status: emergency CT if deterioration.
➤ Monitor blood pressure; treat as indicated.
➤ Admit to intensive care unit.
➤ Hold anticoagulant or antiplatelet treatment for 24 hours.

➤ Initiate supportive therapy as indicated.
➤ Admit the patient.
➤ Consider anticoagulation.
➤ Consider additional conditions needing treatment.
➤ Consider alternative diagnoses.

➤ INDICATIONS FOR FIBRINOLYTIC THERAPY

Not every stroke patient is a candidate for fibrinolytic therapy. The following criteria are used to determine whether a patient should receive this treatment.

Indications

Criteria that must be present for a patient to be considered for fibrinolytic therapy include:
➤ acute ischemic stroke associated with significant neurologic deficit
➤ onset of symptoms less than 3 hours before treatment begins.

Contraindications

In addition to meeting the above criteria, the patient must *not:*
➤ show evidence of intracranial hemorrhage during pretreatment evaluation
➤ exhibit evidence of subarachnoid hemorrhage during pretreatment evaluation
➤ have a history of recent (within 3 months) intracranial or intraspinal surgery, serious head trauma, or previous stroke
➤ have a history of intracranial hemorrhage
➤ have uncontrolled hypertension at the time of treatment
➤ have experienced a seizure at the onset of stroke
➤ have active internal bleeding
➤ have an intracranial neoplasm, arteriovenous malformation, or aneurysm
➤ have a known bleeding condition involving, but not limited to:
  – current use of oral anticoagulants such as warfarin, International Normalized Ratio greater than 1.7, or prothrombin time greater than 15 seconds
  – received heparin within 48 hours before the onset of stroke and presence of elevated partial thromboplastin time
  – platelet count less than 100,000/μl.

➤ Turn the patient often and position him using careful body alignment.
➤ Take steps to prevent skin breakdown.
➤ Provide meticulous eye and mouth care.
➤ Maintain communication with the patient. If he's aphasic, set up a simple method of communicating.
➤ Obtain consultations with a physical therapist, an occupational therapist, and a nutritionist, as appropriate.
➤ Begin exercises as soon as possible. Perform passive range-of-motion exercises for the affected and unaffected sides.
➤ Teach and encourage the patient to use his unaffected side to exercise his affected side.
➤ Modify the patient's diet, as appropriate, such as by increasing fiber.
➤ Provide psychological support.
➤ Prepare the patient for surgery, as indicated.

> **UNDERSTANDING TRANSIENT ISCHEMIC ATTACKS**

Transient ischemic attacks (TIAs) are episodes of neurologic deficit resulting from cerebral ischemia. These recurrent attacks may last from seconds to hours and usually clear within 12 to 24 hours. TIAs are commonly considered a warning sign of stroke; more than half of patients who experience a TIA have a stroke within 2 to 5 years.

Preventive steps

➤ Stress the need to control diseases, such as diabetes or hypertension.
➤ Teach all patients (especially those at high risk) the importance of following a low-cholesterol, low-salt diet; watching their weight; increasing activity; avoiding smoking and prolonged bed rest; and minimizing stress.
➤ Teach at-risk patients how to recognize signs and symptoms of stroke or impending stroke (severe headache, drowsiness, confusion, and dizziness) because seeking prompt treatment is critical to his outcome and survival.
➤ Stress the importance of identifying and seeking treatment for a TIA, which is considered a warning sign of stroke. (See *Understanding transient ischemic attacks.*)

Pathophysiology recap

➤ Stroke results from obstruction of a blood vessel, typically in extracerebral vessels, but occasionally in intracerebral vessels.
➤ The major causes of stroke are thrombosis, embolism, and hemorrhage. (See *Types of stroke,* page 188.)
➤ Thrombosis causes ischemia in brain tissue supplied by the affected vessel as well as congestion and edema; the latter may produce more clinical effects than thrombosis itself, but these symptoms subside with the edema.
➤ Embolism is an occlusion of a blood vessel caused by a fragmented clot, a tumor, fat, bacteria, or air. When an embolus reaches the cerebral vasculature, it cuts off circulation by lodging in a narrow portion of an artery, most commonly the middle cerebral artery, causing necrosis and edema.
➤ Hemorrhage results from chronic hypertension or aneurysms, which cause sudden rupture of a cerebral artery, thereby diminishing the blood supply to the area served by the artery. In addition, blood accumulates deep within the brain, further compressing neural tissue and causing greater damage.

➤ TYPES OF STROKE

Strokes are typically classified as ischemic or hemorrhagic, depending on the underlying cause. This chart describes the major types of strokes.

Type of stroke	Description
Ischemic: Thrombotic	➤ Most common cause of stroke ➤ Frequently the result of atherosclerosis; also associated with hypertension, smoking, diabetes ➤ Thrombus in extracranial or intracranial vessel blocks blood flow to the cerebral cortex ➤ Carotid artery most commonly affected extracranial vessel ➤ Common intracranial sites include bifurcation of carotid arteries, distal intracranial portion of vertebral arteries, and proximal basilar arteries ➤ May occur during sleep or shortly after awakening, during surgery, or after a myocardial infarction
Ischemic: Embolic	➤ Second most common type of stroke ➤ Embolus from heart or extracranial arteries floats into cerebral bloodstream and lodges in middle cerebral artery or branches ➤ Embolus commonly originates during atrial fibrillation ➤ Typically occurs during activity ➤ Develops rapidly
Ischemic: Lacunar	➤ Subtype of thrombotic stroke ➤ Hypertension creates cavities deep in white matter of the brain, affecting the internal capsule, basal ganglia, thalamus, and pons ➤ Lipid-coated lining of the small penetrating arteries thickens and weakens wall, causing microaneurysms and dissections
Hemorrhagic	➤ Third most common type of stroke ➤ Typically caused by hypertension or rupture of aneurysm ➤ Diminished blood supply to area supplied by ruptured artery and compression by accumulated blood

➤ Subdural hematoma

Subdural hematoma is a collection of blood beneath the dura, the outer membrane that covers the brain. Acute subdural hematomas that occur from head trauma are among the most lethal head injuries.

Rapid assessment
➤ Observe the rate, depth, and pattern of spontaneous respirations.

 ALERT *Abnormal respirations and a change in level of consciousness (LOC) may indicate a breakdown in the brain's respiratory center and an impending tentorial herniation — a neurologic emergency.*

➤ Perform a neurologic assessment, noting the patient's LOC, aphasia, slurred speech, and seizure activity.
➤ Obtain the patient's vital signs, noting hypotension, tachycardia, bradypnea or tachypnea, and decreased oxygen saturation.
➤ Obtain the patient's history, including a report of recent injury or trauma to the head followed by loss of consciousness.
➤ Ask about a steady or fluctuating headache, weakness or loss of sensation, lethargy, and nausea and vomiting.
➤ Assess for irritability, anxiety, and behavioral changes, which indicate increased intracranial pressure (ICP).

Immediate actions
➤ Initiate and maintain the patient on bed rest with the head of the bed at 30 degrees. Also institute safety and seizure precautions.
➤ Provide supplemental oxygen and prepare for endotracheal intubation and mechanical ventilation, if necessary.
➤ Insert a intracranial pressure monitoring device, if necessary, and perform continuous monitoring.
➤ Calculate the cerebral perfusion pressure (CPP).
➤ Obtain serum samples for complete blood count, prothrombin time, partial thromboplastin time, International Normalized Ratio, serum electrolytes, and arterial blood gas analysis.
➤ Prepare the patient for a computed tomography scan or magnetic resonance imaging, as ordered, and arrange for neurosurgical consult.
➤ Administer, as ordered:
  – diuretics — to reduce cerebral edema
  – anticonvulsants — to control or prevent seizures
  – continuous infusion of agents, such as midazolam, fentanyl, morphine, or propofol — to help reduce metabolic demand and reduce the risk of increased ICP
  – stool softeners or mild laxatives — to prevent straining, which increases the risk of increased ICP
  – steroids — to reduce inflammation
  – blood products — to treat blood loss or clotting
  – antipyretics — to reduce elevated temperature.

Follow-up actions
➤ Check the patient's vital signs and neurologic status, including LOC and pupil size, every 15 minutes. Notify the physician of changes in the patient's condition.
➤ Carefully observe the patient for cerebrospinal fluid (CSF) leakage by checking the bed sheets for a blood-tinged spot surrounded by a lighter ring (halo sign).
➤ If the patient has CSF leakage or is unconscious, elevate the head of the bed 30 degrees.

➤ If you detect CSF leakage from the nose, place a gauze pad under the nostrils. If CSF leaks from the ear, position the patient so his ear drains naturally — don't pack the ear or nose.

➤ If the patient requires tracheal suctioning, suction him through the mouth, not the nose, to avoid introducing bacteria into the CSF.

➤ If the patient is unconscious, insert an orogastric tube to prevent aspiration.

➤ Monitor intake and output frequently to help maintain a normovolemic state.

➤ Clean and dress superficial scalp wounds using strict sterile technique. (If the skin has been broken, the patient may need tetanus prophylaxis.) Assist with suturing if needed. Carefully cover scalp wounds with a sterile dressing; control bleeding as necessary. Monitor wounds for signs and symptoms of infection.

➤ Prepare the patient for craniotomy, as indicated.

➤ Obtain a consultation with a physical therapist, an occupational therapist, or a nutritionist, if necessary.

➤ Perform passive range-of-motion exercises.

Preventive steps

➤ Although a subdural hematoma isn't preventable after a head injury has occurred, the patient can minimize his risk of head injury by wearing his seatbelt, a helmet when bicycling or motorcycle riding, and other protective equipment while playing sports or during work or recreational activities.

Pathophysiology recap

➤ The tiny blood vessels, called "bridging veins," beneath the dura can rupture with injury or trauma to the head, allowing blood to collect and form a hematoma.

➤ The pressure exerted on the brain from cerebral edema and the presence of the hematoma can rapidly damage the surrounding tissues.

6

Musculoskeletal emergencies

➤ Compartment syndrome

Compartment syndrome occurs when edema or bleeding increases pressure within a muscle compartment (a smaller section of a muscle) to the point of interfering with circulation. It occurs most commonly in the lower arm, hand, lower leg, or foot and is a limb-threatening condition that requires immediate intervention.

Rapid assessment
➤ Obtain the patient's vital signs, noting hypotension and tachycardia.
➤ Ask about intense, deep, throbbing pain out of proportion to the injury that doesn't improve with analgesia, and numbness and tingling distal to the involved muscle.
➤ Ask about a recent injury.
➤ Palpate peripheral pulses, noting absent pulses.
➤ Observe for pallor or mottling in the affected area.
➤ Assess for paralysis or decreased movement.
➤ Test the patient's muscle strength and sensation in the affected extremity, noting a decrease in either or both.

Immediate actions
➤ Remove dressings or constricting coverings or items such as a ring, watch, or cast from the affected area.
➤ Position the affected extremity at heart level.
➤ Monitor the affected extremity and perform neurovascular checks to detect signs and symptoms of impaired circulation.
➤ Prepare the patient for an intracompartmental pressure check and Doppler ultrasound of the affected extremity.
➤ Prepare the patient for emergency fasciotomy, as indicated.
➤ Insert an indwelling urinary catheter.
➤ Administer, as ordered:
  – analgesics — to minimize pain
  – sedatives — to minimize stress and anxiety, which can lead to vasoconstriction
  – blood products — to treat blood loss or to prevent bleeding
  – I.V. fluids — to enhance renal perfusion.

➤ WHAT HAPPENS IN COMPARTMENT SYNDROME

In compartment syndrome, muscle edema compresses nerves and blood vessels, impairing circulation to the affected extremity. This syndrome is characterized by pain that doesn't improve with analgesia or elevation of the extremity. The illustrations below show a cross-section of a normal calf and a cross-section of a calf affected by compartment syndrome.

The illustration on the right shows how a fasciotomy can relieve increased pressure in the extremity by allowing muscular tissue to expand outward. The procedure consists of making two long incisions of the fascia down the affected extremity. These wounds are typically closed in a second surgical procedure 2 to 3 days after the first.

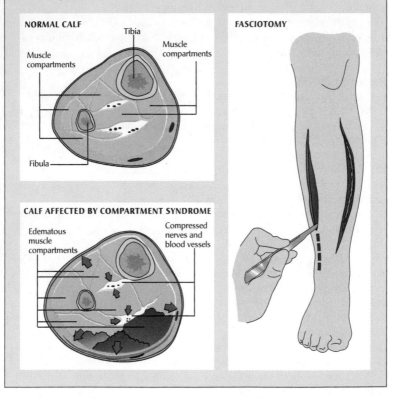

NORMAL CALF

Tibia

Muscle compartments

Muscle compartments

Fibula

FASCIOTOMY

CALF AFFECTED BY COMPARTMENT SYNDROME

Edematous muscle compartments

Compressed nerves and blood vessels

Follow-up actions
➤ Monitor the patient's vital signs frequently.
➤ Perform frequent neurovascular checks of the affected extremity, and report signs and symptoms of impaired circulation.
➤ Measure the circumference of the affected limb every 4 hours, and report any increase in size.

➤ Monitor intake and output, and report signs of decreased kidney function.

➤ Monitor hemoglobin, hematocrit, prothrombin time, International Normalized Ratio, and partial thromboplastin time every 4 hours until the patient is stable.

➤ Perform sterile dressing changes after fasciotomy and reinforce dressings frequently to facilitate monitoring of the extremity. (A large amount of bloody drainage should be expected.)

Preventive steps

➤ Although compartment syndrome can't be prevented, teach all patients in casts the signs and symptoms of the condition because prompt identification and treatment result in the best outcome.

Pathophysiology recap

➤ Compartment syndrome occurs when pressure within a muscle and its surrounding structures increases. If pressure becomes greater than the diastolic blood pressure, circulation can be impaired or interrupted completely. (See *What happens in compartment syndrome.*)

➤ Tissue damage occurs after 30 minutes because of impaired blood flow; after 4 hours, irreversible damage may occur. Permanent nerve damage may occur after 12 to 24 hours of compression.

➤ Compartment syndrome may result from application of a dressing or cast that's too tight, burns, a closed fracture, crushing injury, or muscle swelling after exercise.

➤ Dislocations and subluxations

Dislocations displace joint bones so that their articulating surfaces totally lose contact. (See *Common dislocation,* page 194.) Subluxations partially displace the articulating surfaces. Dislocations and subluxations occur at the joints of the shoulders, elbows, wrists, digits, hips, knees, ankles, and feet.

Rapid assessment

➤ Obtain the patient's history, noting recent incidence of trauma.

➤ Ask about pain. If present, also ask about its intensity and duration, as well as any measures that give relief.

➤ Palpate for peripheral pulses and observe for cyanosis and mottling in the affected extremity.

➤ Observe for deformity around the joint and alterations in the length of the involved extremity by comparing the left and the right side.

➤ Assess for impaired joint mobility, severe pain around the joint, and point tenderness.

➤ Observe for injuries.

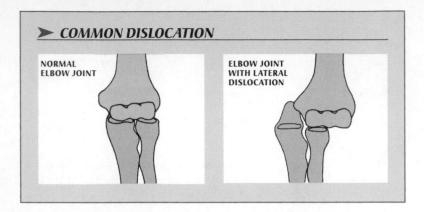

> **COMMON DISLOCATION**

NORMAL ELBOW JOINT

ELBOW JOINT WITH LATERAL DISLOCATION

Immediate actions
➤ Prepare the patient for X-rays to confirm or rule out a fracture.
➤ Until reduction immobilizes the dislocated joint, don't attempt manipulation. (See *Treatment of dislocation and subluxation*.)
➤ Apply ice to ease pain and edema.
➤ Splint and elevate the extremity "as it lies," even if the angle is awkward, unless there's loss of blood flow (no pulse, presence of pallor or cyanosis) distal to the injury.

 ALERT *Check for signs of vascular compromise, such as pallor, pain, loss of pulses, paralysis, and paresthesia. Emergency reduction is necessary if vascular compromise occurs.*

➤ Administer opioid analgesics or benzodiazepines I.V. to relieve pain.

 ALERT *Because a patient who receives opioid analgesics or benzodiazepines I.V. may develop respiratory depression or arrest, keep an airway and a bag-valve mask in the room. Monitor the patient's respirations and pulse rate closely. Also, have opioid and benzodiazepine reversal agents readily available.*

➤ Provide care to accompanying injuries.

Follow-up actions
➤ To avoid injury from a dressing that's too tight, instruct the patient to report numbness, pain, cyanosis, or coldness of the extremity below the cast or splint.
➤ To prevent skin damage, watch for signs of pressure injury (pressure, pain, or soreness) inside and outside the dressing.
➤ Instruct the patient to refrain from scratching his skin under the cast with sharp objects.
➤ Instruct the patient in the use of assistive devices, if necessary.
➤ After the cast or splint is removed, inform the patient that he may gradually return to normal joint activity.

> ### ➤ TREATMENT OF DISLOCATION AND SUBLUXATION
>
> Immediate reduction – before tissue edema and muscle spasm make reduction difficult – can prevent additional tissue damage and vascular impairment from dislocation and subluxation. Reduction may be open or closed. Closed reductions may be performed on the shoulder or knee joint; open reductions may be performed on the wrist and hip.
>
> In closed reduction, the patient is given general anesthesia (or local anesthesia and sedatives) and manual traction is performed. For open reduction procedures, which include wire fixation of the joint, skeletal traction, and ligament repair, the patient is given a regional block or general anesthesia.
>
> After reduction, a splint, a cast, or traction immobilizes the joint. In most cases, digits are immobilized for 2 weeks, hips for 6 to 8 weeks, and other dislocated joints for 3 to 6 weeks, to allow surrounding ligaments to heal. Analgesics can be used to relieve pain, and nonsteroidal anti-inflammatory drugs can be used to decrease inflammation. Physical and occupational therapy can teach the patient to perform activities while the joint is immobilized and after immobilization to prevent pain and a repeat of injury.

➤ For the patient being discharged after a dislocated hip, stress the need for follow-up visits to detect aseptic femoral head necrosis from vascular damage.

Preventive steps
➤ Encourage patients who engage in sports or other strenuous activities to wear protective devices over vulnerable joints, such as wrapped elastic bandages, tape wraps, and knee or shoulder pads, to prevent recurrence or a new injury.

Pathophysiology recap
➤ A dislocation or subluxation may be congenital (as in developmental dysplasia of the hip) or it may follow trauma or disease of surrounding joint tissues.
➤ Dislocation and subluxation injuries may accompany joint fractures or result in fracture fragments depositing between joint surfaces.
➤ Even in the absence of concomitant fractures, the displaced bone may damage surrounding muscles, ligaments, nerves, and blood vessels and may cause bone necrosis, especially if reduction is delayed.

➤ *Fracture of the hip and femur*

Fractures of the hip and femur may occur within the capsule of the femur (intracapsular), outside the capsule of the femur (extracapsular), within the trochanter (intertrochanteric), or below the trochanter (subtrochan-

IN ACTION

➤ *MANAGING HIP FRACTURE*

Agnes Hightower, 85, is brought to your emergency department after falling onto her right hip. She's alert and oriented and appears well nourished. She reports severe pain in her right hip and states that she can't move it.

What's the situation?
Ms. Hightower's right leg is externally rotated and appears shorter than the left leg. Her right posterior tibial and dorsalis pedis pulses are +2. Her right leg is cool to the touch and the range of motion is limited. Her left leg is normal.

An X-ray of the right hip reveals an intertrochanteric fracture (a fracture between the greater and lesser trochanter of the femur). No osteoporotic changes to the bone are seen on X-ray. The physician calls for an orthopedic consultation.

What's your assessment?
Ms. Hightower's fracture needs to be treated promptly to avoid tissue necrosis, blood loss, and infection. Pain management is also a priority.

What must you do immediately?
Start an I.V. line for fluids and keep Ms. Hightower on nothing-by-mouth status before surgery. Administer parenteral analgesics, as prescribed, and a muscle relaxant, if prescribed. Monitor her vital signs and level of consciousness (LOC) frequently, watching for respiratory depression and signs of shock, such as decreases in the LOC and urine output.

To stabilize the fracture, Ms. Hightower's right leg is placed in Buck's traction, which includes a foam boot. A weight attached to the boot pulls the bone fragments into alignment. Buck's traction prevents further traumatic injury and reduces muscle spasms.

However, traction puts a patient (especially an elderly one) at increased risk for complications of immobility, including skin breakdown, deep vein thrombosis (DVT), pulmonary embolism, and pneumonia. Assess Ms. Hightower's skin every 2

teric). These fractures typically result from a fall, trauma due to motor vehicle accident, or a sports-related trauma. (See *Managing hip fracture.*)

Rapid assessment
➤ Palpate peripheral pulses and observe for cyanosis and mottling of the affected extremity.
➤ Test distal movement and sensation in the affected extremity.
➤ Obtain the patient's history, which may include a report of a fall or other trauma to the area.
➤ Ask about pain in the affected hip and leg. If present, determine if it's exacerbated by movement.
➤ Observe for edema in the affected limb.
➤ Observe the affected leg, noting if it's shorter than the contralateral side and rotated outward.

hours. Place her on a pressure-reducing mattress and provide an overhead trapeze bar to help her with bed mobility. Monitor leg sensation and movement every 2 hours; the traction weights put pressure on her peroneal and tibial nerves.

Regularly assess her feet and legs for pain, temperature, pulses, capillary refill, color, and edema. Apply compression stockings to promote venous return and reduce the risk of DVT and pulmonary embolism. Obtain preoperative lab studies and prepare Ms. Hightower for surgery. Although she has fewer reserves than a younger patient, she has no preexisting medical conditions, so her prognosis for successful surgery and functional recovery is good.

Twenty-four hours after her fall, Ms. Hightower undergoes a successful open reduction and internal fixation of her right hip.

What should be done later?
After surgery, Ms. Hightower is transferred to the orthopedic unit where she'll be monitored for complications, such as hemorrhagic shock, neurovascular impairment, and fat embolism (a risk in the patient with long bone fractures). The physician orders low-molecular-weight heparin to prevent DVT and pulmonary embolism. Manage Ms. Hightower's pain, encourage early ambulation and good nutrition, and maintain her fluid balance.

Monitor the amount and character of drainage from the surgical site and her intake and output, assess her vital signs, and monitor the hemoglobin level and hematocrit. She'll have I.V. fluids and a patient-controlled analgesia pump.

Ms. Hightower will have a risk assessment for falls so that the cause of her fall (for example, overmedication) can be determined and she can be educated about fall prevention.

After 4 days in the hospital, she's transferred to a rehabilitation facility and eventually recovers completely.

Sprauve, D. "Action Stat: Hip Fracture," *Nursing* 33(11):88, November 2003. Used with permission.

➤ Assess for limited or abnormal range-of-motion (ROM).
➤ Observe for accompanying injuries.

Immediate actions
➤ Provide supplemental oxygen, if necessary.
➤ Initiate bed rest, keeping the hip extended to prevent further injury and maintain circulation.
➤ Obtain the patient's vital signs, noting hypotension and tachycardia.
➤ Insert an indwelling urinary catheter.
➤ Treat accompanying injuries.
➤ Obtain a computed tomography scan to pinpoint the abnormality and X-rays to reveal a break in the affected bone.
➤ Prepare the patient for Buck's or Russell's skin traction, if necessary.

➤ TOTAL HIP REPLACEMENT

To form a totally artificial hip, the surgeon cements a femoral head prosthesis in place to articulate with a cup, which he then cements into the deepened acetabulum. He may avoid using cement by implanting a prosthesis with a porous coating that promotes bony ingrowth. See illustration at right.

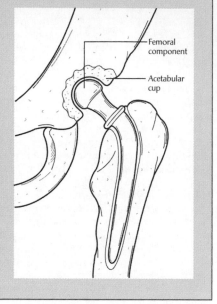

Femoral component

Acetabular cup

➤ Prepare the patient for surgical immobilization or joint replacement. (See *Total hip replacement.*)
➤ Administer, as ordered:
 − analgesics — to relieve pain
 − I.V. fluids — to maintain hydration
 − stool softeners or mild laxatives — to prevent constipation
 − subcutaneous heparin (if the patient isn't undergoing surgery) — to prevent deep vein thrombosis.

Follow-up actions
➤ Monitor the patient's vital signs and the neurovascular status of the affected extremity frequently.
➤ Maintain an abductor splint or trochanter roll between the patient's legs to prevent loss of alignment.
➤ Encourage the patient to perform isometric exercises such as tensing and relaxing the leg muscles.
➤ Arrange for physical therapy to teach the patient non-weight-bearing transfers and to work with changes in weight-bearing status.
➤ Provide skin care and logroll the patient every 2 hours to maintain skin integrity and prevent pressure ulcers. (See *Preventing complications of hip fracture in elderly patients.*)

➤ PREVENTING COMPLICATIONS OF HIP FRACTURE IN ELDERLY PATIENTS

Many elderly people who experience hip fractures never regain their prefracture ambulatory status. Immobility complications are more common in this population due to slowed healing that accompanies aging; these complications can delay rehabilitation, thereby adding to the risk of permanent disability. Preventing complications in elderly patients is a key element of care.

Potential complications
Extended immobility due to slower healing puts the elderly patient at risk for complications, including:
➤ pneumonia
➤ pressure ulcers
➤ venous thrombosis
➤ voiding dysfunction.

Nursing interventions
Use the following interventions to prevent complications in the elderly patient with a hip fracture.
➤ Keep the patient's skin clean and dry.
➤ Turn the patient regularly, and consider using an alternating pressure mattress to prevent skin breakdown.
➤ Provide good nutrition to promote healing and increase resistance to infection. Encourage the patient to eat as much of each meal as possible, and offer high-protein, high-calorie snacks between meals.
➤ As soon as the physician permits, help the patient ambulate. Reassure him that the repaired hip is safe to use. Plan progress in small steps: At the first session, have him walk to a nearby chair, as prescribed. Gradually increase the distance by having him walk in the hallway. The patient's early involvement in physical therapy is vital to successful recovery.

➤ Assist the patient with coughing, deep breathing, and incentive spirometry to maintain his respiratory function and prevent pulmonary infection.
➤ Promote independence in activities of daily living.
➤ Provide active and passive ROM exercises for unaffected limbs to maintain joint mobility.
➤ Provide a trapeze to promote independence in self-care.
➤ Maintain traction at all times to ensure proper body alignment and promote healing.
➤ If the patient is in traction, keep him in a flat position with the foot of the bed raised 25 degrees.
➤ Encourage the patient to increase his intake of fiber and fluids and increase his activity, as allowed, to prevent constipation.
➤ Apply antiembolism stockings to promote venous circulation.
➤ Provide care to accompanying injuries.

Preventive steps

➤ Identify patients at risk for osteoporosis and advise them to obtain bone mineral density testing and to begin treatment to restore bone density and prevent fractures.
➤ Encourage patients to maintain skeletal strength by engaging in regular physical exercise; adopting a diet with sufficient sources of calcium, protein, and vitamin D; and abstaining from alcohol and smoking.

Pathophysiology recap

➤ A fracture occurs when too much stress is placed on the bone. As a result, the bone breaks and local tissue is injured, causing muscle spasm, edema, hemorrhage, compressed nerves, and ecchymosis.
➤ Causes of hip and femur fractures may include aging, bone tumors, Cushing's syndrome, immobility, malnutrition, multiple myeloma, osteomyelitis, osteoporosis, steroid therapy, and trauma.

➤ *Fracture of the long bones*

Arm and leg fractures, or long bone fractures, usually result from trauma; these injuries typically cause substantial muscle, nerve, and other soft-tissue damage.

Rapid assessment

➤ Palpate for bilateral pulses distal to the injury, noting decreased or absent pulses.
➤ Observe for cyanosis and mottling of the affected limb, and palpate the skin, noting cool areas.
➤ Obtain the patient's vital signs, noting hypotension and tachycardia.
➤ Obtain the patient's history, including incidence of traumatic injury.
➤ Gently palpate and assess for such signs as deformity, swelling, and crepitus in the affected area.
➤ Ask about pain and point tenderness.
➤ Test movement and sensation of the affected extremity.
➤ Ask about a tingling feeling distal to the injury.
➤ Assess for obvious skin wounds or accompanying injuries.

Immediate actions

➤ In severe fractures that cause blood loss, apply direct pressure to control bleeding, and administer fluid replacement as soon as possible to prevent or treat hypovolemic shock.

 ALERT *Watch for signs of shock in the patient with a severe open fracture of a large bone such as the femur.*

➤ Splint the limb above and below the suspected fracture, apply a cold pack, and elevate the limb to reduce edema and pain.

➤ CLASSIFYING FRACTURES

One of the best-known systems for classifying fractures uses a combination of terms – such as simple, nondisplaced, and oblique – to describe fractures. An explanation of these terms appears here.

General classification of fractures
➤ *Simple (closed)* – Bone fragments don't penetrate the skin.
➤ *Compound (open)* – Bone fragments penetrate the skin.
➤ *Incomplete (partial)* – Bone continuity isn't completely interrupted.
➤ *Complete* – Bone continuity is completely interrupted.
 Below you'll find definitions of the terms used to describe fractures according to fragment positions and fracture lines.

Classification by fragment position
➤ *Comminuted* – The bone breaks into small pieces.
➤ *Impacted* – One bone fragment is forced into another.
➤ *Angulated* – Fragments lie at an angle to each other.
➤ *Displaced* – Fracture fragments separate and are deformed.
➤ *Nondisplaced* – The two sections of bone maintain essentially normal alignment.
➤ *Overriding* – Fragments overlap, shortening the total bone length.
➤ *Segmental* – Fractures occur in two adjacent areas with an isolated central segment.
➤ *Avulsed* – Fragments are pulled from normal position by muscle contractions or ligament resistance.

Classification by fracture line
➤ *Linear* – The fracture line runs parallel to the bone's axis.
➤ *Longitudinal* – The fracture line extends in a longitudinal (but not parallel) direction along the bone's axis.
➤ *Oblique* – The fracture line crosses the bone at roughly a 45-degree angle to the bone's axis.
➤ *Spiral* – The fracture line crosses the bone at an oblique angle, creating a spiral pattern.
➤ *Transverse* – The fracture line forms a right angle with the bone's axis.

➤ Obtain anteroposterior and lateral X-rays of the suspected fracture as well as X-rays of the joints above and below it to confirm the diagnosis. (See *Classifying fractures*.)
➤ Assist with reduction (restoring displaced bone segments to their normal position) and immobilization by the application of a splint or cast or with traction.
➤ Prepare the patient with an open fracture for thorough wound debridement.
➤ Prepare the patient for surgery (for reduction or internal fixation) to repair soft-tissue damage, if indicated.

➤ Offer reassurance to the patient, who's likely to be frightened and in pain.
➤ Administer, as ordered:
  – I.V. fluids — to increase intravascular volume
  – analgesics — to reduce pain
  – tetanus prophylaxis — to prevent tetanus with open fractures
  – antibiotics — to treat or prevent infection, especially with open fractures
  – stool softeners or mild laxatives — to prevent constipation.

Follow-up actions
After reduction:
➤ Monitor the patient's neurovascular status every 2 to 4 hours for 24 hours, then every 4 to 8 hours, as indicated.
➤ Assess color, motion, sensation, digital movement, edema, capillary refill, and pulses of the affected area.
➤ Compare findings with the unaffected side.
  If the fracture requires long-term immobilization with traction:
➤ Reposition the patient often to increase comfort and prevent pressure ulcers.
➤ Assist with active range-of-motion exercises to prevent muscle atrophy.
➤ Encourage deep breathing and coughing to prevent pneumonia.
➤ Encourage adequate fluid intake to prevent urinary stasis and constipation, and watch for signs of renal calculi (flank pain, nausea, and vomiting).
  For the patient with a cast:
➤ Provide good cast care.
➤ Support the cast with pillows.
➤ Observe for skin irritation near cast edges
➤ Check for foul odors or discharge.
➤ Tell the patient to report signs of impaired circulation (skin coldness, numbness, tingling, or discoloration) immediately.
➤ Warn the patient not to get the cast wet and not to insert foreign objects under the cast.
➤ Encourage the patient to resume ambulation as soon as he can, and provide assistance, if needed. (Remember, a patient who has been bedridden for some time may be dizzy at first.)
➤ Demonstrate the correct use of assistive devices, if necessary.
➤ After cast removal, refer the patient to a physical therapist to restore limb mobility.

Preventive steps
➤ Encourage the patient to maintain maximum bone density by adopting a diet containing adequate sources of calcium, protein, and vitamin D and by engaging in regular physical activity.
➤ Advise the patient to wear required protective gear when playing sports.

COMPLICATIONS

➤ *FAT EMBOLISM*

Although it's typically a complication of long bone fracture, fat embolism may also follow severe soft-tissue bruising and fatty liver injury. Posttraumatic embolization may occur as bone marrow releases fat into the veins. The fat can lodge in the lungs, obstructing the pulmonary vascular bed, or pass into the arteries, eventually disturbing the respiratory and circulatory systems. It typically occurs 12 to 48 hours after an injury.

Signs and symptoms
➤ Altered level of consciousness
➤ Anxiety
➤ Blood-tinged sputum
➤ Coma
➤ Cyanosis
➤ Fever
➤ Petechial rash over the anterior chest, neck, shoulders, and axillae and buccal membranes
➤ Restlessness
➤ Seizures
➤ Tachycardia

Treatment
Treatment measures may include corticosteroids to reduce inflammation, heparin to prevent thrombosis, and oxygen to correct hypoxemia. Expect to immobilize fractures early. As ordered, assist with endotracheal intubation and ventilation.

Nursing considerations
➤ Monitor the patient's vital signs, hemodynamic status, and oxygen saturation.
➤ Assess heart and breath sounds.
➤ Administer prescribed medications and oxygen.
➤ Promote rest and relaxation.
➤ Provide emotional support.
➤ Assess the patient's level of consciousness.
➤ Prepare the patient for diagnostic testing, which may include arterial blood gas analysis, computed tomography, and chest X-ray.
➤ Maintain immobilization and proper alignment of the fractured limb.

Pathophysiology recap
➤ Most arm and leg fractures result from major traumatic injury, such as a fall on an outstretched arm, a skiing accident, or child abuse (suggested by multiple or repeated episodes of fractures).
➤ In a person with a pathologic bone-weakening condition, such as osteoporosis, bone tumors, or metabolic disease, a mere cough or sneeze can produce a fracture.

➤ Prolonged standing, walking, or running can cause stress fractures of the foot and ankle.
➤ Brittle bones make an older person especially prone to fractures. Falling on an outstretched arm or hand or suffering a direct blow to the arm or shoulder is likely to fracture the radius or humerus.
➤ Children's bones usually heal rapidly and without deformity.
➤ Bones of adults in poor health and with impaired circulation may never heal properly.
➤ Severe open fractures, especially of the femoral shaft, may cause substantial blood loss and life-threatening hypovolemic shock and fat embolism. (See *Fat embolism,* page 203.)

➤ Fracture of the pelvis

A pelvic fracture involves a disruption of the bony ring that makes up the pelvis. Because significant force is required to disrupt this structure, organs located in the pelvis are frequently injured as well.

Rapid assessment
➤ Observe the rate, depth, and pattern of respirations.
➤ Palpate pulses, and observe for cyanosis and mottling distal to the injury.
➤ Assess movement and sensation distal to the injury.
➤ Obtain the patient's vital signs, noting hypotension and tachycardia.
➤ Obtain the patient's history, including incidence of blunt trauma to the pelvic region.
➤ Ask about tenderness over the pelvis and pain while moving the hip.
➤ Assess for instability in the hip on adduction.
➤ Assess for damage to the organs within the pelvis (such as the urethra, vagina, and rectum), such as hematuria or blood at the urethral meatus, rectal bleeding, or vaginal bleeding.

Immediate actions
➤ Provide supplemental oxygen, if indicated.
➤ Splint the suspected pelvic injury by tying the patient's legs together with his trousers or a pneumatic antishock garment (which can control bleeding), with a pillow between them.
➤ Try not to move the patient.
➤ Insert an indwelling urinary catheter, if indicated.

 ALERT *Don't insert an indwelling urinary catheter in a patient with suspected urethral damage.*

➤ Prepare the patient for anteroposterior X-rays and a computed tomography scan of the pelvis.

➤ Assist with diagnostic studies to determine the extent of the patient's internal injurioo.
➤ Prepare the patient for emergency fixation of the pelvis.
➤ Administer, as ordered:
  – I.V. fluids — to increase intravascular volume
  – blood products — to replace blood loss or help stop bleeding
  – analgesics — to control pain
  – antibiotics — to treat or prevent infection
  – subcutaneous heparin or Lovenox — to prevent deep-vein thrombosis, if appropriate
  – stool softeners or mild laxatives — to prevent constipation.

Follow-up actions
➤ Monitor neurovascular checks distal to the injury (bilateral lower extremities) frequently.
➤ Monitor the patient's vital signs frequently.
➤ Apply antiembolism stockings.
➤ Assist the patient in performing activities of daily living, as needed.
➤ Obtain consultations from a physical therapist and an occupational therapist.
➤ Provide comfort measures.
➤ Provide emotional support to the patient and his family to facilitate the patient's recovery.

Preventive steps
➤ Advise all patients to wear seat belts and other protective gear.
➤ Encourage all patients to purchase vehicles with airbags, which can also prevent this type of injury.

Pathophysiology recap
➤ The significant force required to fracture the pelvis usually results from motor vehicle accidents, motorcycle accidents, pedestrian-versus-car accidents, falls, and crush injuries in adults; and pedestrian-versus-car accidents and motor vehicle accidents in children.
➤ The organs contained within the pelvis are frequently injured at the same time.
➤ Because the pelvis contains a venous plexus as well as major arteries, significant bleeding may occur.

➤ Herniated disk

Also called a *ruptured* or *slipped disk* and *herniated nucleus pulposus,* a herniated disk occurs when all or part of the nucleus pulposus—the soft, gelatinous, central portion of an intervertebral disk—is forced through the disk's weakened or torn outer ring (anulus fibrosus). The extruded disk may impinge on spinal nerve roots as they exit from the spinal canal or on the spinal cord itself, resulting in back pain and other signs of nerve root irritation.

Rapid assessment

➤ Assess the neurovascular status of the bilateral lower extremities.

 ALERT *During conservative treatment, watch for deterioration in the patient's neurologic status (especially during the first 24 hours after admission), which may indicate an urgent need for surgery.*

➤ Ask about severe lower back pain that radiates to the buttocks, legs, and feet (usually unilaterally), which may have a sudden onset that subsides in a few days and recurs at shorter intervals with progressive intensity.

➤ Ask about sciatic pain that begins as a dull pain in the buttocks.

➤ Ask if Valsalva's maneuver, coughing, sneezing, or bending intensifies the pain, because these actions cause muscle spasms.

➤ Observe the patient's gait.

➤ Assess for sensory and motor loss in the area innervated by the compressed spinal nerve root and, in later stages, weakness and atrophy of leg muscles.

➤ Perform the straight-leg–raising test: Have the patient assume a supine position. Place one hand on the patient's ilium (to stabilize the pelvis) and the other hand under the ankle; slowly raise the patient's leg. The test is positive only if the patient complains of posterior leg (sciatic) pain rather than back pain.

➤ Perform the Lasègue test: Have the patient lie flat while the thigh and knee are flexed to a 90-degree angle. Resistance and pain as well as loss of ankle or knee-jerk reflex indicate spinal root compression.

➤ Ask about allergies to iodides, iodine-containing substances, or seafood in case the patient may need a diagnostic test that requires dye.

Immediate actions

➤ Initiate bed rest, if necessary.

➤ Prepare the patient for magnetic resonance imaging, computed tomography scans, or myelography, as ordered.

➤ Prepare the patient for surgery, such as microdiskectomy, laminectomy, chemonucleolysis, if necessary.

➤ Apply antiembolism stockings, as prescribed.

➤ Assist with a regimen of leg- and back-strengthening exercises.

➤ Instruct the patient in the use of assistive devices, if necessary.

➤ Encourage the patient to move his legs, as allowed.

➤ Provide high-topped sneakers to prevent footdrop.

➤ Instruct the patient to cough, deep breathe, and use an incentive spirometer to prevent pulmonary complications.

➤ Assess bowel function.

➤ Provide a fracture bedpan for the patient on complete bed rest.

➤ Encourage adequate fluid intake to prevent renal stasis.

➤ Provide good skin care.

➤ Administer, as ordered:
 – analgesics   to treat pain
 – steroids — to decrease inflammation
 – I.V. fluids — to prevent renal stasis and enhance the excretion of dye after computed tomography or myelography
 – stool softeners or mild laxatives — to prevent constipation
 – muscle relaxers — to prevent and treat muscle spasms.

Follow-up actions
➤ Assess the patient's vital signs and the neurovascular status of the legs frequently.
➤ Use the logrolling technique to turn the patient.
➤ Administer analgesics, as ordered, especially 30 minutes before initial attempts at sitting or walking.
➤ Give the patient assistance during his first attempt to walk.
➤ Provide the patient with a straight-backed chair for limited sitting.
➤ Monitor for bowel sounds and abdominal distention.
➤ Warn the patient taking muscle relaxants to avoid activities that require alertness until he has developed a tolerance to the drug's sedative effects.
➤ Provide emotional support and encouragement.
➤ If the patient requires chemonucleolysis, make sure that he isn't allergic to meat tenderizers (chymopapain is a similar substance).

 ALERT *An allergy to meat tenderizers contraindicates the use of the enzyme chymopapain, which can produce severe anaphylaxis in a sensitive patient.*

After chemonucleolysis:
➤ Enforce bed rest.
➤ Administer analgesics.
➤ Apply heat.
➤ Urge the patient to cough and deep breathe.
➤ Assist with special exercises, and instruct the patient to continue these exercises after discharge.
   After surgery:
➤ Enforce bed rest.
➤ If a blood drainage system (Hemovac or Jackson Pratt drain) is in use, check the tubing frequently for kinks and a secure vacuum, and empty it at the end of each shift, recording the amount and color of drainage.
➤ Report colorless moisture on dressings (possible cerebrospinal fluid leakage) or excessive drainage immediately.
➤ Instruct the patient on how to wear a brace.
➤ Assist with straight-leg raising and toe-pointing exercises.
   Before discharge:
➤ Teach proper body mechanics —bending at the knees and hips (never at the waist), standing straight, and carrying objects close to the body.
➤ Advise the patient to lie down when tired.

> ## WHAT HAPPENS WHEN A DISK HERNIATES?

The spinal column is made of vertebrae that are separated by cartilage called *disks*. Within each disk is a soft, gelatinous center that acts as a cushion during vertebral movement. When severe trauma, strain, or intervertebral joint degeneration occur, the outer fibrous ring can weaken or tear, the pulpy nucleus can be forced through, and the extruded disk can impinge on the spinal nerve root or the spinal column itself.

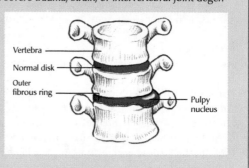

Vertebra
Normal disk
Outer fibrous ring
Pulpy nucleus

> Instruct the patient to sleep on his side (never on his abdomen) on an extra-firm mattress or a bed board.
> Urge maintenance of proper weight to prevent lordosis caused by obesity.

Preventive steps

> Encourage the patient to maintain an appropriate body weight, and discuss proper nutrition.
> Reinforce proper body mechanics.

Pathophysiology recap

> The ligament and posterior capsule of the disk are usually torn, allowing the nucleus pulposus to extrude, compressing the nerve root.
> Occasionally, the injury tears the entire disk loose, causing protrusion onto the nerve root or compression of the spinal cord.
> Large amounts of extruded nucleus pulposus or complete disk herniation of the capsule and nucleus pulposus may compress the spinal cord. (See *What happens when a disk herniates?*)
> Herniated disks may result from severe trauma or strain or may be related to intervertebral joint degeneration.

> Osteomyelitis, acute

Acute osteomyelitis is a pyogenic bone infection that commonly results from a combination of local trauma—usually trivial but resulting in hematoma formation—and an acute infection originating elsewhere in the body. Although acute osteomyelitis typically remains localized, it can spread through the bone to the marrow, cortex, and periosteum. Acute osteomyelitis is usually a blood-borne disease and typically affects rapidly growing children. (Chronic osteomyelitis is rare and is characterized by multiple draining sinus tracts and metastatic lesions.)

Rapid assessment

➤ Obtain the patient's vital signs, noting tachycardia and fever.
➤ Ask about pain or tenderness.
➤ Palpate for heat and swelling in the affected area.
➤ Test for restricted movement of the affected area.
➤ Observe for erythema in the affected area.

Immediate actions

➤ Begin treatment immediately—don't wait for the diagnosis to be confirmed.
➤ Obtain a serum sample for blood cultures to identify the causative organism and a complete blood count.
➤ Prepare the patient for a bone scan (indicates infected bone) and a bone lesion biopsy or culture (may reveal causative organism).
➤ Assist with immobilization of the affected bone by plaster cast, traction, or bed rest.
➤ Prepare the patient with an abscess for incision and drainage (submit a sample of the drained fluid for culture).
➤ Administer, as ordered:
 – antibiotics — to treat the infection, after blood cultures are drawn
 – analgesics — to relieve pain
 – I.V. fluids — to increase intravascular volume.

Follow-up actions

➤ Monitor the patient's vital signs and for signs and symptoms of infection frequently.
➤ Use strict sterile technique when changing dressings and irrigating wounds.
➤ Support the affected limb with firm pillows, keeping the limb level with the body; don't let it sag.
➤ Carefully monitor suctioning equipment and document the amount of solution instilled and suctioned.
➤ Provide good skin care.
➤ Turn the patient gently every 2 hours and watch for signs of developing pressure ulcers.
➤ Provide a diet high in protein and vitamin C.
➤ Report sudden pain, crepitus, or deformity immediately.
➤ Watch for a sudden malposition of the limb, which may indicate fracture.
➤ Provide wound and cast care: Support the cast with firm pillows and smooth rough cast edges by petaling with pieces of adhesive tape or moleskin. Check circulation and drainage; if a wet spot appears on the cast, circle it with a marking pen and note the time of appearance (on

the cast). Be aware of how much drainage is expected. Check the circled spot at least every 4 hours. Report an enlargement immediately.
➤ If the patient is in skeletal traction for compound fractures, cover insertion points of pin tracks with small, dry dressings, and tell him not to touch the skin around the pins and wires.
➤ Assess the patient's vital signs, the wound's appearance, and new pain every day; these may indicate secondary infection.
➤ Provide emotional support and appropriate diversions.
➤ Before discharge, teach the patient how to protect and clean the wound and, most importantly, how to recognize signs of recurring infection (increased temperature, redness, localized heat, and swelling).
➤ Stress the need for follow-up examinations.

Preventive steps
➤ Encourage patients at risk for osteomyelitis to seek prompt treatment for primary bacterial infections to prevent bacterial seeding of the bone from the infected blood.

Pathophysiology recap
➤ Virtually any pathogenic bacteria can cause osteomyelitis under the right circumstances. The most common pyogenic organism in osteomyelitis is *Staphylococcus aureus.*
➤ Typically, the offending organism finds a culture site in a hematoma from recent trauma or in a weakened area, such as the site of local infection (for example, furunculosis), and spreads directly to bone.
➤ As the organisms grow and form pus within the bone, tension builds within the rigid medullary cavity, forcing pus through the haversian canals. This forms a subperiosteal abscess that deprives the bone of its blood supply and may eventually cause necrosis.
➤ In turn, necrosis stimulates the periosteum to create new bone (involucrum); the old bone (sequestrum) detaches and works its way out through an abscess or the sinuses. By the time sequestrum forms, osteomyelitis is chronic.

➤ Septic arthritis

Septic, or infectious, arthritis occurs when bacterial invasion of a joint causes inflammation of the synovial lining, effusion and pyogenesis, and destruction of bone and cartilage. Septic arthritis can lead to ankylosis and fatal septicemia. However, prompt antibiotic therapy and joint aspiration or drainage cures most patients.

Rapid assessment
➤ Obtain the patient's vital signs, noting hypotension, tachycardia, and increased temperature.
➤ Ask about intense pain.

➤ Observe for inflammation, swelling of the affected joint, and erythoma.

Immediate actions
➤ Initiate and maintain isolation precautions as determined by the facility.
➤ Immobilize the affected joint with a splint or traction as ordered until the patient can tolerate movement.
➤ Prepare the patient for needle aspiration (arthrocentesis), reminding him that it will be extremely painful.
➤ Obtain a Gram stain or culture of synovial fluid, a biopsy of the synovial membrane, or two sets of positive cultures and Gram stain smears of skin exudates, sputum, urethral discharge, stools, urine, or nasopharyngeal discharge.
➤ Instruct the patient that arthrocentesis is performed daily under sterile conditions to remove grossly purulent joint fluid until fluid appears normal.
➤ Carefully evaluate the patient's condition after joint aspiration.
➤ Obtain a serum sample for complete blood count and serum electrolytes.
➤ Provide emotional support throughout the diagnostic tests and procedures.
➤ Administer, as ordered:
 – analgesics (opioid, non-opioid) — to treat pain
 – antipyretics — to reduce fever
 – corticosteroids — to reduce inflammation, keeping in mind that they may mask signs of infection
 – antibiotics — to treat the infection, after synovial cultures have been sent to the laboratory
 – I.V. fluids — to increase intravascular volume.

 ALERT _Don't administer aspirin to treat pain because it causes a misleading reduction in swelling, hindering accurate monitoring of progress._

Follow-up actions
➤ Monitor the patient's vital signs frequently.
➤ Keep the joint in proper alignment but avoid prolonged immobilization.
➤ Start passive range-of-motion exercises immediately, and progress to active exercises as soon as the patient can move the affected joint and put weight on it.
➤ Medicate for pain before exercise; keep in mind that the pain of septic arthritis is easy to underestimate.
➤ Apply heat or ice packs to reduce pain.
➤ Assist with frequent joint fluid cultures, synovial fluid leukocyte counts, and glucose determinators.
➤ Assist with open surgical drainage (usually arthrotomy with lavage of the joint, if indicated.

Preventive steps
➤ Practice strict sterile technique with all procedures.
➤ Prevent contact between immunosuppressed patients and infected patients.

Pathophysiology recap
➤ In most cases of septic arthritis, bacteria spread from a primary site of infection—usually in adjacent bone or soft tissue—through the bloodstream to the joint.
➤ Various factors can predispose a person to septic arthritis: concurrent bacterial infection, chronic illness (malignancy, renal failure, rheumatoid arthritis, systemic lupus erythematosus, diabetes, or cirrhosis), diseases that depress the immune system, immunosuppressive therapy, I.V. drug abuse, recent articular trauma, joint surgery, intra-articular injections, and local joint abnormalities.

➤ Sprains

A sprain is a complete or incomplete tear in the supporting ligaments surrounding a joint that usually follows a sharp twist. A sprained ankle is the most common joint injury, followed by sprains of the wrist, elbow, and knee.

Rapid assessment
➤ Palpate pulses and observe for cyanosis and mottling distal to the injury.
➤ Assess motor functioning and sensation at the site and distal to the injury, noting decreased movement (which may not occur until several hours after the injury) and sensation.
➤ Observe for swelling and a black-and-blue discoloration from blood extravasating into surrounding tissues.
➤ Obtain the patient's history, including his report of feeling a stretch or tear of the affected joint followed by localized pain.
➤ Observe for accompanying injuries.

Immediate actions
➤ Initiate and maintain a nonweight-bearing status, and rest the injured joint.
➤ Elevate the joint above heart level.
➤ Apply ice using a towel between the ice pack and the skin to prevent a cold injury. (See *Using the RICE protocol.*)
➤ Support and immobilize the joint using an elastic bandage or splint, if the injury is severe.
➤ Obtain stress radiography (used to visualize the injury in motion), as indicated.
➤ Treat accompanying injuries.

> **USING THE RICE PROTOCOL**

Most sprains and strains can be treated for the first 24 to 48 hours using the rest, ice, compression, and elevation (RICE) protocol, which promotes healing, decreases pain, and reduces swelling. Here's what to do:

Rest: Rest the affected extremity; avoid the activity that caused the injury.

Ice: Apply cold packs to the affected extremity for 20-minute intervals several times per day.

Compression: Apply an elastic compression bandage to help immobilize the joint and prevent additional swelling.

Elevation: Elevate the affected area at a level higher than the heart to reduce swelling.

➤ Administer, as ordered, analgesics to reduce pain, and nonsteroidal anti-inflammatory drugs to decrease inflammation and reduce pain.

Follow-up actions
➤ Monitor the neurovascular status of the affected limb frequently.
➤ Maintain joint elevation for 48 to 72 hours after the injury (pillows can be used while sleeping).
➤ Apply ice intermittently for 24 to 48 hours after the injury.
➤ Teach the patient to reapply the elastic bandage by wrapping from below to above the injury, forming a figure eight.
➤ Instruct the patient to remove the bandage before going to sleep and to loosen it if it causes the leg to become pale, numb, or painful.
➤ Instruct the patient in the use of assistive devices, if necessary.
➤ Instruct the patient to call the physician if the pain worsens or persists; if so, an additional X-ray may reveal a previously undetected fracture.

Preventive steps
➤ Advise patients to tape their wrists and ankles before sports activities to prevent sprains.

Pathophysiology recap
➤ A sprain is usually caused by sharply twisting with a force stronger than that of the ligament, inducing joint movement beyond the normal range of motion. A sprain may also occur concurrently with fractures or dislocations.
➤ When a ligament is torn, an inflammatory exudate develops in the hematoma between the torn ends, initiating the healing process.
➤ Granulation tissue and collagen formation at the site of injury are the foundations for new ligament tissue.
➤ Eventually, the new tissue becomes strong enough to withstand normal muscle tension.

➤ *Strains*

A strain is a muscle or tendon injury due to sudden, forced motion that causes stretching beyond normal capacity. Strains may be acute, due to vigorous muscle overuse or overstress or traumatic rupture caused by a knife or gunshot wound, or chronic due to repeated overuse.

Rapid assessment
➤ Palpate the pulses and observe for cyanosis and mottling distal to the injury.
➤ Assess movement and sensation at the injury site and distal to it.
➤ Ask if the patient heard a snapping sound. If so, ask him if it was followed by severe pain and rapid swelling.
➤ Observe for muscle tenderness, ecchymosis, and swelling in the affected area.
➤ For the patient with a chronic strain, ask about stiffness, soreness, and generalized tenderness several hours after the injury.

Immediate actions
For acute strains:
➤ Institute the RICE protocol.
➤ Administer analgesics, as ordered.
   For chronic strains:
➤ Apply heat to the affected area.
➤ Administer nonsteroidal anti-inflammatory drugs, such as ibuprofen, or analgesic muscle relaxants, as needed.

Follow-up actions
➤ Follow the neurovascular status of the affected area frequently.
➤ After ice application for 48 hours, heat may be applied to the affected area of an acute strain to enhance blood flow, reduce cramping, and promote healing.
➤ Instruct the patient in the use of assistive devices, if necessary.
➤ Prepare the patient with complete muscle rupture for surgery, as indicated. (See *Muscle-tendon rupture.*)

Preventive steps
➤ Advise patients to stretch and warm up muscles before engaging in physical activity; warming up increases range of motion and reduces stiffness.
➤ Advise patients to preserve muscle conditioning by engaging in regular physical activity.

Pathophysiology recap
➤ Bleeding into the muscle and surrounding tissue occurs if a muscle is torn.

> ## MUSCLE-TENDON RUPTURE

Perhaps the most serious muscle-tendon injury is a rupture of the muscle-tendon junction. This type of rupture may occur at any junction, but it's most common at the Achilles tendon, extending from the posterior calf muscle to the foot. An Achilles tendon rupture produces a sudden, sharp pain and, until swelling begins, a palpable defect. Such a rupture typically occurs in men between ages 35 and 40, especially during physical activities, such as jogging or tennis.

To distinguish an Achilles tendon rupture from other ankle injuries, the physician performs this simple test: With the patient prone and his feet hanging off the foot of the table, squeeze the calf muscle. The response establishes the diagnosis:

> Plantar flexion – The tendon is intact.
> Ankle dorsiflexion – The tendon is partially intact.
> No flexion of any kind – The tendon is ruptured.

An Achilles tendon rupture usually requires surgical repair, followed first by a long leg cast for 4 weeks, then by a short cast for an additional 4 weeks.

> An inflammatory exudate develops between the torn ends, initiating the healing process.
> Granulation tissue and collagen formation lay the groundwork for new tissue development.
> Eventually, the new tendon or muscle tissue becomes strong enough to withstand normal muscle strain.
> In chronic strains, calcium may deposit into a muscle, limiting movement by causing stiffness and muscle fatigue.

> *Traumatic amputation*

Traumatic amputation is the accidental loss of a body part, usually a finger, toe, arm, or leg. In a complete amputation, the member is totally severed; in a partial amputation, some soft-tissue connection remains.

Rapid assessment
> Observe the rate, pattern, and depth of respirations, and auscultate breath sounds.
> Determine the patient's level of consciousness.
> In partial amputation, palpate pulses distal to the injury and observe for cyanosis and mottling.
> Observe for hemorrhagic bleeding.
> Obtain the patient's vital signs, noting hypotension, tachycardia, and decreased oxygen saturation.

➤ CARING FOR AN AMPUTATED BODY PART

After traumatic amputation, a surgeon may be able to reimplant the severed body part through microsurgery. The chance of successful reimplantation is much greater if the amputated part has received proper care.

   If a patient arrives at the hospital with a severed body part, first make sure that bleeding at the amputation site has been controlled. Then follow these guidelines to preserve the body part.

➤ Put on sterile gloves. Place several sterile gauze pads and an appropriate amount of sterile roller gauze in a sterile basin, and pour sterile normal saline over them. Don't try to scrub or debride the part.

➤ Holding the body part in one gloved hand, carefully pat it dry with sterile gauze. Place moist saline gauze pads over the stump, then wrap the whole body part with moist saline roller gauze. Wrap the gauze with a sterile towel, if available. Then put this package in a watertight container or bag and seal it.

➤ Fill another plastic bag with ice and place the part, still in its watertight container, inside. Seal the outer bag. (Always protect the part from direct contact with ice to prevent irreversible tissue damage, which would make the part unsuitable for reimplantation. Never use dry ice.) Keep this bag cold until the physician is ready to do the reimplantation surgery. Don't allow the part to freeze.

➤ Label the bag with the patient's name, identification number, identification of the amputated part, the hospital identification number, and the date and time when cooling began.

   Note: The body part must be wrapped and cooled quickly because irreversible tissue damage occurs after only 6 hours at ambient temperature. However, hypothermic management seldom preserves tissues for more than 24 hours.

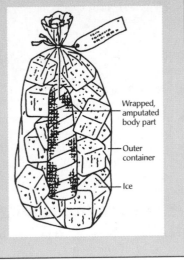

Wrapped, amputated body part

Outer container

Ice

➤ Obtain serum samples for complete blood count, serum electrolytes, prothrombin time, International Normalized Ratio, and partial thromboplastin time.

➤ Assess for other traumatic injuries.

➤ Obtain a patient history and determine whether the patient or family has brought the amputated body part with them.

Immediate actions

➤ Provide supplemental oxygen and prepare for endotracheal intubation and mechanical ventilation, if necessary.

➤ Control the bleeding using pressure or elevation.

➤ Monitor the neurovascular status of the limb frequently before surgery.
➤ Obtain a serum sample for complete blood count, type and crossmatch, prothrombin time, International Normalized Ratio, partial thromboplastin time, and serum electrolytes.
➤ Clean the wound by flushing it with sterile saline solution, and apply a sterile dressing.
➤ After a partial amputation, position the limb in normal alignment, drape it with towels or a moist sterile normal saline dressing, and contact the surgical team to determine if the amputated part can be reattached.
➤ After a complete amputation, prepare the amputated part for reimplantation. (See *Caring for an amputated body part.*)

Follow-up actions
➤ Postoperatively, perform dressing changes using sterile technique to help prevent skin infection and elevate and wrap the stump to prepare it for a prosthesis, if necessary.
➤ Help the amputee cope with his altered body image. Encourage the patient to perform prescribed exercises while taking care to prevent stump trauma.
➤ Obtain consultations from a physical therapist and an occupational therapist, if necessary.
➤ Monitor the amputation or surgical site for signs and symptoms of infection.

Preventive steps
➤ Advise patients to use caution and appropriate protective gear when working with machinery, equipment, or tools that can cause this type of injury.
➤ Encourage the use of seat belts whenever driving or riding in a motor vehicle.

Pathophysiology recap
➤ Traumatic amputations usually result directly from accidents involving factory, farm, or power tools, or from motor vehicle accidents.
➤ Profuse bleeding that may occur with the injury can further complicate the patient's condition.

7

Endocrine and metabolic emergencies

➤ *Adrenal crisis*

Adrenal crisis, also called *addisonian crisis,* is a critical deficiency of mineralocorticoids and glucocorticoids. It's a medical emergency that necessitates immediate, vigorous treatment. Adrenal crisis is the most serious complication of Addison's disease.

Rapid assessment
➤ Assess the patient's vital signs, noting hypotension, tachypnea, and tachycardia.
➤ Observe the patient for profound weakness and fatigue.
➤ Watch for nausea and vomiting and assess for signs of dehydration.
➤ Observe the patient for excessive sweating and darkening of the skin.
➤ Obtain the patient's history, noting a history of Addison's disease.

Immediate actions
➤ Administer 100 mg of hydrocortisone via I.V. bolus.
➤ Administer I.V. fluid therapy—usually dextrose 5% and normal saline solution.
➤ Administer vasopressors as needed to treat hypotension uncorrected by initial treatment with hydrocortisone and fluid therapy; titrate according to blood pressure.

 ALERT *Because of hormonal deficiencies, patients in acute adrenal crisis have a decreased response to catecholamines, vasopressors, and inotropic agents. Therefore, these agents may not be as effective as they would be for patients with adequate adrenal gland function.*

Follow-up actions
➤ Monitor the patient's vital signs frequently.
➤ Obtain serum samples to determine cortisol, fasting blood sugar, potassium, and sodium levels.
➤ Perform a corticotropin stimulation test to determine whether the patient's cortisol level is low.

➤ ADRENAL CRISIS: HOW IT HAPPENS

Acute adrenal crisis, the most serious complication of Addison's disease, involves a critical deficiency of glucocorticoids and mineralocorticoids. This life-threatening event requires prompt assessment and immediate treatment. The flowchart below highlights the underlying mechanisms responsible for adrenal crisis.

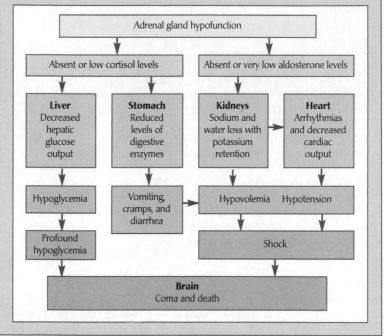

➤ Administer 50- to 100-mg doses (up to 300 mg/day) of I.M. or I.V. hydrocortisone (diluted with dextrose in saline solution) until the patient's condition stabilizes.

➤ Monitor the patient for hyperglycemia and electrolyte imbalances (especially hyponatremia and hyperkalemia) during steroid replacement therapy.

➤ Monitor intake and output.

➤ Monitor the patient for complications such as shock or coma.

Preventive steps

➤ Explain to patients with Addison's disease that stressors may precipitate an adrenal crisis. (See *Adrenal crisis: How it happens*.)

➤ Remind the patient to contact the physician immediately, give himself an injection of hydrocortisone, or increase his oral dose, as instructed, during a stressful event.

Pathophysiology recap
➤ Adrenal crisis occurs as a result of insufficient glucocorticoids and mineralocorticoids.
➤ Factors that trigger adrenal crisis include a deteriorating adrenal gland, injury to the pituitary gland, and abrupt withdrawal of corticosteroid therapy.
➤ Other precipitating factors may include acute stress, sepsis, trauma, and surgery.

➤ Diabetes insipidus

Diabetes insipidus is a water metabolism disorder caused by a deficiency of antidiuretic hormone (ADH) or vasopressin. The absence of ADH allows filtered water to be excreted in urine instead of being reabsorbed.

Rapid assessment
➤ Assess for a change in the patient's level of consciousness.
➤ Assess the patient's vital signs, noting hypotension and tachycardia.
➤ Obtain the patient's history; inquire about extreme thirst and monitor for a fluid intake of 5 to 20 L/day.
➤ Monitor for the abrupt onset of increased urine output, sometimes producing 4 to 16 L of dilute urine per day.
➤ Assess the patient for dizziness and weakness.
➤ Assess the patient for signs of dehydration, such as fever and dry skin and mucous membranes.

Immediate actions
➤ Administer subcutaneous (S.C.) or I.M. vasopressin aqueous preparations as well as S.C., I.V., or nasal spray desmopressin acetate to maintain fluid volume.

 ALERT *Vasopressin administration can cause hypertension, angina, and myocardial infarction because of the vasoconstrictive effects of the drug. Monitor the patient's cardiac status closely, including vital signs, cardiac rhythm, and hemodynamic status.*

➤ Administer hypotonic I.V. solution (1 ml for every 1 ml of urine output) to replace free water loss.
➤ Give thiazide diuretics if the patient has nephrogenic diabetes insipidus.

Follow-up actions
➤ Monitor the patient's vital signs frequently.
➤ Obtain urine samples to confirm colorless urine, low osmolality, and decreased specific gravity.
➤ Obtain blood samples to confirm increased serum osmolality and an increased sodium level.

➤ Monitor intake and output and urine specific gravity hourly.
➤ Prepare the patient with a pituitary tumor for a transphenoidal hypophysectomy.

Preventive steps

➤ Prompt and aggressive treatment of causative disorders may help prevent some cases of nephrogenic diabetes insipidus.
➤ Prompt and aggressive treatment of infections, tumors, and injuries may help to reduce the risk of diabetes insipidus.

Pathophysiology recap

➤ Diabetes insipidus is a syndrome resulting from a lack of ADH secretion.
➤ ADH is a hormone released by the posterior pituitary gland in response to increased serum osmolality; it also controls the body's ability to retain water.
➤ Diabetes insipidus is classified as neurogenic, nephrogenic, or psychogenic.
➤ Neurogenic (or central) diabetes insipidus is an acute-onset form caused by inadequate synthesis or release of ADH. It occurs when an organic lesion of the hypothalamus, infundibular stem, or posterior pituitary partially or completely blocks ADH synthesis, transport, or release.
➤ Nephrogenic diabetes insipidus is caused by inadequate renal response to ADH.
➤ Psychogenic diabetes insipidus is caused by extremely large fluid intake, which may be idiopathic or related to psychosis or sarcoidosis. Polydipsia and resultant polyuria deplete ADH, resulting in immediate excretion of large volumes of dilute urine and consequent plasma hyperosmolality.

➤ Diabetic ketoacidosis

Diabetic ketoacidosis (DKA) is an acute complication of hyperglycemic crisis in patients with diabetes mellitus. It's a life-threatening complication that's most common in patients with type 1 diabetes and is sometimes the first evidence of the disease.

Rapid assessment

➤ Obtain the patient's vital signs, noting an increased respiratory rate and decreased oxygen saturation.
➤ Observe for the rapid onset of drowsiness, stupor, and coma.
➤ Assess the patient for signs of severe dehydration.
➤ Monitor for polyuria, polydipsia, and polyphagia.
➤ Obtain the patient's history; inquire about weight loss, vision changes, abdominal and leg cramps, recurrent infections, nausea, and vomiting.
➤ Assess for a fruity breath odor due to acetone.

➤ Monitor the patient for rapid and deep breathing (Kussmaul's respirations).

Immediate actions

➤ If the patient is comatose, provide airway support; assist with endotracheal intubation and mechanical ventilation.
➤ Perform a bedside blood glucose test to determine blood glucose level (typically higher than 200 mg/dl).
➤ Obtain a sample for a serum glucose level (typically 200 to 800 mg/dl).
➤ Obtain a sample for arterial blood gas (ABG) analysis to confirm metabolic acidosis.
➤ Administer non-dextrose-based I.V. fluids.
➤ Provide I.V. regular insulin therapy (usually as an initial bolus, followed by continuous infusion) based on laboratory test results.

 ALERT *Blood glucose levels must be reduced gradually to prevent cerebral fluid shifting and subsequent cerebral edema.*

➤ Administer fluid and electrolyte replacements based on laboratory test results.

Follow-up actions

➤ Monitor the patient's vital signs frequently.
➤ Monitor blood glucose levels every 15 to 30 minutes until stable, then every hour.

 ALERT *As blood glucose decreases to approach 250 mg/dl, give dextrose-based fluid I.V. to prevent hypoglycemia.*

➤ Monitor for an increased serum ketone level, positive urine acetone, and elevated serum osmolality.
➤ Monitor ABG results.
➤ Monitor the serum potassium level, which will be elevated initially, but will decrease until it becomes normal or low.
➤ Obtain an electrocardiogram and monitor for changes consistent with the patient's potassium level. (Hyperkalemia produces a tall, tented T wave and widened QRS complex; hypokalemia produces a flattened T wave and a U wave.)

Preventive steps

➤ Measure urine ketones in patients with infections to give early warning of DKA.
➤ Teach patients with diabetes to recognize early warning signs and symptoms of DKA.

Pathophysiology recap

➤ The production and release of glucose into the blood is increased or uptake of glucose by cells is decreased.

➤ In the absence of endogenous insulin, the body breaks down fats for en
ergy.
➤ Fatty acids develop too rapidly and are converted to ketones, resulting
in severe metabolic acidosis.
➤ Acidosis also affects potassium levels: for every 0.1 change in pH,
there's a reciprocal 0.6 change in potassium.
➤ Blood glucose levels increase, and hyperkalemia and acidosis worsen.
➤ The cycle continues until coma and death occur.
➤ The liver responds to the lack of fuel (glucose) in cells by converting
glycogen to glucose for release into the bloodstream.
➤ Excess glucose molecules in the serum trigger osmosis resulting in fluid
shifts.

➤ Hyperaldosteronism

In hyperaldosteronism, also called *Conn's syndrome,* hypersecretion of the
mineralocorticoid aldosterone by the adrenal cortex causes excessive reabsorption of sodium and water and excessive renal excretion of potassium.

Rapid assessment
➤ Assess the patient's vital signs, noting hypertension.
➤ Obtain the patient's history; inquire about vision disturbances, fatigue,
and headache.
➤ Assess for increased neuromuscular irritability, muscle weakness, inter-
mittent flaccid paralysis, paresthesia and, possibly, tetany.
➤ Monitor for polyuria and polydipsia, which result in a loss of renal con-
centrating ability.
➤ Assess for edema.

Immediate actions
➤ Institute and maintain safety precautions.
➤ Obtain a blood sample to determine the serum potassium level, which
will reveal hypokalemia.
➤ Administer a potassium-sparing diuretic (spironolactone).

 ALERT *Monitor the patient taking potassium-sparing diuretics for
hyperkalemia.*

➤ Initiate and observe sodium restrictions.

Follow-up actions
➤ Monitor the patient's vital signs frequently.
➤ Prepare the patient for a 3-day suppression test to differentiate between
primary and secondary hyperaldosteronism. (Plasma aldosterone levels
and urinary metabolites are normal in primary disease but decreased in
secondary disease.)

➤ Watch for signs of tetany (muscle twitching, Chvostek's sign) and for hypokalemia-induced arrhythmias, paresthesia, or weakness.
➤ Monitor potassium levels and supplement as needed.
➤ Keep I.V. calcium gluconate available.
➤ Provide a low-sodium, high-potassium diet.
➤ Prepare the patient with primary hyperaldosteronism for a unilateral adrenalectomy.

Preventive steps
➤ Prevention of hyperaldosteronism involves prompt, aggressive treatment of causative disorders.

Pathophysiology recap
➤ In primary hyperaldosteronism, chronic aldosterone excess is independent of the renin-angiotensin system and, in fact, suppresses plasma renin activity.
  – Aldosterone excess enhances sodium reabsorption by the kidneys, which leads to mild hypernatremia, hypokalemia, and increased extracellular fluid volume.
  – Expansion of intravascular fluid volume also occurs and results in volume-dependent hypertension and increased cardiac output.
➤ Secondary hyperaldosteronism results from an extra-adrenal abnormality that stimulates the adrenal gland to increase aldosterone production. Other causes include:
  – conditions that reduce renal blood flow—such as renal artery stenosis, and extracellular fluid volume—or that produce a sodium deficit that activates the renin-angiotensin system and increases aldosterone secretion
  – conditions that induce hypertension through increased renin production such as Wilm's tumor
  – ingestion of hormonal contraceptives
  – pregnancy
  – heart failure.

➤ Hypercalcemia

Hypercalcemia occurs when the serum calcium level rises above 10.5 mg/dl, and the rate of calcium entry into extracellular fluid exceeds the rate of calcium excretion by the kidneys.

Rapid assessment
➤ Determine the patient's level of consciousness.
➤ Observe the rate, depth, and pattern of spontaneous respirations.
➤ Assess the patient's vital signs, noting hypertension.
➤ Obtain the patient's history; inquire about anorexia, nausea and vomiting, fatigue, and lethargy.

➤ Assess the patient for confusion or personality changes.
➤ Auscultate for decreased bowel sounds and ask about abdominal pain.
➤ Assess the patient for muscle weakness, hypoactive deep tendon reflexes, and decreased muscle tone.
➤ Obtain an electrocardiogram and assess for arrhythmias.
➤ Monitor the patient for polyuria and signs of dehydration.

Immediate actions
➤ Assist with endotracheal intubation and mechanical ventilation, if necessary.
➤ Obtain a blood sample to measure the serum calcium level (level initially is above 10.5 mg/dl).
➤ Prepare the patient with life-threatening hypercalcemia for hemodialysis or peritoneal dialysis to increase calcium excretion.
➤ Administer I.V. normal saline solution, as ordered, to inhibit renal tubular reabsorption of calcium and loop diuretics to promote calcium excretion.

 ALERT *While administering normal saline solution at rapid rates, watch the patient for signs of pulmonary edema, such as crackles and dyspnea.*

Follow-up actions
➤ Monitor the patient's vital signs frequently.
➤ Monitor serum electrolyte levels, especially calcium, and treat abnormalities.
➤ Obtain a blood sample to measure digoxin level and monitor for toxicity.
➤ Monitor the patient for lethargy that may progress to a coma.
➤ Monitor intake and output.
➤ Encourage the patient to drink 3 to 4 L/day to stimulate calcium excretion from the kidneys and decrease the risk of calculi formation.
➤ Strain the urine for calculi.
➤ Prepare the patient for radiologic studies to look for pathologic fractures and kidney stones.
➤ Decrease dietary calcium and decrease or discontinue medications containing calcium.
➤ Encourage activity, as tolerated, and implement measures to prevent pathologic fractures.
➤ Administer corticosteroids (I.V. initially, then orally), etidronate disodium, pamidronate disodium, mithramycin, or calcitonin to block bone resorption.

Preventive steps
➤ Caution patients to consult a physician when taking calcium or vitamin A or D supplements without a prescription.

Pathophysiology recap

➤ Hypercalcemia usually results from increased resorption of calcium from bone. It may develop as a result of any of the following conditions:
 – Hyperparathyroidism is the most common cause of hypercalcemia. In this disorder, the body excretes excessive amounts of parathyroid hormone (PTH), greatly strengthening its effects. Calcium resorption from bone and reabsorption from the kidneys are also increased as well as calcium absorption from the intestines.
 – Cancer is the second most common cause of hypercalcemia. Malignant cells invade the bones, causing bone destruction and triggering the release of a substance similar to PTH, which, in turn, causes elevated serum calcium levels. Because the kidneys can't excrete the excess calcium, serum calcium levels remain elevated. (Regardless of the cause, there's an increase in the absorption of calcium by the GI tract and a decrease in the excretion of calcium by the kidneys).
 – Hyperthyroidism can cause an increased calcium release from bone.
 – Multiple fractures or prolonged immobilization can also cause an increase in calcium release from bone.
 – Hypophosphatemia and acidosis increase calcium ionization.
 – Drugs may also cause hypercalcemia—for example, antacids that contain calcium can cause milk-alkali syndrome, a condition in which calcium and alkali are combined, increasing the calcium level. Lithium or thiazide diuretics can decrease calcium excretion by the kidneys. Vitamin A and D overdose can lead to increased bone resorption of calcium.

➤ Hyperglycemia

Hyperglycemia is an increase in serum blood sugar. A blood glucose level greater than 300 mg/dl—if it isn't treated promptly and adequately—can lead to coma. Hyperglycemia is usually the first sign of diabetes mellitus. (See *Classifying blood glucose levels*.)

Rapid assessment

➤ Assess the patient for an altered level of consciousness, including drowsiness and irritability.
➤ Observe the rate, pattern, and depth of the patient's spontaneous respirations.
➤ Obtain the patient's history; inquire about blurred vision, recent infections, and wounds that were slow to heal. Also inquire about polyuria, polydipsia, and polyphagia.

> ## CLASSIFYING BLOOD GLUCOSE LEVELS

The American Diabetes Association classifies fasting blood glucose levels as follows:
- normal: less than 100 mg/dl
- impaired fasting glucose: 100 to 125 mg/dl
- diabetes: 126 mg/dl or more, confirmed by a repeat test on another day.

Immediate actions
- Provide supplemental oxygen and prepare the patient for endotracheal intubation and mechanical ventilation, if necessary.
- Initiate safety measures.
- Initiate continuous cardiac monitoring.
- Perform a bedside blood glucose test.
- Obtain a serum blood glucose sample to confirm the diagnosis.
- Discontinue parenteral administrations that contain dextrose, if possible.
- Administer I.V. regular insulin.

Follow-up actions
- Monitor the patient's vital signs frequently.
- Monitor blood glucose levels every 15 to 30 minutes until stable and then every hour; some patients develop hypoglycemia after treatment.
- Monitor the patient for hyperkalemia due to a lack of insulin.
- If the patient has diabetes, assess his current insulin or oral antidiabetic medication regimen and make changes, as necessary and as ordered.
- Initiate a diabetic diet regimen with individualized meal planning designed to meet nutritional needs, control blood glucose and lipid levels, and maintain appropriate body weight.

Preventive steps
- Monitor blood glucose levels carefully in at-risk patients.
- Observe careful administration of glucocorticoids, I.V. solutions containing glucose, and total parenteral nutrition (TPN).
- Teach patients with diabetes to follow the individualized meal plan.
- Advise the patient to engage in physical activity, as tolerated.
- Remind the patient with diabetes that timely blood glucose monitoring and timely and accurate administration of insulin and oral antidiabetic medications will prevent hyperglycemia.
- Caution the patient to consult a physician during periods of illness, which may necessitate a higher dose of insulin than usual.
- Teach the patient with diabetes stress management techniques.

Pathophysiology recap
➤ Hyperglycemia usually happens slowly.
➤ Causes of hyperglycemia include glucocorticoid administration, excess administration of I.V. solutions containing glucose, and long-term TPN.
➤ In patients with diabetes, hyperglycemia can result from excessive food intake, inadequate insulin or oral hypoglycemic administration, lack of exercise, infections, and stress.
➤ Prolonged hyperglycemia can cause eye, heart, and kidney damage.

 ALERT *In a patient with type 1 diabetes, hyperglycemia can lead to ketoacidosis, a serious diabetic emergency.*

➤ Hyperosmolar hyperglycemic nonketotic syndrome

Hyperosmolar hyperglycemic nonketotic syndrome (HHNS) is an acute hyperglycemic crisis accompanied by hyperosmolality and severe dehydration without ketoacidosis. If not treated properly, it can cause coma or death.

Rapid assessment
➤ Assess the patient for a decreased level of consciousness. HHNS, which is an acute complication of diabetes, shares some similarities with diabetic ketoacidosis. (See *Comparing HHNS and DKA*.)
➤ Observe the rate, pattern, and depth of the patient's spontaneous respirations, noting tachypnea.
➤ Assess the patient's vital signs, noting hypotension and tachycardia.
➤ Assess the patient for diaphoresis and signs of dehydration.
➤ Monitor for polyuria, polydipsia, and polyphagia.
➤ Obtain the patient's history; inquire about vision changes.

Immediate actions
➤ Provide airway support and assist with endotracheal intubation and mechanical ventilation, if necessary.
➤ Administer isotonic fluids or half-normal saline solution I.V. to correct dehydration.

 ALERT *When the patient's blood glucose level approaches 250 mg/dl, add dextrose to the fluid to prevent hypoglycemia.*

➤ Give I.V. regular insulin by continuous infusion, titrating the dose based on the patient's blood glucose levels, which should be checked at least every hour.

 ALERT *The patient with HHNS typically secretes some insulin and may be sensitive to additional doses.*

➤ COMPARING HHNS AND DKA

Hyperosmolar hyperglycemic nonketotic syndrome (HHNS) and diabetic ketoacidosis (DKA) are acute complications of diabetes. They share some similarities, but are two distinct conditions. Use the flowchart below to determine which condition your patient has.

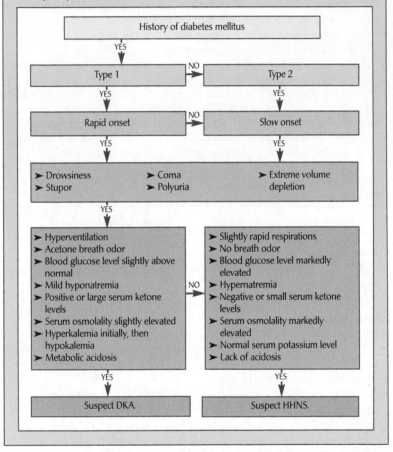

➤ Initiate electrolyte replacement therapy based on the patient's laboratory test results.

Follow-up actions
➤ Obtain blood samples to confirm initially elevated blood glucose level (800 to 2,000 mg/dl), hypernatremia, normal potassium level, negative or small ketone levels, and elevated serum osmolality.
➤ Follow and treat blood glucose levels and serum electrolytes until they normalize.

Preventive steps
➤ Caution patients who have experienced HHNS to practice careful monitoring and control of blood sugar levels, especially during periods of stress, illness, or infection.

Pathophysiology recap
➤ When cells don't receive fuel (glucose), the liver responds by converting glycogen to glucose for release into the bloodstream.
➤ When all excess glucose molecules remain in the serum, osmosis causes fluid shifts.
➤ The cycle continues until fluid shifts in the brain cause coma and death.
➤ HHNS is most common in patients with type 2 diabetes (usually middle-aged or older), but can occur in anyone whose insulin tolerance is stressed and in patients who have received such therapeutic procedures as peritoneal dialysis, hemodialysis, or total parenteral nutrition.
➤ In those with type 2 diabetes, glucose production and release into the blood is increased or glucose uptake by cells is decreased.

➤ Hyperkalemia

Hyperkalemia occurs when the serum potassium level rises above 5 mEq/L.

 ALERT *Because the normal serum potassium range is so narrow (3.5 to 5 mEq/L), a slight increase can have profound consequences.*

Rapid assessment
➤ Determine the patient's level of consciousness.
➤ Observe the rate, pattern, and depth of the patient's spontaneous respirations, noting bradypnea and shallow respirations.
➤ Assess the patient's vital signs.
➤ Evaluate the patient for neuromuscular signs and symptoms, such as paresthesia, irritability, skeletal muscle weakness that spreads from the legs to the trunk and involves the respiratory muscles (may lead to flaccid paralysis), and smooth muscle hyperactivity (especially in the GI tract) leading to nausea, abdominal cramping, and diarrhea.
➤ Assess for cardiac signs and symptoms, such as bradycardia, an irregular pulse, decreased cardiac output, hypotension and, ultimately, cardiac arrest.
➤ Obtain an electrocardiogram (ECG); observe for the presence of tall, tented T waves.

> ## VERIFYING SERUM POTASSIUM LEVEL RESULTS

If you suspect a laboratory test result indicating that a high serum potassium level is incorrect, verify the result by submitting another sample for analysis. Potential causes of falsely high potassium levels include:
> ➤ drawing the sample above an I.V. infusion containing potassium
> ➤ using a recently exercised extremity for the venipuncture site
> ➤ causing hemolysis (cell damage) as the specimen is obtained.

Immediate actions
➤ Administer 10 units of regular insulin I.V. to move potassium into the cells and lower the serum level.

 ALERT *When I.V. regular insulin is used to treat hyperkalemia, it's given with I.V. 10% to 50% hypertonic dextrose to prevent hypoglycemia.*

➤ Obtain serum electrolyte levels to confirm hyperkalemia. (See *Verifying serum potassium level results.*)
➤ Obtain arterial blood gas levels; if the patient has acidosis, give sodium bicarbonate (usually 50 ml) I.V. to help shift potassium into the cells.
➤ Provide airway support and prepare the patient for endotracheal intubation and mechanical ventilation, if necessary.
➤ Initiate continuous ECG monitoring and monitor for cardiac arrhythmias.
➤ Initiate safety measures.
➤ Perform a 12-lead ECG and look for tall, tented T waves, flattened P waves, prolonged PR intervals, widened QRS complexes, and depressed ST segments.

 ALERT *Hyperkalemia can also lead to heart block, ventricular arrhythmias, and asystole. The more serious arrhythmias become especially dangerous when serum potassium levels reach 7 mEq/L.*

➤ If the patient has renal failure, prepare him for hemodialysis.
➤ Administer sodium polystyrene sulfonate (a cation-exchange resin) orally, via nasogastric tube, or as a retention enema.
➤ Give loop diuretics to increase potassium loss from the body or to resolve acidosis.
➤ Administer 10% calcium gluconate (usually 10 ml) I.V. over 3 minutes to counteract the myocardial effects of hyperkalemia.

Follow-up actions
➤ Monitor the patient's vital signs and the ECG tracing frequently.
➤ Monitor arterial blood gas levels.

➤ CLINICAL EFFECTS OF POTASSIUM IMBALANCE

Dysfunction	Hypokalemia	Hyperkalemia
Acid–base balance	➤ Metabolic alkalosis	➤ Metabolic acidosis
Cardiovascular	➤ Dizziness, hypotension, arrhythmias, electrocardiogram (ECG) changes (flattened T wave, elevated U wave, depressed ST segment), cardiac arrest (with serum potassium levels < 2.5 mEq/L)	➤ Tachycardia and later brady-cardia, ECG changes (tented and elevated T wave, widened QRS complex, prolonged PR interval, flattened or absent P wave, depressed ST segment), cardiac arrest (with levels > 7 mEq/L)
Gastrointestinal	➤ Nausea, vomiting, anorexia, diarrhea, abdominal distention, paralytic ileus or decreased peristalsis	➤ Nausea, diarrhea, abdominal cramps
Genitourinary	➤ Polyuria	➤ Oliguria, anuria
Musculoskeletal	➤ Muscle weakness and fatigue, leg cramps	➤ Muscle weakness, flaccid paralysis
Neurologic	➤ Malaise, irritability, confu-sion, mental depression, speech changes, decreased reflexes, respiratory paralysis	➤ Hyperreflexia progressing to weakness, numbness, tingling, and flaccid paralysis

➤ Monitor electrolyte levels and watch the patient for signs of hypo-kalemia after treatment. (See *Clinical effects of potassium imbalance*.)
➤ Monitor intake and output.
➤ Monitor for hyperactive bowels sounds, which may occur due to the body's attempt to maintain homeostasis by excreting surplus potassium through the bowels.
➤ Administer antidiarrheals, as necessary.
➤ Restrict dietary potassium.
➤ Readjust or discontinue medications that cause high potassium levels such as potassium-sparing diuretics.

Preventive steps
➤ Closely monitor the potassium levels of at-risk patients.
➤ Restrict potassium intake in at-risk patients.
➤ Provide regular dialysis in patients with renal failure.

Pathophysiology recap

➤ Potassium is gained through intake and lost through excretion by the kidneys, which are vital in preventing a toxic buildup of the electrolyte.
➤ Hyperkalemia may result from excessive potassium intake in the patient's diet (especially with decreased urine output), excessive use of salt substitutes (most of which use potassium as a substitute for sodium), or ingestion of oral or I.V. potassium supplements.
➤ Transfusion can cause hyperkalemia if the patient is given a large volume of donated blood nearing its expiration date because serum potassium levels increase the longer donated blood is stored.
➤ Drugs that can cause or contribute to hyperkalemia include beta-adrenergic blockers, which inhibit potassium shifts into cells; potassium-sparing diuretics, which prevent its excretion; and antibiotics such as penicillin G potassium. Angiotensin-converting enzyme inhibitors and nonsteroidal anti-inflammatory drugs influence aldosterone secretion, which promotes potassium excretion in the kidneys. Nephrotoxic drugs, such as aminoglycosides, cause renal injury, which may lead to decreased potassium excretion and hyperkalemia.
➤ Chemotherapy causes cell death, which leads to hyperkalemia.
➤ Hyperkalemia may also occur if potassium excretion is diminished with acute or chronic renal failure. Diseases that cause kidney damage, such as diabetes, sickle cell disease, or systemic lupus erythematosus, and conditions, such as Addison's disease and hypoaldosteronism, can lead to decreased potassium excretion.
➤ Injury to cells from a burn, severe infection, trauma, crush injury, or intravascular hemolysis causes potassium to leave the cells.
➤ In acidosis, potassium moves outside the cell as hydrogen ions shift into the cell, resulting in hyperkalemia.

➤ Hypernatremia

Hypernatremia refers to an excess of sodium relative to body water. It occurs when the serum sodium level rises above 145 mEq/L. Severe hypernatremia can lead to seizures, coma, and permanent neurologic damage.

Rapid assessment

➤ Assess the patient for neurologic signs and symptoms, such as restlessness or agitation, weakness, lethargy, confusion, stupor, seizures, and coma.
➤ Assess for muscle twitching.
    If sodium gain is suspected, observe for signs of hypervolemia:
➤ Observe for dyspnea.
➤ Assess the patient's vital signs, noting a low-grade fever, elevated blood pressure, and bounding pulse.

If water loss is suspected, observe for signs of hypovolemia:
➤ Assess the patient's vital signs, noting orthostatic hypotension.
➤ Observe for dry mucous membranes and oliguria.

Immediate actions
➤ Prepare the patient for endotracheal intubation and mechanical ventilation, if necessary.
➤ Initiate safety measures and seizure precautions.
➤ Obtain samples for serum sodium, urine specific gravity, and serum osmolality to confirm the diagnosis.
➤ In hypernatremia due to dehydration, encourage oral fluids and administer I.V. fluid replacement with salt-free solutions, such as dextrose 5% in water, followed by half-normal saline solution.

 ALERT *Fluids should be given gradually over 48 hours to avoid shifting water into brain cells. If too much water is introduced to the body too quickly, water moves into brain cells, causing swelling and cerebral edema.*

➤ In hypernatremia due to excess sodium, restrict sodium intake and administer diuretics along with oral or I.V. fluid replacement to increase sodium loss.
➤ In hypernatremia due to diabetes insipidus, administer vasopressin, hypertonic I.V. fluids, and thiazide diuretics.

Follow-up actions
➤ Monitor the patient's vital signs frequently.
➤ Monitor fluid delivery and the patient's response to therapy.
➤ Watch for signs of cerebral edema during fluid delivery.
➤ Measure intake and output every hour.
➤ Monitor serum sodium and electrolyte levels and urine specific gravity.

Preventive steps
➤ Ensure adequate hydration in patients at risk for hypernatremia related to dehydration.
➤ Institute dietary salt restriction for patients at risk for increased sodium intake.
➤ Monitor sodium levels carefully in at-risk patients due to medications or parenteral I.V. fluid administration.

Pathophysiology recap
➤ The body typically maintains sodium balance with high serum osmolality (increased solute concentrations in the blood), which stimulates the hypothalamus to initiate the sensation of thirst—the body's main defense against hypernatremia. Antidiuretic hormone is secreted by the posterior pituitary gland, allowing water to be retained, which also keeps sodium levels normalized.

➤ In hypernatremia, increased serum osmolality causes cells to shed fluid in an attempt to balance the concentration. Fluid loss dehydrates cells, which may lead to neurologic impairment or hypervolemia from increased extracellular fluid volume in the blood vessels.

➤ Hypothalamic disorders, in which a lesion on the hypothalamus causes a disturbance of the thirst mechanism, are potential—although rare—causes of hypernatremia.

➤ Other potential causes of hypernatremia include dehydration due to insensible water loss from fever and heatstroke; extensive burns; severe, watery diarrhea; or diabetes insipidus.

➤ Pulmonary infections, with loss of water vapor from the lungs due to hyperventilation, may also result in hypernatremia.

➤ Hyperosmolar hyperglycemic nonketotic syndrome due to osmotic diuresis can lead to hypernatremia.

➤ Excessive sodium levels due to ingestion of salt tablets or heavily salted foods is another potential cause.

➤ Administration of medications, such as sodium polystyrene sulfonate (Kayexalate), and excessive parenteral administration of sodium solutions can also cause hypernatremia.

➤ Hypervolemia

Hypervolemia is an excess of isotonic fluid (water and sodium) in the extracellular compartment. Osmolality is usually unaffected because fluid and solutes are gained in equal proportions. The body has compensatory mechanisms to deal with hypervolemia, but when they fail, signs and symptoms of hypervolemia develop.

Rapid assessment
➤ Observe the rate, pattern, and depth of the patient's spontaneous respirations, noting labored breathing; auscultate the lungs, noting crackles.

➤ Assess the patient's vital signs, noting elevated blood pressure, central venous pressure, and pulmonary artery pressure, and decreased oxygen saturation.

➤ Obtain the patient's history; inquire about dyspnea, tachypnea, and a cough that produces frothy secretions.

➤ Auscultate for an S_3 gallop.

➤ Observe for distended jugular and hand veins.

➤ Assess for edema in dependent areas or for generalized edema or anasarca.

Immediate actions
➤ Raise the head of the bed to facilitate the patient's breathing.

➤ Provide supplemental oxygen and prepare the patient for endotracheal intubation and mechanical ventilation, if necessary.

➤ Maintain the patient on bed rest.

➤ *UNDERSTANDING CRRT*

Continuous renal replacement therapy (CRRT) is used to manage fluid and electrolyte imbalances in a hemodynamically unstable patient who can't tolerate hemodialysis. In CRRT, a dual-lumen venous catheter provides access to the patient's blood and propels it through a tubing circuit.

The illustration shows the standard setup for one type of CRRT called *continuous venovenous hemofiltration*. The patient's blood enters the hemofilter from a line connected to one lumen of the venous catheter, flows through the hemofilter, and returns to the patient through the second lumen of the catheter.

At the first pump, an anticoagulant may be added to the blood. A second pump moves dialysate through the hemofilter. A third pump adds replacement fluid, if needed. The ultrafiltrate (plasma water and toxins) removed from the blood drains into a collection bag.

Advantages
➤ Allows immediate access to the patient's blood via a dual-lumen venous catheter
➤ Conserves cellular and protein components of blood
➤ Doesn't create dramatic changes in the patient's blood pressure, which commonly occurs with hemodialysis

Disadvantages
➤ Must be performed by a specially trained critical care or nephrology nurse
➤ Must take place on a critical care unit
➤ Requires CRRT equipment and supplies
➤ May pose issues of staff competency if CRRT is rarely used
➤ Is time-consuming

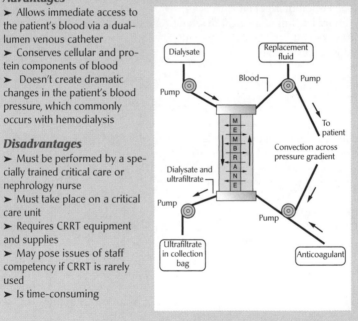

➤ Restrict the patient's fluid intake and monitor fluid balance.
➤ Administer diuretics to promote the loss of excess fluid.
➤ If the patient has pulmonary edema, administer morphine and nitroglycerin to dilate blood vessels and reduce pulmonary congestion.
➤ If the patient has heart failure, give digoxin to strengthen cardiac contractions and slow the heart rate.
➤ Administer angiotensin-converting enzyme inhibitors or beta-adrenergic blockers, as ordered, to improve cardiac function.

Follow-up actions

➤ Monitor the patient's vital signs and hemodynamic status frequently.
➤ Prepare the patient for a chest X-ray to determine the presence of pulmonary congestion.
➤ Monitor arterial blood gas values to assess oxygenation.
➤ Monitor serum electrolyte levels, especially potassium, that may change with diuretic administration.
➤ Restrict the patient's sodium intake.
➤ Insert an indwelling urinary catheter.
➤ Monitor intake and output hourly.
➤ Prepare the patient with compromised kidney function that doesn't respond to diuretics for hemodialysis or continuous renal replacement therapy. (See *Understanding CRRT.*)
➤ Watch for signs of hypovolemia due to overcorrection.
➤ Weigh the patient daily.

Preventive steps

➤ Hypervolemia can be prevented by careful administration of saline, lactated Ringer's, and hypertonic solutions.
➤ Institute a low-sodium, high-protein diet.
➤ Provide aggressive management of causative disorders.
➤ Ensure timely administration of prescribed diuretics.

Pathophysiology recap

➤ Extracellular fluid volume may increase in either the interstitial or intravascular compartments. The body can usually compensate and restore fluid balance by adjusting circulating levels of aldosterone, antidiuretic hormone, and atrial natriuretic peptide, causing the kidneys to release additional water and sodium.
➤ If hypervolemia is prolonged or severe or if the patient has poor heart function, the body can't compensate for the extra volume. Heart failure and pulmonary edema result. Fluid is forced out of blood vessels and into the interstitial space, causing tissue edema.
➤ Hypervolemia may occur due to excessive fluid or sodium intake, I.V. replacement therapy using normal saline or lactated Ringer's solution, blood or plasma replacement, or excessive intake of dietary sodium.
➤ Fluid and sodium retention occur due to heart failure, cirrhosis of the liver, nephrotic syndrome, corticosteroid therapy, hyperaldosteronism, and low intake of dietary protein.
➤ Fluid shifts from the intravascular space occur in remobilization of fluids after burn treatment; administration of hypertonic fluids, such as mannitol or hypertonic saline solution; and administration of plasma proteins such as albumin.
➤ Elderly patients and those with impaired renal or cardiovascular function are especially prone to hypervolemia.

> ## CHECKING FOR TROUSSEAU'S AND CHVOSTEK'S SIGNS

Testing for Trousseau's and Chvostek's signs can aid in the diagnosis of tetany associated with hypocalcemia. Here's how to check for these important signs.

Trousseau's sign

To check for Trousseau's sign, apply a blood pressure cuff to the patient's upper arm and inflate it to a pressure 20 mm Hg above the systolic pressure. Trousseau's sign (carpal spasm) may appear after 1 to 4 minutes. The patient will experience an adducted thumb, flexed wrist and metacarpophalangeal joints, and extended interphalangeal joints (with fingers together) indicating tetany, a major sign of hypocalcemia.

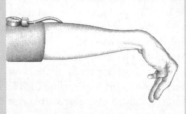

Chvostek's sign

You can induce Chvostek's sign by tapping the patient's facial nerve adjacent to the ear. A brief contraction of the upper lip, nose, or side of the face indicates Chvostek's sign.

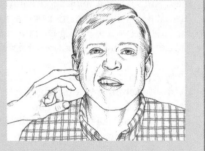

➤ Hypocalcemia

Hypocalcemia occurs when calcium levels fall below 8.5 mg/dl.

Rapid assessment

- ➤ Assess the patient's respirations, listening for stridor.
- ➤ Obtain the patient's vital signs, noting hypotension and decreased oxygen saturation.
- ➤ Assess the patient for neurologic effects, such as anxiety, confusion, irritability, and seizures.
- ➤ Obtain the patient's history; inquire about paresthesia of the toes, fingers, or face, especially around the mouth.
- ➤ Assess the patient for muscle twitching, cramps, and tremors.
- ➤ Check for Trousseau's and Chvostek's signs. (See *Checking for Trousseau's and Chvostek's signs.*)
- ➤ Test for hyperactive deep tendon reflexes.

➤ ADMINISTERING I.V. CALCIUM SAFELY

The patient who has symptomatic hypocalcemia may require parenteral calcium administration. Always determine whether the physician's order specifies calcium gluconate or calcium chloride. Doses vary according to the specific drug. Note the type and dosage of each calcium preparation carefully, and follow these steps for administration.

Preparing
Dilute the prescribed I.V. calcium preparation in dextrose 5% in water. Never dilute calcium in solutions containing bicarbonate because precipitation will occur. Avoid giving the patient calcium diluted in normal saline solution because sodium chloride increases renal calcium loss.

Administering
Always administer I.V. calcium slowly, according to the physician's order or your facility's established protocol. Rapid administration may result in syncope, hypotension, or cardiac arrhythmias. Initially, calcium may be given as a slow I.V. bolus. If hypocalcemia persists, the initial bolus may be followed by a slow I.V. drip using an infusion pump.

Monitoring
Because overcorrection can cause hypercalcemia, watch for anorexia, nausea, vomiting, lethargy, and confusion. Institute cardiac monitoring, and observe the patient for arrhythmias, especially if he's receiving digoxin. Observe the I.V. site for signs of infiltration; calcium can cause tissue sloughing and necrosis. Closely monitor serum calcium levels.

Immediate actions
➤ Provide supplemental oxygen and prepare the patient for endotracheal intubation and mechanical ventilation, if necessary.
➤ Place a tracheotomy tray and handheld resuscitation bag at the bedside of a patient who has just had parathyroid or thyroid surgery in case of laryngospasm.
➤ Initiate safety and seizure precautions.
➤ Initiate continuous cardiac monitoring and monitor for cardiac arrhythmias such as heart block.
➤ Obtain a sample for a serum calcium level to confirm the diagnosis.
➤ Administer I.V. calcium gluconate or I.V. calcium chloride. (See *Administering I.V. calcium safely.*)
➤ Give magnesium sulfate.
➤ Administer aluminum hydroxide for hyperphosphatemia.

Follow-up actions
➤ Monitor the patient's vital signs frequently.
➤ Perform a 12-lead ECG, noting prolonged ST-segment and QT intervals.

ALERT *A prolonged QT interval places the patient at risk for torsades de pointes.*

➤ Continue cardiac monitoring of the patient for arrhythmias such as heart block.

ALERT *Carefully watch the patient who's taking calcium and digoxin; these agents have similar effects on the heart.*

➤ Monitor serum calcium and electrolyte levels and treat abnormalities.
➤ Prepare the patient for X-rays to check for fractures.
➤ Handle the patient carefully to prevent fractures.
➤ Administer vitamin D supplements for chronic hypocalcemia to facilitate GI absorption of calcium, and oral calcium supplements (1 to 1½ hour after meals to prevent GI upset) to help increase calcium levels.
➤ Provide a diet high in calcium, vitamin D, and protein.

Preventive steps
➤ Explain the importance of adequate vitamin D intake and exposure to sunlight to mothers who are breast-feeding.
➤ Keep calcium gluconate at the bedside of a patient who has undergone parathyroid or thyroid surgery to allow for rapid treatment if signs and symptoms of hypocalcemia develop.

Pathophysiology recap
➤ Hypocalcemia occurs due to insufficient calcium intake, calcium malabsorption, or excessive calcium loss.
➤ Hypocalcemia may occur when burned or diseased tissues trap calcium ions from extracellular fluid.
➤ A decrease in the intestinal absorption of calcium results from diarrhea, laxative abuse, or chronic malabsorption syndrome.
➤ Renal failure harms the kidney's ability to activate vitamin D.
➤ Some anticonvulsants interfere with vitamin D metabolism and calcium absorption.
➤ Reduced gastric acidity can decrease the solubility of calcium salts.
➤ Excessive calcium loss may result from pancreatic insufficiency, which can cause malabsorption and loss of calcium in stool.
➤ Reduced or eliminated parathyroid hormone secretion from thyroid surgery, surgical removal of the parathyroid gland, removal of a parathyroid tumor, or injury or disease of the parathyroid gland such as hypoparathyroidism cause decreased serum sodium levels.
➤ Medications that decrease calcium resorption from bone, such as calcitonin and mithramycin, may result in hypocalcemia.
➤ Hypocalcemia may result from excessive calcium excretion caused by administration of some loop diuretics.

➤ Patients who have received transfusions may develop hyperphosphatemia, in which citrate added to stored blood to prevent clotting binds with calcium and renders it unavailable for use.

➤ Those at risk for hypocalcemia include alcoholics who have poor nutritional intake, poor calcium absorption, and low magnesium levels and infants being breast-fed by mothers with low calcium and vitamin D intake.

➤ Hypoglycemia

Hypoglycemia is an abnormally low glucose level (less than 50 mg/dl) that occurs when glucose is used too quickly, when its release falls below the demands of tissues, or when excessive insulin enters the bloodstream.

Rapid assessment

➤ Observe the rate, pattern, and depth of the patient's spontaneous respirations.

➤ Assess the patient for mental status changes, such as a decreased level of consciousness, seizures, and coma.

➤ Assess the patient's vital signs, noting tachycardia.

➤ Obtain the patient's history; inquire about food intake for the past 24 hours, hunger, drug and alcohol use, history of diabetes mellitus or hepatic disease, and recent surgery.

➤ Inquire about dizziness, headache, cloudy vision, and palpitations.

➤ Assess the patient for diaphoresis, pallor, anxiety, nervousness, and weakness.

➤ Inspect for tremors and loss of fine motor skills.

Immediate actions

➤ Provide supplemental oxygen, if necessary.

➤ Initiate safety measures and seizure precautions.

➤ Perform bedside blood glucose testing.

➤ Obtain a sample to measure the serum blood glucose level to confirm the diagnosis.

➤ Administer 25 or 50 g of 50% dextrose solution via I.V. bolus.

➤ Maintain a continuous glucose infusion until the patient can have a meal.

Follow-up actions

➤ Monitor blood glucose levels carefully to avoid hyperglycemia.

➤ If the patient is receiving hypertonic glucose solutions, monitor him for fluid overload.

➤ Prepare the patient for a 5-hour glucose tolerance test to induce reactive hypoglycemia.

➤ Prepare the patient for a 12-hour fast and plasma insulin and glucose levels to diagnose fasting hypoglycemia.

If the patient has reactive hypoglycemia:
- ➤ Provide small, frequent, high-protein, high-fiber meals without simple carbohydrates to delay glucose absorption and gastric emptying.
- ➤ Administer anticholinergic drugs to slow gastric emptying and decrease intestinal motility.

If the patient has pharmacologic hypoglycemia:
- ➤ Titrate the dosage of, or discontinue, the causative drug. Insulin or anti-diabetic drugs may need dosage adjustments for patients with diabetes mellitus.

If the patient has fasting hypoglycemia:
- ➤ Prepare him for surgery to remove the insulin-secreting or insulin-like-secreting tumor.
- ➤ Administer diazoxide or octreotide for inoperable insulinomas.
- ➤ Initiate hormone replacement therapy for pituitary or adrenal disorders.

Preventive steps
- ➤ Advise patients to avoid fasting and not to delay meals.
- ➤ Suggest nutritional counseling for patients at risk for hypoglycemia.
- ➤ Instruct patients with diabetes mellitus in the strict management of the disease. Teach about signs and symptoms of hypoglycemia. Advise patients to carry a high-glucose snack for emergency use.

Pathophysiology recap
- ➤ An abnormally low glucose level deprives the brain of energy, causing deterioration in brain function.

 ALERT *Tissue damage—or even death—can occur as a result of prolonged hypoglycemia or blood glucose levels of 20 mg/dl or less.*

- ➤ Reactive hypoglycemia is linked to the timing of meals; blood glucose usually falls 2 to 4 hours after meals. This type of hypoglycemia may result from alimentary hyperinsulinism due to dumping syndrome, fructose or galactose intolerance, or type 2 diabetes mellitus.
- ➤ Pharmacologic hypoglycemia is a response to a drug that increases the amount of insulin in the bloodstream, enhances the action of insulin, or hinders the liver's ability to break down stored glycogen to glucose. Insulin, oral sulfonylureas, and beta-adrenergic blockers can cause pharmacologic hypoglycemia. It may also result from excessive alcohol ingestion.
- ➤ Fasting hypoglycemia is caused by periods of abstinence from food. It typically occurs at least 5 hours after a meal, usually during the night.
- ➤ Nonendocrine causes of hypoglycemia include hepatitis, hepatic cancer, cirrhosis, and liver congestion with heart failure.
- ➤ Endocrine causes include damage to the islet cells of the pancreas, insulinomas, adrenocortical insufficiency, and pituitary insufficiency.

➤ Hypokalemia

Hypokalemia is a potentially dangerous electrolyte imbalance because it can lead to respiratory and cardiac arrest. It's denoted by a serum potassium level below 3.5 mEq/L.

 ALERT *Because the normal range for the serum potassium is narrow (3.5 to 5.0 mEq/L), a slight decrease has profound consequences.*

Rapid assessment

➤ Observe the rate, pattern, and depth of the patient's spontaneous respirations, noting shallow respirations and tachypnea.

 ALERT *Paralysis in severe hypokalemia could involve the respiratory muscles. Notify the physician immediately if respirations become shallow and rapid. Keep a manual resuscitation bag at the bedside of a patient with severe hypokalemia.*

➤ Palpate for a weak and irregular pulse.
➤ Assess the patient's vital signs, noting orthostatic hypotension.
➤ Assess the patient for skeletal muscle weakness, paresthesia, leg cramps, and paralysis.
➤ Test for decreased or absent deep tendon reflexes.
➤ Obtain the patient's history; inquire about polyuria, constipation, anorexia, nausea, and vomiting.
➤ Assess for paralytic ileus by auscultating for decreased bowel sounds.

Immediate actions

➤ Provide supplemental oxygen and prepare the patient for intubation and mechanical ventilation, if necessary.
➤ Initiate continuous electrocardiogram (ECG) monitoring and obtain a 12-lead ECG, noting flattened T waves, depressed ST segments, and characteristic U waves.
➤ Obtain a sample for serum potassium level analysis (less than 3.5 mEq/L) to confirm the diagnosis.
➤ Administer oral potassium supplements, using potassium salts or I.V. infusion potassium replacement therapy. (See *Guidelines for I.V. potassium administration,* page 244.)

Follow-up actions

➤ Monitor the patient's vital signs frequently.
➤ Monitor serum potassium levels after supplementation.
➤ If the patient is being given digoxin, monitor blood levels.

 ALERT *A patient taking digoxin, especially if he's also taking a diuretic, should be watched closely for hypokalemia, which can potentiate digoxin's action and cause toxicity.*

➤ Monitor intake and output.

➤ *GUIDELINES FOR I.V. POTASSIUM ADMINISTRATION*

Below are some guidelines for administering I.V. potassium and for monitoring the patient receiving it. Remember, potassium only needs to be replaced via I.V. infusion if hypokalemia is severe or if the patient can't take oral potassium supplements.

Administration
➤ When adding the potassium preparation to an I.V. solution, mix it well. Don't add the preparation to a hanging container – the potassium will pool, causing the patient to receive a highly concentrated bolus. Use premixed potassium, if available.
➤ To reduce or prevent toxic effects, I.V. infusion concentrations shouldn't exceed 40 to 60 mEq/L. Although 10 mEq/hour is the typical infusion rate, more rapid infusion may be used in severe cases. The maximum adult dose generally shouldn't exceed 200 mEq/24 hours, unless prescribed.
➤ Use infusion devices when administering potassium solutions to control the flow rate.
➤ *Remember:* Never administer potassium by I.V. push or bolus; doing so can cause cardiac arrhythmias and cardiac arrest, which could be fatal.

Patient monitoring
➤ Monitor the patient's cardiac rhythm during I.V. potassium administration, especially during rapid infusion. A rapid rise in serum potassium levels can lead to hyperkalemia, resulting in cardiac complications. Immediately report any irregularities.
➤ Evaluate the results of treatment by checking serum potassium levels and assessing the patient for signs and symptoms of toxic reaction, such as muscle weakness and paralysis.
➤ Watch the I.V. site for signs and symptoms of infiltration, phlebitis, or tissue necrosis.
➤ Monitor the patient's urine output and notify the physician if the volume is inadequate. Urine output should exceed 30 ml/hour to avoid hyperkalemia.
➤ Repeat potassium level measurements as ordered.

   ALERT *About 40 mEq of potassium is lost in each liter of urine. Diuresis can put the patient at risk for potassium loss.*

➤ Instruct the patient to eat foods rich in potassium.
➤ Administer sustained-release oral potassium supplements.
➤ If necessary, switch the patient from a potassium-wasting diuretic to a potassium-sparing diuretic.

Preventive steps
➤ Provide sufficient dietary potassium.
➤ Observe cautious and monitored administration of potassium-deficient I.V. fluids.

➤ Initiate potassium supplementation.
➤ Observe close monitoring and supplementation for at-risk patients such as those taking loop diuretics.

Pathophysiology recap
➤ The body can't conserve potassium.
➤ In certain situations, potassium shifts from the extracellular space to the intracellular space and hides in the cells, causing less potassium to be measured in the blood.
➤ Hypokalemia may result from inadequate dietary intake or administration of potassium-deficient I.V. fluids.
➤ GI loss of potassium may occur due to suctioning, lavage, prolonged vomiting, diarrhea, fistulas, or laxative abuse.
➤ Severe diaphoresis can cause potassium loss.
➤ Losses through the kidney occur with diuresis following kidney transplant or osmotic diuresis due to high urine glucose levels.
➤ Drugs that can deplete potassium include diuretics, corticosteroids, cisplatin, and antibiotics such as amphotericin.
➤ Excessive insulin secretion causes potassium to shift into cells.

➤ Hyponatremia

Hyponatremia, a common electrolyte imbalance, is a sodium deficiency in relation to body water. Body fluids are diluted and cells swell due to decreased extracellular fluid osmolality. Severe hyponatremia can lead to seizures, coma, and permanent neurologic damage. Hyponatremia occurs when serum sodium levels fall below 13.5 mEq/L.

Rapid assessment
In the patient with suspected *hyponatremia:*
➤ Observe the patient for changes in his level of consciousness, such as shortened attention span, progressive lethargy, confusion, stupor, seizures, and coma.
➤ Observe the rate, pattern, and depth of the patient's spontaneous respirations, noting respiratory difficulty.
➤ Obtain the patient's history; inquire about headache, abdominal cramps, and nausea.
   In a patient with *hypovolemia:*
➤ Assess the patient's vital signs, noting hypotension or orthostatic hypotension; a weak, rapid pulse; and decreased central venous pressure (CVP), pulmonary artery pressure (PAP), and pulmonary artery wedge pressure.
➤ Assess for poor skin turgor and dry, cracked mucous membranes.
   In a patient with *hypervolemia:*
➤ Assess the patient's vital signs, noting hypertension, a rapid bounding pulse, and an elevated CVP and PAP.

➤ Assess for edema and weight gain.

Immediate actions
➤ Assist with endotracheal intubation and mechanical ventilation, if necessary.
➤ Initiate safety measures and seizure precautions.
➤ Obtain a serum sodium level analysis (less than 135 mEq/L) to confirm the diagnosis.
➤ Infuse hypertonic saline solution, such as 3% or 5% saline, except in hypervolemic patients.
➤ In patients with hypovolemia, administer isotonic I.V. fluids, such as normal saline solution, to restore volume.

 ALERT *A hypertonic saline solution causes water to shift out of cells, which may lead to intravascular volume overload and serious brain damage (osmotic demyelination), especially in the pons. To prevent overload, the hypertonic saline solution is infused slowly and in small volumes. Furosemide is usually administered at the same time.*

➤ If the patient has hypervolemia or isovolemia, restrict fluid intake.

Follow-up actions
➤ Monitor the patient's vital signs frequently.
➤ Monitor serum sodium and electrolyte levels.
➤ Watch the patient receiving hypertonic saline solution for signs of circulatory overload or worsening neurologic status.
➤ Monitor intake and output hourly.
➤ Weigh the patient daily.
➤ Monitor urine specific gravity.
➤ For the patient with hypovolemia, institute a high-sodium diet.
➤ For patients with hypervolemia or isovolemia, administer oral sodium supplements.

Preventive steps
➤ Recognize patients who are at risk for hyponatremia and monitor sodium levels closely.
➤ Initiate prompt, aggressive treatment of causative disorders.

Pathophysiology recap
➤ Hyponatremia occurs when the body can't get rid of excess water by secreting less antidiuretic hormone (ADH).
➤ Less ADH causes diuresis.
➤ Serum sodium levels decrease and more water moves into the blood vessels.
➤ Fluid moves by osmosis from the extracellular area into the more concentrated intracellular area.

➤ More fluid in the cells and less in the blood vessels causes cerebral edoma and hypovolemia.

➤ In hypovolemic hyponatremia, sodium loss is greater than water loss. Nonrenal causes of this condition include vomiting, diarrhea, fistulas, gastric suctioning, excessive sweating, cystic fibrosis, burns, and wound drainage. Renal causes include osmotic diuresis, salt-losing nephritis, adrenal insufficiency, and diuretic use.

➤ In hypervolemic hyponatremia, water and sodium levels increase in the extracellular area, but the water gain is greater. Serum sodium levels are diluted and edema occurs. This condition is caused by heart failure, liver failure, nephrotic syndrome, excessive administration of hypotonic I.V. fluids, and hyperaldosteronism.

➤ In isovolemic hyponatremia, sodium levels may appear low due to the presence of excess fluid. There are no physical signs of fluid volume excess, and total body sodium remains stable. Isovolemic hyponatremia is caused by glucocorticoid deficiency (causing inadequate fluid filtration by the kidneys), hypothyroidism (causing limited water excretion), and renal failure.

➤ Syndrome of inappropriate antidiuretic hormone secretion causes excessive release of ADH and disturbs fluid and electrolyte balance.

➤ *Metabolic acidosis*

Metabolic acidosis is characterized by a pH below 7.35 and a bicarbonate (HCO_3^-) level below 22 mEq/L. This disorder depresses the central nervous system. Left untreated, it may lead to ventricular arrhythmias, coma, and cardiac arrest.

Rapid assessment

➤ Assess the patient's level of consciousness, noting confusion, stupor, and coma.

➤ Assess the patient for hyperventilation (as acid builds up in the bloodstream, the lungs compensate by increased exhalation of carbon dioxide) with rapid and deep breaths or Kussmaul's respirations.

➤ Assess the patient's vital signs, noting decreased cardiac output and hypotension.

➤ Obtain the patient's history; inquire about weakness, a dull headache, anorexia, nausea, and vomiting.

➤ Assess the patient with diabetes for a fruity breath odor from the catabolism of fats and excretion of acetone through the lungs.

➤ Obtain an electrocardiogram (ECG) and assess for arrhythmias.

➤ Assess the patient for warm and dry skin.

➤ Assess the patient for decreased muscle tone and deep tendon reflexes.

> ## ➤ *ANION GAP*

The anion gap is the difference between concentrations of serum cations and anions – determined by measuring one cation (sodium) and two anions (chloride and bicarbonate [HCO_3^-]). The normal concentration of sodium is 140 mEq/L; of chloride, 102 mEq/L; and of bicarbonate HCO_3^-, 26 mEq/L. Thus, the anion gap between *measured* cations (actually sodium alone) and *measured* anions is about 12 mEq/L (140 minus 128).

Concentrations of potassium, calcium, and magnesium (*unmeasured* cations), or proteins, phosphate, sulfate, and organic acids (*unmeasured* anions) aren't needed to measure the anion gap. Added together, the concentration of unmeasured cations would be about 11 mEq/L; of unmeasured anions, about 23 mEq/L. Thus, the normal anion gap between unmeasured cations and anions is about 12 mEq/L (23 minus 11) – plus or minus 2 mEq/L for normal variation. An anion gap over 14 mEq/L indicates *metabolic acidosis*. It may result from the accumulation of excess organic acids or from the retention of hydrogen ions, which chemically bond with HCO_3^- and decrease HCO_3^- levels.

Immediate actions
- ➤ Initiate safety measures.
- ➤ Elevate the head of the bed to promote chest expansion and facilitate breathing.
- ➤ Provide airway support and prepare the patient for endotracheal intubation and mechanical ventilation, if necessary, to provide respiratory compensation.
- ➤ Initiate continuous cardiac monitoring.
- ➤ Obtain a blood sample for arterial blood gas (ABG) analysis. (A pH below 7.35, HCO_3^- level below 22 mEq/L and, possibly, carbon dioxide less than 35 mm Hg indicate compensatory attempts by the lungs to rid the body of excess carbon dioxide.)
- ➤ If the patient has diabetes, administer rapid-acting regular insulin to reverse diabetic ketoacidosis (DKA) and drive potassium back into the cells.
- ➤ If the patient has a pH lower than 7.1 and HCO_3^- loss, administer I.V. sodium bicarbonate to neutralize blood acidity.

 ALERT *Remember to flush the I.V. line with normal saline solution before and after giving HCO_3^- because that chemical can inactivate many drugs or can cause them to precipitate.*

- ➤ Administer antibiotics to treat infections and antidiarrheals to treat diarrhea-induced HCO_3^- loss.

Follow-up actions
- ➤ Monitor the patient's vital signs frequently.
- ➤ Monitor ABG results frequently.

➤ Monitor the 12-lead ECG for changes due to hyperkalemia, such as tall 'T' waves, prolonged PR intervals, and wide QRS complexes.
➤ Monitor intake and output hourly.
➤ Prepare the patient with renal failure or a toxic reaction to a drug for hemodialysis, if necessary.
➤ Monitor the patient for signs of shock, including cold and clammy skin.
➤ Monitor the patient for hyperkalemia (hydrogen ions move into the cells and potassium moves out) and increased plasma lactate levels.
➤ Monitor the patient with DKA for hyperglycemia and increased serum ketone levels.

Preventive steps
➤ Explain the need for strict management of type 1 diabetes mellitus.
➤ Initiate prompt, aggressive treatment of causative disorders.
➤ Caution patients to avoid ingesting or inhaling toxic materials.

Pathophysiology recap
➤ Metabolic acidosis consists of a loss of HCO_3^- from extracellular fluid, an accumulation of metabolic acids, or a combination of both.
➤ If the patient's anion gap is greater than 14 mEq/L, the acidosis is due to an accumulation of metabolic acids; if the anion gap is normal (8 to 14 mEq/L), loss of HCO_3^- may be the cause. (See *Anion gap.*)
➤ Acid gain with base loss can lead to metabolic acidosis due to overproduction of ketone bodies from the conversion of fatty acids when glucose supplies have been used and the body draws on fat stores for energy. Such overproduction of ketone bodies may result from diabetes mellitus, chronic alcoholism, severe malnutrition or starvation, poor dietary intake of carbohydrates, hyperthyroidism, and severe infection with fever.
➤ Kidney malfunction may cause metabolic acidosis due to a decrease in the kidneys' ability to excrete acids. This may occur in renal insufficiency or renal failure with acute tubular necrosis.
➤ Excessive GI losses leading to metabolic acidosis include diarrhea, intestinal malabsorption, a draining fistula of the pancreas or liver, urinary diversion to the ileum, hyperaldosteronism, and use of potassium-sparing diuretics.
➤ Inhalation of toluene or ingestion of a salicylate, methanol, ethylene glycol, paraldehyde, hydrochloric acid, or ammonium chloride may cause metabolic acidosis.

➤ *Metabolic alkalosis*

Metabolic alkalosis is characterized by a blood pH above 7.45 and is accompanied by a bicarbonate (HCO_3^-) level above 26 mEq/L. In acute metabolic alkalosis, the HCO_3^- level may be as high as 50 mEq/L. With early diagnosis and prompt treatment, the prognosis for recovery is good. Left untreated, metabolic alkalosis can result in coma, arrhythmias, and death.

Rapid assessment
➤ Assess the patient's vital signs, noting hypotension.
➤ Obtain the patient's history; inquire about anorexia, nausea, vomiting, polyuria, and numbness and tingling in the fingers, toes, and mouth area.
➤ Observe for hypoventilation with slow, shallow respirations (the compensatory mechanism until hypoxemia stimulates ventilation).
➤ Assess the patient for muscle twitching, weakness, and tetany.
➤ Assess for hyperactive deep tendon reflexes.
➤ Assess the patient for an altered level of consciousness, including apathy, confusion, seizures, stupor, and coma.
➤ Obtain an electrocardiogram (ECG) and assess for arrhythmias.

Immediate actions
➤ Raise the head of the bed to promote chest expansion and ease breathing.
➤ Administer supplemental oxygen and prepare the patient for endotracheal intubation and mechanical ventilation, if necessary.
➤ Initiate safety measures and seizure precautions.
➤ Initiate cardiac monitoring.
➤ Discontinue thiazide diuretics and nasogastric (NG) suctioning.
➤ Obtain a sample for arterial blood gas (ABG) analysis, which will reveal a blood pH above 7.45 and a HCO_3^- level above 26 mEq/L, to confirm the diagnosis. (If the underlying cause is excessive acid loss, the HCO_3^- level may be normal, while the partial pressure of arterial carbon dioxide [$PaCO_2$] level may be above 45 mm Hg, indicating respiratory compensation.)
➤ Administer an antiemetic to treat underlying nausea and vomiting and acetazolamide to increase renal excretion of HCO_3^-.
➤ Give potassium supplements, as indicated by serum potassium levels.

Follow-up actions
➤ Monitor the patient's vital signs frequently.
➤ Monitor ABG values frequently.
➤ Monitor serum electrolytes for hypokalemia, hypocalcemia, hypochloremia, and an increased HCO_3^- level.
➤ Perform a 12-lead ECG, noting low T waves that merge with the P waves.
➤ Monitor intake and output.

Preventive steps
➤ Monitor patients at risk for metabolic alkalosis.
➤ Initiate prompt, aggressive treatment of causative disorders.

➤ Observe careful administration of medications that contain sodium bicarbonate and thiazide and loop diuretics.
➤ Provide close monitoring during the treatment of acidosis.

Pathophysiology recap
➤ Metabolic alkalosis consists of a loss of hydrogen ions (acid), a gain in HCO_3^-, or both.
➤ $PaCO_2$ greater than 45 mm Hg indicates that the lungs are compensating for the alkalosis.
➤ Renal compensation is more effective, but slower.
➤ Metabolic alkalosis is commonly associated with hypokalemia, hypochloremia, and hypocalcemia.
➤ Metabolic alkalosis may result from excessive acid loss from the GI tract due to vomiting or NG suctioning, which cause loss of hydrochloric acid.
➤ Thiazide and loop diuretics can lead to a loss of hydrogen, potassium, and chloride ions from the kidneys.
➤ Hypokalemia causes hydrogen ion excretion from the kidneys as they try to conserve potassium.
➤ Potassium moves out of the cells as hydrogen moves in, resulting in alkalosis.
➤ Cushing's disease can cause metabolic alkalosis due to sodium retention and chloride and urinary loss of potassium and hydrogen.
➤ Rebound alkalosis can occur following the correction of acidosis, such as after cardiac arrest and sodium bicarbonate administration.
➤ Renal artery stenosis causes increased mineralocorticoid activity, resulting in the reabsorption of sodium in the distal tubule and the excretion of potassium and hydrogen ions.
➤ Milk-alkali syndrome caused by chronic ingestion of calcium carbonate may lead to metabolic alkalosis.

➤ Myxedema coma

Myxedema coma is a life-threatening disorder that progresses from hypothyroidism.

Rapid assessment
➤ Assess the patient for decreased mental ability—slight mental-slowing to severe obtundation.
➤ Listen for a hoarse voice and slow, slurred speech.
➤ Assess the patient's vital signs, noting hypotension, bradycardia, and severe hypothermia without shivering.
➤ Observe for periorbital edema; dry, flaky skin; thick, brittle nails; a thick, dry tongue; and sacral or peripheral edema. (See *Facial signs of myxedema coma,* page 252.)

➤ FACIAL SIGNS OF MYXEDEMA COMA

Characteristic myxedematous signs in adults include dry, flaky, inelastic skin, a puffy face, and upper eyelid droop.

➤ Auscultate for muffled or S_3 heart sounds.
➤ Observe for significantly depressed respirations and auscultate for adventitious breath sounds.
➤ Obtain an electrocardiogram and assess for arrhythmias.

Immediate actions
➤ Maintain a patent airway, provide supplemental oxygen, and prepare the patient for endotracheal intubation and mechanical ventilation, if necessary.
➤ Initiate continuous cardiac monitoring.
➤ Check for hypoglycemia by obtaining a bedside blood glucose level.
➤ Apply a warming blanket, if necessary.
➤ Send serum samples to check for decreased triiodothyronine and thyroxine levels and increased thyroid-stimulating hormone (TSH) level to help confirm the diagnosis.
➤ Administer I.V. hydrocortisone and levothyroxine, I.V. fluids, and serum electrolyte supplements.

Follow-up actions
➤ Monitor the patient's vital signs frequently.
➤ Monitor arterial blood gas values.
➤ Administer maintenance thyroid replacement.
➤ Obtain blood, sputum, and urine samples to send for culture to identify possible sources of infection.
➤ Provide meticulous skin care.
➤ Prepare the patient for radioisotope scanning of thyroid tissue to identify ectopic thyroid tissue.
➤ Prepare the patient for a computed tomography scan, magnetic resonance imaging, or a skull X-ray to disclose an underlying cause such as pituitary or hypothalamic lesions.

Preventive steps

➤ Initiate prompt administration of maintenance thyroid hormone replacement therapy.

 ALERT *Hormone replacement therapy is a lifelong therapy that must be taken exactly as prescribed and must not be discontinued abruptly.*

➤ Counsel the patient about stress reduction therapy.
➤ Caution the patient to seek prompt, aggressive treatment of infections.
➤ Practice caution when using sedatives in patients with hypothyroidism.

Pathophysiology recap

➤ Primary hypothyroidism originates as a disorder of the thyroid gland.
➤ Secondary hypothyroidism is caused by a failure to stimulate normal thyroid function or an inability to synthesize thyroid hormone due to an iodine deficiency (usually dietary) or use of antithyroid medications.
➤ Myxedema coma results from either primary or secondary hypothyroidism. It progresses slowly and gradually.
➤ Causes of myxedema coma include pituitary failure to produce TSH, hypothalamic failure, chronic autoimmune thyroiditis (*Hashimoto's disease*), amyloidosis and sarcoidosis, an inability to synthesize hormone, use of antithyroid medications, postthyroidectomy effects, and postradiation effects.
➤ Myxedema coma is precipitated by infection, exposure to cold, or sedative use.
➤ Cellular metabolism decreases to a fatal level in untreated myxedema coma.

➤ *Pheochromocytoma*

Pheochromocytoma is a chromaffin-cell tumor of the adrenal medulla that secretes an excess of the catecholamines epinephrine and norepinephrine, which results in severe hypertension, increased metabolism, and hyperglycemia. This disorder is potentially fatal, but the prognosis is generally good with treatment. Pheochromocytoma-induced kidney damage is irreversible.

Rapid assessment

➤ Assess the patient's vital signs, noting persistent or paroxysmal hypertension and orthostatic hypotension, tachypnea, and tachycardia.
➤ Obtain the patient's history; inquire about headache, dizziness, lightheadedness, palpitations, visual blurring, nausea, vomiting, feelings of impending doom, and abdominal pain.
➤ Observe the patient for severe diaphoresis and pallor or flushing.
➤ Observe the patient for tremors or seizures.
➤ Palpate for moist, cool hands and feet.

➤ Palpate for the tumor.

 ALERT *The tumor is rarely palpable; when it is, palpation of the surrounding area may induce an acute attack and help confirm the diagnosis.*

Immediate actions
➤ Provide supplemental oxygen and prepare the patient for endotracheal intubation and mechanical ventilation, if necessary.
➤ Initiate safety and seizure precautions.
➤ Administer I.V. phentolamine (push or drip) to normalize blood pressure and nitroprusside to decrease blood pressure.

Follow-up actions
➤ Monitor the patient's vital signs frequently.
➤ Monitor blood glucose levels.
➤ Prepare the patient for a 24-hour urine collection to test for increased excretion of total free catecholamines and their metabolites, vanillylmandelic acid and metanephrine.

 ALERT *To ensure the reliability of this test, instruct the patient to avoid foods high in vanillin, such as coffee, nuts, chocolate, and bananas, for 2 days before urine collection.*

➤ Prepare the patient for a clonidine suppression test, which will cause decreased plasma catecholamine levels in normal patients but don't change in those with pheochromocytoma.
➤ The patient may also require a computed tomography scan or magnetic resonance imaging of the abdomen or 131-I metaiodobenzylguanidine nuclear scan to confirm the diagnosis.
➤ If the patient will undergo surgical removal of the tumor, administer preoperative alpha-adrenergic blockers or metyrosine for 1 to 2 weeks before surgery and beta-adrenergic blockers (propranolol) after achieving alpha blockade.
➤ Postoperatively, monitor for hypertension due to the stress of surgery and manipulation of the adrenal glands, which stimulate catecholamine secretion.
➤ Monitor the patient for hypotension and treat with I.V. fluids, plasma volume expanders, vasopressors and, possibly, transfusions.
➤ Provide a quiet, calm environment.
➤ Check dressings and monitor the patient's vital signs for indication of hemorrhage.
➤ Administer analgesics.

Preventive steps
➤ Pheochromocytoma can't be prevented.
➤ Suggest genetic counseling if autosomal dominant transmission of pheochromocytoma is suspected.

Pathophysiology recap

- Pheochromocytoma may result from an inherited autosomal dominant trait.
- The tumor is usually benign, but may be malignant in 10% of patients.
- Pheochromocytoma stems from a chromaffin-cell tumor in the adrenal medulla (more commonly in the right adrenal medulla than the left) or sympathetic ganglia.
- Similar tumors in the abdomen, thorax, bladder, neck, and near the ninth and tenth cranial nerves are called extra-adrenal pheochromocytomas.
- Epinephrine overproduction occurs with adrenal pheochromocytomas; norepinephrine overproduction occurs with adrenal or extra-adrenal pheochromocytomas.
- Pheochromocytoma produces complications similar to severe, persistent hypertension: stroke, retinopathy, heart disease, and kidney damage.
- Attacks may be caused by the shifting of abdominal contents and increased pressure on the tumor during heavy lifting, exercise, bladder distention, or pregnancy.
- Administration of opioids, histamine, glucagon, and corticotropin may precipitate a severe crisis.

➤ Syndrome of inappropriate antidiuretic hormone

Syndrome of inappropriate antidiuretic hormone (SIADH) is a complication of surgery or critical illness. It results in high sodium levels, fluid shifts into the cells, and thirst.

Rapid assessment

- Assess the patient's vital signs, noting tachycardia.
- Obtain the patient's history; inquire about excessive thirst, anorexia, nausea, and vomiting, as well as weight gain.
- Assess the patient for neurologic changes, such as lethargy, headache, and emotional and behavioral changes.
- Test for decreased deep tendon reflexes.
- Assess the patient for signs of increased fluid volume (crackles, dyspnea, and jugular vein distention).
- Obtain an electrocardiogram and assess for arrhythmias.

Immediate actions

- Initiate and maintain safety precautions.
- Obtain a serum sodium sample (which will reflect hyponatremia).
- Restrict fluid intake to 500 to 1,000 ml/day.
- Initiate continuous cardiac monitoring.

➤ *WHAT HAPPENS IN SIADH*

This flowchart shows the events that occur in syndrome of inappropriate anti-diuretic hormone (SIADH).

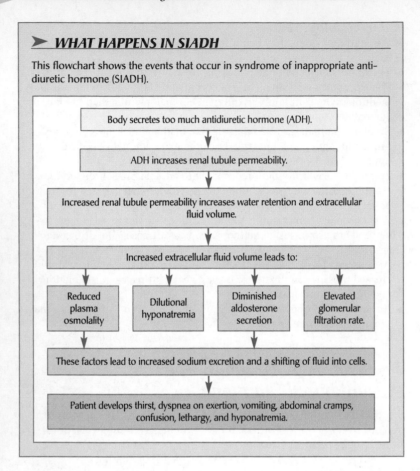

Body secretes too much antidiuretic hormone (ADH).

⬇

ADH increases renal tubule permeability.

⬇

Increased renal tubule permeability increases water retention and extracellular fluid volume.

⬇

Increased extracellular fluid volume leads to:

⬇   ⬇   ⬇   ⬇

| Reduced plasma osmolality | Dilutional hyponatremia | Diminished aldosterone secretion | Elevated glomerular filtration rate. |

These factors lead to increased sodium excretion and a shifting of fluid into cells.

⬇

Patient develops thirst, dyspnea on exertion, vomiting, abdominal cramps, confusion, lethargy, and hyponatremia.

➤ Administer 200 to 300 ml of 3% to 5% sodium chloride solution, followed by loop diuretics (usually furosemide).

 ALERT *Avoid rapid administration of hypertonic saline to prevent volume overload and pulmonary edema.*

➤ Monitor the patient's vital signs frequently.
➤ Monitor intake and output.
➤ Weigh the patient daily.
➤ Monitor serum osmolality, urine sodium, and serum antidiuretic hormone (ADH) level.

Preventive steps
➤ Initiate prompt, aggressive treatment of causative disorders.

Pathophysiology recap
➤ In SIADH, excessive secretion of ADH leads to water retention.
➤ Fluid shifts cause decreased serum osmolality. (See *What happens in SIADH.*)
➤ SIADH may result from oat-cell lung cancer, which secretes ADH or a vasopressor-like substance that the body responds to as if ADH were secreted.
➤ Other neoplastic diseases that can lead to SIADH include Hodgkin's disease, thymoma, and pancreatic, brain, and prostate tumors.
➤ Brain abscess, stroke, Guillain-Barré syndrome, and pulmonary disorders can also lead to SIADH.
➤ Medications, such as chlorpropamide, tolbutamide, vincristine, cyclophosphamide, haloperidol, carbamazepine, clofibrate, morphine, and thiazides, can also cause SIADH.
➤ Adrenal insufficiency and anterior pituitary insufficiency can lead to SIADH.

➤ Thyroid storm

Thyroid storm, also called *thyrotoxic crisis,* is a life-threatening emergency in a patient with hyperthyroidism. It may be the initial symptom in a patient with hyperthyroidism that hasn't been diagnosed.

Rapid assessment
➤ Assess the patient's vital signs, noting tachycardia and fever.

 ALERT *Fever, typically above 100.4° F (38° C), begins insidiously and rises rapidly to a lethal level.*

➤ Observe the patient for irritability, restlessness, and stupor.
➤ Obtain the patient's history; inquire about angina, shortness of breath, heat intolerance, vomiting, and visual disturbances such as diplopia.
➤ Assess the patient for muscle weakness, tremors, and swollen extremities.
➤ Observe for a cough.
➤ Palpate for an enlarged thyroid gland.
➤ Obtain an electrocardiogram and assess for arrhythmias.

Immediate actions
➤ Initiate safety measures.
➤ Prepare the patient for endotracheal intubation and mechanical ventilation, if necessary.
➤ Institute continuous cardiac monitoring.
➤ Perform cooling measures such as using the hypothermia blanket.
➤ Administer beta-adrenergic blockers, propylthiouracil and methimazole to block thyroid hormone synthesis, antipyretics and, possibly, cortico-

steroids to block conversion of triiodothyronine (T3) to thyroxine (T4). Avoid aspirin because salicylates block binding of T3 and T4.

Follow-up actions
➤Monitor the patient's vital signs closely.
➤Monitor serum T_3 and T_4 levels (elevated initially) and the thyroid-stimulating hormone (TSH) level (decreased initially).
➤Monitor electrolyte levels and treat abnormalities.
➤Watch for hyperglycemia; excessive thyroid activity can lead to glycogenolysis.
➤Provide a quiet environment.
➤Prepare the patient for radioisotope scanning to test for increased uptake and a computed tomography scan or magnetic resonance imaging to reveal an underlying cause such as a pituitary lesion.

Preventive steps
➤Initiate prompt, aggressive treatment of causative disorders.
➤Advise patients to practice good hygiene, including thorough handwashing, to prevent infection.
➤Counsel patients about the importance of careful management of hyperthyroidism.

Pathophysiology recap
➤The onset is almost always abrupt and evoked by a stressful event, such as trauma, surgery, or infection.
➤Other causes include metastatic carcinoma of the thyroid, a pituitary tumor that secretes TSH, and diabetic ketoacidosis.
➤It develops because of a surge of thyroid hormones.
➤Hyperthyroidism can result from genetic or immunologic factors.
➤Grave's disease is the most common form of hyperthyroidism. It's an autoimmune process in which the body manufactures an antibody similar to TSH and the thyroid responds to it.
➤Overproduction of T_3 and T_4 increases adrenergic activity.
➤Severe hypermetabolism results, which can rapidly lead to cardiac, sympathetic nervous system, and GI collapse.

8
Obstetric and gynecologic emergencies

➤ *Abruptio placentae*

In abruptio placentae, or *placental abruption,* the placenta prematurely separates from the uterine wall (usually after 20 weeks' gestation), resulting in hemorrhage. It may be mild, moderate, or severe. Abruptio placentae is most common in multigravida females older than age 35 and is a typical cause of bleeding during the second half of pregnancy. The condition may necessitate termination of the pregnancy. Fetal prognosis depends on gestational age and amount of blood lost; maternal prognosis is good if hemorrhage is controlled.

Rapid assessment
➤For all types of abruptio placentae, obtain maternal vital signs, noting hypotension and tachycardia, and the patient's history.

In mild abruptio placentae:
➤Assess for mild to moderate bleeding.
➤Obtain the patient's history; inquire about vague lower abdominal discomfort, mild to moderate abdominal tenderness, and uterine irritability.
➤Auscultate for fetal heart tones.

In moderate abruptio placentae:
➤Obtain the patient's history; inquire about continuous abdominal pain.
➤Assess for moderate, dark-red vaginal bleeding.
➤Palpate for a tender uterus that remains firm between contractions.
➤Auscultate for fetal heart tones (may be barely audible or irregular and bradycardic).
➤Watch for rapidly progressing labor within the next 2 hours.

In severe abruptio placentae:
➤Obtain the patient's history; inquire about agonizing, unremitting uterine pain described as tearing or knifelike.
➤Palpate for a boardlike, tender uterus.
➤Assess for moderate vaginal bleeding.
➤Auscultate for fetal heart tones, which may be absent at this stage. (See *Degrees of placental separation in abruptio placentae,* page 260.)

> ## DEGREES OF PLACENTAL SEPARATION IN ABRUPTIO PLACENTAE

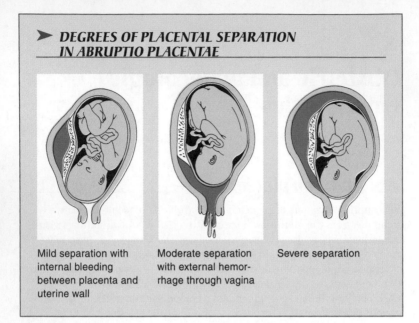

| Mild separation with internal bleeding between placenta and uterine wall | Moderate separation with external hemorrhage through vagina | Severe separation |

Immediate actions

➤ Start a large-bore I.V. line and administer normal saline solution or lactated Ringer's to combat hypovolemia.
➤ Provide supplemental oxygen and monitor oxygen saturation.
➤ Insert an indwelling urinary catheter.
➤ Obtain serum samples for complete blood count (CBC), coagulation studies, and typing and crossmatching.
➤ Initiate external fetal monitoring. (See *Managing abruptio placentae*.)

Follow-up actions

➤ Monitor maternal vital signs and fetal heart rate frequently.
➤ Assist with central venous catheter insertion to monitor central venous pressure as an indicator of fluid balance.
➤ Assist with a vaginal speculum examination, if necessary.
➤ Prepare the patient for ultrasonography.
➤ Prepare the patient for cesarean delivery if the fetus is in distress. (See *Fetal distress*, page 263.)

 ALERT *Because of possible fetal blood loss through the placenta, a pediatric team should be ready at delivery to assess and treat the neonate for shock, blood loss, and hypoxia.*

➤ Monitor CBC for decreased hemoglobin level, hematocrit, and platelets.
➤ Monitor serum studies for fibrin split products to detect disseminated intravascular coagulation.

IN ACTION

➤ *MANAGING ABRUPTIO PLACENTAE*

Kathleen Cramer, 38, who's 30 weeks' pregnant, arrives in your clinic complaining of sharp abdominal pains and vaginal spotting that started about an hour ago. She's pale, anxious, and slightly diaphoretic. You place her on a stretcher in a left-side-lying position and administer oxygen at 4 L/minute using a nasal cannula.

What's the situation?
Ms. Cramer's vital signs are blood pressure, 160/94 mm Hg; pulse, 112 beats/minute; respirations, 28 breaths/minute; and temperature, 100.9° F (37.3° C). Using an ultrasound device, you check the fetal heart rate; it's in the 160s (normal range is 120 to 160). Her abdomen is tender to touch and rigid. You notice a large amount of dark vaginal bleeding.

Ms. Cramer says she has one child and this is her second pregnancy. She hasn't sought medical care during this pregnancy. She takes no medications. Although she admits using crack cocaine in the past, she says she stopped when she found out she was pregnant.

What's your assessment?
Ms. Cramer's signs and symptoms and her history lead you to suspect abruptio placentae, or separation of a normally placed placenta from the uterine wall. If the separation is complete or occurs along the lower edge of the placenta, the patient will notice vaginal bleeding. If the placental separation is in the middle, the hemorrhage will be concealed.

Possible causes of abruptio placentae include maternal hypertension, trauma, diabetes, cocaine use, alcohol abuse, cigarette smoking, premature rupture of the amniotic sac, or an abnormally short umbilical cord that causes placental separation during birth. Other risk factors include advanced maternal age and retroplacental bleeding from a needle puncture such as during amniocentesis. Abruptio placentae can also occur spontaneously, without an identifiable cause.

Because of the risks — fetal anoxia or death and maternal hemorrhage, shock, or death — an emergency cesarean delivery is usually indicated.

What must you do immediately?
Immediately notify the obstetrician and arrange for Ms. Cramer to be transported to the labor and delivery (L&D) unit. Explain to Ms. Cramer what's happening and note the last time she ate or drank; withhold fluids and solids for surgery. Administer supplemental oxygen, start a large-bore I.V. line, and infuse lactated Ringer's or normal saline solution at 150 ml/hour. Obtain a fetal ultrasound immediately. Collect specimens for complete blood cell count, prothrombin time, partial thromboplastin time, fibrinogen level, fibrin split products, thrombin time, bleeding time, d-dimer, and typing and crossmatching. Insert an indwelling urinary catheter and send a urine sample for immediate urinalysis and a drug screen.

(continued)

> **MANAGING ABRUPTIO PLACENTAE** *(continued)*

The L&D nurse attaches Ms. Cramer to an external fetal/uterine monitor, which shows contractions every 2 to 3 minutes lasting 40 to 60 seconds each. The ultrasound shows placental separation. The fetal heart rate dropped into the 100s with the last contraction.

What should be done later?
The neonate, a male, is delivered via an emergency cesarean. He'll be monitored in the neonatal intensive care unit for problems related to prematurity and possible drug withdrawal. Ms. Cramer is transferred to the obstetric unit and will be monitored closely for such complications as hemorrhagic shock, coagulopathy, and uterine rupture.

To prevent abruptio placentae in future pregnancies, Ms. Cramer should be treated for hypertension, if indicated; assessed for possible domestic partner abuse; and encouraged to stop smoking and discontinue substance abuse. If Ms. Cramer has no complications, she and her son will be discharged home after 5 days.

Korby, J. "Action Stat: Abruptio Placentae," *Nursing* 34(2);96, February 2004. Used with permission.

> Monitor maternal intake and output, noting urine output.

 ALERT *Urine output of 30 ml/hour is a sign of impending renal failure.*

> Provide emotional support for the patient and her family.
> Contact spiritual support personnel, if necessary.

Preventive steps
> Instruct patients to avoid drinking alcohol, smoking, or using drugs during pregnancy.
> Encourage patients to obtain early and adequate prenatal care.
> Initiate prompt, aggressive treatment of preexisting and newly diagnosed conditions, such as diabetes and hypertension.

Pathophysiology recap
> Blood vessels at the placental bed rupture spontaneously due to a lack of resiliency or abnormal changes in uterine vasculature.
> Hypertension and an enlarged uterus complicate the condition because the uterus can't contract sufficiently to seal off torn vessels.
> Bleeding continues and the placenta sheers off partially or completely.
> Blood enters the muscle fibers.
> Complete relaxation of the uterus becomes impossible, increasing uterine tone and irritability.
> If bleeding is profuse, the accumulated blood prevents normal uterine contractions after delivery.

COMPLICATIONS

➤ *FETAL DISTRESS*

Usually discovered during late pregnancy or childbirth, fetal distress refers to indications that the fetus is deprived of oxygen, fatigued, or otherwise endangered. Potential causes of fetal distress include placental malfunction; strong contractions; maternal hypotension due to local or regional anesthesia, which, in turn, decreases oxygen supply to the fetus; and a pinched, kinked, or flattened umbilical cord.

Signs and symptoms
➤ Fetal tachycardia or bradycardia, especially during and after a contraction
➤ Decreased fetal movement as reported by the mother or as seen on a nonstress test
➤ Meconium staining of the amniotic fluid
➤ Fetal scalp blood samples that reveal fetal acidosis and elevated fetal blood lactate, indicating lactic acidosis

Treatment
Treatment includes:
➤ supplemental oxygen and I.V. fluids
➤ placing the mother in a left side-lying position to enhance blood flow to the fetus
➤ internal examination to determine whether the umbilical cord has dropped into the vagina
➤ discontinuation of oxytocin if it's being used to induce labor
➤ medication to relax the uterus
➤ immediate delivery.

Nursing considerations
➤ Monitor the mother's vital signs, including oxygen saturation.
➤ Maintain an internal or external fetal monitoring device.
➤ Provide emotional support.
➤ Allow the parents to verbalize their feelings.

➤ Predisposing factors include trauma (a direct blow to the uterus), placental site bleeding from a needle puncture during amniocentesis, chronic or pregnancy-induced hypertension, multiparity, smoking, and cocaine use.

➤ *Ectopic pregnancy*

An ectopic pregnancy is the implantation of the fertilized ovum outside the uterine cavity.

Rapid assessment

➤ Assess for enlarged breasts and a soft cervix (signs of pregnancy).

 ALERT *Be aware that the patient with an ectopic pregnancy may have no other symptoms other than mild abdominal pain, making diagnosis difficult.*

➤ In suspected fallopian tube implantation, obtain the patient's history; inquire about amenorrhea or abnormal menses, followed by slight vaginal bleeding, and unilateral pelvic pain on the suspected side.
   In suspected fallopian tube rupture:
➤ Assess the patient's vital signs, noting hypotension, tachycardia, tachypnea, and fever.
➤ Assess the patient for a rigid, boardlike abdomen, which may indicate peritonitis.
➤ Obtain the patient's history; inquire about sharp lower abdominal pain (possibly radiating to the shoulders and neck) that's typically precipitated by activities that increase abdominal pressure, such as lifting or a bowel movement.
➤ Perform a pelvic examination, assessing for extreme pain upon motion of the cervix and palpation of the adnexa.

Immediate actions

➤ Obtain a serum pregnancy test to detect human chorionic gonadotropin.
➤ Obtain a sample for hemoglobin level and hematocrit, noting decreased levels.
➤ Prepare the patient for ultrasonography to determine extrauterine pregnancy if the pregnancy test is positive.
➤ Administer analgesics.

Follow-up actions

➤ Monitor the patient's vital signs frequently.
➤ Monitor complete blood count values.
➤ Prepare the patient for culdocentesis to detect free or nonclotting blood in the peritoneum.
➤ Prepare the patient for laparoscopy or laparotomy to diagnose and treat an ectopic pregnancy.
➤ If the pregnancy is interstitial, prepare the patient for hysterectomy, if necessary.
➤ Provide the patient with emotional support and a quiet, relaxing environment.
➤ Administer transfusions of whole blood and packed red blood cells to replace excessive blood loss, broad-spectrum I.V. antibiotics for septic infection, and I.M. or oral iron supplements.
➤ If the patient's condition is stable, the ectopic pregnancy is in the fallopian tube and is very small, and surgery isn't required, give methotrexate as ordered.

➤ IMPLANTATION SITES OF ECTOPIC PREGNANCY

In 90% of patients with ectopic pregnancy, the ovum implants in the fallopian tube, either in the fimbria, ampulla, or isthmus. Other possible sites include the interstitium, tubo-ovarian ligament, ovary, abdominal viscera, and internal cervical os.

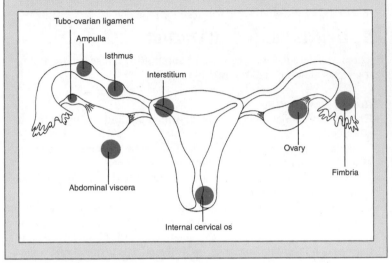

Preventive steps
➤ Advise patients to avoid risk factors for pelvic inflammatory disease (PID) which include multiple partners, sexual intercourse without a condom, and sexually transmitted diseases (STDs).
➤ Teach patients the importance of early diagnosis and prompt, aggressive treatment of STDs, salpingitis, and PID.

Pathophysiology recap
➤ Ectopic pregnancy occurs when passage of the fertilized ovum through the fallopian tube is prevented or slowed, causing the ovum to implant in the tube or outside the uterine cavity.
➤ The most common site for ectopic pregnancy is the fallopian tube; however, other sites include the interstitium, tubo-ovarian ligament, ovary, abdominal viscera, and internal cervical os. (See *Implantation sites of ectopic pregnancy.*)
➤ Ectopic pregnancy may result from congenital defects in the reproductive tract or ectopic endometrial implants in the tubal mucosa.
➤ The increased incidence of sexually transmitted tubal infection may be a factor.
➤ The prognosis is good with prompt diagnosis, appropriate surgical intervention, and control of bleeding.

➤Ectopic pregnancy may result from diverticula, the formation of blind pouches that cause tubal abnormalities.

➤Ectopic pregnancy may also occur due to endometriosis, endosalpingitis, PID, previous surgery (tubal ligation or resection, or adhesions from previous abdominal or pelvic surgery), or tumors pressing against the tube.

➤ *Hyperemesis gravidarum*

Hyperemesis gravidarum is severe and unremitting nausea and vomiting that persists after the first trimester of pregnancy.

Rapid assessment

➤Observe the patient for confusion, delirium, lassitude, stupor and, possibly, coma.

➤Observe the rate, pattern, and depth of the patient's spontaneous respirations, noting bradypnea and shallow respirations.

➤Assess the patient's vital signs, noting a subnormal or an elevated temperature and tachycardia.

➤Obtain the patient's history; inquire about headache, substantial weight loss, and unremitting nausea and vomiting. (The vomitus initially contains undigested food, mucus, and small amounts of bile; later it contains only bile and mucus; and, finally, blood and material that resembles coffee grounds.)

➤Assess the patient for emaciation, dry mucous membranes, and pale, dry, waxy, and possibly jaundiced skin.

➤Assess for a fetid, fruity breath odor from acidosis.

➤Obtain an electrocardiogram and assess for arrhythmias.

Immediate actions

➤Provide supplemental oxygen and prepare the patient for endotracheal intubation and mechanical ventilation, if necessary.

➤Administer I.V. fluids to treat dehydration and parenteral nutrition to maintain electrolyte balance and prevent starvation until the patient can eat.

Follow-up actions

➤Encourage the patient to eat and to remain upright for 45 minutes after eating to decrease reflux.

➤Progress the patient slowly to a clear liquid, than a full liquid diet and, finally, to small, frequent meals of high-protein solid foods.

➤Serve a midnight snack to help stabilize blood glucose levels.

➤Administer vitamin B supplements to help correct vitamin deficiency.

➤Provide emotional support and a quiet, relaxing environment.

Preventive steps

➤Hyperemesis gravidarum can't be prevented.

➤Teach patients methods to reduce vomiting, such as maintaining a healthy diet, getting adequate rest, managing stress, eating dry foods, decreasing liquid intake during meals, remaining upright after meals, eating soda crackers in the morning to prevent morning sickness, discontinuing iron supplements until the sickness subsides, and eating small, frequent meals.

Pathophysiology recap

➤The cause of hyperemesis gravidarum is unknown.

➤Hyperemesis gravidarum commonly affects females with conditions that produce high levels of human chorionic gonadotropin, such as hydatidiform mole or multiple pregnancy.

➤Other possible causes include pancreatitis, biliary tract disease, drug toxicity, inflammatory obstructive bowel disease, vitamin deficiency (especially vitamin B_6), and psychological factors such as ambivalence toward pregnancy.

➤ Ovarian cyst, rupture

An ovarian cyst is a fluid-filled mass. It develops on the ovary when an egg isn't released at ovulation and the follicle fills with fluid and grows in size, eventually weakening and rupturing.

Rapid assessment

➤Assess the patient's vital signs, noting fever, tachycardia, and hypotension.

➤Obtain the patient's history; inquire about nausea, vomiting, diarrhea, and severe, knifelike pelvic pain (indicates bleeding into the ovary or uterus).

➤Observe for tremors.

➤Assess for a rigid, boardlike abdomen or back pain, which may indicate internal bleeding.

Immediate actions

➤Prepare the patient for ultrasonography to visualize the ruptured cyst and fluid in the pelvic cavity behind the uterus.

➤Obtain serum samples for hemoglobin level and hematocrit to assess for internal bleeding.

➤Administer blood products, as necessary; I.V. fluids to treat hypovolemia; vasopressors to treat hypotension; and analgesics, as indicated.

➤Perform cooling measures; apply a hypothermia blanket, if necessary.

Follow-up actions

➤Monitor the patient's vital signs frequently.

➤ Monitor for decreased hemoglobin level and hematocrit.
➤ If the pain is subsiding, administer analgesics and continue to monitor pain levels.
➤ If pain doesn't improve in a few hours, prepare the patient for surgery (may include laparoscopy, cystectomy, oophorectomy, or hysterectomy).

Preventive steps
➤ Inform patients that hormonal contraceptives can decrease the size of existing cysts and help prevent new cysts from forming by preventing ovulation.

Pathophysiology recap
➤ The ovaries develop follicular cysts that are filled with a fluid that nourishes developing eggs.
➤ The fluid is usually absorbed into the pelvic cavity after ovulation.
➤ If the egg isn't released, the follicle fills with more fluid and enlarges.
➤ Eventually, the walls of the follicle may weaken and the fluid leaks out; the follicle ruptures.
➤ The fluid can irritate the pelvic lining and cause pain.
➤ Most ruptured cysts dissolve naturally over time, but some may continue to bleed.

➤ Placenta previa

In placenta previa, the placenta is implanted in the lower uterine segment, where it encroaches on the internal cervical os. It's one of the most common causes of bleeding in the second half of pregnancy and occurs in 1 in every 200 pregnancies, more commonly in multigravidas than in primigravidas.

 ALERT *Placenta previa — especially in females who have had one or more cesarean births — is associated with placenta accrete, a dangerous condition in which the placenta grows into the myometrium.*

Rapid assessment
➤ Obtain maternal vital signs, noting hypotension and tachycardia.
➤ Obtain the patient's history; inquire about painless third-trimester bleeding.
➤ Palpate for fetal activity.
➤ Auscultate for fetal heart tones.

Immediate actions
➤ Insert a large-bore I.V. line.
➤ Initiate external fetal monitoring.

➤ Obtain a serum sample for complete blood count and typing and cross-matching.
➤ Administer blood transfusions, as necessary.
➤ Prepare the patient for a transvaginal ultrasound scan to determine placental position.

Follow-up actions

➤ If the fetus is premature, expect to monitor the patient and fetus while allowing the fetus additional time to mature.
➤ If the examination reveals complete placenta previa, observe for signs of hemorrhage.
➤ Assist with a pelvic examination immediately before delivery to confirm the diagnosis.
➤ If the fetus is sufficiently mature, or in case of intervening severe hemorrhage, prepare the patient for immediate cesarean delivery.
➤ Prepare the patient for a vaginal delivery if the bleeding is minimal and the placenta previa is marginal or if the labor is rapid.
➤ Contact a pediatric team to be on hand during delivery because fetal blood loss through the placenta can cause neonatal shock, blood loss, and hypoxia.
➤ Provide emotional support.

Preventive steps

➤ Placenta previa isn't preventable.

Pathophysiology recap

➤ The placenta may cover all (total, complete, or central), part (partial or incomplete), or a fraction (marginal or low-lying) of the internal os. (See *Three types of placenta previa,* page 270.)
➤ The degree of placenta previa depends largely on the extent of cervical dilation at the time of examination because the dilating cervix gradually uncovers the placenta.
➤ The specific cause is unknown.
➤ Factors that may affect the site of the placenta's attachment to the uterine wall include defective vascularization of the decidua, multiple pregnancy (the placenta requires a larger surface for attachment), previous uterine surgery, multiparity, and advanced maternal age.
➤ The lower segment of the uterus fails to provide as much nourishment as the fundus does.
➤ The placenta spreads out, seeking the blood supply it needs, and becomes larger and thinner than normal.
➤ Eccentric insertion of the umbilical cord commonly develops for unknown reasons.
➤ Hemorrhage occurs as the internal cervical os effaces and dilates, tearing the uterine vessels.

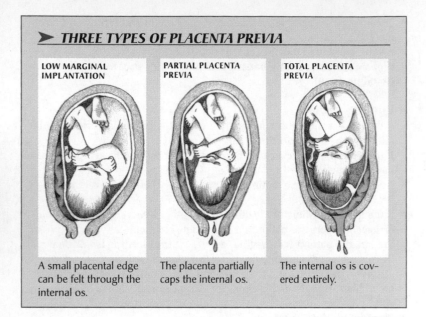

THREE TYPES OF PLACENTA PREVIA

LOW MARGINAL IMPLANTATION	PARTIAL PLACENTA PREVIA	TOTAL PLACENTA PREVIA
A small placental edge can be felt through the internal os.	The placenta partially caps the internal os.	The internal os is covered entirely.

➤ Generally, termination of pregnancy is necessary when the diagnosis is made in the presence of life-threatening maternal bleeding.
➤ Maternal prognosis is good if hemorrhage is controlled; fetal prognosis depends on gestational age and the amount of blood lost.

➤ *Pregnancy-induced hypertension*

Pregnancy-induced hypertension (PIH) is a potentially life-threatening disorder that usually develops late in the second trimester or in the third trimester. Preeclampsia is the nonconvulsive condition; it develops in about 7% of pregnancies. Eclampsia is the convulsive condition. About 5% of patients with preeclampsia develop eclampsia and, of these, 15% die from PIH or its complications.

Rapid assessment
➤ Assess fetal status by instituting electronic fetal monitoring.
  If the patient has mild preeclampsia:
➤ Assess maternal vital signs, noting a blood pressure of 140 mm Hg systolic or a rise of 30 mm Hg or greater above the patient's normal systolic pressure, measured on two occasions, at least 6 hours apart; or 90 mm Hg diastolic or a rise of 15 mm Hg or greater above the patient's normal diastolic pressure, measured on two occasions, at least 6 hours apart.
➤ Assess for generalized edema and sudden weight gain of more than 3 lb (1.4 kg) per week during the second trimester or more than 1 lb (0.5 kg) per week during the third trimester.

➤ Test a urine sample for proteinuria.
  If the patient has severe preeclampsia:
➤ Assess maternal vital signs, noting a blood pressure of 160/110 mm Hg or higher on two occasions, at least 6 hours apart on bed rest, with the patient lying on her left side.
➤ Test a urine sample for proteinuria.
➤ Obtain the patient's history; inquire about oliguria, severe frontal headache, and epigastric pain or heartburn. Also, ask about blurred vision and perform ophthalmoscopic examination to observe for retinal arteriolar spasms.
➤ Assess for hyperactive deep tendon reflexes.
  If the patient has eclampsia:
➤ Assess for the signs and symptoms of preeclampsia.
➤ Observe for seizures and coma.
➤ Assess for signs of premature labor.
➤ Perform ophthalmoscopic examination (may reveal vascular spasm, papilledema, retinal edema or detachment, and arteriovenous nicking or hemorrhage).

Immediate actions
➤ Provide supplemental oxygen, if necessary.
➤ Place the patient in a left lateral position to increase venous return, cardiac output, and renal blood flow.
➤ Initiate safety measures and seizure precautions.
➤ Administer magnesium sulfate and maintain strict bed rest to produce an anticonvulsant effect, relieve anxiety, and reduce hypertension.

 ALERT *Antihypertensive therapy doesn't alter the potential for developing eclampsia, and diuretics aren't appropriate during pregnancy.*

➤ If the patient has mild preeclampsia, initiate a 24-hour hour urine collection to measure protein (which will be more than 300 mg but less than 5 g/24 hours).
➤ If the patient has severe preeclampsia, initiate a 24-hour urine collection to measure protein (which will be more than 5 g/24 hours).

 ALERT *Monitor the patient with severe preeclampsia for HELLP syndrome, a severe variant that includes Hemolysis, Elevated Liver enzymes, and Low Platelets.*

  If the patient has eclampsia:
➤ Monitor for increased blood urea nitrogen and creatinine levels and intake and output for indications of renal failure (urine output of 400 ml/24 hours or less).
➤ Monitor for increased liver enzymes, which indicate liver failure.
➤ If the patient has seizures, administer oxygen; also administer magnesium sulfate via I.V. drip.

Follow-up actions
- Assess maternal vital signs and electronic fetal monitoring frequently.
- Assess for absence of patellar reflexes (may indicate magnesium sulfate toxicity).

 ALERT *Keep calcium gluconate at the bedside for administration to counteract the toxic effects of magnesium sulfate.*

- Prepare the patient for ultrasonography to evaluate fetal health.
- Prepare the patient for stress and nonstress tests to evaluate fetal status.
- Measure intake and output.
- If the hypertension doesn't respond to bed rest and sedation and rises over 160/100 mm Hg, or if central nervous system irritability increases or seizures develop, prepare the patient for cesarean delivery or oxytocin induction to deliver the fetus or terminate the pregnancy.

 ALERT *Depending on the gestational age of the fetus and its potential statistical viability, a decision will be made to deliver the fetus or terminate the pregnancy. If a delivery is possible, notify the pediatric emergency team and place them on standby.*

- Provide emotional support.

Preventive steps
- Instruct patients to obtain adequate nutrition as well as early and regular prenatal care and to control preexisting hypertension during pregnancy.
- Early recognition and prompt treatment of preeclampsia can prevent progression to eclampsia.

Pathophysiology recap
- The cause of PIH is unknown.
- Geographic, ethnic, racial, nutritional, immunologic, familial factors, preexisting vascular disease, and maternal age over 35 may contribute to the development of PIH.
- Neonates of mothers with PIH are usually small for gestational age but sometimes fare better than other premature neonates of the same weight, possibly because they developed adaptive responses to stress in utero.

➤ *Premature labor*

Premature labor, also called *preterm labor,* is the onset of rhythmic uterine contractions that produce cervical change after fetal viability but before fetal maturity. It usually occurs between 20 and 37 weeks' gestation.

Rapid assessment
➤ Observe the rate, depth, and pattern of the patient's spontaneous respirations, noting hyperventilation.
➤ Obtain a prenatal history.
➤ Assess for rhythmic uterine contractions.
➤ Assess the fetus's status through electronic fetal monitoring.
➤ Assess the position of the fetus in relation to the mother's pelvis.
➤ Assist with a vaginal examination and assess for progressive cervical effacement and dilation and rupture of the membranes.
➤ Observe for the cervical mucus plug and for bloody discharge.

Immediate actions
➤ Administer oxygen.
➤ Prevent maternal hyperventilation by using a rebreathing bag.
➤ Place the patient in a left lateral position to prevent vena cava compression, which can cause supine hypotension and subsequent fetal hypoxia.
➤ Suppress premature labor if tests show immature fetal pulmonary development and if cervical dilation is less than 4 cm and the patient doesn't exhibit factors that contraindicate continuation of pregnancy.
➤ Maintain bed rest.
➤ Administer beta-adrenergic stimulants to inhibit uterine contractions.

 ALERT *Adverse effects of beta-adrenergic stimulants include maternal tachycardia and hypotension and fetal tachycardia.*

➤ Give magnesium sulfate to relax the muscle of the myometrium.

 ALERT *Monitor for maternal adverse effects of magnesium sulfate administration, which include drowsiness, slurred speech, flushing, decreased reflexes, decreased GI motility, and decreased respirations. Fetal and neonatal adverse effects may include central nervous system depression, decreased respirations, and decreased sucking reflex.*

➤ If the patient has an infection, abruptio placentae, placental insufficiency, or severe preeclampsia, prepare her for premature delivery.

Follow-up actions
➤ Assess maternal vital signs and electronic fetal monitoring frequently.
➤ Provide comfort measures, such as frequent repositioning and good perineal and back care.

 ALERT *Give sedatives and analgesics sparingly, staying mindful of their potentially harmful effects on the fetus.*

➤ Offer emotional support.
➤ In the event of a delivery, contact the prenatal intensive care team.

Preventive steps

> ➤ Advise patients to obtain early and regular prenatal care, adequate nutrition, and proper rest.
> ➤ Some patients may require insertion of a purse-string (cerclage) to reinforce an incompetent cervix at 14 to 16 weeks' gestation.

Pathophysiology recap

> ➤ About 5% to 10% of pregnancies end prematurely.
> ➤ About 75% of neonatal deaths and a great many birth defects stem from premature labor.
> ➤ Fetal prognosis depends on birth weight and length of gestation: neonates weighing less than 1 lb 10 oz (750 g) and of less than 26 weeks' gestation have a survival rate of 40% to 50%; neonates weighing 1 lb 10 oz to 2 lb 3 oz (750 to 1,000 g) and of 27 to 28 weeks' gestation have a survival rate of 70% to 80%; those weighing 2 lb 3 oz to 2 lb 11 oz (1,000 to 1,250 g) and of 28 weeks' gestation have an 85% to 97% survival rate.
> ➤ Possible causes of premature labor include:
>   – premature rupture of the membranes (30% to 50% of premature labor cases)
>   – preeclampsia
>   – chronic hypertensive vascular disease
>   – hydramnios
>   – multiple pregnancy
>   – placenta previa
>   – abruptio placentae
>   – incompetent cervix
>   – abdominal surgery
>   – trauma
>   – structural anomalies of the uterus
>   – infections, such as rubella and toxoplasmosis
>   – congenital adrenal hyperplasia
>   – fetal death.
> ➤ Premature labor may also result from fetal stimulation, as when genetically imprinted information tells the fetus that nutrition is inadequate and a change in environment is required for well-being, which provokes the onset of labor.
> ➤ If the myometrium becomes hypersensitive to oxytocin, the hormone that normally induces uterine contractions, premature labor may occur.
> ➤ In myometrial oxygen deficiency, the fetus becomes increasingly proficient in obtaining oxygen, depriving the myometrium of the oxygen and energy it needs to function normally, thereby irritating the myometrium and triggering premature labor.
> ➤ Maternal genetics may also play a role if a genetic defect in the mother shortens gestation.

➤ *Premature rupture of the membranes*

Premature rupture of the membranes is a spontaneous break or tear in the amniochorial sac before the onset of regular contractions, resulting in progressive cervical dilation. It occurs in nearly 10% of all pregnancies over 20 weeks' gestation, and labor usually starts within 24 hours; more than 80% of these neonates are mature.

Rapid assessment
➤ Observe for blood-tinged amniotic fluid containing vernix particles gushing or leaking from the vagina.
➤ Assess fetal status by observing electronic fetal monitoring or auscultating fetal heart rate.
➤ Determine the fetus's gestational age using the date of the last menstrual period or ultrasound aging.
➤ Palpate (using Leopold's maneuver) to assess for fetal presentation and size.
➤ Assess for signs of maternal infection, such as fever, foul-smelling vaginal discharge, and fetal tachycardia.
➤ Determine whether the fluid is amniotic fluid by treating nitrazine paper with a sample of fluid from the posterior fornix and observing for color change (paper turns blue with alkaline pH).
➤ A smear of fluid can also be placed on a slide and allowed to dry; amniotic fluid will dry in a fernlike pattern due to high sodium and protein content.

Immediate actions
➤ With a term pregnancy, await spontaneous labor.
➤ Obtain samples for a lecithin/sphingomyelin ratio and a foam stability test (shake test) to determine fetal pulmonary maturity.
➤ With a preterm pregnancy of 28 to 34 weeks when infection is suspected, prepare the patient for induction of labor and administer I.V. antibiotics.

 ALERT *A culture should be made of gastric aspirate or a swabbing from the infant's ear because antibiotic therapy may be indicated for the neonate as well. At such a delivery, have resuscitative equipment available to treat neonatal distress.*

➤ Prepare the patient for a cesarean hysterectomy if a gross uterine infection is present.

Follow-up actions
➤ Assess maternal vital signs and electronic fetal monitoring frequently.
➤ Make sure that the patient doesn't engage in sexual intercourse or douche after membranes rupture.

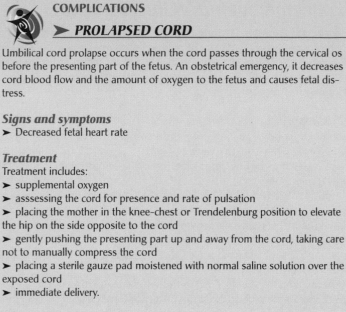

COMPLICATIONS

➤ PROLAPSED CORD

Umbilical cord prolapse occurs when the cord passes through the cervical os before the presenting part of the fetus. An obstetrical emergency, it decreases cord blood flow and the amount of oxygen to the fetus and causes fetal distress.

Signs and symptoms
➤ Decreased fetal heart rate

Treatment
Treatment includes:
➤ supplemental oxygen
➤ asssessing the cord for presence and rate of pulsation
➤ placing the mother in the knee-chest or Trendelenburg position to elevate the hip on the side opposite to the cord
➤ gently pushing the presenting part up and away from the cord, taking care not to manually compress the cord
➤ placing a sterile gauze pad moistened with normal saline solution over the exposed cord
➤ immediate delivery.

Nursing considerations
➤ Monitor maternal vital signs.
➤ Maintain internal or external fetal monitoring.
➤ Provide emotional support; allow the parents to verbalize their feelings.

➤ Monitor the patient for a prolapsed cord. (See *Prolapsed cord.*)
➤ In term pregnancy without suspected infection, if spontaneous labor and vaginal delivery haven't occurred within 24 hours, prepare the patient for induction of labor with oxytocin or cesarean delivery if induction fails.
➤ When infection is suspected, obtain a sample of amniotic fluid for culture and Gram stain to determine the infectious organism.
➤ Provide emotional support.

Preventive steps
➤ Advise patients to obtain adequate nutrition and avoiding cigarette smoking during pregnancy.

Pathophysiology recap
➤ The latent period (between membrane rupture and onset of labor) is generally brief when the membranes rupture near term. If the pregnancy isn't near term, this period is prolonged, which increases the risk of mortality from maternal infection (amnionitis and endometritis), fetal infection (pneumonia and septicemia), and prematurity.
➤ The cause is unknown.

➤ Malpresentation and a contracted pelvis commonly accompany the rupture.
➤ Predisposing factors include infection (including uterine infection), an
incompetent cervix, smoking, poor nutrition and hygiene, lack of proper prenatal care, increased intrauterine tension due to hydramnios or
multiple pregnancies, and defects in the amniochorial membranes' ten-
sile strength.

➤ Toxic shock syndrome

Toxic shock syndrome (TSS) is an acute bacterial infection. It primarily affects menstruating females younger than age 30 and is associated with
continuous use of tampons during the menstrual period.

Rapid assessment
➤ Observe the patient's rate, depth, and pattern of spontaneous respira-
tions, noting tachypnea or shallow respirations.
➤ Assess the patient for a decreased level of consciousness and rigors.
➤ Assess the patient's vital signs, noting a fever over 104° F (40° C), tachy-
cardia, and severe hypotension, which are indicators of hypovolemic
shock.
➤ Obtain the patient's history; inquire about intense myalgia, vomiting, di-
arrhea, and headache.
➤ Observe for vaginal hyperemia and discharge.
➤ Assess for conjunctival hyperemia and a red rash, especially on the
palms and soles.

Immediate actions
➤ Provide supplemental oxygen and prepare the patient for endotracheal
intubation and mechanical ventilation, if necessary.
➤ Initiate safety measures.
➤ Initiate fever-reducing methods, such as a hypothermia blanket, if necessary.
➤ Obtain samples of vaginal discharge or swabs of vaginal lesions for culture and Gram stain.
➤ Administer I.V. beta-lactamase–resistant antistaphylococcal antibiotics,
normal saline solution to treat hypotension and shock, colloids to treat
hypovolemia, and antipyretics.

Follow-up actions
➤ Monitor the patient's vital signs frequently.
➤ Ensure that the patient doesn't use tampons.
➤ Practice strict infection control precautions.
➤ Obtain a sample to determine creatine kinase level, which will be in-
creased initially.

➤ *TOXIC SHOCK SYNDROME: HOW IT HAPPENS*

Toxic shock syndrome is an acute bacterial infection caused by toxin-producing, penicillin-resistant strains of *Staphylococcus aureus*. It's primarily associated with continuous use of tampons during the menstrual period, although some cases unrelated to tampon use have been reported. Toxin-producing bacterial pathogens are introduced into the vagina by way of contaminated fingers or tampon applicator, and the menstrual flow provides a medium for bacterial growth.

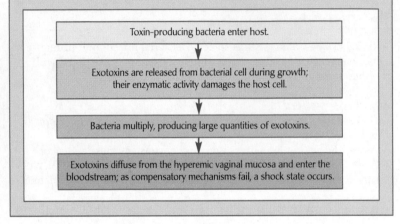

Toxin-producing bacteria enter host.

⬇

Exotoxins are released from bacterial cell during growth; their enzymatic activity damages the host cell.

⬇

Bacteria multiply, producing large quantities of exotoxins.

⬇

Exotoxins diffuse from the hyperemic vaginal mucosa and enter the bloodstream; as compensatory mechanisms fail, a shock state occurs.

➤ Monitor for increased blood urea nitrogen and creatinine levels and liver enzymes (indicate renal and hepatic involvement, respectively).

Preventive steps
➤ Advise all patients to avoid the continuous use of tampons during menstrual periods.
➤ Stress the need for thorough hand washing before insertion and removal of tampons, diaphragms, or contraceptive sponges.
➤ Advise patients who have had TSS to avoid tampons completely.
➤ Instruct patients about careful and minimal use of diaphragms and sponges.
➤ Provide meticulous postoperative wound care.

Pathophysiology recap
➤ TSS is caused by toxin-producing, penicillin-resistant strains of *Staphylococcus aureus,* such as TSS toxin-1 and staphylococcal enterotoxins B and C. (See *Toxic shock syndrome: How it happens.*)
➤ Tampons contribute to the development of TSS by introducing *S. aureus* into the vagina during insertion, absorbing toxins from the vagina, traumatizing the vaginal mucosa during insertion (leading to infection), and providing a favorable environment for the growth of *S. aureus.*
➤ The withdrawal of high-absorbency tampons from the market since the 1980s has decreased the incidence of TSS.

9
Genitourinary emergencies

➤ *Acute poststreptococcal glomerulonephritis*

Acute poststreptococcal glomerulonephritis (APSGN), also known as *acute glomerulonephritis,* is a relatively common bilateral inflammation of the glomeruli.

Rapid assessment
➤ Assess the patient's vital signs, noting mild to severe hypertension from sodium or water retention (due to a decreased glomerular filtration rate [GFR]) or inappropriate renin release.
➤ Obtain the patient's history; inquire about oliguria (less than 400 ml/ 24 hours), fatigue, and incidence of untreated pharyngitis within the preceding 1 to 3 weeks.
➤ Assess for mild to moderate edema.
➤ Test for proteinuria and observe and test for hematuria.
➤ In children, observe for seizures and focal neurologic deficits.

 ALERT *Hypervolemia associated with APSGN can lead to heart failure and pulmonary edema.*

Immediate actions
➤ Initiate bed rest.
➤ Initiate fluid restriction.
➤ Obtain a blood sample to measure creatinine, blood urea nitrogen (BUN), and electrolyte levels.
➤ Administer diuretics to reduce extracellular fluid overload and anti-hypertensives.
➤ If staphylococcal or streptococcal infection is confirmed, give antibiotics for 7 to 10 days.
➤ Provide electrolyte supplementation.

Follow-up actions
➤ Monitor the patient's vital signs frequently.
➤ Assess renal function through BUN and creatinine level analysis.
➤ Monitor intake and output.
➤ Watch the patient for signs of acute renal failure—oliguria, azotemia, and acidosis.

➤ Monitor electrolyte levels and treat abnormalities.
➤ Obtain a throat culture to detect group A beta-hemolytic streptococcus.
➤ Prepare the patient for renal ultrasound, renal biopsy, or dialysis (rare), if necessary.
➤ Provide a diet high in calories and low in protein, sodium, and potassium; maintain fluid restriction.
➤ Make sure that health care providers prevent secondary infection by using good hygienic technique when examining or caring for the patient.
➤ Instruct the patient to resume activity gradually after the acute phase of the disease.
➤ Provide emotional support.

Preventive steps
➤ Counsel patients to seek prompt, aggressive treatment of streptococcal infections.

Pathophysiology recap
➤ APSGN results from the entrapment and collection of antigen-antibody (produced as an immunologic mechanism in response to streptococcus) in the glomerular capillary membranes.
➤ This entrapment induces inflammatory damage and impedes glomerular function.
➤ The immune complex can also damage the glomerular membrane.
➤ The damaged and inflamed glomerulus loses the ability to be selectively permeable and allows red blood cells and proteins to filter through as the GFR falls.
➤ Uremic poisoning may result.
➤ APSGN usually follows a streptococcal infection of the respiratory tract or, less commonly, a skin infection such as impetigo.
➤ APSGN is most common in males ages 3 to 7, but can occur at any age.
➤ Up to 95% of children and up to 70% of adults with APSGN recover fully, usually within 2 weeks; the rest may progress to chronic renal failure within months.

➤ *Acute pyelonephritis*

Acute pyelonephritis, also known as *acute infective tubulointerstitial nephritis,* is a sudden inflammation caused by bacteria that primarily affects the interstitial area and renal pelvis or, less commonly, the renal tubules.

Rapid assessment
➤ Assess the patient's vital signs, noting a temperature of 102° F (38.9° C) or higher and shaking chills.
➤ Obtain the patient's history; inquire about flank pain, anorexia, general fatigue, dysuria, nocturia, urinary urgency and frequency, and burning during urination.

ALERT *Although these symptoms may disappear within days, even without treatment, residual bacterial infection is likely and may cause symptoms to recur later.*

➤ Observe for gross hematuria or cloudy urine with an ammonia-like or fishy odor.
➤ In elderly patients, observe for GI or pulmonary signs and symptoms.
➤ In children younger than age 2, assess for fever, vomiting, nonspecific abdominal complaints, or failure to thrive.

Immediate actions
➤ Obtain a urine sample and test for hematuria, leukocytes in clumps, casts, low specific gravity and osmolality, alkaline pH, proteinuria, glycosuria, and ketonuria.
➤ Obtain a sterile urine sample for culture.
➤ Administer antibiotics (appropriate to the infecting organism if known or broad spectrum until identified) for 10 to 14 days.
➤ Give urinary analgesics, such as phenazopyridine, and antipyretics for fever.
➤ Administer I.V. fluids to achieve urine output of more than 2,000 ml/day to help empty the bladder of contaminated urine.

ALERT *Don't encourage the intake of more than 2 to 3 qt (2 to 3 L) of fluid because this may decrease the effectiveness of the antibiotics.*

Follow-up actions
➤ Prepare the patient for a computed tomography scan.
➤ Reculture a urine sample 1 week after drug therapy stops, and periodically for the next year to detect residual or recurring infection.
➤ Provide an acid-ash diet to prevent stone formation.

ALERT *It's important to perform follow-up care on patients with acute pyelonephritis, because it can lead to chronic pyelonephritis. (See* Chronic pyelonephritis, *page 282.)*

➤ In infection from obstruction or vesicoureteral reflux, prepare the patient for surgery, if necessary.

Preventive steps
➤ Observe strict sterile technique during catheter insertion and care.
➤ Instruct females to prevent bacterial contamination by wiping the perineum from front to back after defecation.
➤ Advise routine checkups for patients with a history of urinary tract infections. Teach them to recognize signs of infection — such as cloudy urine, burning on urination, urgency, and frequency — especially when accompanied by a low-grade fever.

> ## CHRONIC PYELONEPHRITIS

Persistent kidney inflammation in chronic pyelonephritis can scar the kidneys and may lead to chronic renal failure. Its etiology may be bacterial, metastatic, or urogenous. The disease is most common in patients who are predisposed to recurrent acute pyelonephritis, such as those with urinary obstructions or vesicoureteral reflux.

Patients with chronic pyelonephritis may have a childhood history of unexplained fevers or bedwetting. Clinical effects may include flank pain, anemia, low urine specific gravity, proteinuria, leukocytes in urine and, especially in late stages, hypertension. Uremia rarely develops from chronic pyelonephritis unless structural abnormalities exist in the excretory system. Bacteriuria may be intermittent. When no bacteria are found in urine, diagnosis depends on excretory urography (renal pelvis may appear small and flattened) and renal biopsy.

Effective treatment of chronic pyelonephritis requires control of hypertension, elimination of the existing obstruction (when possible), and long-term antimicrobial therapy.

Pathophysiology recap

➤ Acute pyelonephritis is one of the most common renal diseases. It results from a bacterial infection of the kidneys by normal intestinal and fecal flora that grow readily in urine.

➤ The most common causative organism is *Escherichia coli*, but *Proteus, Pseudomonas, Staphylococcus aureus*, and *Enterococcus faecalis* may also cause this disease.

➤ Infection may result from vesicoureteral reflux, instrumentation (catheterization, cystoscopy, or urologic surgery), hematogenic infection (septicemia or endocarditis), lymphatic infection, an inability to empty the bladder (neurogenic bladder), urinary stasis, or urinary obstruction.

➤ The infection spreads from the bladder to the ureters, and then to the kidneys.

➤ With treatment and continued follow-up care, the prognosis is good and extensive permanent damage is rare.

➤ Acute pyelonephritis occurs more commonly in females due to a shorter urethra and the proximity of the urinary meatus to the vagina and rectum, which allows bacteria to reach the bladder more easily.

➤ Incidence increases with age and is more common in sexually active females, pregnant females, patients with diabetes, and those with other renal diseases.

➤ Acute renal failure

Acute renal failure is the sudden interruption of kidney function due to obstruction, reduced circulation, or renal parenchymal disease. It's usually reversible with medical treatment; otherwise, it may progress to end-stage renal disease, uremic syndrome, and death.

Rapid assessment

➤ Assess the patient's vital signs, noting early hypotension and later hypertension.

➤ Obtain the patient's history; inquire about headache, anorexia, nausea, vomiting, and diarrhea from electrolyte imbalance.

➤ Assess the patient for drowsiness, irritability, confusion, peripheral neuropathy, seizures, and coma secondary to altered cerebral perfusion.

➤ Assess the patient for early signs, such as oliguria, azotemia and, rarely, anuria from decreased renal blood flow.

➤ Observe for dry skin, pruritus, pallor, purpura, dry mucous membranes and, rarely, uremic frost.

➤ Observe the electrocardiogram for arrhythmias; tall, peaked T waves; and a widening QRS complex.

➤ Auscultate the lungs for crackles and observe for dyspnea.

➤ Assess for peripheral edema.

Immediate actions

➤ Administer supplemental oxygen and prepare the patient for endotracheal intubation and mechanical ventilation, if necessary.

➤ Initiate safety measures and seizure precautions.

➤ Obtain a blood sample for arterial blood gas analysis and evaluate for metabolic acidosis.

➤ Obtain a serum sample and monitor for electrolyte imbalances (especially hyperkalemia), abnormal clotting times, and increased blood urea nitrogen and creatinine levels.

➤ Administer I.V. hypertonic glucose, regular insulin infusions, sodium bicarbonate, and calcium chloride to treat severe hyperkalemia.

➤ Administer sodium polystyrene sulfonate by mouth or enema to treat mild hyperkalemia.

➤ Give low-dose dopamine to enhance renal perfusion.

Follow-up actions

➤ Monitor the patient's vital signs closely.

➤ Monitor for cardiac arrhythmias.

➤ Monitor serum electrolyte levels frequently and assess the patient for signs and symptoms of hyperkalemia (malaise, anorexia, paresthesia, or muscle weakness).

➤ Monitor for low hemoglobin level and hematocrit and administer packed red blood cells as needed.

➤ Obtain a urine sample to assess for casts, cellular debris, decreased specific gravity and, possibly, proteinuria and urine osmolality close to serum osmolality.

➤ Check urine sodium. (Less than 20 mEq/L is due to decreased perfusion; greater than 40 mEq/L is due to an intrinsic problem.)

➤ Monitor intake and output.

➤ Assess the patient for signs and symptoms of fluid overload and heart failure.

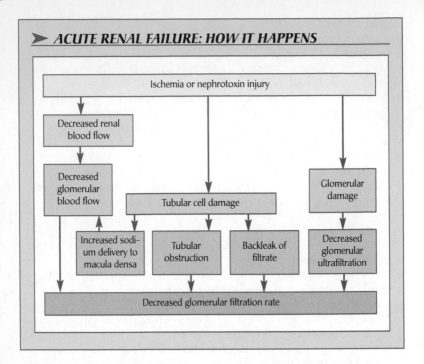

> ➤ **ACUTE RENAL FAILURE: HOW IT HAPPENS**

Ischemia or nephrotoxin injury

Decreased renal blood flow

Decreased glomerular blood flow

Tubular cell damage

Glomerular damage

Increased sodium delivery to macula densa

Tubular obstruction

Backleak of filtrate

Decreased glomerular ultrafiltration

Decreased glomerular filtration rate

➤ Prepare the patient for renal ultrasonography, kidney-ureter-bladder X-rays, excretory urography, renal scan, or nephrotomography.
➤ Prepare the patient for hemodialysis, peritoneal dialysis, or continuous renal replacement therapy, as necessary.
➤ Provide a diet that's high in calories and low in protein, sodium, and potassium, with supplemental vitamins and fluid restriction.
➤ Weigh the patient daily.
➤ Use aseptic technique because the patient with acute renal failure is highly susceptible to infection.
➤ Provide good mouth care.

Preventive steps
➤ Initiate prompt, aggressive treatment of causative disorders.

Pathophysiology recap
➤ Ischemia or nephrotoxic injury causes a decreased glomerular filtration rate. (See *Acute renal failure: How it happens.*)
➤ Acute renal failure may be associated with diminished blood flow to the kidneys.
➤ Diminished blood flow can result from hypovolemia, shock, embolism, blood loss, sepsis, severe anaphylaxis, pooling of fluid in ascites or burns, or cardiovascular disorders, such as heart failure, arrhythmias, and tamponade.

➤ Intrinsic acute renal failure results from damage to the kidneys themselves. It's usually due to acute tubular necrosis, but it may result from poststreptococcal glomerulonephritis, systemic lupus erythematosus, periarteritis nodosa, vasculitis, sickle cell disease, bilateral renal vein thrombosis, nephrotoxins, ischemia, renal myeloma, and acute pyelonephritis.
➤ Postrenal acute renal failure results from bilateral obstruction of urinary outflow. Its causes include kidney calculi, blood clots, papillae from papillary necrosis, tumors, benign prostatic hyperplasia, strictures, and ureteral edema from catheterization.

➤ Acute tubular necrosis

Acute tubular necrosis, also known as *acute tubulointerstitial nephritis,* accounts for about 75% of all cases of acute renal failure and is the most common cause of acute renal failure in critically ill patients.

Rapid assessment
➤ Observe for decreased urine output, generally the first recognizable effect.
➤ Obtain an electrocardiogram (ECG) and assess for changes due to hyperkalemia.
➤ Assess the patient for dry mucous membranes and skin.
➤ Assess the patient for lethargy, twitching, or seizures.
➤ Watch for uremic syndrome, such as oliguria or, rarely, anuria, and confusion, which may progress to uremic coma.

Immediate actions
➤ Obtain a sample for serum potassium, creatinine, and blood urea nitrogen levels (all elevated).
➤ Obtain a urine sample, noting sediment containing red blood cells (RBCs) and casts, and dilute urine of low specific gravity, low osmolality, and high sodium level.
➤ Administer diuretics and a large volume of fluids to flush tubules of cellular casts and debris and replace fluid loss.
➤ Give I.V. 50% glucose, regular insulin, sodium bicarbonate, and calcium gluconate to treat hyperkalemia.
➤ Administer polystyrene sulfonate with sorbitol by mouth or enema to treat hyperkalemia.

Follow-up actions
➤ Obtain a 12-lead ECG, noting arrhythmias and, with hyperkalemia, widening QRS segments, disappearing P waves, and tall, peaked T waves.
➤ Monitor complete blood count and administer RBCs to treat anemia and epogen to stimulate RBC production, as needed.

► UNDERSTANDING ACUTE TUBULAR NECROSIS

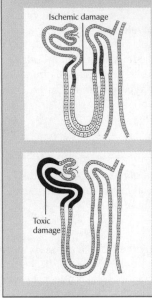

Ischemic damage

Acute tubular necrosis results from ischemia or nephrotoxic injury. When caused by ischemia, necrosis typically develops as patches in straight portions of the proximal tubules, creating deep lesions that destroy the tubular epithelium and basement membrane. In areas without lesions, tubules usually are dilated.

Toxic damage

With nephrotoxic injury, necrosis occurs only in the epithelium of the tubules, leaving the basement membrane of the nephrons intact. Consequently, the damage may be reversible. The tubules maintain a more uniform appearance.

➤ Monitor electrolyte levels and treat abnormalities.
➤ Provide daily fluid replacement for projected and calculated fluid losses, including insensible loss.
➤ Monitor intake and output.
➤ Watch the patient for signs and symptoms of fluid overload.
➤ Weigh the patient daily.
➤ Enforce dietary sodium, potassium, and protein restrictions.
➤ Prepare the patient for hemodialysis or peritoneal dialysis, if necessary.

Preventive steps
➤ Make sure that patients are well hydrated before surgery or after X-rays that use contrast medium.
➤ Administer mannitol, as ordered, to high-risk patients before and during these procedures.
➤ Carefully monitor patients receiving blood transfusions to detect early signs of a transfusion reaction (fever, rash, and chills).

 ALERT *If the patient develops signs of a transfusion reaction, discontinue the blood transfusion immediately and follow your facility's transfusion reaction policy and procedure guidelines.*

Pathophysiology recap
➤ Acute tubular necrosis results from ischemia or nephrotoxic injury. (See *Understanding acute tubular necrosis.*)

In ischemic injury:
➤ Blood flow to the kidneys is interrupted.
➤ Necrosis develops as patches in straight portions of the proximal tubules.
➤ The development of deep lesions destroys the tubular epithelium and basement membrane.
➤ In areas without lesions, the tubules are usually dilated.
➤ Causes of acute tubular necrosis due to ischemic injury include circulatory collapse, severe hypotension, trauma, hemorrhage, severe dehydration, cardiogenic or septic shock, surgery, anesthetics, or transfusion reactions.

In nephrotoxic injury:
➤ Necrosis occurs in the epithelium of the tubules.
➤ The basement membrane of the nephron remains intact.
➤ The damage may be reversible.
➤ Its causes include ingesting or inhaling toxic chemicals, a hypersensitivity reaction of the kidneys to antibiotics, and radiographic contrast agents.
➤ Acute tubular necrosis due to nephrotoxic injury usually affects debilitated patients, such as those who are critically ill or have undergone extensive surgery.

➤ *Bladder trauma, blunt*

Blunt trauma to the bladder is an uncommon occurrence. Traumatic injury to the bladder can lead to perforation; the extent of the injury depends on how full the bladder is at the time of the injury and the mechanism of the injury.

Rapid assessment
➤ Observe the patient for a decreased level of consciousness, pallor, and diaphoresis.
➤ Assess the patient's vital signs, noting hypotension and tachycardia.
➤ Obtain the patient's history; inquire about injury to the pelvic area. Ask about lower abdominal or pelvic pain, difficulty initiating a urine stream, pain on urination, inability to void, and a small, weak urine stream.
➤ Observe for blood in the urine or at the urethral meatus.
➤ Observe for abdominal pain and tympany over the abdomen.

Immediate actions
➤ Provide supplemental oxygen and prepare the patient for endotracheal intubation and mechanical ventilation, if necessary.
➤ Prepare the patient for ultrasonography to confirm the diagnosis.
➤ Prepare the patient for surgery to repair the bladder and drain urine from the abdominal cavity.

ALERT *If injury to the bladder is suspected, consult a urologist before attempting to insert an indwelling urinary catheter.*

➤ Administer I.V. fluids, blood products, analgesics, and antibiotics to treat peritonitis and prevent urinary tract infection (UTI).

Follow-up actions
➤ Monitor the patient's vital signs frequently.
➤ Monitor intake and output.
➤ Maintain the patency of the urinary drainage catheter, which will be inserted through the abdominal wall.
➤ Monitor serum blood urea nitrogen and creatinine levels to determine kidney function.
➤ Monitor hemoglobin level and hematocrit and treat low levels with blood products, as necessary.
➤ Monitor white blood cells to track the progress in treating peritonitis or UTI.

Preventive steps
➤ Instruct patients to practice safety precautions and use safety equipment at work and during recreation, such as seat belts and protective sports gear.

Pathophysiology recap
➤ The bladder is located within the pelvis and is protected from external forces by the pelvic bones.
➤ A force that's strong enough to break the pelvic bones can lead to penetration of the bladder wall by bone fragments.
➤ After the bladder is penetrated, urine leaks into the abdomen, leading to peritonitis.
➤ Severe bleeding and fluid imbalance can occur.
➤ Scarring or swelling can develop in the area of injury, leading to urinary stricture, obstruction, or retention.
➤ This can cause vesicoureteral reflux or kidney damage.
➤ The risk of UTIs is increased due to urinary stasis and retention.
➤ Causes of bladder penetration include a severe blow from a sports injury (or assault), a motor vehicle accident, and pelvic or groin surgery, such as a hernia repair or an abdominal hysterectomy.

➤ Epididymitis

Epididymitis is an infection of the epididymis, the testicle's cordlike excretory duct. It's one of the most common infections of the male reproductive tract. It may spread to the testicle itself, causing orchitis; bilateral epididymitis may cause sterility. (See *Orchitis*.)

COMPLICATIONS

➤ *ORCHITIS*

Orchitis, an infection of the testicles, is a serious complication of epididymitis. If orchitis results from mumps, it may lead to sterility. Rarely, orchitis may also result from another systemic infection, testicular torsion, or severe trauma.

Signs and symptoms
➤ Nausea and vomiting
➤ Swelling of the scrotum and testicles (affected testicle may be red)
➤ Sudden onset of pain
➤ Testicular ischemia (indicated by sudden cessation of pain), which may result in permanent damage to one or both testicles
➤ Unilateral or bilateral tenderness

Treatment
Treatment consists of immediate antibiotic therapy or, in mumps orchitis, diethylstilbestrol, which may relieve pain, swelling, and fever. Severe orchitis may require surgery to incise and drain the hydrocele and to improve testicular circulation. Additional treatment is similar to that for epididymitis.

Nursing considerations
➤ Maintain the patient on bedrest.
➤ Apply a scrotal support and ice packs to decrease the swelling and pain.
➤ Administer analgesics as needed and as ordered.
➤ To prevent mumps orchitis, stress the need for prepubertal males to receive mumps vaccine (or gamma globulin injection after contracting mumps).

Rapid assessment
➤ Assess the patient's vital signs, noting a high fever.
➤ Obtain the patient's history; inquire about pain and tenderness in the groin.
➤ Observe for swelling and erythema in the groin and scrotum and a characteristic waddle—an attempt to protect the groin and scrotum during walking.
➤ Observe the patient for malaise.

Immediate actions
➤ Initiate and maintain the patient on bed rest.
➤ Elevate the scrotum on towel rolls or adhesive strapping.
➤ Apply an ice bag to the area to reduce swelling and relieve pain.

 ALERT *Heat is contraindicated because it may damage germinal cells, which are viable only at or below normal body temperature.*

➤ Administer broad-spectrum antibiotics and analgesics.
➤ Although controversial, some physicians may prescribe corticosteroids to help counteract inflammation.

➤ Provide cooling measures, such as a hypothermia blanket, if necessary.

Follow-up actions
➤ Obtain urine samples to detect an increased leukocyte count and urine culture to identify the causative organism.
➤ Obtain a serum sample to assess the patient's white blood cell count (more than 10,000/cells/mm^3 in infection).
➤ Prepare the patient for scrotal ultrasonography to help diagnose acute epididymitis.
➤ When pain and swelling subside, encourage ambulation with an athletic support in place.
➤ Watch the patient closely for abscess formation or extension of infection into the testes.
➤ If sterility is a possibility, encourage the patient to seek counseling.

Preventive steps
➤ Inform patients that they'll be given prophylactic antibiotics prior to any surgical procedure that increases the risk of epididymitis.
➤ Educate patients about safe sexual practices (monogamous relationships and condom use), which may prevent epididymitis associated with sexually transmitted diseases.

Pathophysiology recap
➤ Epididymitis is usually a complication of pyogenic bacterial infection of the urinary tract (urethritis or prostatitis).
➤ The pyrogenic pathogens reach the epididymis through the lumen of the vas deferens or the lymphatics of spermatic cord.
➤ Rarely, epididymitis results from a distant infection, such as pharyngitis or tuberculosis, which spreads through the lymphatic system or, less commonly, the bloodstream.
➤ Other causes include trauma, gonorrhea, syphilis, chlamydial infection, prostatectomy, and chemical irritation by extravasation of urine through the vas deferens.
➤ Trauma may reactivate a dormant infection or initiate a new one.

➤ Incarcerated inguinal hernia

An inguinal hernia occurs when a portion of the small intestine protrudes through an opening in the membrane that encloses the abdominal cavity. When the herniated portion of intestine becomes trapped or incarcerated, it becomes a medical emergency.

Rapid assessment
➤ Obtain the patient's history; inquire about nausea, vomiting, and loss of appetite.
➤ Assess for a firm, extremely painful bulge in the groin.

➤ If a hernia is suspected but isn't visible, palpate the abdomen to attempt to make it appear or have the patient stand and bear down with his abdominal muscles.
➤ Assess for anorexia, vomiting, groin pain, and irreducible and diminished bowel sounds with strangulation, and partial bowel obstruction.
➤ Assess for shock, high fever, and absent bowel sounds with strangulation and complete bowel obstruction.
➤ In males, assess for painful scrotal swelling; in females, assess for a painful bulge in the labia.

Immediate actions
➤ Prepare the patient for emergency surgery to reposition the protruding portion of the intestine and secure and reinforce (usually with mesh) the weakened muscles in the abdomen.
➤ Administer analgesics, as indicated.

Follow-up actions
➤ Monitor the patient's vital signs, including temperature.
➤ Encourage activity (excluding heavy lifting) as tolerated in the immediate postoperative period.
➤ Monitor the incision for signs and symptoms of infection.
➤ Provide snug-fitting undergarments to reduce swelling near the surgical site.
➤ Advance diet from clear liquids to solid foods, as tolerated.

Preventive steps
➤ Incarcerated inguinal hernias can't be prevented.
➤ Counsel patients who have experienced incarcerated inguinal hernias to drink eight glasses of water per day, eat a high-fiber diet to prevent constipation, and avoid heavy lifting or use proper technique if heavy lifting is necessary.

Pathophysiology recap
➤ An inguinal hernia occurs when the large or small intestine, omentum, or bladder protrudes through an opening in the membrane that encloses the abdominal cavity.
➤ An incarcerated inguinal hernia is one that becomes trapped and can't be manually reduced.
➤ Intestinal flow becomes obstructed and the blood supply to the herniated portion of intestine is cut off, which causes gangrene and necrosis.
➤ Incarcerated inguinal hernias occur due to failure of the peritoneum (the membranous lining of the abdominal cavity) to close fully during fetal development, weak abdominal muscles (caused by congenital malformation, trauma, or aging), or increased abdominal pressure (due to heavy lifting, pregnancy, obesity, or straining).
➤ An indirect inguinal hernia results from weakness in the fascial margin of the internal inguinal ring. Abdominal viscera leave the abdomen through the inguinal ring and follow the spermatic cord (in males) or

round ligament (in females). They emerge at the external ring and extend down the inguinal canal, typically into the scrotum or labia.

➤ A direct inguinal hernia results from a weakness in the fascial floor of the inguinal canal. It passes through the posterior inguinal wall, protrudes directly through the transverse fascia of the canal (Hesselbach's triangle), and comes out at the external ring.

➤ Inguinal hernias are more common in infancy and childhood and are also more common in males.

➤ *Renal calculi*

Renal calculi, commonly called *kidney stones,* may form anywhere in the urinary tract but usually develop in the renal pelvis or the calyces of the kidneys.

Rapid assessment
➤ Assess the patient's vital signs, noting a fever.
➤ Assess for chills and abdominal distention.
➤ Obtain the patient's history; inquire about nausea and vomiting. Ask specific questions about pain, including its pattern (classic renal colic travels from the costovertebral angle to the flank, the suprapubic region, and the external genitalia), its quality (constant and dull pain may indicate calculi that are in the renal pelvis and calyces), and its location (back pain results from calculi that obstruct a kidney, abdominal pain occurs with calculi traveling down a ureter).
➤ Observe for hematuria from calculi that abrade a ureter.
➤ Assess for anuria.

Immediate actions
➤ Strain all urine and submit solid material recovered for analysis.
➤ Administer vigorous hydration (orally or I.V.), antimicrobial therapy to treat and prevent infection, and analgesics, as indicated.
➤ Give diuretics to prevent urinary stasis and further calculus formation, allopurinol for uric acid calculi, and ascorbic acid to acidify urine.

Follow-up actions
➤ Prepare the patient for a computed tomography scan, excretory urography, kidney-ureter-bladder X-rays, and kidney ultrasonography.
➤ Obtain a midstream urine sample for culture.
➤ Obtain a urine sample for urinalysis (may show hematuria, pyuria, increased specific gravity, acid or alkaline pH that identify stone formation, or casts or crystals, such as urate, calcium, or cystine).
➤ Prepare the patient with small calculi for natural passage.
➤ Encourage ambulation and sufficient intake of fluids (including juices to acidify the urine) to maintain a urine output of 3 to 4 L/day.

COMPLICATIONS

► *HYDRONEPHROSIS*

In hydronephrosis, a backup of urine causes distention or swelling of the kidney.

Signs and symptoms
- ► Abdominal mass
- ► Dysuria
- ► Fever
- ► Flank pain
- ► Nausea and vomiting
- ► Urinary frequency and urgency

Treatment
- ► Placement of a ureteral stent or nephrostomy tube allows the kidney to drain by bypassing the ureter.
- ► Antibiotics may be ordered to prevent and treat urinary tract infection (UTI).

Nursing considerations
- ► Monitor intake and output.
- ► Maintain the urinary drainage catheter and system.
- ► Promote adequate fluid intake.
- ► Perform patient teaching regarding care of the urinary drainage catheter.
- ► Monitor the patient for signs and symptoms of UTI.

- ► Prepare the patient with calculi too large for natural removal for surgical removal through cystoscopy, open surgery, percutaneous ultrasonic lithotripsy, or extracorporeal shock wave lithotripsy.
- ► Monitor the patient for hydronephrosis. (See *Hydronephrosis*.)
- ► Monitor serial serum calcium and phosphorus levels to detect hyperparathyroidism and an increased calcium level in proportion to normal serum protein.
- ► Prepare the patient with hyperparathyroidism for a parathyroidectomy.

Preventive steps
- ► Institute a low-calcium diet for at-risk patients.
- ► Advise the patient with a history of calculi to consume six to eight glasses of water per day to produce adequate amounts of dilute urine.
- ► Instruct the patient to take diuretics, phosphate solutions, allopurinol (for uric acid calculi), antibiotics (for struvite calculi), and medications that alkalinize the urine, such as sodium bicarbonate or sodium citrate.

Pathophysiology recap
- ► Calculi formation follows precipitation of substances normally dissolved in urine (calcium oxalate, calcium phosphate, magnesium ammonium phosphate or, occasionally, urate or cystine).

➤ Calculi vary in size and may be solitary or multiple.
➤ Calculi may remain in the renal pelvis or enter the ureter and may damage renal parenchyma.
➤ Large calculi cause pressure necrosis.
➤ In certain locations, calculi cause obstruction, with resultant hydronephrosis.
➤ Predisposing factors include dehydration, infection, obstruction, and metabolic factors.

➤ *Renal vein thrombosis*

Renal vein thrombosis is clotting in the renal vein. It may affect both kidneys and may be acute or chronic.

Rapid assessment
In the patient with rapid-onset renal vein thrombosis:
➤ Obtain the patient's history; inquire about severe lumbar pain and tenderness in the epigastric region and costovertebral angle.
➤ Assess the patient's vital signs, noting fever.
➤ Assess the patient for pallor and peripheral edema.
➤ Observe the patient for hematuria.
➤ Palpate for enlarged kidneys.
   In the patient with gradual onset:
➤ Obtain the patient's history; inquire about pain, which may not be present.
➤ Assess the patient for peripheral edema.
   In infants, palpate for enlarged kidneys and assess for oliguria.

Immediate actions
➤ Prepare the patient for a computed tomography scan with contrast, excretory urography, and renal arteriography and biopsy.
➤ Obtain a urinalysis (may reveal gross or microscopic hematuria, proteinuria, casts, and oliguria).
➤ Administer anticoagulation therapy (heparin initially for 5 to 7 days, then warfarin for long-term therapy, and streptokinase or urokinase in the early stage) to reduce the incidence of new thrombus formation and reverse the deterioration of renal function.
➤ Give diuretics for edema and analgesics for pain.

Follow-up actions
➤ Monitor the patient's vital signs.
➤ Initiate sodium and potassium restrictions.
➤ Prepare the patient for surgery (within 24 hours of thrombosis) to remove the clot.

 ALERT *Although rare, some patients with extensive intrarenal bleeding require nephrectomy.*

➤ Monitor the patient for signs of pulmonary emboli.
➤ Monitor intake and output.
➤ Maintain bleeding precautions and monitor clotting times for patients receiving anticoagulants.

Preventive steps
➤ Renal vein thrombosis can't usually be prevented.
➤ Preventing dehydration can reduce the risk.

Pathophysiology recap
➤ Clotting occurs in the renal vein, resulting in renal congestion, engorgement, and possible infarction.
➤ Chronic thrombosis usually impairs renal function, causing nephrotic syndrome.
➤ Abrupt onset with extensive damage may precipitate rapidly fatal renal infarction.
➤ Less severe thrombosis (affecting only one kidney) or gradual progression (allowing circulation to develop) may preserve partial renal function.
➤ Causes of renal vein thrombosis include heart failure, periarteritis, a tumor that obstructs the renal vein, and thrombophlebitis of the inferior vena cava or blood vessels of the legs.
➤ In infants, diarrhea that causes severe dehydration may lead to renal vein thrombosis.
➤ Causes of chronic renal vein thrombosis include amyloidosis, systemic lupus erythematosus, diabetic nephropathy, and membranoproliferative glomerulonephritis.

➤ Testicular torsion

Testicular torsion is an abnormal twisting of the spermatic cord due to rotation of a testis or the mesorchium (a fold in the area between the testis and epididymis), which causes strangulation and, if untreated, eventual infarction of the testis.

Rapid assessment
➤ Obtain the patient's history; inquire about excruciating pain in the affected testis or iliac fossa.
➤ Observe for a tense, tender swelling in the scrotum or inguinal canal and hyperemia of the overlying skin.

Immediate actions
➤ Prepare the patient for Doppler ultrasonography to aid in diagnosis.
➤ Prepare the patient for immediate surgical repair by orchiopexy (fixation of a viable testis to the scrotum) or orchiectomy (excision of a nonviable testis).
➤ Administer analgesics, as indicated.

➤ *EXTRAVAGINAL TORSION*

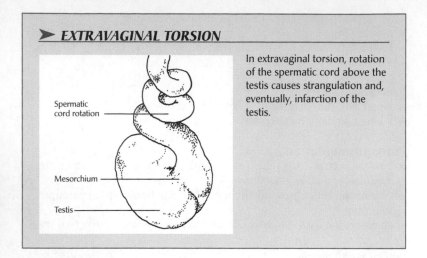

Spermatic cord rotation

Mesorchium

Testis

In extravaginal torsion, rotation of the spermatic cord above the testis causes strangulation and, eventually, infarction of the testis.

Follow-up actions
Postoperatively:
➤ Monitor urinary output.
➤ Administer analgesics.
➤ Apply an ice bag with a cover to reduce edema.
➤ Protect the wound from contamination.
➤ Allow the patient to perform as many normal daily activities as possible.

Preventive steps
➤ Most cases of testicular torsion aren't preventable.
➤ Advise patients to avoid trauma to the scrotum.

Pathophysiology recap
➤ Normally, the tunica vaginalis envelops the testis and attaches to the epididymis and spermatic cord.
➤ It's almost always (90%) unilateral.
➤ The prognosis is good with early detection and treatment.
➤ In intravaginal torsion, the most common type of torsion in adolescents, testicular twisting may result from an abnormality of the tunica, in which the testis is abnormally positioned, or from a narrowing of the mesentery support.
➤ In extravaginal torsion, which is most common in neonates, loose attachment of the tunica vaginalis to the scrotal lining causes spermatic cord rotation above the testis. A sudden, forceful contraction of the cremaster muscle may precipitate this condition. (See *Extravaginal torsion*.)
➤ Testicular torsion is most common between ages 12 and 18, but it may occur at any age.

10

Hematologic emergencies

➤ *Anticoagulant-induced coagulopathy*

Anticoagulants are used to reduce the blood's clotting ability. The primary adverse reaction to these agents is bleeding; this condition is called *anticoagulant-induced coagulopathy*. (See *Anticoagulants and their actions,* page 298.)

Rapid assessment
➤ Obtain the patient's history; ask about fatigue, weakness, lethargy, and malaise. Also ask about a sudden onset of ecchymosis or petechiae.
➤ Examine the patient, noting shortness of breath, ecchymosis and petechiae over the skin, and large, blood-filled bullae in the mouth.
➤ Check the patient's vital signs, noting tachycardia or hypotension.
➤ Examine for obvious signs of hemorrhage.
➤ Assess the patient's level of consciousness (LOC), noting a decreased LOC or a loss of consciousness.

Immediate actions
➤ Treatment includes discontinuing the drug or reducing the dosage.
➤ Institute measures to identify and control sources of bleeding.
➤ Administer corticosteroids and platelet transfusions, as ordered. Be prepared to administer platelet stimulating factors to halt bleeding, protamine sulfate for severe bleeding caused by heparin, and vitamin K to treat frank bleeding caused by warfarin.
➤ Administer I.V. fluid replacement.
➤ Monitor blood samples for the prothrombin time (PT), International Normalized Ratio (INR), and partial thromboplastin time closely.
➤ Monitor the patient's vital signs and his blood samples for hemoglobin level and hematocrit closely. Administer blood products (whole blood, fresh frozen plasma, or plasma concentrates), as ordered.
➤ Monitor the patient closely for further bleeding. Assess his urine, stools, and vomitus for blood.

Follow-up actions
➤ Maintain bleeding precautions for the duration of treatment with anticoagulants. Watch the patient for signs of bleeding, including tachycardia,

➤ ANTICOAGULANTS AND THEIR ACTIONS

This chart shows the classes of anticoagulants and how they work to reduce the blood's ability to clot.

Drugs	Actions
HEPARIN DERIVATIVES	
Heparin and low-molecular-weight heparins (dalteparin, enoxaparin, and tinzaparin)	➤ Accelerate formation of an antithrombin III–thrombin complex ➤ Inactivate thrombin and prevent conversion of fibrinogen to fibrin
COUMARIN DERIVATIVE	
Warfarin	➤ Inhibits vitamin K–dependent activation of clotting factors II, VII, IX, and X, which are formed in the liver
THROMBIN INHIBITORS	
Argatroban Bivalirudin	➤ Directly bind to thrombin and inhibit its action
SELECTIVE FACTOR Xa INHIBITOR	
Fondaparinux	➤ Binds to antithrombin III, which in turn initiates the neutralization of factor Xa

hypotension, hematuria, bleeding from the nose or gums, ecchymosis, petechiae, and tarry stools.

➤ Urge the patient taking an anticoagulant to take the drug exactly as prescribed. If he's taking warfarin, tell him to take it at night and to have blood drawn for PT or INR in the morning for accurate results.

➤ Teach the patient and his family signs of bleeding, and stress the importance of immediately reporting the first sign of excessive bleeding.

➤ Advise the patient to consult his physician before taking other drugs, including over-the-counter medications and herbal remedies.

Preventive steps

➤ Review bleeding prevention precautions the patient needs to take. Advise him to use an electric razor and soft toothbrush and to avoid trauma. Urge the patient to remove safety hazards from the home to reduce the risk of injury.

➤ Advise the patient not to increase his intake of green, leafy vegetables because vitamin K may antagonize anticoagulant effects.

➤ Encourage the patient to keep appointments for follow-up examinations and blood tests to monitor therapy.

Pathophysiology recap

➤ Fldorly patients are at greater risk for hemorrhage because of altered hemostatic mechanisms or age-related deterioration of hepatic and renal functions.

➤ The risk of anticoagulant-induced coagulopathy also increases with higher doses of these drugs or with the addition of antiplatelet drugs such as aspirin.

➤ *Autoimmune thrombocytopenic purpura*

Autoimmune thrombocytopenic purpura, also known as *idiopathic thrombocytopenic purpura,* results from immunologic platelet destruction. This chronic disorder mainly affects adults younger than age 50, especially females between ages 20 and 40. Prognosis is good; remissions lasting weeks or years are common, especially among females.

Rapid assessment

➤ Obtain the patient's history; ask about clinical features common to all forms of thrombocytopenia, such as epistaxis, oral bleeding, and the development of purpura and petechiae. Also ask the female patient about menorrhagia.

➤ Ask about a sudden onset of bleeding. Remember, however, that with the chronic form, the onset of bleeding may be insidious.

➤ Assess the patient for petechiae, ecchymosis, and mucosal bleeding from the mouth, nose, or GI tract. Generally, hemorrhage is a rare physical finding.

➤ Palpate for splenomegaly.

Immediate actions

➤ Monitor the patient's vital signs and cardiopulmonary status and assess him for signs of bleeding. Test stool, urine, and vomitus for blood.

➤ Obtain blood samples for hematologic studies; a platelet count of less than 20,000/mm^3 and a prolonged bleeding time suggest autoimmune thrombocytopenic purpura.

➤ Administer glucocorticoids, immunoglobulin, or corticosteroids (prednisone), as ordered.

➤ Administer platelets for patients with severe bleeding.

➤ Protect all areas of petechiae and ecchymosis from further injury.

 ALERT *During active bleeding, maintain the patient on strict bed rest. Elevate the head of the bed to prevent gravity-related pressure increases, possibly leading to intracranial bleeding.*

Follow-up actions

➤ Guard against bleeding by protecting the patient from trauma. Keep the bed's side rails raised and pad them, if possible. Promote the use of an electric razor and soft toothbrush.

➤ Monitor the patient receiving immunosuppressants for signs of bone marrow depression, infection, mucositis, GI ulcers, and severe diarrhea or vomiting. Tell the patient to avoid aspirin and ibuprofen.

➤ Prepare the patient for surgery, if indicated. (Patients who don't respond or can't tolerate corticosteroid therapy may be treated with splenectomy.)

Preventive steps

➤ Teach the patient methods to prevent bleeding, including:
  – avoiding aspirin and other drugs that impair coagulation
  – using a humidifier at night if he experiences frequent nosebleeds
  – using a stool softener, as needed, to prevent constipation (passage of hard stools can tear the rectal mucosa and cause bleeding).

➤ Teach the patient how to observe for petechiae, ecchymosis, and other signs of recurrence.

Pathophysiology recap

➤ In autoimmune thrombocytopenic purpura, the platelet membrane is coated with immunoglobulin G or other antibody and these sensitized platelets are then destroyed. Their destruction is brought about by the reticuloendothelial system of the liver and spleen.

➤ Chronic autoimmune thrombocytopenic purpura seldom follows infection and is commonly linked to immunologic disorders such as systemic lupus erythematosus. It's also linked to drug reactions and may occur with alcohol abuse.

➤ Disseminated intravascular coagulation

Disseminated intravascular coagulation (DIC) is a grave coagulopathy that accelerates clotting, causing small blood vessel occlusion, organ necrosis, depletion of circulating clotting factors and platelets, and activation of the fibrinolytic system. This, in turn, can provoke severe hemorrhage. Clotting in the microcirculation usually affects the kidneys and extremities, but may occur in the brain, lungs, pituitary and adrenal glands, and GI mucosa. The prognosis depends on early detection and treatment, the severity of the hemorrhage, and treatment of the underlying disease or condition.

Rapid assessment

➤ Obtain the patient's vital signs and oxygen saturation level, noting tachycardia, hypotension, and decreased oxygen saturation.

➤ Ask about nausea, vomiting, dyspnea, epistaxis, and severe muscle, back, abdominal, and chest pain.
➤ Assess the patient for cutaneous oozing, petechiae, ecchymosis, and hematomas caused by bleeding into the skin. Evaluate him for bleeding from surgical or I.V. sites and from the GI tract, acrocyanosis (cyanosis of the extremities), and signs of acute tubular necrosis. Be aware that abnormal bleeding without a history of serious hemorrhagic disorder is a significant feature of DIC.
➤ Evaluate the patient for hypotension, oliguria, shock, major organ failure, and hemoptysis.
➤ Palpate for reduced peripheral pulses.
➤ Perform a neurologic assessment, noting changes in mental status, including confusion, which may progress to seizures and coma.

Immediate actions
➤ Monitor the patient's cardiac, respiratory, and neurologic status closely, at least every 30 minutes initially. Assess his breath sounds and monitor his vital signs and cardiac rhythm.

 ALERT *Assess the patient for signs of hemorrhage and hypovolemic shock. Observe his skin color and check peripheral circulation and capillary refill time. Inspect the skin and mucous membranes for signs of bleeding.*

➤ Use pressure to control bleeding. To avoid dislodging clots and causing fresh bleeding, don't scrub bleeding areas.
➤ Obtain blood samples for hematologic studies; initial laboratory findings may reveal a decreased platelet count (less than $100,000/mm^3$) and fibrinogen level (less than 150 mg/dl) an an increased D-dimer assay.
➤ As the excessive clot breaks down, hemorrhagic diathesis occurs and serum test results reflect a prolonged prothrombin time (more than 15 seconds), a prolonged partial thromboplastin time (more than 60 seconds), and an increase in fibrin degradation products (usually more than 100 μg/ml).
➤ Assess the patient's renal status, noting a reduced urine output (less than 30 ml/hour) and elevated serum blood urea nitrogen (more than 25 mg/dl) and serum creatinine (more than 1.3 mg/dl) levels.
➤ Administer blood, fresh frozen plasma, platelets, or packed red blood cells, as ordered. (See *Understanding DIC and its treatment,* page 302.)
➤ Check all I.V. and venipuncture sites frequently for bleeding. Apply pressure to injection sites for 3 to 5 minutes, then apply a pressure dressing. Apply pressure for at least 15 minutes to arterial puncture sites. Afterward, apply a pressure dressing. Alert other personnel to the patient's tendency to hemorrhage.
➤ Administer supplemental oxygen, as ordered. Monitor oxygen saturation and blood gas results, assess for signs of hypoxemia, and anticipate the need for endotracheal intubation and mechanical ventilation.

➤ UNDERSTANDING DIC AND ITS TREATMENT

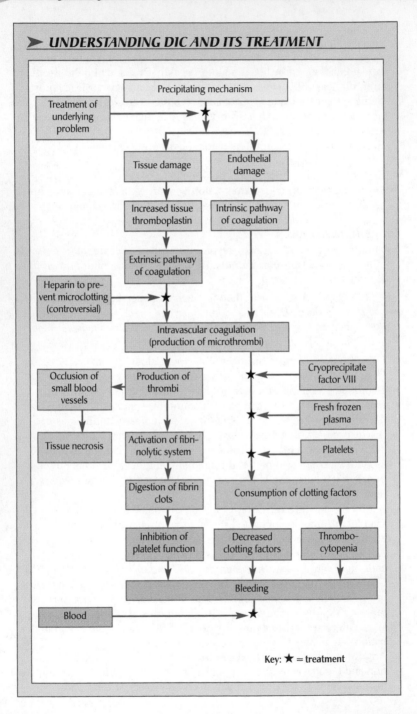

Key: ★ = treatment

➤ Monitor intake and output hourly in acute DIC, especially when administering blood products. Watch for transfusion reactions and signs of fluid overload. Weigh dressings and linens and record drainage to measure the amount of blood lost.

➤ Monitor for bleeding from the GI and genitourinary tracts. If you suspect intra-abdominal bleeding, measure the patient's abdominal girth at least every 4 hours, and monitor him closely for signs of shock.

➤ Monitor the results of serial blood studies (particularly hematocrit, hemoglobin level, and coagulation time).

➤ Explain all diagnostic tests and procedures. Allow time for questions.

Follow-up actions

➤ Keep the patient as quiet and comfortable as possible to minimize oxygen demands. Place him in semi-Fowler's position, as tolerated, to maximize chest expansion.

 ALERT *Assess the patient for potential complications of DIC, including pulmonary emboli caused by accelerated clotting, acute tubular necrosis, or multiple organ dysfunction syndrome. (See* Multiple organ dysfunction syndrome, *page 304.)*

➤ Enforce complete bed rest during bleeding episodes to prevent injury. If the patient is agitated, pad the side rails.

➤ Weigh the patient daily, particularly if there's renal involvement.

➤ Inform the patient's family of his progress, and provide emotional support to the patient and his family. As needed, enlist the aid of a social worker, chaplain, and other members of the health care team in providing such support.

Preventive steps

➤ DIC can't be prevented; however, inform patients about conditions that may cause it and stress the importance of prompt recognition and early treatment of underlying conditions.

Pathophysiology recap

➤ DIC may result from infection, obstetric complications, neoplastic disease, disorders that produce necrosis (such as extensive burns and trauma and transplant rejection), heatstroke, shock, cirrhosis, poisonous snakebite, and incompatible blood transfusion.

➤ Regardless of how DIC begins, the typical accelerated clotting results in generalized activation of prothrombin and a consequent excess of thrombin.

➤ Excess thrombin converts fibrinogen to fibrin, producing fibrin clots in the microcirculation. This process consumes large amounts of coagulation factors, causing hypofibrinogenemia, hypoprothrombinemia, thrombocytopenia, and deficiencies in factors V and VIII.

➤ Circulating thrombin activates the fibrinolytic system, which lyses fibrin clots into fibrin degradation products. Hemorrhage may be the result

COMPLICATIONS

➤ MULTIPLE ORGAN DYSFUNCTION SYNDROME

Multiple organ dysfunction syndrome (MODS) occurs when two or more organs or organ systems can't function in their role of maintaining homeostasis. Intervention is necessary to support and maintain organ function.

MODS develops when widespread systemic inflammation, a condition known as *systemic inflammatory response syndrome (SIRS)*, overtaxes a patient's compensatory mechanisms. SIRS can be triggered by infection, ischemia, trauma, reperfusion injury, or multisystem injury. If allowed to progress, SIRS can lead to organ inflammation and, ultimately, MODS.

Signs and symptoms
Early findings may include fever; tachycardia; narrowed pulse pressure; tachypnea; decreased pulmonary artery pressure (PAP), pulmonary artery wedge pressure (PAWP), and central venous pressure; and increased cardiac output.

Findings progress to reflect impaired perfusion of the tissues and organs and may include a decreased level of consciousness, respiratory depression, diminished bowel sounds, jaundice, oliguria or anuria, increased PAP and PAWP, and decreased cardiac output.

Treatment
Treatment focuses on supporting the patient's respiratory and circulatory function. This may include:
➤ supplemental oxygen
➤ endotracheal intubation and mechanical ventilation
➤ I.V. fluids (crystalloids and colloids), vasopressors, dialysis, or antimicrobial agents.

Nursing considerations
Keep in mind that nursing care for the patient with MODS is primarily supportive.
➤ Maintain the patient's airway and breathing with the use of mechanical ventilation and supplemental oxygen.
➤ Monitor the patient's vital signs, oxygen saturation, and hemodynamic parameters.
➤ Monitor the patient's cardiac rhythm for arrhythmias.
➤ Administer I.V. fluids and medications, as ordered.
➤ Monitor laboratory values and intake and output.
➤ Explain diagnostic tests and treatments to the patient and his family.
➤ Provide emotional support to the patient and his family.

of the anticoagulant activity of fibrin degradation products as well as the depletion of plasma coagulation factors.

➤ Hemophilia

Hemophilia is a hereditary bleeding disorder occurring in males that results from a deficiency of specific clotting factors. After a person with hemophilia forms a platelet plug at a bleeding site, the clotting factor deficiency impairs the blood's capacity to form a stable fibrin clot. Bleeding occurs primarily into large joints, especially after trauma or surgery. Spontaneous intracranial bleeding can occur and may be fatal.

Hemophilia A (classic hemophilia), which accounts for over 80% of all those with the disease, results from a factor VIII deficiency. Hemophilia B (Christmas disease), which accounts for approximately 15% of patients with hemophilia, results from a factor IX deficiency. Advances in treatment have greatly improved the prognosis for patients with hemophilia.

Rapid assessment
➤ Obtain the patient's history; ask about episodes of prolonged bleeding after surgery (including dental extractions) or trauma or spontaneous bleeding into muscles or joints.
➤ Ask about pain and swelling in a weight-bearing joint, such as the hip, knee, or ankle. Note reports of postoperative bleeding that continues as a slow ooze or ceases and starts again up to 8 days after surgery.
➤ Ask about spontaneous or severe bleeding after minor trauma and pain, swelling, and extreme tenderness. Examine the patient for large subcutaneous and deep intramuscular hematomas.
➤ Assess for deformity caused by bleeding into joints and muscles.
➤ Assess for peripheral neuropathy, pain, paresthesia, and muscle atrophy.

 ALERT *If bleeding impairs blood flow through a major vessel, it can cause ischemia and gangrene. Pharyngeal, lingual, intracardial, intracerebral, and intracranial bleeding may all lead to shock and death.*

Immediate actions
➤ Obtain blood samples for hematologic studies. Characteristic findings in hemophilia A include factor VIII-C assay (0% to 30% of normal), a prolonged partial thromboplastin time (PTT), and normal platelet count and function, bleeding time, and prothrombin time. Characteristics of hemophilia B include deficient factor IX-C, baseline coagulation results similar to hemophilia A, with normal factor VIII. (See *Factor replacement products,* page 306.)

➤ *FACTOR REPLACEMENT PRODUCTS*

Treatment of hemophilia aims to stop bleeding by increasing plasma levels of deficient clotting factors. Halting bleeding quickly helps prevent disabling deformities that result from repeated bleeding into muscles and joints.

Treating hemophilia A

Desmopressin administered I.V. or intranasally is usually sufficient to manage bleeding episodes in children and adolescents with mild hemophilia A. Patients with moderate to severe hemophilia A require commercially prepared factor VIII concentrates to treat bleeding episodes. Concentrates derived from human plasma are virally attenuated by one or more available methods, significantly minimizing the risk of human immunodeficiency virus (HIV)-1, HIV-2, hepatitis B, and hepatitis C contamination. However, no currently available method has been successful in eradicating parvovirus B19 from blood products.

Multiple clinical trials suggest that factor VIII concentrate derived from recombinant technology (rFVIII) is as effective as virally attenuated plasma-derived concentrate. The risk of viral contamination is essentially nonexistent in preparations of rFVIII in which human serum albumin isn't used as a stabilizer.

Treating hemophilia B

In hemophilia B, administration of factor IX concentrate during bleeding episodes increases factor IX levels.

The U.S. National Hemophilia Foundation first recommended prophylaxis with factor concentrates in 1994 after investigators in Sweden demonstrated repeated success with this approach. The ultimate goal is to prevent irreversible destructive arthritis that results from repeated joint bleeding and synovial hypertrophy. Prophylaxis may be administered to patients with hemophilia A or B as early as age 1 or 2.

Managing hemophilia during surgery

A patient with hemophilia who undergoes surgery needs careful management by a hematologist with expertise in treating hemophilia. The patient will require replacement of the deficient factor before and after surgery; he may require factor replacement even for such minor surgery as a dental extraction. In addition, epsilon-aminocaproic acid is commonly used for oral bleeding to inhibit the active fibrinolytic system present in the oral mucosa.

During bleeding episodes:
➤ Administer clotting agents, as ordered. The body uses up antihemophilic factor in 48 to 72 hours; therefore, repeat infusions, as ordered, until the bleeding stops.
➤ Apply cold compresses or ice bags and raise the injured extremity.
➤ Restrict the patient's activity for 48 hours after bleeding is under control to prevent bleeding recurrence.

➤ Control pain with an analgesic, such as acetaminophen, propoxyphene, codeine, or meperidine, as ordered. Avoid I.M. injections because of possible hematoma formation at the injection site. Aspirin and aspirin-containing medications are contraindicated because they decrease platelet adherence and may increase bleeding. Caution should be used when using other nonsteroidal anti-inflammatory drugs, such as ibuprofen or ketoprofen.

If the patient has bled into a joint:
➤ Immediately elevate and immobilize the joint.
➤ Begin range-of-motion exercises, if ordered, at least 48 hours after the bleeding is controlled to restore joint mobility. Tell the patient to avoid weight bearing until the bleeding stops and swelling subsides.

Follow-up actions
➤ Watch the patient closely for such signs and symptoms of continued bleeding as increased pain and swelling, fever, or symptoms of shock.
➤ Closely monitor PTT.
➤ Teach parents special precautions to prevent bleeding episodes, signs of internal bleeding, and how to administer emergency first aid. (See *Helping parents manage their child's hemophilia,* pages 308 and 309.)
➤ Refer new patients to a hemophilia treatment center for evaluation. The center will devise a treatment plan for such patients' primary physicians and is a resource for other medical and school personnel, dentists, and others involved in their care.
➤ Persons who have been exposed to HIV through contaminated blood products need special support.
➤ Refer patients and carriers for genetic counseling.

Preventive steps
➤ Teach patients how to avoid trauma, manage minor bleeding, and recognize bleeding that requires immediate medical intervention.
➤ Suggest genetic counseling.

Pathophysiology recap
➤ Hemophilia A and B are inherited as X-linked recessive traits. Female carriers have a 50% chance of transmitting the gene to each daughter, who would then be a carrier, and a 50% chance of transmitting the gene to each son, who would be born with hemophilia.

➤ HELPING PARENTS MANAGE THEIR CHILD'S HEMOPHILIA

Teach parents how to care for their child with hemophilia by explaining the following information and answering any questions they may have.

Risk of injury and bleeding
➤ Instruct parents to notify the physician immediately after even a minor injury, but especially after an injury to the head, neck, or abdomen. Such injuries may require special blood factor replacement. Also, tell them to check with the physician before allowing dental extractions or other surgery.
➤ Stress the importance of regular, careful toothbrushing to prevent the need for dental surgery. The child should use a soft-bristled toothbrush.
➤ Teach parents to stay alert for signs of serious internal bleeding, such as extreme pain or swelling in a joint or muscle, stiffness, decreased joint movement, severe abdominal pain, blood in urine, black tarry stools, and severe headache.

Risk of other disorders
➤ Because the child receives blood components, he's at risk for hepatitis. Early signs — headache, fever, decreased appetite, nausea, vomiting, abdominal tenderness, and pain over the liver — may appear 3 weeks to 6 months after treatment with blood components. Advise parents to ask the physician about hepatitis vaccination.
➤ Discuss the increased risk of human immunodeficiency virus (HIV) infection if the child received a blood product before routine screening of blood products for HIV began. Advise his parents to ask the physician about periodic testing for HIV.

Precautions and treatment
➤ Urge parents to make sure that their child wears a medical identification bracelet at all times.

➤ Sickle cell crisis

A congenital hemolytic anemia that occurs primarily but not exclusively in blacks, sickle cell anemia results from a defective hemoglobin (Hb) molecule (Hb S) that causes red blood cells (RBCs) to roughen and become sickle-shaped. Such cells impair circulation, resulting in chronic ill health (fatigue, dyspnea on exertion, and swollen joints), periodic crises, long-term complications, and premature death. A sickle cell crisis occurs when sickled cells block oxygen-rich blood from reaching organs and tissues. Infection, stress, dehydration, and conditions that provoke hypoxia — strenuous exercise, high altitude, unpressurized aircraft, cold, and vasoconstrictive drugs — may all provoke such a crisis. (See *Understanding sickle cell crisis*, page 310.)

➤ Warn parents never to give their child aspirin, which can aggravate the tendency to bleed. Advise them to give acetaminophen instead.

➤ Instruct parents to protect their child from injury, but to avoid unnecessary restrictions that impair his normal development. For example, they can sew padded patches into the knees and elbows of a toddler's clothing to protect these joints during falls. They must forbid an older child to participate in contact sports, such as football, but can encourage him to swim or to play golf.

➤ Teach parents to elevate and apply cold compresses or ice bags to an injured area and to apply light pressure to a bleeding site. Advise parents to restrict the child's activity for 48 hours after bleeding is under control to prevent bleeding recurrence.

➤ If parents have been trained to administer blood factor components at home to avoid frequent hospitalizations, make sure that they know how to perform proper venipuncture and infusion techniques. Warn them not to delay treatment during bleeding episodes.

➤ Instruct parents to keep blood factor concentrate and infusion equipment on hand at all times, even while on vacation.

➤ Emphasize the importance of having the child keep routine medical appointments at the local hemophilia center.

Importance of genetic screening
➤ Daughters of patients with hemophilia should undergo genetic screening to determine whether they're hemophilia carriers. Affected males should undergo counseling as well. If they mate with a noncarrier, all of their daughters will be carriers; if they mate with a carrier, each male or female child has a 25% chance of being affected.

➤ For more information, refer parents to the National Hemophilia Foundation.

Rapid assessment
➤ Assess the patient's vital signs, noting body temperature over 104° F (40° C) or a temperature of 100° F (37.8° C) that has persisted for 2 or more days.
➤ Obtain the patient's history; ask about sleepiness with difficulty awakening, severe pain, and hematuria.
➤ Assess the patient for lethargy, listlessness, irritability, and pale lips, tongue, palms, and nail beds.
➤ Evaluate the patient for severe abdominal, thoracic, muscular, or bone pain and, possibly, worsening jaundice, dark urine, and a low-grade fever (vaso-occlusive or infarctive crisis).

 ALERT *Autosplenectomy, in which splenic damage and scarring is so extensive that the spleen shrinks and becomes impalpable, occurs in long-term disease. It can lead to increased susceptibility to* Streptococcus pneumoniae *sepsis, which can be fatal without prompt*

➤ UNDERSTANDING SICKLE CELL CRISIS

Infection, overexertion, or exposure to cold, high altitudes, or other factors that cause cellular oxygen deprivation may trigger a sickle cell crisis. The deoxygenated, sickle-shaped red blood cells stick to the capillary wall and each other, blocking blood flow and causing cellular hypoxia. The crisis worsens as tissue hypoxia and acidic waste products cause more sickling and cell damage. With each new crisis, organs and tissues are slowly destroyed; the spleen and kidneys are particularly likely to be affected.

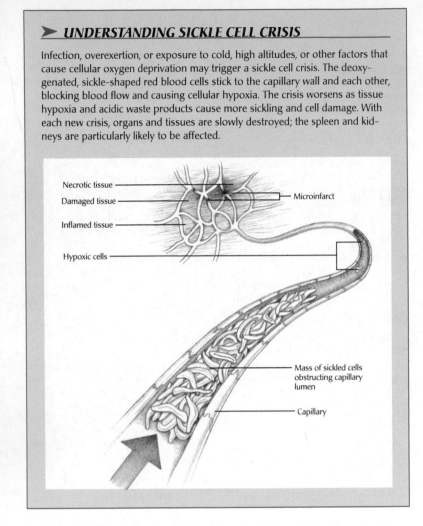

treatment. Infection may develop after the crisis subsides (in 4 days to several weeks), so watch for lethargy, sleepiness, fever, or apathy.

➤ Assess the patient for pallor, lethargy, sleepiness, dyspnea, possible coma, markedly decreased bone marrow activity, and RBC hemolysis (aplastic or megaloblastic crisis).

➤ If the patient is an infant between ages 8 months and 2 years, inspect for lethargy or pallor, which may progress to hypovolemic shock (acute sequestration crisis).

➤ Inspect the patient for jaundice, and palpate for hepatomegaly (hemolytic crisis).

➤ If the patient is a young child, palpation may reveal splenomegaly.

Immediate actions
➤ If the patient's Hb level drops suddenly or if his condition deteriorates rapidly, he'll need to be hospitalized for a transfusion of packed RBCs.
➤ In a sequestration crisis, treatment may include sedation, administration of analgesics, a blood transfusion, oxygen administration, and large amounts of oral or I.V. fluids.
➤ Apply warm compresses to painful areas, and cover the child with a blanket. (Never use cold compresses because they aggravate the condition.)
➤ Administer an analgesic–antipyretic such as aspirin or acetaminophen. Additional pain relief, such as an opioid, may be required during an acute crisis.
➤ Encourage bed rest, and place the patient in a sitting position. If dehydration or severe pain occurs, hospitalization may be necessary.
➤ When cultures indicate, administer antibiotics as ordered.

Follow-up actions
➤ Advise the patient to avoid tight clothing that restricts circulation.
➤ Warn against strenuous exercise, vasoconstricting medications, cold temperatures (including drinking large amounts of ice water and swimming), unpressurized aircraft, high altitude, and other conditions that provoke hypoxia.
➤ Stress the importance of normal childhood immunizations, meticulous wound care, good oral hygiene, regular dental checkups, and a balanced diet as safeguards against infection.
➤ Emphasize the need for prompt treatment of infection.
➤ Inform the patient about the need to increase fluid intake to prevent dehydration because of the impaired ability to concentrate urine properly. Tell parents to encourage the child to drink more fluids, especially in the summer, by offering such fluids as milkshakes, ice pops, and eggnog.
➤ During general anesthesia, a patient with sickle cell anemia requires optimal ventilation to prevent a hypoxic crisis. Make sure that the surgeon and anesthesiologist know that the patient has sickle cell anemia. Provide a preoperative transfusion of packed RBCs, as needed.

Preventive steps
➤ Refer parents of children with sickle cell anemia for genetic counseling to answer their questions about the risk to future offspring. Recommend screening other family members to determine whether they're heterozygote carriers. (See *Managing sickle cell anemia,* page 312.)
➤ Penicillin prophylaxis can decrease morbidity and mortality from bacterial infections.
➤ Electrophoresis should be done on umbilical cord blood samples at birth to provide sickle cell disease screening for all neonates at risk.

> ## ➤ MANAGING SICKLE CELL ANEMIA

Before discharge, the patient must learn how to live with sickle cell anemia to prevent recurrences of sickle cell crisis. Review with the patient and his family the need to:
> ➤ eat a well-balanced, healthy diet
> ➤ keep up-to-date on immunizations
> ➤ get adequate rest
> ➤ take all medications as prescribed
> ➤ drink plenty of fluids
> ➤ contact the physician at the first sign of infection or pain
> ➤ keep telephone numbers for the physician handy
> ➤ plan ahead for emergencies
> ➤ contact national support groups, local groups, genetic counselors, and sickle cell treatment centers for up-to-date information on treatment and research.

Pathophysiology recap
➤ Sickle cell anemia results from autosomal recessive inheritance (homozygous inheritance of the gene that produces Hb S).
➤ The abnormal Hb S found in RBCs of patients with sickle cell anemia become insoluble whenever hypoxia occurs. As a result, RBCs become rigid, rough, and elongated, forming a crescent or sickle shape.
➤ Sickling may result in hemolysis; sickled cells may also accumulate in capillaries and smaller blood vessels, making blood more viscous.
➤ Normal circulation is impaired, causing pain, tissue infarction, and swelling. The blockage causes anoxic changes that lead to further sickling and obstruction.

➤ Transfusion reaction, hemolytic

A transfusion reaction accompanies or follows I.V. administration of blood components. A hemolytic transfusion reaction follows the transfusion of mismatched blood.

Rapid assessment
➤ Obtain the patient's history; ask about a recent (minutes to hours) transfusion, chills, nausea, vomiting, chest tightness, and chest, flank, and back pain.
➤ Assess the patient's vital signs, noting fever, tachycardia, and hypotension.
➤ Evaluate the patient for dyspnea and anxiety. Inspect the skin for urticaria and angioedema.
➤ Auscultate the lungs for wheezing.

➤ Assess the patient for signs of anaphylaxis, shock, heart failure, and pulmonary edema.

➤ If the patient reports having had a transfusion several weeks before presenting to the emergency department, assess him for fever, an unexpected decrease in serum hemoglobin level, and jaundice.

Immediate actions

ALERT *Blood transfusion should be stopped immediately if a hemolytic reaction develops. Change all I.V. tubing and begin administration of I.V. fluids with normal saline solution.*

➤ Obtain blood samples for proof of blood incompatibility and evidence of hemolysis, such as hemoglobinuria, anti-A or anti-B antibodies in the serum, a decreased serum hemoglobin level, and an elevated serum bilirubin level. If a hemolytic reaction is suspected, retype and crossmatch the patient's blood with that of the donor. Send unused blood and tubing to the laboratory for analysis.

➤ Maintain a patent I.V. line with normal saline solution, and insert an indwelling urinary catheter. Monitor intake and output.

➤ Administer osmotic or loop diuretics to prevent acute tubular necrosis and maintain urinary tract function.

➤ If ordered, administer vasopressors and normal saline solution to combat shock, epinephrine to treat dyspnea and wheezing, diphenhydramine to combat cellular histamine released from mast cells, and corticosteroids to reduce inflammation.

➤ Monitor the patient's vital signs every 15 to 30 minutes, watching for signs of shock.

➤ Cover the patient with blankets to ease chills.

➤ Provide respiratory support and administer supplemental oxygen at a low flow rate through a nasal cannula or handheld resuscitation bag.

ALERT *Dialysis may be necessary if acute tubular necrosis occurs.*

Follow-up actions

➤ Monitor blood and urine laboratory results.

➤ Assess the patient for signs of complications, such as acute renal failure, anaphylactic shock, vascular collapse, and disseminated intravascular coagulation.

➤ Report early signs of complications.

➤ Fully document the transfusion reaction on the patient's chart, noting the duration of the transfusion and the amount of blood absorbed. Provide a complete description of the reaction and interventions.

➤ Complete the transfusion reaction report according to your facility's policy and procedures.

Preventive steps

➤ Follow your facility's policy for administering a blood transfusion.
➤ Check and double-check the patient's name, identification number, ABO group, and Rh status. Most facilities require confirmation of this information by a second nurse before initiating the transfusion.
➤ Don't start the transfusion if you find a discrepancy. Notify the blood bank immediately and return the unopened unit.

Pathophysiology recap

➤ Transfusion with serologically incompatible blood triggers a serious reaction, marked by intravascular agglutination of red blood cells (RBCs).
➤ The recipient's antibodies (immunoglobulin [Ig] G or IgM) attach to the donor RBCs, leading to widespread clumping and destruction of the recipient's RBCs.

11

Eye, ear, nose, and throat emergencies

➤ *Chemical burns to the eye*

Chemical burns to the eye result from splashing or spraying hazardous materials into the eyes. These injuries may be work-related or may occur while using common household products. Chemical injury to the eye may also result from exposure to fumes or aerosols. Chemical burns may be caused by an acidic or alkaline substance or by an irritant. Alkaline substances have a high pH and tend to cause the most severe ocular damage. Examples include lye, cement, lime, and ammonia. Acidic substances have a low pH and tend to cause less severe damage. (However, hydrofluoric acid, found in rust removers, aluminum brighteners, and heavy-duty cleaners, is an exception and causes severe burns.) An automobile battery explosion, causing a sulfuric acid burn, is the most common injury to the eye involving an acidic substance. Other common acids that can cause chemical burns include sulfurous acid, hydrochloric acid, nitric acid, acetic acid, and chromic acid. Irritant substances have a neutral pH and tend to cause discomfort rather than ocular damage. Examples of irritants include pepper spray and many household detergents.

Rapid assessment
➤ Obtain the patient's history; ask about a chemical spraying or splashing in the face or exposure to fumes or aerosols. Also, ask about the use of cleaning solutions, solvents, or lawn and garden chemicals.
➤ Ask the patient about pain, irritation, an inability to keep his eyes open, blurred vision, and a sensation of having something in the eye.
➤ Assess the patient's eye pH before irrigating the eye with sterile saline solution. Assessing the patient's visual acuity can be delayed until after irrigation.
➤ After irrigation, inspect for conjunctival and scleral redness and tearing and for corneal opacification.
➤ Arrange for a full ophthalmologic examination.

➤ EYE IRRIGATION FOR CHEMICAL BURNS

The patient's eye may be irrigated using either of these methods.

Morgan lens
Connected to irrigation tubing, a Morgan lens permits continuous lavage and also delivers medication to the eye. Use an adapter to connect the lens to the I.V. tubing and the solution container. Begin the irrigation at the prescribed flow rate. To insert the device, ask the patient to look down as you insert the lens under the upper eyelid. Then have her look up as you retract and release the lower eyelid over the lens.

I.V. tube
If a Morgan lens isn't available, set up an I.V. bag and tubing without a needle. Direct a constant, gentle stream at the inner canthus so that the solution flows across the cornea to the outer canthus. Flush the eye for at least 15 minutes.

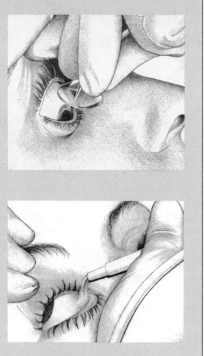

Immediate actions
➤ Flush the patient's eyes with large amounts of sterile isotonic saline solution for at least 15 to 30 minutes. Intermittently check the pH of the eye. (Ocular pH may be increased if the offending chemical is alkali, decreased if it's acidic, or neutral if it's an irritant.) Continue to irrigate until the pH returns to a normal level. (See _Eye irrigation for chemical burns._)
➤ Prepare the patient for an ophthalmologic examination.
➤ Provide analgesics, as needed, for pain.
➤ Administer other medications—topical or oral antibiotics, cycloplegics to prevent ciliary spasms and reduce inflammation, and topical lubricants, as ordered.
➤ Be prepared to administer beta-adrenergic blockers or alpha agonists to lower intraocular pressure if secondary glaucoma develops.

 ALERT _If the patient has burns on the face from an alkaline substance, assess him for tracheal or esophageal burns; these can be life-threatening injuries._

ALERT *Because burns resulting from hydrofluoric acid may cause severe hypocalcemia, monitor serum calcium levels, as ordered.*

Follow-up actions
➤ Apply eye dressings or patches, as needed, to reduce eye movement.
➤ Teach the patient how to apply ophthalmic medications, as necessary.

Preventive steps
➤ Strongly advise patients to wear protective goggles or eyewear when working with toxic substances.
➤ Instruct patients to keep all toxic home products out of the reach of children.

Pathophysiology recap
➤ The severity of chemical injury to the eye depends on the chemical's pH, the duration of contact with the chemical, the amount of chemical causing the injury, and the chemical's ability to penetrate the eye.
➤ Alkaline substances can penetrate the surface of the eye into the anterior chamber within 5 to 15 minutes, causing damage to such internal structures as the iris, ciliary body, lens, and trabecular network.
➤ Acidic substances can't penetrate the corneal epithelial layer of the eye, which limits injury to superficial, nonprogressive damage. However, because hydrofluoric acid has properties similar to alkaline substances, it can cause more progressive and severe damage.

➤ Corneal abrasion

A corneal abrasion is a scratch on the surface epithelium of the cornea. An abrasion, or foreign body in the eye, is the most common eye injury. With treatment, prognosis is usually good.

Rapid assessment
➤ Obtain the patient's history; ask about eye trauma or wearing contact lenses for a prolonged period. Ask about a sensation of something in the eye, sensitivity to light, decreased visual acuity (if the abrasion occurs in the pupillary region), and pain.
➤ Inspect the patient's eye for redness, increased tearing and, possibly, a foreign body on the cornea or under the eyelid.
➤ Stain the cornea with fluorescein stain to confirm the diagnosis. (The physician will use a cobalt-blue light and slit-lamp examination; the injured area will appear green when examined.)

COMPLICATIONS

➤ *CORNEAL ULCERATION*

A major cause of blindness worldwide, corneal ulcers result in corneal scarring or perforation. They occur in the central or marginal areas of the cornea, vary in shape and size, and may be singular or multiple. Prompt treatment (within hours of onset) can prevent visual impairment.

Corneal ulcers generally result from bacterial, protozoan, viral, or fungal infections, but other causes may include ocular trauma, exposure, toxins, and allergens.

Signs and symptoms

Typically, corneal ulceration begins with pain (aggravated by blinking) and photophobia, followed by increased tearing. Eventually, central corneal ulceration produces pronounced visual blurring. The eye may appear injected (red). Purulent discharge is possible if a bacterial ulcer is present.

Treatment

Prompt treatment is essential for all forms of corneal ulcer to prevent complications and permanent visual impairment. Treatment aims to eliminate the underlying cause of the ulcer and to relieve pain.

A corneal ulcer should never be patched because patching creates the dark, warm, moist environment ideal for bacterial growth. However, it should be protected with a perforated shield. Antibiotics, antivirals, or antifungals are prescribed based on culture and sensitivity findings. Artificial tears and lubricating ointments may be prescribed as needed.

Nursing considerations

➤ Because corneal ulcers are quite painful, give analgesics as needed.
➤ Watch for signs of secondary glaucoma (transient vision loss and halos around lights).
➤ The patient may be more comfortable in a darkened room or when wearing dark glasses.

Immediate actions

➤ Assist with the eye examination. Check visual acuity before beginning treatment.
➤ If a foreign body is visible, carefully irrigate the eye with normal saline solution.
➤ Instill topical anesthetic eyedrops in the affected eye before assisting the physician, who will be using a foreign body spud to remove a superficial foreign body.
➤ If the foreign body is a rust ring, it must be removed by the physician with an ophthalmic burr. When only partial removal is possible, reep-

ithelialization will lift what remains of the ring to tho surface so that removal can be completed the next day.

➤ Instill broad-spectrum antibiotic eyedrops in the affected eye every 3 to 4 hours.

➤ Reassure the patient that the corneal epithelium usually heals in 24 to 48 hours.

➤ Provide tetanus prophylaxis.

Follow-up actions

➤ If a patch is ordered, tell the patient to leave it in place for 6 to 12 hours. Warn him that a patch alters depth perception and advise caution in performing daily activities, such as climbing stairs or stepping off a curb. (Patching is no longer routinely recommended in the treatment of corneal abrasions.)

➤ Stress the importance of instilling antibiotic eyedrops as ordered because an untreated corneal abrasion, if infected, can lead to a corneal ulcer and permanent vision loss. Teach the patient the proper way to instill eye medications. (See *Corneal ulceration.*)

➤ Advise the patient who wears contact lenses to abstain from wearing the lenses until the corneal abrasion heals.

Preventive steps

➤ Urge patients to wear safety glasses to protect the eyes from flying fragments.

➤ Review instructions for wearing and caring for contact lenses with the patient to prevent further trauma.

➤ Taping the patient's eyelids closed during surgical procedures helps prevent corneal abrasion, which is a common perioperative ocular injury in the patient who receives general anesthesia.

Pathophysiology recap

➤ A corneal abrasion usually results from a foreign body, such as a cinder or a piece of dust, dirt, or grit that becomes embedded under the eyelid.

➤ Small pieces of metal that get in the eyes of workers who don't wear protective glasses quickly form a rust ring on the cornea and cause corneal abrasion. Such abrasions also commonly occur in the eyes of people who fall asleep wearing hard contact lenses or whose lenses are not fitted properly.

➤ A corneal scratch caused by a fingernail, a piece of paper, or other organic substance may cause a persistent lesion. The epithelium doesn't always heal properly, and a recurrent corneal erosion may develop, with delayed effects more severe than the original injury.

➤ Epistaxis

Epistaxis, or *nosebleed,* may be a primary disorder or may occur secondary to another condition. Such bleeding in children generally originates in the anterior nasal septum and tends to be mild. In adults, such bleeding is most likely to originate in the posterior septum and can be severe.

Rapid assessment

➤ Obtain the patient's history; ask about trauma to the nose or a predisposing factor, such as anticoagulant therapy, hypertension, chronic aspirin use, high altitudes and dry climate, sclerotic vessel disease, Hodgkin's disease, vitamin K deficiency, or blood dyscrasias.

➤ Use a bright light and nasal speculum to locate the site of bleeding; assess for bright red blood oozing from the nostrils (originates in the anterior nose). Blood visible in the back of the throat originates in the posterior area and may be dark or bright red (it's commonly mistaken for hemoptysis because of expectoration).

➤ Determine whether epistaxis is unilateral (typical) or bilateral (in dyscrasia or severe trauma).

➤ Inspect for blood seeping behind the nasal septum, in the middle ear, and in the corners of the eyes.

Immediate actions

➤ Compress the soft portion of the nostrils against the septum continuously for 5 to 10 minutes. Apply an ice collar or cold compresses to the nose. Bleeding should stop after 10 minutes.

➤ Assist with treatment for anterior bleeding, including the application of a cotton ball saturated with 4% topical cocaine solution or a solution of 4% lidocaine and topical epinephrine (1:10,000) to the bleeding site and external pressure, followed by cauterization with electrocautery or a silver nitrate stick. If these measures don't control the bleeding, petroleum gauze nasal packing may be needed. (See *Types of nasal packing.*)

➤ Assist with treatment for posterior bleeding, including the use of a nasal balloon catheter to control bleeding effectively, gauze packing inserted through the nose, or postnasal packing inserted through the mouth, depending on the bleeding site. (Gauze packing generally remains in place for 24 to 48 hours; postnasal packing remains in place for 3 to 5 days.)

➤ Administer oxygen, as needed.

➤ Monitor the patient's vital signs and skin color; record blood loss.

➤ Tell the patient to breathe through his mouth and not to swallow blood, talk, or blow his nose.

➤ Monitor oxygen saturation levels.

➤ Keep vasoconstrictors, such as phenylephrine, on hand.

➤ TYPES OF NASAL PACKING

Nosebleeds may be controlled with anterior or posterior nasal packing.

Anterior nasal packing

The physician may treat an anterior nosebleed by packing the anterior nasal cavity with a strip of antibiotic-impregnated petroleum gauze strip (shown at right) or with a nasal tampon.

A nasal tampon is made of tightly compressed absorbent material with or without a central breathing tube. The physician inserts a lubricated tampon along the floor of the nose and, with the patient's head tilted backward, instills 5 to 10 ml of antibiotic or normal saline solution. This caus-

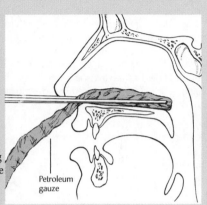

Petroleum gauze

es the tampon to expand, stopping the bleeding. The tampon should be moistened periodically, and the central breathing tube should be suctioned regularly.

In a patient with blood dyscrasias, the physician may fashion an absorbable pack by moistening a gauzelike, regenerated cellulose material with a vasoconstrictor. Applied to a visible bleeding point, this substance will swell to form a clot. The packing is absorbable and doesn't need removal.

Posterior nasal packing

Posterior packing consists of a gauze roll shaped and secured by three sutures (one suture at each end and one in the middle) or a balloon-type catheter. To insert the packing, the physician advances one or two soft catheters into the patient's nostrils (shown at right). When the catheter tips appear in the nasopharynx, the physician grasps them with a Kelly clamp or bayonet forceps and pulls them forward through the mouth. He secures the two end sutures to the catheter tip and draws the catheter back through the nostrils.

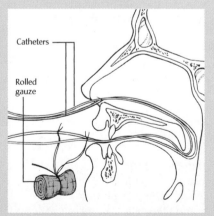

Catheters

Rolled gauze

(continued)

> **TYPES OF NASAL PACKING** *(continued)*

This step brings the packing into place with the end sutures hanging from the patient's nostril. (The middle suture emerges from the patient's mouth to free the packing, when needed.)

The physician may weight the nose sutures with a clamp. Then he'll pull the packing securely into place behind the soft palate and against the posterior end of the septum (nasal choana).

After he examines the patient's throat (to ensure that the uvula hasn't been forced under the packing), he inserts anterior packing and secures the whole apparatus by tying the posterior pack strings around rolled gauze or a dental roll at the nostrils (shown below).

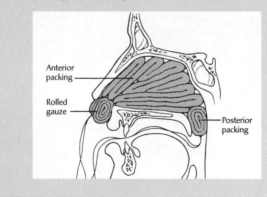

> Reassure the patient and his family that epistaxis usually looks worse than it is. (See *Managing epistaxis*.)

Follow-up actions
> If local measures fail to control bleeding, assist with additional treatment, which may include supplemental vitamin K and, for severe bleeding, blood transfusions and surgical ligation or embolization of a bleeding artery.
> Administer antibiotics, as ordered, if packing must remain in place for longer than 24 hours.

Preventive steps
> Instruct the patient not to insert foreign objects into his nose and to avoid bending and lifting.
> Instruct the patient to sneeze with his mouth open.
> Emphasize the need for follow-up examinations and periodic blood studies after an episode of epistaxis. Advise the patient to seek prompt treatment for nasal infection or irritation.
> Suggest a humidifier if the patient lives in a dry climate or at a high elevation or if his home is heated with circulating hot air.

IN ACTION

➤ *MANAGING EPISTAXIS*

As you walk down the hall of the medical-surgical unit, you're approached by Mrs. Bell, who shouts, "My husband is bleeding!" Following her into his room, you find Mr. Bell sitting up on the edge of the bed and leaning forward. The front of his gown is covered with blood, and you see a small puddle of fresh blood on the floor. Mrs. Bell says her husband sneezed, and then started bleeding profusely from his left nostril.

What's the situation?

Mr. Bell, 55, was admitted from the emergency department (ED) with a hypertensive emergency after experiencing chest pain at work. His blood pressure is now under control with hydrochlorothiazide, carvedilol, and enalapril, and he's scheduled for discharge later today.

Besides hypertension, Mr. Bell has a history of coronary heart disease and hyperlipidemia. His medications include one baby aspirin daily. He had a severe nosebleed requiring a visit to the ED 2 years ago.

What's your assessment?

Based on Mr. Bell's medical and drug history—particularly the hypertension and use of aspirin, which increases bleeding risk—you suspect that sneezing triggered the epistaxis. Vessels of the nasal capillary bed can be very fragile in the patient with chronic hypertension and may be damaged by the force of nose blowing or a sneeze. About 90% of nosebleeds originate in the anterior nasal septum. Bleeding in the posterior nasal septum is less common and is more difficult to treat.

Other risk factors for epistaxis include local or facial trauma, anticoagulant use, chronic alcohol use, smoking, cocaine abuse, nasal septal deviation, hereditary or acquired coagulopathies, vascular abnormalities, nasal tumor, nasal foreign bodies, chronic nasal spray usage, and environmental factors that dry nasal passages.

What must you do immediately?

Reassure the Bells. Put on protective gear and check Mr. Bell's airway, breathing, circulation, and vital signs. Monitor him for hypotension from volume loss and have a colleague notify Mr. Bell's physician.

Ask Mr. Bell to remain sitting upright to prevent aspiration of blood; lowering the head can increase bleeding. Tell him to firmly grasp and pinch his entire nose between the thumb and fingers for at least 10 minutes. He should breathe slowly through his mouth. Prepare to apply ice over the bridge of the nose to promote vasoconstriction and slow bleeding.

Every 10 minutes, have Mr. Bell release the pressure on his nose so you can check for bleeding. Monitor his vital signs until he's stable.

If the bleeding doesn't stop, Mr. Bell's physician will examine him with a nasal speculum to determine the location of the bleeding. Be prepared to assist

(continued)

> ➤ *MANAGING EPISTAXIS* (continued)

with application of topical anesthetic vasoconstrictor solution such as a 4% lidocaine and topical epinephrine, topical chemical cauterization with silver nitrate, nasal tampon insertion, or insertion of up to 36" to 72" (90 to 180 cm) of ½" petroleum gauze packing into the nostril.

If these measures don't stop the bleeding, suspect posterior nasal epistaxis, a relatively serious condition that may require intervention by an otolaryngologist. Treatment may include placement of a double-lumen posterior epistaxis balloon catheter and packing.

What should be done later?

Mr. Bell's bleeding stops after 10 minutes of nose pinching and ice application. Tell the physician how long the nosebleed lasted, which side was involved, how it was treated, and how the patient responded to treatment, including his vital signs. Remind the physician that Mr. Bell is taking aspirin and has a history of epistaxis.

Keep the head of the bed elevated 30 to 45 degrees for the next 4 hours. Tell Mr. Bell not to blow his nose for several hours and to avoid lifting objects or bending at the waist for the next 24 hours.

As long as he's stable and the nosebleed doesn't recur, Mr. Bell can be discharged this afternoon as planned. He'll have a follow-up appointment with an ear, nose, and throat specialist. Teach him what to do if the nosebleed recurs and when to call his physician.

McErlane, K., and Pence, C. "Action Stat: Epistaxis," *Nursing* 34(8):88, August 2004. Used with permission.

➤ Caution the patient against inserting cotton or tissues into the nose on his own because these objects are difficult to remove and may further irritate nasal mucosa.

Pathophysiology recap

➤ Epistaxis usually follows trauma from external or internal causes, such as a blow to the nose, nose picking, or insertion of a foreign body.
➤ Less commonly, it results from polyps, inhalation of chemicals that irritate the nasal mucosa, vascular abnormalities, or acute or chronic infections, such as sinusitis or rhinitis, that cause congestion and eventual bleeding from capillary blood vessels.
➤ Epistaxis may also follow sudden mechanical decompression (caisson disease) and strenuous exercise.

➤ Facial fractures

A facial fracture refers to any injury that results in a broken bone or bones of the face. Facial fractures may involve damage to almost any of the bone structures of the face, including the nose, zygoma (cheekbone), mandible, frontal region, maxilla, and supraorbital rim. Nasal bone fractures are the most common type of facial fracture.

Rapid assessment

➤ Obtain the patient's history; ask about blunt trauma or a severe blow to the head. Ask about pain, numbness, blurred or double vision or, in cases of jaw fracture, jaw pain or numbness and an inability to open the jaw.

➤ Inspect for areas of obvious trauma indicated by facial lacerations, swelling, ecchymosis, or areas of depression. Inspect the oral pharynx for loose or missing teeth and lacerations.

➤ Assess for subconjunctival hemorrhage and ecchymosis and edema of the eyelids (suggests orbital fractures).

➤ Inspect for epistaxis, crepitus, obstructed nasal passages, and periorbital ecchymosis (suggests nasal fractures).

➤ Assess for depression of the inferior orbital rim and diplopia (suggests zygomatic fractures).

➤ Evaluate the patient for an elongated facial appearance and a mobile maxilla, which suggests a fractured maxilla.

➤ Assess the patient for an inability to grasp a tongue blade between his teeth, facial asymmetry, malocclusion, and an inability to open the jaw, which indicates mandibular fractures.

➤ Perform cranial nerve assessment.

Immediate actions

ALERT *Because a head injury commonly involves the patient's airway, immediately assess airway, breathing, and circulation. If the patient has sustained severe facial trauma, oral airway insertion or endotracheal intubation and mechanical ventilation may be necessary.*

ALERT *Immobilize the cervical spine until spinal injury is ruled out. Because of the force needed to cause a facial fracture, cervical spine injury may be present in 1% to 4% of those with facial fractures.*

➤ Obtain a computed tomography scan of the face to locate the fracture and determine the level of severity.

➤ Initiate measures to reduce swelling and control bleeding; this may include elevating the patient's head if cervical spine injury has been ruled out.

➤ Administer analgesics and other medications, including tetanus prophylaxis, as ordered.

➤ Prepare the patient for surgery, as indicated.

Follow-up actions
➤ Provide postoperative care, as indicated.

ALERT *Make sure that you can access the patient's airway at all times. If the patient's jaw is wired for maxilla or mandibular fractures, keep a pair of wire clippers at the bedside to cut the wires in an emergency—for instance, to prevent aspiration if the patient vomits. When the patient becomes ambulatory, have him keep wire clippers available at all times, and make sure that he knows which wires to cut if an emergency should occur.*

➤ Administer analgesics and antibiotics, as ordered.
➤ If the patient has trouble talking because of edema or the method of repair, provide him with a dry erase board or pencil and paper for communication. Also, suggest appropriate diversionary activities.
➤ Encourage the patient to keep follow-up appointments so that the progress of healing can be monitored properly.

Preventive steps
➤ Encourage athletes to wear appropriate protective gear when engaging in sporting activities.
➤ Advise patients to wear seat belts whenever driving or riding as a passenger in a motor vehicle.

Pathophysiology recap
➤ Many facial fractures result from sports-related injuries. Other mechanisms of injury may include motor vehicle accidents, manual blows to the face, and falls.
➤ The amount of force necessary to fracture bones of the face varies depending on the bone. Nasal fractures require the least amount of force, while fractures of the supraorbital rim require the greatest amount of force.

➤ Glaucoma, acute angle-closure

Glaucoma is a group of disorders characterized by abnormally high intraocular pressure (IOP), which can damage the optic nerve. Acute angle-closure glaucoma is a medical emergency that requires immediate referral to the ophthalmologist; if untreated, it can lead to gradual peripheral vision loss and, ultimately, blindness.

Acute angle-closure glaucoma, also known as *closed-angle* or *narrow-angle glaucoma*, occurs when the angle formed by the cornea and the iris narrows or becomes blocked, obstructing the outflow of aqueous humor through the eye and resulting in a rapid elevation in IOP. (See *What happens in angle-closure glaucoma.*)

➤ WHAT HAPPENS IN ANGLE-CLOSURE GLAUCOMA

Normally, aqueous humor, a plasmalike fluid produced by the ciliary epithelium of the ciliary body, flows from the posterior chamber to the anterior chamber through the pupil. Here it flows peripherally and filters through the trabecular meshwork to the canal of Schlemm, through which the fluid ultimately enters venous circulation.

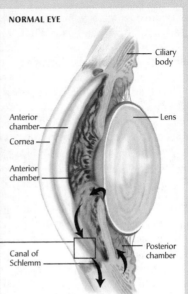

NORMAL EYE

Ciliary body

Anterior chamber

Cornea

Lens

Anterior chamber

Canal of Schlemm

Posterior chamber

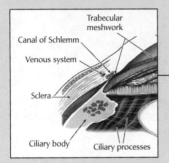

Trabecular meshwork

Canal of Schlemm

Venous system

Sclera

Ciliary body

Ciliary processes

In angle-closure glaucoma, the normal flow of aqueous humor through and out of the eye becomes obstructed by a narrowed angle between the iris and the cornea, causing a rapid rise in intraocular pressure.

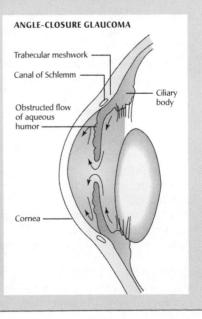

ANGLE-CLOSURE GLAUCOMA

Trabecular meshwork

Canal of Schlemm

Ciliary body

Obstructed flow of aqueous humor

Cornea

Rapid assessment

➤ Obtain the patient's history; ask about rapid onset of unilateral pain and pressure over the eye, blurred vision, decreased visual acuity, seeing halos around lights, and nausea and vomiting (from increased IOP).

➤ Inspect for unilateral eye inflammation, a cloudy cornea, and a moderately dilated pupil that's nonreactive to light. Loss of peripheral vision and disk changes confirm that glaucoma is present.

➤ Palpate for increased IOP by applying gentle fingertip pressure to the patient's closed eyelids. With acute angle-closure glaucoma, one eye may feel harder than the other.

➤ Assist with tonometry measurement of IOP. Normal IOP ranges from 8 to 21 mm Hg, but it may increase to 40 mm Hg or greater with acute angle-closure glaucoma.

Immediate actions

➤ Give medications, as ordered, and prepare the patient for laser iridotomy or surgery.

➤ Administer analgesics, as needed, for pain. Severe pain may require opioid analgesics.

➤ Stress the importance of meticulous compliance with prescribed drug therapy to prevent an increase in IOP, resulting in disk changes and vision loss.

Follow-up actions

➤ Postoperative care after peripheral iridectomy includes cycloplegic eyedrops to relax the ciliary muscle and decrease inflammation, thus preventing adhesions.

 ALERT *Cycloplegics must be used only in the affected eye. The use of these drops in the normal eye may precipitate an attack of acute angle-closure glaucoma in this eye, threatening the patient's residual vision.*

➤ Encourage ambulation immediately after surgery.

➤ Teach the patient signs and symptoms that require immediate medical attention, such as sudden vision changes or eye pain.

Preventive steps

➤ Inform patients that prophylactic iridectomy on the unaffected eye may be indicated.

➤ Stress the importance of glaucoma screening for early detection and prevention. All people older than age 35, especially those with family histories of glaucoma, should have an annual tonometric examination.

Pathophysiology recap

➤ Acute angle-closure glaucoma results from obstruction to the outflow of aqueous humor due to anatomically narrow angles between the anterior iris and the posterior corneal surface, shallow anterior chambers, a thickened iris that causes angle closure on pupil dilation, or a bulging iris that presses on the trabeculae, closing the angle (peripheral anterior synechiae).

➤ IOP rises rapidly as the aqueous humor can't drain properly from the eye. If left untreated, increased IOP will cause damage to the optic nerve.

➤ *Ocular trauma, penetrating*

Penetrating ocular trauma occurs when a foreign object enters the intraocular space. The object may not remain in the eye, it may remain and be visible externally (such as a fishhook), or it may enter the eye and not be visible externally (such as small shards of metal).

Rapid assessment
➤ Obtain the patient's history; ask about a traumatic event and about irritation or the feeling that something entered the eye.
➤ Inspect the affected eye for an obvious foreign object, tearing, conjunctival injection, and edema. Note a disruption in the smooth surface of the cornea, indicating the entry point of the foreign object.
➤ Note conjunctival injection or an area of darker pigmentation, indicating that the object entered through the sclera.
➤ Assess for decreased visual acuity.
➤ Arrange for slit-lamp examination and a full ophthalmologic examination to reveal the location of the foreign object.

Immediate actions
➤ If the object is visible externally, don't manipulate it. Protect the site with a metal shield or a small styrofoam cup placed over the eye until it can be examined by an ophthalmologist. (See *Protective eye covering,* page 330.)
➤ Encourage the patient to avoid eye movements. This can be accomplished by lightly covering both eyes with gauze.
➤ Prepare the patient for surgical removal of the foreign object, as indicated. Before surgery, the patient should have restricted activity and avoid straining and Valsalva's maneuver.

Follow-up actions
➤ Assess the patient's tetanus immunization history and administer tetanus prophylaxis, as necessary.
➤ Administer medications, which may include antibiotics, corticosteroids, and cycloplegics, as ordered.
➤ Monitor the patient closely for complications, such as corneal opacity, cataracts, endophthalmitis, retinal detachment, siderosis, and optic neuropathy.

➤ *PROTECTIVE EYE COVERING*

Provide a protective cover for the eye until it can be examined by an ophthalmologist. To do this, make padding by wrapping gauze loosely around your hand several times to form a "donut" with a central opening diameter large enough to avoid pressure on the globe. Secure with an over and under wrap of gauze to form a firm edge.

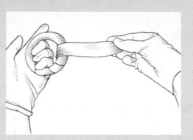

Apply the donut over the orbit of eye, avoiding contact with the globe.

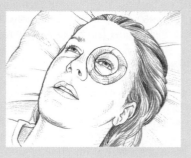

Lay an eye shield (or styrofoam cup) on top of the donut.

Apply an eye patch to the unaffected eye to prevent consensual movement of and further trauma to the affected eye. Secure the eye patch and the eye shield by wrapping 4" gauze around the head several times.

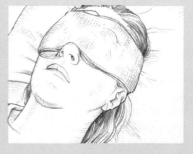

Preventive steps
➤ Advise the patient to always wear protective eyewear when working with machinery or power tools.

Pathophysiology recap
➤ The location of the foreign object and extent of damage depend on the type of foreign body (its size, shape, and composition) and the momentum of the object at the time of impact.
➤ Some intraocular foreign objects may settle inferiorly in the eye due to gravity.

➤ Orbital cellulitis

Orbital cellulitis is an acute infection of the orbital tissues and eyelids that doesn't involve the eyeball. It typically occurs in childhood and, with treatment, prognosis is good; if cellulitis isn't treated, infection may spread to the cavernous sinus or meninges, where it can be life-threatening.

Rapid assessment
➤ Obtain the patient's history; ask about severe orbital pain, chills, fever, and malaise.
➤ Inspect for unilateral eyelid edema, hyperemia of the orbital tissues, reddened eyelids, and matted lashes.
➤ Assess for impaired eye movement, chemosis, and purulent discharge from indurated areas.

Immediate actions
➤ Prepare the patient for diagnostic testing, such as computed tomography or magnetic resonance imaging, as ordered.
➤ Administer systemic antibiotics (I.V. or oral), as ordered.
➤ Monitor the patient's vital signs every 4 hours, and maintain fluid and electrolyte balance.
➤ Instill antibiotic eyedrops or ointment, as ordered.
➤ Apply compresses every 3 to 4 hours to localize inflammation and relieve discomfort. Give pain medication, as ordered, after assessing pain level.
➤ If an orbital abscess is present, prepare the patient as needed for surgical incision and drainage.

Follow-up actions
➤ Teach the patient or, if the patient is a child, his parents, how to apply eye compresses.
➤ Before discharge, stress the importance of completing prescribed antibiotic therapy. Also, teach the patient or, if the patient is a child, his parents, how to instill eyedrops or apply eye ointment.

Preventive steps
➤ Advise patients to maintain good general hygiene and to carefully clean abrasions and cuts that occur near the orbit.
➤ Urge patients to seek early treatment of orbital cellulitis to prevent the spread of infection.
➤ Encourage parents to keep their child up-to-date with immunizations; the *Haemophilus influenzae* type b vaccine can help prevent *H. influenzae* infections.

Pathophysiology recap
➤ Orbital cellulitis may result from bacterial, fungal, or parasitic infection. It can develop from direct inoculation, via the bloodstream, or spread from adjacent structures.
➤ Periorbital tissues may be inoculated as a result of surgery, foreign body trauma, and even animal or insect bites.
➤ The most common pathogens in children are *H. influenzae, Streptococcus pneumoniae,* and *Staphylococcus aureus.*
➤ In young children, infection is spread from adjacent sinuses (especially the ethmoid air cells) and accounts for the majority of postseptal cellulitis cases. Immunosuppressed patients are also susceptible.

➤ Otitis media, acute

Acute otitis media is an inflammation of the middle ear with a rapid onset of symptoms and clinical signs. Otitis media is the most commonly diagnosed illness in childhood. It usually occurs in children ages 6 months to 3 years and is uncommon after age 8. The incidence is higher during the winter months. Breast-fed infants have a lower incidence than formula-fed infants because breast milk provides an increased immunity that protects the eustachian tube and middle ear mucosa from pathogens.

Rapid assessment
➤ Obtain the patient's history; ask the parents about ear pain that may present as pulling at the ears in younger children or difficulty eating or lying down due to ear pressure and pain. Ask about fever, irritability, loss of appetite, nasal congestion and cough, and vomiting and diarrhea.
➤ Perform an otoscopic examination, noting purulent drainage in the external ear canal, tympanic membrane injection (sometimes bright red), and a bulging tympanic membrane (dull, with no visible landmarks or light reflex).
➤ Perform pneumatic otoscopy (with air insufflation), noting diminished mobility of the tympanic membrane.

Immediate actions
➤ Administer antibiotics, as ordered. (See *Treating acute otitis media.*)

➤ TREATING ACUTE OTITIS MEDIA

In early 2004, the American Academy of Pediatrics and the American Academy of Family Physicians issued new guidelines for treating acute otitis media to help inhibit the development of antibiotic-resistant organisms and contain the escalating costs of otitis media, both direct (treatment) and indirect (lost time from school and work). These guidelines are intended for otherwise healthy children without underlying medical conditions that may complicate otitis media, such as cleft palate, Down syndrome, and other genetic or immune system disorders, and include:

➤ using analgesics, such as ibuprofen and acetaminophen, to relieve pain, especially in the first 24 hours of infection (Inform parents that analgesics — not antibiotics — will relieve the ear pain of acute otitis media.)

➤ giving parents the option of allowing their child's immune system to fight the infection for 48 to 72 hours and starting antibiotics only if the child's condition doesn't improve after that time

➤ encouraging the prevention of otitis media by breast-feeding for the first 6 months of life, avoiding "bottle-propping," and eliminating the child's exposure to tobacco smoke.

The guidelines also recommend that antibiotics should be used without a waiting period for infants younger than age 6 months, children ages 6 months to 2 years with a confirmed diagnosis of acute otitis media, and children ages 2 and older with severe symptoms. With antibiotic therapy, the child should experience symptom resolution within 48 to 72 hours.

After antibiotic therapy is completed, the child should be reevaluated to make sure that treatment was effective and no complications occurred. Other treatments for repeated or complicated infections may include:

➤ myringotomy, which is an incision in the posterior inferior aspect of the tympanic membrane, may be necessary to promote drainage of exudate and release pressure

➤ tympanoplasty ventilating tubes, or pressure-equalizing tubes, which may be surgically inserted into the middle ear to create an artificial auditory canal that equalizes pressure on both sides of the tympanic membrane.

➤ Relieve pain by administering analgesics, offering liquid or soft foods to limit the need for chewing, and applying local heat or a cool compress over the affected ear.

➤ Reduce fever by administering antipyretics and removing extra clothing.

➤ Facilitate ear drainage by having the child lie with the affected ear in a dependent position.

Follow-up actions

➤ Help prevent skin breakdown by keeping the external ear clean and dry; apply zinc oxide or petroleum jelly to protect the skin, if needed.

➤ Assess the patient for hearing loss and refer him for audiology testing, if necessary.

➤ *CHARACTERISTICS OF A CHILD'S EAR*

The three major differences between an infant's or young child's ear and an adult's ear make the infant and young child more susceptible to ear infection.

➤ A child's tympanic membrane slants horizontally rather than vertically.
➤ A child's external canal slants upward.
➤ A child's eustachian tube slants horizontally, which causes fluid to stagnate and act as a medium for bacteria.

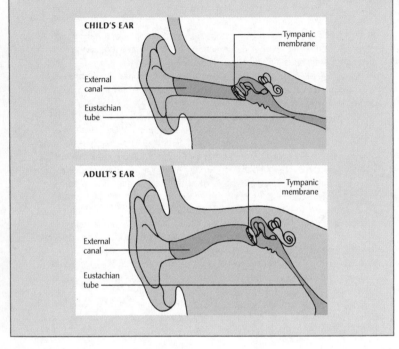

➤ Administer prescribed medications as ordered, including prophylactic antibiotic treatment with low-dose amoxicillin.
➤ Provide appropriate preoperative and postoperative teaching if the child requires surgical intervention.
➤ Educate parents about the indications for and use of earplugs postoperatively for bathing and swimming.

Preventive steps
➤ Encourage breast-feeding for at least the first 6 months of life.
➤ Advise parents to avoid "bottle-propping" or feeding an infant in the supine position.
➤ Encourage parents to eliminate the child's exposure to tobacco smoke.
➤ Advise parents to keep the child up-to-date on immunizations.

Pathophysiology recap

➤ Infants and young children are predisposed to acute otitis media because they have short, horizontally positioned eustachian tubes, allowing fluid to stagnate and act as a medium for bacteria. (See *Characteristics of a child's ear*.)

➤ When swelling or other predisposing factors cause eustachian tube dysfunction, secretions remain in the middle ear. Air also can't escape through the obstructed tubes and causes negative pressure within the middle ear. If the tube opens, the difference in pressure causes bacteria to be drawn into the middle ear chamber where they proliferate and invade the mucosa, causing infection.

➤ Perforated eardrum

A perforated eardrum is a ruptured tympanic membrane. If left untreated, a perforated eardrum can cause infection and permanent hearing loss.

Rapid assessment

➤ Obtain the patient's history; ask about mild or severe trauma to the ear or middle ear infection. Also ask whether the patient has introduced a foreign object into the ear.

➤ Ask about a sudden onset of a severe earache and bleeding from the ear, hearing loss, tinnitus, and vertigo.

➤ Observe the patient for signs of hearing loss such as the patient turning his unaffected ear toward you when you speak.

➤ Inspect the outer ear for drainage, noting its color and odor. Purulent otorrhea within 24 to 48 hours of injury signals infection.

➤ An otoscopic examination reveals the perforated tympanic membrane.

➤ A neurologic examination of the facial nerves should reveal normal voluntary facial movements if no facial nerve damage occurred from the injury.

Immediate actions

➤ Use a sterile, cotton-tipped applicator to absorb blood from the ear and check for purulent drainage or evidence of cerebrospinal fluid leakage (clear fluid).

➤ Apply a sterile dressing over the outer ear.

➤ Administer prescribed analgesics, as necessary.

➤ Administer prescribed antibiotics.

➤ If the patient has difficulty hearing, face him, speak distinctly and slowly, and try to provide a quiet environment.

➤ If the patient has a large perforation with uncontrolled bleeding, prepare him for immediate surgery (myringoplasty or tympanoplasty) to approximate the ruptured edges.

Follow-up actions
➤ Make sure that the patient understands the ordered treatment. If he needs surgery, reinforce the physician's explanation and answer any questions the patient has.
➤ Warn against irrigating the ear.
➤ Caution the patient not to clean the external ear canal with a cotton-tipped applicator. Explain that this may injure the eardrum further.
➤ Advise the patient and his family to exercise care when washing the patient's hair. Water may enter the middle ear and cause infection.
➤ Tell the patient to avoid swimming unless the physician gives him permission, and to use earplugs when swimming to prevent water from entering the ears.
➤ Stress the importance of completing the course of antibiotic therapy as prescribed.

Preventive steps
➤ Teach the patient and his family about using proper safety equipment in the workplace and at home to prevent injuries to the ear.

Pathophysiology recap
➤ The usual cause of a perforated eardrum is trauma: the deliberate or accidental insertion of a sharp object, such as a hair pin, or a sudden excessive change in pressure from an explosion, a blow to the head, flying, or diving.
➤ The injury may also result from untreated otitis media and, in children, from acute otitis media.

➤ Retinal detachment

Retinal detachment occurs when the outer retinal pigment epithelium splits from the neural retina, creating a subretinal space. This space then fills with fluid, called *subretinal fluid.* (See *Understanding retinal detachment.*) Retinal detachment usually involves only one eye, but may later involve the other eye. Surgical reattachment is typically successful. However, the prognosis for good vision depends on which area of the retina has been affected.

Rapid assessment
➤ Obtain the patient's history; ask about floating spots and recurrent flashes of light (photopsia). Ask about gradual, painless vision loss, which the patient may describe as a veil, curtain, or cobweb that eliminates a portion of the visual field (indicates progression of the detachment).
➤ Assist with ophthalmoscopic examination, which shows the usually transparent retina as gray and opaque; in severe detachment, it reveals folds in the retina and ballooning out of the area.

➤ UNDERSTANDING RETINAL DETACHMENT

Traumatic injury or degenerative changes cause retinal detachment by allowing the retina's sensory tissue layers to separate from the retinal pigment epithelium. This permits fluid — for example, from the vitreous — to seep into the space between the retinal pigment and the rods and cones of the tissue layers.

The pressure, which results from the fluid entering the space, balloons the retina into the vitreous cavity away from choroidal circulation. Separated from its blood supply, the retina can't function. Without prompt repair, the detached retina can cause permanent vision loss.

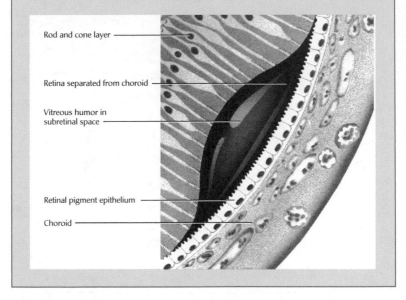

Rod and cone layer

Retina separated from choroid

Vitreous humor in subretinal space

Retinal pigment epithelium

Choroid

Immediate actions

➤ Provide emotional support because the patient may be distraught about his vision loss.

➤ Maintain complete bed rest and instruct the patient to restrict eye movements until surgical reattachment is done.

➤ Avoid pressure to the globe of the eye, which could cause further extrusion of intraocular contents into the subretinal space. This can be accomplished with goggles or a metallic eye shield.

➤ To prepare for surgery, wash the patient's face with no-tears shampoo. Give antibiotics and cycloplegic-mydriatic eyedrops.

➤ Prepare the patient for cryothermy to repair a hole in the peripheral retina or laser therapy to repair a hole in the posterior portion, as indicated.

➤ Prepare the patient for a scleral buckling procedure, pneumatic retinopexy (insertion of an intraocular gas bubble to compress the retina to the

➤ SCLERAL BUCKLING PROCEDURE

In scleral buckling, cryothermy (cold therapy), photocoagulation (laser therapy), or diathermy (heat therapy) creates a sterile inflammatory reaction that seals the retinal hole and causes the retina to readhere to the choroid. The surgeon then places a silicone plate or sponge – called an *explant* – over the site of reattachment and holds it in place with a silicone band. The pressure exerted on the explant indents (buckles) the eyeball and gently pushes the choroid and retina closer together.

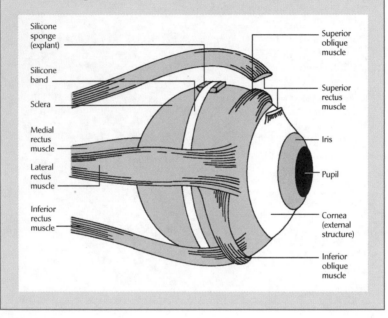

choroid), or a vitrectomy to reattach the retina, as indicated. (See *Scleral buckling procedure.*)

Follow-up actions

➤ Postoperatively, position the patient facedown on his right or left side and with the head of the bed raised. Discourage straining at stool, bending down, forceful coughing, sneezing, or vomiting, which can increase intraocular pressure. Antiemetics may be indicated.

➤ Position the patient facedown if gas has been injected to maintain pressure on the retina.

➤ Protect the eye with a shield or glasses.

➤ Apply ice packs, as ordered, to reduce edema and discomfort.

➤ Administer analgesics, as ordered, for eye pain.

➤ After removing the eye shield, gently clean the eye with cycloplegic eyedrops and administer steroid-antibiotic eyedrops, as ordered. Use cold compresses to decrease swelling and pain.

➤ Administer analgesics, as needed, and report persistent pain. Teach the patient how to properly instill eyedrops, and emphasize compliance and follow-up care. Suggest dark glasses to compensate for light sensitivity caused by cycloplegia.

Preventive steps

➤ Review early symptoms of retinal detachment and emphasize the need for immediate treatment to prevent permanent vision loss.

Pathophysiology recap

➤ A retinal tear or hole allows the liquid vitreous to seep between the retinal layers, separating the retina from its choroidal blood supply.

➤ Predisposing factors include myopia, intraocular surgery, and trauma.

➤ In adults, retinal detachment usually results from degenerative changes of aging, which cause a spontaneous retinal hole.

➤ Retinal detachment may also result from seepage of fluid into the subretinal space because of inflammation, tumors, or systemic diseases or from traction that's placed on the retina by vitreous bands or membranes due to proliferative diabetic retinopathy, posterior uveitis, or a traumatic intraocular foreign body.

➤ Retinal detachment is rare in children, but occasionally can develop as a result of retinopathy of prematurity, tumors (retinoblastomas), trauma, or myopia, which tends to run in families.

12

Dermatologic emergencies

➤ Cellulitis

Cellulitis is an acute infection of the dermis and subcutaneous tissue that causes cell inflammation. It may follow damage to the skin, such as a bite or wound. Prognosis is usually good with prompt treatment. Patients who have comorbidities, such as diabetes, are at an increased risk for developing or spreading cellulitis.

Rapid assessment
➤ Assess the patient's vital signs, noting fever.
➤ Obtain the patient's history; ask about risk factors, tenderness, pain at the site and (possibly) surrounding area, erythema and warmth, edema and, possibly, chills and malaise.
➤ Inspect the affected area for a well-demarcated, tender, warm, erythematous, swollen area; note the presence of a warm, red, tender streak following the course of a lymphatic vessel.
➤ Palpate for regional lymph node enlargement and tenderness.

Immediate actions
➤ Immediately immobilize and elevate the affected extremity.
➤ Monitor the patient's vital signs, especially temperature, frequently.
➤ Obtain specimens for culture; a Gram stain may indicate the causative organism.
➤ Administer antibiotics and analgesics, and apply warm soaks to the affected area, as ordered.
➤ Prepare the patient for surgical debridement and incision and drainage of surrounding tissue if gangrene (gas-forming cellulitis) is present.

Follow-up actions
➤ Monitor the patient for complications, including sepsis, deep vein thrombosis, progression of cellulitis, local abscesses, thrombophlebitis, and lymphangitis. (See Deep vein thrombosis.)
➤ Teach the patient how to apply warm compresses.
➤ Advise the patient to keep the affected extremity elevated to reduce swelling.
➤ Instruct the patient to limit activity until his condition improves.

COMPLICATIONS

➤ *DEEP VEIN THROMBOSIS*

Deep vein thrombosis (DVT) is characterized by inflammation and thrombus formation in the deep (intermuscular or intramuscular) veins. This disorder is frequently progressive, leading to pulmonary embolism, a potentially lethal complication.

DVT may be idiopathic, but it usually results from endothelial damage, accelerated blood clotting, and reduced blood flow. Predisposing factors include prolonged bed rest, trauma, surgery, childbirth, and use of hormonal contraceptives such as estrogen.

Signs and symptoms
DVT may produce severe pain, fever, chills, malaise and, possibly, swelling and cyanosis of the affected arm or leg. Some patients, however, are asymptomatic.

Treatment
Symptomatic measures include:
➤ bed rest, with elevation of the affected arm or leg
➤ warm, moist soaks to the affected area
➤ analgesics.
Treatment may also include anticoagulants to prolong clotting time and thrombolytics for lysis of acute, extensive DVT.

Nursing considerations
➤ Enforce bed rest and elevate the affected extremity.
➤ Apply warm soaks to increase circulation to the affected area and to relieve pain and inflammation. Give analgesics to relieve pain.
➤ Measure and record the circumference of the affected arm or leg daily, and compare this measurement to the other arm or leg as well as to previous measurements of the same extremity.
➤ Stay alert for signs of pulmonary emboli (crackles, dyspnea, hemoptysis, sudden changes in mental status, restlessness, and hypotension).
➤ Teach the patient how to properly apply and use antiembolism stockings.
➤ Tell the patient to avoid prolonged sitting or standing to help prevent recurrence.

➤ Encourage a well-balanced diet and adequate fluid intake.
➤ Instruct the patient to complete the antibiotic course and follow-up with his family physician.

Preventive steps
➤ Emphasize the importance of complying with treatment to prevent relapse.
➤ Instruct patients to avoid injury to the skin by wearing appropriate protective gear when participating in work or sporting activities.
➤ Teach patients to carefully clean breaks in the skin and to watch injured areas for redness, pain, drainage, or other signs of infection.

➤ Advise patients to maintain a good state of health and to keep chronic conditions well-controlled; a healthy body is more able to fight off infection.

Pathophysiology recap

➤ Cellulitis is caused by bacterial infections (usually *Staphylococcus aureus* and group A beta-hemolytic streptococci), fungal infections, extension of a skin wound or ulcer, or furuncles or carbuncles.
➤ A break in skin integrity almost always precedes infection.
➤ As the offending organism invades the compromised area, it overwhelms the defensive cells, including neutrophils, eosinophils, basophils, and mast cells that normally contain and localize the inflammation.
➤ As cellulitis progresses, the organism invades tissue around the initial wound site.
➤ Risk factors may include venous and lymphatic compromise, edema, diabetes mellitus, an underlying skin lesion, or previous trauma to the affected area.

➤ Necrotizing fasciitis

Most commonly known as *flesh-eating bacteria,* necrotizing fasciitis is a progressive, rapidly spreading inflammatory infection of the deep fascia. Necrotizing fasciitis is also called *hemolytic streptococcal gangrene, acute dermal gangrene, suppurative fasciitis,* and *synergistic necrotizing cellulitis.* Mortality for this condition is high—70% to 80%.

Rapid assessment

➤ Obtain the patient's history; ask about risk factors and a history of trauma to the skin or other tissue injury. Ask about pain, which the patient will report as out of proportion to the size of the wound or injury.
➤ Inspect the affected area, noting rapidly progressing erythema at the injury site and fluid-filled blisters and bullae.
➤ Assess the patient for fever, sepsis, hypovolemia, hypotension, respiratory insufficiency, and deterioration in level of consciousness.
➤ By days 4 and 5, inspection will reveal large areas of gangrenous skin.
➤ By days 7 to 10, extensive necrosis of the subcutaneous tissue will have occurred.

Immediate actions

➤ Monitor the patient's vital signs, and report changes in trends immediately.
➤ Administer antibiotic therapy immediately.
➤ Assist with exploration and debridement of suspected necrotizing fasciitis.

➤ Obtain specimens for cultures of microorganisms from the periphery of the spreading infection or from deeper tissues during surgical debridement to identify the causative organism.

➤ Assist with tissue biopsy, which may show infiltration of the deep dermis, fascia, and muscular planes with bacteria and polymorphonuclear cells as well as necrosis of fatty and muscular tissue.

➤ Conduct accurate and frequent assessments of the patient's level of pain, mental status, wound status, and vital signs to determine the progression of wounds or the development of new signs and symptoms. Report and document changes immediately.

➤ Provide supportive care, such as endotracheal intubation, cardiac monitoring, fluid replacement, and supplemental oxygen, as appropriate.

➤ Prepare the patient for surgical debridement, fasciectomy, or amputation.

➤ Prepare the patient for hyperbaric oxygen therapy, if ordered.

Follow-up actions
➤ Maintain the patient on bed rest until treatment is effective.

 ALERT *Stay alert for signs and symptoms of complications, including shock, acute respiratory distress syndrome, renal impairment, and bacteremia, any of which can lead to sudden death.*

➤ Encourage the patient to eat a high-protein, high-calorie diet and to increase his fluid intake.

➤ Refer the patient for follow-up with an infectious disease specialist and surgeon, as indicated.

➤ Refer the patient for physical rehabilitation, if indicated.

➤ For education and support, refer the patient to organizations such as the National Necrotizing Fasciitis Foundation.

Preventive steps
➤ Explain to the patient and his family that postoperative care as well as care for trauma wounds requires strict aseptic technique, good hand washing, and barriers between health care providers and patients to prevent contamination.

➤ Urge health care workers with sore throats to see their physician to determine if they have streptococcal infection. If they are diagnosed positive, they should stay home from work for at least 24 hours after initiation of antibiotic therapy.

Pathophysiology recap
➤ Group A beta-hemolytic streptococcus (GAS) and *Staphylococcus aureus,* alone or together, are the most common primary infecting bacteria. (More than 80 types of the causative bacteria, *Streptococcus pyogenes,* make epidemiology of GAS infections complex.)

➤ Infecting bacteria enter the host through a local tissue injury or a breach in a mucous membrane barrier.

➤ Organisms proliferate in an environment of tissue hypoxia caused by trauma, recent surgery, or a medical condition that compromises the patient.

➤ Necrosis of the surrounding tissue results, accelerating the disease process by creating a favorable environment for organisms.

➤ The fascia and fat tissues are destroyed, with secondary necrosis of subcutaneous tissue.

➤ *Pemphigus vulgaris*

Pemphigus vulgaris (PV) is a rare autoimmune disorder characterized by blistering of the skin and mucous membranes. The lesions of PV almost always start in the mouth, but never progress to internal organs—the disorder is limited to the skin and mucous membranes. If untreated, PV is usually fatal as the patient succumbs to generalized infection secondary to contamination of open skin lesions. However, with the widespread use of corticosteroids to treat PV, mortality has decreased to 5% to 15%.

Rapid assessment

➤ Obtain the patient's history; ask about lesions on the skin, oral mucosa, or mucous membranes.

➤ Inspect for fragile, flaccid blisters that may drain, ooze, and crust. As the disorder progresses, the lesions become widespread and may cover the scalp, trunk, or other skin areas. (See *Pemphigus vulgaris lesions*.)

➤ Palpate for a positive Nikolsky's sign—superficial skin that peels or detaches when the surface of the unaffected skin near the lesions is rubbed with a cotton swab or finger.

Immediate actions

➤ Obtain a tissue biopsy; examination under immunofluorescence confirms the diagnosis.

➤ Administer medications, such as corticosteroids, antibiotics, and analgesics, as ordered.

➤ Provide local care of blisters and lesions, including soothing or drying lotions and wet dressings.

➤ Monitor the patient closely for signs of generalized infection.

➤ Administer I.V. fluids if the patient has severe oral lesions. Provide him with anesthetic mouth lozenges, which may relieve the pain associated with mild to moderate oral lesions.

➤ Be prepared to administer immunosuppressants if corticosteroids are ineffective or the patient can't tolerate them.

➤ Prepare the patient for transfer to a burn center or an intensive care unit if PV is severe.

➤ PEMPHIGUS VULGARIS LESIONS

Pemphigus vulgaris (PV) is a rare autoimmune skin disorder in which autoantibodies attack the cells that bind adjacent skin cells together. The disorder produces fragile, flaccid blisters that rupture easily.

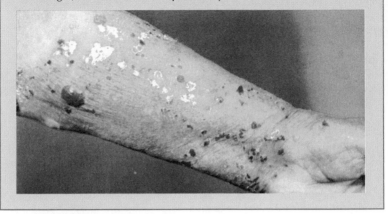

Follow-up actions
➤ Monitor the lesions for signs of secondary bacterial, fungal, or viral infection.
➤ Monitor the patient for complications of long-term corticosteroid use, including weight gain, emotional lability, osteoporosis, glaucoma, cataracts, and type 2 diabetes.
➤ Teach the patient about the importance of medication compliance.

Preventive steps
➤ Advise the patient with oral lesions to avoid spicy foods, tomatoes, orange juice, or hard foods (nuts, chips, and hard vegetables or fruits) that may cause further damage to the oral epithelium.
➤ Teach the patient to minimize activities that cause trauma to the skin such as contact sports.

Pathophysiology recap
➤ The specific cause of PV is unknown, but patients with a genetic history of the disease and those with other autoimmune disorders, such as myasthenia gravis, are at increased risk.
➤ PV may also be an adverse reaction to angiotensin-converting enzyme inhibitors or chelating agents.
➤ PV occurs when autoantibodies (antibodies that attack one's own cells) bind to desmoglein, a keratinocyte cell that attaches adjacent skin cells. This binding prevents cell-to-cell adhesion (a process called *acantholysis*), causing a separation of epidermal skin cells.

➤ *Stevens-Johnson syndrome*

Stevens-Johnson syndrome (SJS) is the maximal variant of erythema multiforme, an acute inflammatory skin disease that develops as a result of drug sensitivity or infection. Also known as *erythema multiforme major,* SJS is a multisystem disorder that may involve mucous membranes of the mouth, nose, eyes, lower respiratory tract, GI tract, vagina, and urethra. SJS can occasionally be fatal, with a mortality of 3% to 15%.

Rapid assessment

- ➤ Obtain the patient's history; ask about coughing, vomiting, diarrhea, coryza, epistaxis, and exposure to a drug or recent history of infection or malignancy. Ask about sore throat and blisters on the lips, tongue, and buccal mucosa.
- ➤ Assess the patient for fever, prostration, difficulty with oral intake due to mouth and lip lesions, conjunctivitis due to ulceration, vulvitis, and balanitis.
- ➤ Inspect for macules, papules, vesicles, bullae, urticarial plaques, or large areas of erythema. The center of these lesions may be vesicular, purpuric, or necrotic, giving them a "target" appearance.
- ➤ Assess for fragile bullae that rupture, leaving large areas of denuded skin susceptible to secondary infection.
- ➤ Assess for tachypnea, chest pain, malaise, muscle or joint pain, and a weak, rapid pulse.

Immediate actions

- ➤ Discontinue the drug suspected of causing SJS, or promptly treat underlying conditions that may have prompted the disorder.
- ➤ Maintain a patent airway. Assist with endotracheal intubation, if necessary.
- ➤ Monitor the patient's vital signs and hemodynamic parameters closely.
- ➤ Assess the patient's pain level and provide analgesics, as appropriate.
- ➤ Insert an I.V. line and administer fluid and electrolyte replacement.
- ➤ Treat the lesions as burns; if the patient is critically ill, arrange a transfer to a burn center or an intensive care unit.
- ➤ Assist with skin biopsy sampling to confirm the diagnosis.
- ➤ Cover areas of denuded skin where blisters have ruptured with sterile warm saline compresses.

Follow-up actions

- ➤ Monitor the patient closely for signs of secondary infection and sepsis. Administer antibiotics, as ordered, for specific identified infections.
- ➤ Provide the patient with analgesic mouthwashes for oral lesions to reduce pain and allow the patient to consume oral fluids.
- ➤ Teach the patient about SJS. Tell him that individual lesions should heal within 1 to 2 weeks, but that residual scarring is possible.

Preventive steps

➤ Because recurrence is possible, advise the patient that he must avoid future exposure to the agent (drug or microorganism) suspected of causing SJS.

➤ Advise the patient to wear a medical alert bracelet indicating that he has a drug allergy.

Pathophysiology recap

SJS is an immune-complex-mediated hypersensitivity disorder. Its etiology may be attributed to one of four possible causes:

➤ infection—viral, bacterial, fungal, or protozoal infections

➤ drug-induced—penicillins, sulfa drugs, phenytoin, carbamazepine, or barbiturates

➤ malignancies—various carcinomas or lymphomas

➤ idiopathic—almost one-half of all cases.

➤ Toxic epidermal necrolysis

Also called *scalded skin syndrome,* toxic epidermal necrolysis is a rare, severe skin disorder that causes epidermal erythema, superficial necrosis, and skin erosions. Mortality is high (40%), especially among debilitated and elderly patients. Reepithelialization is slow, and residual scarring is common.

Rapid assessment

➤ Obtain the patient's history; ask about prodromal signs and symptoms, such as mucous membrane inflammation, a burning sensation in the conjunctivae, malaise, fever, and generalized skin tenderness.

➤ Assess for a diffuse, erythematous rash (first phase), vesiculation and blistering (second phase), or large-scale epidermal necrolysis and desquamation (third phase).

➤ Inspect for large, flaccid bullae that rupture easily to expose extensive areas of denuded skin.

➤ Assess the patient for systemic complications, such as bronchopneumonia, pulmonary edema, GI and esophageal hemorrhage, shock, renal failure, sepsis, and disseminated intravascular coagulation—these conditions markedly increase the likelihood of mortality.

➤ Assess for Nikolsky's sign (skin sloughs off with slight friction) in erythematous areas.

Immediate actions

 ALERT *Toxic epidermal necrolysis is treated in the same manner as severe burns. Cover the lesions with dry, sterile coverings. Monitor the patient's fluid and respiratory status closely. Administer fluid replacement to maintain fluid and electrolyte balance.*

➤ Monitor the patient's vital signs, central venous pressure, and urine output. Watch for signs of renal failure (decreased urine output) and bleeding. Report fever immediately, and obtain blood cultures and sensitivity tests promptly, as ordered, to detect and treat sepsis.

➤ Frequently assess hematocrit and hemoglobin, electrolyte, serum protein, and blood gas levels.

➤ Administer medications, as ordered.

➤ Prepare the patient for transfer to a burn center or an intensive care unit.

➤ Prepare the patient for a xenograft procedure, as indicated.

Follow-up actions

➤ Maintain skin integrity as much as possible. The patient shouldn't wear clothing and should be covered loosely to prevent friction and sloughing of skin. A low-air-loss or air-fluidized bed is helpful.

➤ Administer analgesics, as needed. Wounds will be virtually pain-free after the dermis is covered by the xenograft.

➤ Provide eye care hourly to remove exudate. Because ocular lesions are common, an ophthalmologist should examine the patient's eyes daily.

Preventive steps

➤ Prevent secondary infection with appropriate precautions. Use systemic antibiotics for specific identified infections only.

Pathophysiology recap

➤ The immediate cause of this life-threatening skin disease is still obscure, but about one-third of cases are attributable to drug reactions — most commonly sulfonamides, penicillins, barbiturates, hydantoins, procainamide, isoniazid, nonsteroidal anti-inflammatory drugs, or allopurinol.

➤ Toxic epidermal necrolysis may reflect an immune response or it may be related to overwhelming physiologic stress (coexisting sepsis, neoplastic diseases, and drug treatments).

➤ Urticaria and angioedema

Urticaria and angioedema are common allergic reactions that may occur separately or simultaneously. Urticaria is an episodic, rapidly occurring, usually self-limiting skin reaction. It involves only the superficial portion of the dermis, which erupts with local wheals surrounded by an erythematous flare.

Angioedema involves additional skin layers and produces deeper, larger wheals (usually on the hands, feet, lips, genitalia, and eyelids). It causes diffuse swelling of loose subcutaneous tissue and may affect the upper respiratory and GI tracts.

Rapid assessment

➤ Obtain the patient's history; ask about the source of the offending substance. Check the patient's drug history, including use of over-the-counter preparations, such as vitamins, aspirin, and antacids.
➤ Investigate potential allergies to such foods as strawberries, milk products, and seafood. Also investigate environmental allergens, such as pets, clothing (wool or down), soap, inhalants (hairsprays), cosmetics, hair dyes, and insect bites or stings.
➤ Ask the patient about exposure to physical factors, such as cold, sunlight, exercise, and trauma.
➤ Ask about abdominal colic with or without nausea and vomiting, which is indicative of GI involvement.
➤ Inspect the skin, noting distinct, raised, evanescent dermal wheals surrounded by a reddened flare (urticaria). The lesions vary in size and typically erupt on the extremities, external genitalia, and face, particularly around the eyes and lips. In cholinergic urticaria, the wheals may appear tiny and blanched with an erythematous rim.
➤ Assess for angioedema—nonpitted swelling of deep subcutaneous tissue on the eyelids, lips, genitalia, and mucous membranes. Usually, these swellings don't itch but may burn and tingle.
➤ Auscultate for upper respiratory tract involvement, including respiratory stridor and hoarseness caused by laryngeal obstruction. The patient may appear anxious, gasp for breath, and have difficulty speaking.

Immediate actions

➤ Maintain a patent airway and perform emergency measures as needed for anaphylactic reactions.
➤ Administer drug therapy, as prescribed. Antihistamines, such as diphenhydramine, may be ordered to ease itching and swelling.
➤ Monitor the patient's vital signs, with attention to his respiratory status and response to treatment.
➤ Monitor the patient closely for complications, such as laryngeal edema and respiratory arrest. (See *Laryngeal edema,* page 350.)
➤ Inspect the skin for signs of secondary infection caused by scratching.

Follow-up actions

➤ Advise the patient to prevent or limit contact with triggering factors; explain that desensitization to the triggering antigen may be an option.
➤ Teach the patient how to keep a diary to record exposure to suspected offending substances and signs and symptoms that appear after the exposure.
➤ If the patient modifies his diet to exclude food allergens, teach him how to monitor his nutritional status. Provide him with a list of food replacements for nutrients lost by excluding allergy-provoking foods and beverages.

COMPLICATIONS

➤ *LARYNGEAL EDEMA*

Laryngeal edema is a life-threatening complication that may result from an allergic reaction to a drug, food, irritant, or other trigger. As the tissue in the larynx expands due to edema, the airway becomes dangerously obstructed.

Signs and symptoms
Early signs of hoarseness, dysphagia, dyspnea, tachypnea, and stridor may progress to complete airway obstruction.

Treatment
If the airway appears to be becoming compromised, early intubation should be performed because as laryngeal edema progresses, endotracheal (ET) intubation may become increasingly difficult. If laryngeal edema becomes severe, an airway must be surgically created through cricothyrotomy or tracheotomy.

Nursing considerations
➤ Assess the patient's cardiopulmonary status and provide supplemental oxygen with cool humidification. Assist with ET intubation, if necessary.
➤ Continuously monitor the patient's vital signs and oxygen saturation.
➤ Insert a large-bore I.V. line, and administer I.V. fluids and medications, as ordered. Medications may include I.V. corticosteroids and racemic epinephrine.
➤ Reassure the patient, who may be frightened by the breathing difficulties he's experiencing.

➤ Instruct the patient to keep his fingernails short to avoid abrading the skin when scratching.
➤ Review signs and symptoms that indicate a skin infection. Explain hygiene measures for managing minor infection, and direct the patient to seek medical attention as needed.

Preventive steps
➤ Reduce or minimize environmental exposure to offending allergens and irritants, such as wool clothing and harsh detergents.
➤ If the offending substance hasn't been identified, inform the patient that his physician will likely begin to gradually eliminate suspected substances, monitoring his condition to document improvement.
➤ Advise the patient to check food labels on products for the allergy-provoking food.

Pathophysiology recap
➤ Causes may include drug allergy, food allergy, insect bites, occupational skin exposure, inhalant allergens (animal dander or cosmetics), viral in-

fection, hormones, thyroid abnormality, rheumatologic disease, or a cholinergic trigger (heat, exercise, or stress).

➤ Several mechanisms and disorders may provoke urticaria and angioedema, including immunoglobulin (Ig) E-induced release of mediators from cutaneous mast cells and binding of IgG or IgM to antigen, resulting in complement activation.

13

Environmental emergencies

➤ *Burns*

A burn is a tissue injury resulting from contact with fire, a thermal chemical, or an electrical source. It can cause cellular skin damage and a systemic response that leads to altered body function.

Rapid assessment
➤ Assess the patient's vital signs, noting hypotension (which may indicate shock) and decreased oxygen saturation.

 ALERT *To obtain the patient's blood pressure if all extremities are burned, place a 4″ × 4″ sterile gauze pad or sterile towel on the extremity before applying the blood pressure cuff.*

➤ Obtain the patient's history, noting the cause of the burn.
➤ Auscultate the lungs to ensure the presence of bilateral breath sounds and note the presence of crackles, rhonchi, and signs of respiratory disress, such as tachypnea, nasal flaring, retractions, wheezing, and stridor.
➤ Auscultate the apical heart rate, noting abnormal heart sounds, such as a S_3 or S_4, gallop or murmur, signs of myocardial injury, or decompression.

 ALERT *If the patient has an electrical burn, stay alert for ventricular fibrillation and cardiac and respiratory arrest caused by electrical shock. Begin cardiopulmonary resuscitation immediately.*

➤ Determine the depth of tissue damage.
➤ If a first-degree burn is suspected, assess for pain and erythema, usually without blisters in the first 24 hours; if a more severe first-degree burn is suspected, assess for chills, headache, localized edema, nausea, and vomiting.
➤ If a second-degree superficial partial-thickness burn is suspected, assess for thin-walled, fluid-filled blisters appearing within minutes of the injury with mild to moderate edema and pain; if a second-degree deep partial-thickness burn is suspected, assess for a white, waxy appearance to the damaged area.

➤ If a third-degree burn is suspected, assess for white, brown, or black leathery tissue and visible thrombosed vessels due to destruction of skin elasticity, without blisters.
➤ If an electrical burn is suspected, assess for a silver-colored raised area, usually at the site of electrical contact.
➤ Suspect smoke inhalation and pulmonary damage if the patient has singed nasal hairs, mucosal burns, voice changes, coughing, wheezing, soot in his mouth or nose, and darkened sputum.
➤ Assess the configuration of the burn.

 ALERT *If the patient has a circumferential burn, he's at risk for edema, which can occlude circulation in his extremity. If he has burns on his neck, he may suffer airway obstruction; burns on the chest can lead to restricted respiratory excursion.*

➤ Palpate for edema and peripheral pulses and assess for other signs of vascular compromise.
➤ Auscultate the abdomen for bowel sounds.
➤ Use the Rule of Nines or the Lund-Browder chart to determine the size and classification of the patient's wounds. (See *Using the Rule of Nines and the Lund-Browder chart,* pages 354 and 355.)

Immediate actions
➤ Provide 100% oxygen, and prepare the patient for endotracheal intubation and mechanical ventilation, if necessary.

 ALERT *If the patient has facial or neck burns, anticipate the need for early intubation to reduce the risk of airway obstruction.*

➤ Place the patient in semi-Fowler's position to maximize chest expansion.
➤ Initiate continuous cardiac monitoring.
  For minor burns:
➤ Immerse the burned area in cool water (55° F [12.8° C]) or apply cool compresses.
➤ Prepare the patient for bedside or surgical debridement, as needed.
➤ Cover the area with an antimicrobial agent and a nonstick bulky dressing after debridement.
➤ Provide a prophylactic tetanus injection as needed.
  For moderate or major burns:
➤ Control active bleeding.
➤ Cover partial-thickness burns over 30% of the body surface area (BSA) or full-thickness burns over 5% of BSA with a clean, dry, sterile bed sheet.

 ALERT *Because of a drastic reduction in body temperature, don't cover large burns with saline-soaked dressings.*

(Text continues on page 356.)

➤ USING THE RULE OF NINES AND THE LUND-BROWDER CHART

You can quickly estimate the extent of an adult patient's burn by using the Rule of Nines. To use this method, which divides an adult's body surface area (BSA) into percentages, visualize your patient's burns on the body chart shown below, and then add the corresponding percentages for each burned body section. The total, an estimate of the extent of the burn, can be entered into the formula to determine the patient's initial fluid replacement needs.

The Rule of Nines isn't accurate for measuring the extent of burns in infants or children because their body section percentages differ from those of adults. For example, an infant's head accounts for about 17% of the total BSA compared with 9% for an adult. Instead, use the Lund-Browder chart.

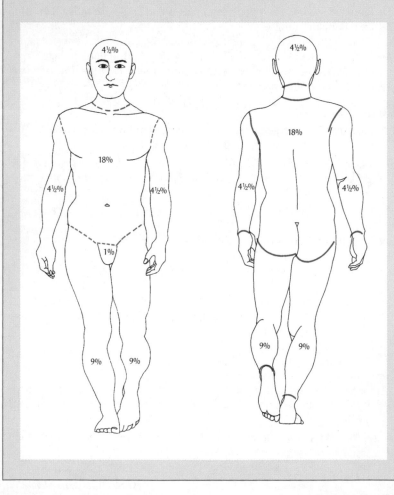

Lund-Browder chart

To determine the extent of an infant's or child's burns, use the Lund-Browder chart shown here.

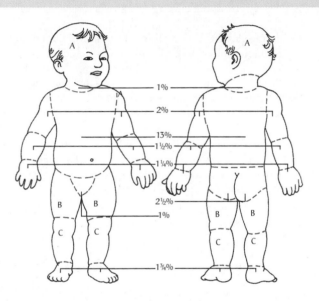

1%

2%

13%
1½%
1¼%

2½%
1%

1¾%

Relative percentages of areas affected by growth

	Birth	0 to 1 year	1 to 4 years	5 to 9 years	10 to 15 years	Adult
A: HALF OF HEAD						
	9½%	8½%	6½%	5½%	4½%	3½%
B: HALF OF THIGH						
	2¾%	3¼%	4%	4¼%	4½%	4¾%
C: HALF OF LEG						
	2½%	2½%	2¾%	3%	3¼%	3½%

> ## ➤ *FLUID REPLACEMENT AFTER A BURN*

The Parkland formula is generally used for fluid replacement in burn patients. Administer 4 ml/kg of crystalloid × the percentage of total burn surface area; give half of the solution over the first 8 hours (calculated from the time of the injury) and the balance over the next 16 hours. Vary the specific infusions according to the patient's response, especially urine output.

➤ Remove smoldering clothing (first soaking it in saline solution if the clothing is stuck to the patient's skin), rings, and other constricting items.
➤ Prepare the patient for emergency escharotomy of the chest and neck for deep burns or circumferential injuries to promote lung expansion.
➤ Assist with central venous or pulmonary artery catheter placement as needed.
➤ Administer an analgesic and anti-inflammatory medications as needed.

 ALERT *Expect to administer analgesics I.V. rather than I.M. because tissue damage associated with the burn injury may impair drug absorption when given I.M.*

➤ Administer lactated Ringer's solution or a fluid replacement formula to prevent hypovolemic shock and maintain cardiac output. (See *Fluid replacement after a burn.*)
➤ If indicated, administer antimicrobial therapy.
➤ Administer bronchodilators and mucolytics, if indicated, to aid in the removal of secretions.
➤ Prepare the patient for transfer to a burn center, if appropriate.

Follow-up actions
➤ Monitor the patient's vital signs and cardiac, respiratory, neurovascular, and neurologic status closely.
➤ Perform oropharyngeal suctioning as needed.
➤ Monitor blood tests, such as complete blood count and electrolyte, glucose, blood urea nitrogen, and serum creatinine levels.

 ALERT *Stay alert for hypokalemia, which may occur 3 to 4 days after the initial burn. Potassium levels — initially elevated due to cell lysis, increased cell permeability, and fluid shifts — may decrease during this time because of restoration of cell membrane integrity and a subsequent decrease in cell permeability and diuresis. Monitor serum potassium levels and electrocardiogram waveforms closely for changes.*

➤ Monitor arterial blood gas levels.
➤ Obtain a urinalysis to check for myoglobinuria and hemoglobinuria.
➤ Insert an indwelling urinary catheter.

➤ Monitor intake and output.
➤ Insert a nasogastric tube to decompress the stomach and prevent aspiration of stomach contents.
➤ Withhold oral fluids and solids.
➤ Watch the patient for signs and symptoms of infection.
➤ For chemical burns, provide frequent wound irrigation with copious amounts of normal saline solution.
➤ Prepare the patient for surgical intervention, including skin grafts and more thorough surgical debridement for major burns.
➤ Weigh the patient daily.
➤ Consult a nutritional therapist to help promote healing and recovery.
➤ Provide a calm, quiet environment.

Preventive steps
➤ Advise parents to keep matches and chemicals out of the reach of children and to use safety covers on all electrical outlets, including those in use and those not being used.
➤ Instruct parents to make sure that stove knobs are protected and not in the reach of children.
➤ Caution the patient not to smoke in bed or near curtains or other loose fabrics.
➤ Advise the patient to report a gas smell to the gas company immediately.
➤ Instruct the patient on the safe use of candles, propane tanks, and portable heaters.
➤ Caution the patient not to cook with loose hanging sleeves.
➤ Remind the patient to read and follow directions on all household products and to purchase potentially dangerous substances in safety containers when available. Urge him to store toxic or otherwise hazardous substances in the original container and to make sure that the label is attached and legible.
➤ Instruct the patient to check electrical cords for fraying and to stop using questionable or obviously damaged devices immediately.
➤ Teach the patient the proper use, placement, and maintenance of smoke and fire detectors and fire extinguishers in the home.

Pathophysiology recap
➤ The injuring agent denatures cellular proteins.
➤ Some cells die because of traumatic or ischemic necrosis.
➤ Loss of collagen cross-linking also occurs with denaturation, creating abnormal osmotic and hydrostatic pressure gradients that cause intravascular fluid to shift into interstitial spaces.
➤ Cellular injury triggers the release of mediators of inflammation, contributing to local and, in the case of major burns, systemic increases in capillary permeability.

➤ VISUALIZING BURN DEPTH

The most widely used system of classifying burn depth and severity categorizes burns by degree. However, it's important to remember that most burns involve tissue damage of multiple degrees and thicknesses. This illustration may help you visualize burn damage at the various degrees.

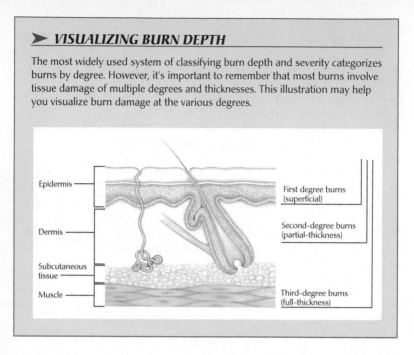

- ➤ Thermal burns, the most common type of burn, commonly result from residential fires; automobile accidents; playing with matches; improper handling of firecrackers; scalding and kitchen accidents, such as a child climbing on top of a stove or grabbing a hot iron; parental abuse (in children and the elderly); and clothes that have caught fire.
- ➤ Chemical burns result from contact, ingestion, inhalation, or injection of acids, alkalis, or vesicants.
- ➤ Electrical burns usually result from contact with faulty electrical wiring or high-voltage power lines.
- ➤ First-degree burns are limited to the epidermis; these burns cause localized injury or destruction to the skin by direct or indirect contact. The barrier function of the skin remains intact. (See *Visualizing burn depth*.)
- ➤ Second-degree superficial partial-thickness burns involve destruction to the epidermis and some dermis. Thin-walled, fluid-filled blisters develop within a few minutes of the injury. As these blisters break, the nerve endings become exposed to the air. Pain and tactile responses remain intact, causing treatments to be very painful. The barrier function of the skin is lost.
- ➤ In second-degree deep partial-thickness burns, destruction of the epidermis and dermis occur, producing blisters and mild to moderate edema and pain. The hair follicles remain intact. These burns are less painful than second-degree superficial partial-thickness burns because the sensory neurons have undergone extensive destruction. The areas

around the burn are sensitive to pain because the barrier function of the skin is lost.

➤ Third-degree full-thickness burns extend through the epidermis and dermis and into the subcutaneous tissue layer. These burns may also involve muscle, bone, and interstitial tissues. Within hours, fluids and protein shift from capillary to interstitial spaces, causing edema.

 ALERT *Immunologic response to a burn is immediate, making burn wound sepsis a potential threat. There's an increase in calorie demand after a burn increases the metabolic rate.*

➤ *Carbon monoxide poisoning*

Carbon monoxide is a gas produced by the incomplete combustion of fossil fuels (gas, oil, coal, and wood). Carbon monoxide poisoning is a toxic response to the inhalation of this gas.

Rapid assessment

➤ Assess the patient's vital signs, noting hypotension, signs and symptoms of shock, and his level of consciousness.
➤ Assess the patient's neurologic status, noting irritability, confusion, impaired judgment, bizarre behavior, hyperactivity, seizures, and coma.
➤ Obtain the patient's history; ask about headache, fainting, nausea, vomiting, and chest pain.
➤ Observe for shortness of breath and rapid or no respirations.
➤ Palpate and auscultate for a rapid or abnormal pulse and heart rate, respectively.

Immediate actions

➤ Place the patient in semi-Fowler's position to enhance respirations.
➤ Provide humidified 100% oxygen by a tight-fitting face mask and prepare the patient for endotracheal intubation and mechanical ventilation as needed.
➤ Provide safety measures and implement seizure precautions.
➤ Initiate continuous cardiac monitoring, noting arrhythmias, such as heart blocks or premature ventricular contractions (PVCs).
➤ Obtain a serum sample for carboxyhemoglobin analysis.
➤ Prepare the patient with severe poisoning to be transferred for hyperbaric oxygen therapy.
➤ Administer normal saline solution I.V.; be prepared to administer diazepam for seizures.

Follow-up actions

➤ Monitor the patient's vital signs closely.
➤ Watch the patient for signs and symptoms of cerebral edema.

➤ Obtain a 12-lead electrocardiogram, noting arrhythmias, such as heart blocks or PVCs.
➤ Monitor arterial blood gas levels.

Preventive steps
➤ Advise the patient to install carbon monoxide detectors on each floor of his home, with an additional detector near any gas-burning appliances.
➤ Remind the patient to perform regular inspection and maintenance of gas-burning appliances.

Pathophysiology recap
➤ Carbon monoxide—a tasteless, odorless gas—is emitted from a combustion engine (including automobile engines), portable propane heaters, charcoal-burning barbecues, and portable or nonvented natural gas appliances, furnaces, or water heaters.
➤ Dangerous amounts of carbon monoxide can accumulate as a result of improper fuel burning, poor ventilation, or the improper installation or maintenance of, damage to, or malfunction of an appliance.
➤ Poisoning occurs when carbon monoxide enters the lungs through normal breathing.
➤ Carbon monoxide causes tissue hypoxia by displacing oxygen with carboxyhemoglobin, which affects the supply of oxygen to the heart, brain, and other vital organs.
➤ People with heart or respiratory conditions, infants, small children, pregnant females, and house pets may be the first to show signs and symptoms of poisoning.

➤ Caustic substance ingestion

Ingestion of caustic substances, such as household cleaners, strong acids, and strong bases, may occur as an accident (typically in children) or as a deliberate action to cause self-harm (usually in adolescents and adults).

Rapid assessment
➤ Assess the patient's vital signs, noting hypotension, fever, level of consciousness, airway patency, and rate, depth, and pattern of respirations.
➤ Auscultate the lungs and heart sounds.
➤ Obtain an electrocardiogram and note arrhythmias, if present.
➤ Obtain the patient's history; ask about the substance and the amount ingested, chest pain, and vomiting.
➤ Listen to the patient's voice to detect laryngitis, hoarseness, and dysphasia.
➤ Inspect the oropharyngeal cavity for burns and injury.
➤ Observe for drooling and dysphagia.
➤ Observe for stridor.
➤ Auscultate bowel sounds.

➤ Assess for abdominal pain; a boardlike, rigid abdomen; and other signs of peritonitis.

 ALERT *Signs and symptoms of peritonitis, fever, chest pain, and hypotension suggest a full-thickness gastric injury or perforation, which requires immediate surgical intervention.*

Immediate actions
➤ Provide supplemental oxygen, and prepare the patient for emergency endotracheal intubation, cricothyroidotomy, or tracheostomy and mechanical ventilation, if necessary.
➤ Initiate suicide precautions, if necessary.
➤ Withhold oral fluids and solids.

 ALERT *Don't induce vomiting or perform gastric intubation and lavage, which may cause vomiting. Inducing vomiting reintroduces the caustic substance to the upper GI tract.*

➤ Contact Poison Control or a toxicology center to get quick and accurate information, suggestions, and recommendations, if necessary.
➤ Wash the patient's mouth and face to remove particles of the ingested substance.
➤ Administer broad-spectrum antibiotics, antireflux medication, and sucralfate.
➤ Be prepared to administer corticosteroids; however, their use in this indication is controversial.

Follow-up actions
➤ Monitor serum electrolyte levels and provide supplements to correct abnormalities.
➤ Contact Child Protective Services if abuse or neglect is suspected.
➤ Administer total parenteral nutrition or tube feedings to allow for gastric or esophageal rest, respectively, and advance diet, as tolerated.
➤ Prepare the patient for:
– flexible nasopharyngoscopy, laryngoscopy, or endoscopy to visualize the patient's injuries
– chest X-ray to check the mediastinal width and to detect free air in the mediastinum or abdomen, or neck X-ray if the patient has stridor
– surgical intervention, such as an exploratory laparotomy or thoracotomy with possible esophagectomy, esophagogastrectomy, or gastrectomy (for a full-thickness injury)
– periodic esophagography (with a water-soluble contrast) and possible esophageal stenting or dilatation with contrast to detect and correct dysphagia.

Preventive steps
➤ Advise the patient to keep cleaning supplies in their original, closed containers in a locked cabinet out of the reach of children.
➤ Refer the patient with known suicidal impulses for counseling.

Pathophysiology recap

➤ The extent of the injury is determined by the amount of the ingested material, its concentration and form, and whether the patient has vomited or aspirated.

➤ After ingestion, there's an extreme inflammatory reaction that results in erythema and edema of the superficial layers.

➤ Ingestion of caustic substances can cause esophageal stricture and laryngeal stenosis and increase the risk of esophageal cancer.

➤ Alkaline agents, such as drain cleaner, are generally tasteless and odorless, which allows larger amounts to be ingested. These substances typically cause injury to the mucosa and submucosa of the esophagus. Alkaline substances cause liquification necrosis, a process in which necrosis continues from the superficial layers into the deeper tissues.

➤ Acidic agents, such as chlorinated household cleaners, undergo oxygenation reactions and form hydrochloric acid which, if ingested, causes gastric injury. These agents cause coagulation necrosis, a process in which a protective layer forms at the site of the injury, limiting its depth.

➤ Cyanide poisoning

Cyanide can occur in the form of hydrocyanic gas, such as in smoke inhalation; a liquid, such as in hydrocyanic acid and hydrogen cyanide; or as a solid such as potassium cyanide. It's used to make paper, cloth, and plastic; develop photographs; clean metal; and remove gold and silver from ore. It's present in foods, such as apricot and wild cherry pits, and in cigarettes. It's dangerous in any form and is one of the most lethal poisons.

Rapid assessment

➤ Assess the patient's vital signs, noting tachycardia and hypertension (early signs), bradycardia and hypotension (later signs), and a decreased respiratory rate and oxygen saturation.

➤ Assess the patient's neurologic status, noting a staggering gait, loss of consciousness, convulsions, paralysis, and coma.

➤ Obtain the patient's history; ask about nausea, vomiting, dizziness, headache, faintness, vertigo, excitement, and anxiety. Also ask about a burning sensation in the mouth and throat and shortness of breath.

➤ Observe for diaphoresis.

➤ Assess for a bitter almond breath odor.

Immediate actions

➤ Provide high-dose supplemental oxygen, and prepare the patient for endotracheal intubation and mechanical ventilation, if necessary.

➤ Initiate continuous cardiac monitoring.

➤ Administer an antidote to cyanide, such as amyl nitrite, by inhalation, as ordered, until I.V. access is established. Then, administer I.V. sodium nitrite, as ordered.
➤ If the poison was ingested, prepare the patient for insertion of a naso-gastric tube and gastric lavage.

Follow-up actions
➤ Obtain a blood sample for serum cyanide level analysis.

 ALERT *Cyanide levels take time to be confirmed. Treatment should start without the laboratory confirmation to ensure the best possible prognosis.*

➤ Monitor the patient's vital signs closely.
➤ Monitor the patient's respiratory, neurologic, and cardiovascular status frequently.
➤ Monitor arterial blood gas and serum lactic acid levels, noting lactic acidosis.
➤ Take suicide precautions, including one-on-one surveillance of the patient who intended to harm himself or who is suicidal.
➤ Arrange a follow-up appointment with a neurologist 7 to 10 days after discharge to assess for complications.

Preventive steps
➤ Counsel the patient about the safe storage of substances that contain or may have been contaminated by cyanide; reinforce these precautions if he has children.
➤ Explain safety regulations to prevent occupational exposure.
➤ Teach the patient the proper use and maintenance of smoke detectors and practice of fire prevention techniques.
➤ Refer the patient who's suicidal to a suicide prevention hotline or center for counseling.

Pathophysiology recap
➤ Poisoning occurs within seconds of inhaling hydrogen cyanide or within 30 minutes of ingesting the salts of hydrogen cyanide.
➤ Cyanide is rapidly absorbed from the stomach, lungs, mucosa, and skin.
➤ Cyanide inhibits cellular aerobic metabolism and causes cell death.
➤ Death can occur immediately after ingesting only 200 to 300 mg of potassium or sodium cyanide or inhaling 100 mg of hydrogen cyanide.
➤ If the dose of cyanide isn't lethal, the body detoxifies it to form sulfo-cyanides, which are nontoxic.
➤ Complete recovery usually follows if the antidote is administered promptly.

➤ *Decompression sickness*

A rapid change in pressure, such as that experienced by a deep sea diver who surfaces too quickly, causes decompression sickness.

Rapid assessment
➤ Assess the patient's vital signs, noting dyspnea and a dry cough.
➤ Assess the patient for confusion, memory loss, scotoma, tunnel vision, double vision, seizures, and unconsciousness.
➤ Assess for muscle weakness, ascending weakness, or paralysis.
➤ Test to determine if active and passive motion of the painful joints intensifies the pain.
➤ Assess for mottled or marble-looking skin around the abdomen, chest, and shoulders and for pitting edema.
➤ Obtain the patient's history; ask about localized, mild to excruciating deep pain. Ask about headache, blurry vision, vertigo, and nausea and vomiting. Also ask about itching around the ears, face, neck, arms, and upper torso.
➤ Ask about abdominal or chest pain and incontinence (bladder and bowel). Ask about numbness, tingling, burning, or twitching in the peripheral muscles. Ask about burning and tingling in the lower chest and back area. Ask about a deep, burning chest pain located near or under the sternum that's intensified by breathing.

Immediate actions
➤ Provide 100% oxygen via face mask.
➤ Perform cardiopulmonary resuscitation, and prepare the patient for endotracheal intubation and mechanical ventilation, if necessary.
➤ Keep the patient flat to prevent inert gas bubbles from traveling to the brain.
➤ Maintain the patient on bed rest.
➤ If the patient has joint pain, keep the affected joint still.

Follow-up actions
➤ Monitor the patient's vital signs, including oxygen saturation, frequently.
➤ Monitor arterial blood gas values.
➤ Encourage fluid intake or initiate I.V. hydration.
➤ Prepare the patient for a chest X-ray.
➤ Prepare the patient for hyperbaric oxygen treatment—100% oxygen delivered in a high-pressure chamber.
➤ Monitor pain and provide pain medication as needed.
➤ Monitor the patient for decreasing signs and symptoms.
➤ Instruct the patient not to fly or dive again until he's cleared by a physician.

Preventive steps

If decompression resulted from flying, advise the patient:
- not to fly in an unpressurized aircraft above 18,000 feet (5,486 m)
- to avoid strenuous physical activity before flying in an unpressurized aircraft above 18,000 feet and for 24 hours after the flight
- to prebreathe 100% oxygen before a high-altitude flight and continue to do so during the flight.

If decompression resulted from diving, advise the patient:
- to use decompression tables and dive computers to determine the depth and duration of the necessary decompression stops for particular dive depths
- to avoid long and deep dives
- to ascend slowly
- not to fly at high altitudes shortly after a dive.

If decompression resulted from tunnel work, advise the patient to perform a gradual ascent to sea level, making decompression stops.

Pathophysiology recap

- Decompression results from a rapid ascent from scuba diving at depths greater than 33′ (10 m) or a rapid ascent or decompression in an airplane. It can also occur when flying at a high altitude soon after scuba diving. Tunnel work can also result in decompression (in this case, it's sometimes called *caisson disease*).
- In decompression, a relatively rapid decrease in environmental pressure causes inert gases (usually nitrogen), to release into the body tissues.
- In one type of decompression sickness, *the bends,* large joints and limbs—the elbows, shoulders, hip, wrists, knees, and ankles—are affected. Gas is deposited in the tissues and causes localized pain in the limbs and joints, most commonly the shoulder.
- In the patient with neurologic effects of decompression *(cerebral bends)*, an arterial gas embolism causes strokelike signs and symptoms; cerebral bends also affects the spinal cord and peripheral nerves. In the spinal cord, paresis is caused by venous thrombosis, which leads to necrosis and edema of the spinal cord. Embolus formation can also cause damage to peripheral nerves.
- Decompression that affects the lungs is also called *chokes.* Bronchoconstriction and irritation of pulmonary tissue occur as a result of venous gas bubbles that release vasoactive substances.
- Decompression that affects the skin is also called *skin bends.* An embolism causes decreased oxygenated blood flow and decreased venous return.
- Repetitive episodes of decompression sickness can cause cell death in the long bones and in brittle bones.
- Death can occur from larger bubbles that prevent oxygenated blood from getting to the central nervous system and other vital body organs.

➤ *Electric shock*

Injury to the skin or internal organs that results from exposure to an electrical current is called an *electric shock*. Electric shock causes approximately 1,000 deaths annually in the United States.

Rapid assessment
➤ Assess the patient's vital signs, noting spontaneous respirations; if present, assess the rate, depth, and pattern of breathing. Assess the patient's level of consciousness, auscultate for an apical pulse, and palpate for a peripheral pulse.
➤ Obtain the patient's history; ask about headache, numbness, tingling, and muscle pain as well as the date of his last tetanus shot.
➤ Observe the patient for seizures. Examine the skin for burns. Assess for muscle weakness and contraction and signs of bone fractures.

Immediate actions
➤ Initiate continuous cardiac monitoring and observe for arrhythmias such as ventricular fibrillation.
➤ Initiate cardiopulmonary resuscitation, if necessary.
➤ If the patient *isn't* in shock, place him in an upright position to facilitate breathing.

 ALERT *If the patient shows signs of shock, place him in a supine position, with his head slightly lower than his body.*

➤ Administer supplemental oxygen and prepare the patient for endotracheal intubation and mechanical ventilation, if necessary.
➤ Implement seizure and safety precautions.
➤ If the patient has a burn, remove clothing that comes off easily and provide burn care.
➤ Administer I.V. fluids, vasopressors (if indicated), and analgesics.

Follow-up actions
➤ Monitor the patient's vital signs frequently.
➤ Obtain a 12-lead electrocardiogram.
➤ Provide tetanus prophylaxis to the patient with a burn.
➤ Obtain a serum sample to assess complete blood count and cardiac enzymes; obtain a urine myoglobin sample to assess muscle injury.
➤ Observe the patient for signs and symptoms of wound or systemic infection.
➤ Insert an indwelling urinary catheter.
➤ Assess kidney function by monitoring intake and output and blood urea nitrogen and creatinine levels.
➤ Prepare the patient for X-rays to visualize fractures or dislocations.
➤ Prepare the patient for a computed tomography scan of the affected area.

IN ACTION

➤ *MANAGING LIGHTNING STRIKE*

After your softball game is canceled because of a thunderstorm, you start putting your equipment in your car. Suddenly you see a flash of lightning in the next field and hear someone shout that a player is down. Hurrying to help, you find Pete Dunn, 33, lying on the field unconscious. You keep his back and neck as straight as possible and help his teammates carefully move him to the shelter of a nearby concession stand, out of the storm.

What's the situation?

Checking his airway, breathing, and circulation, you find that Mr. Dunn isn't breathing; you also note that he's unresponsive. His uniform is shredded and torn in several places around his right arm. One of his teammates has called 911.

What's your assessment?

Lightning strike – whether direct or indirect (in which lightning passes through the ground or a tree, for example) – can cause severe injuries. Cardiac arrest is the most common cause of death related to lightning strike. Respiratory arrest may persist even after a cardiac rhythm has been established.

Because lightning usually passes over the body's surface rather than through the body, even in a direct hit, tissue damage and elevated levels of potassium, creatine kinase, and myoglobin are relatively rare. Burns, if present, are usually mild and superficial.

What must you do immediately?

Use a jaw-thrust maneuver to open Mr. Dunn's airway and deliver two rescue breaths. You see no signs of spontaneous circulation, so you start chest compressions. After a minute, you assess for signs of spontaneous breathing or circulation. Finding none, you continue with cardiopulmonary resuscitation.

The paramedics arrive and attach a portable monitor-defibrillator to Mr. Dunn. After determining that he's in ventricular fibrillation, they deliver two rapid defibrillations. Mr. Dunn's heart responds with sinus bradycardia followed by sinus tachycardia. He has a carotid pulse, but still isn't attempting to breathe, so the paramedics intubate and manually ventilate him. They also establish I.V. access, draw blood for laboratory studies, and start an infusion of normal saline solution. Mr. Dunn is taken to the local hospital.

When continuous electrocardiogram (ECG) monitoring is started in the emergency department (ED), it reveals sinus tachycardia. A 12-lead ECG rules out cardiac conduction defects. Mr. Dunn is having vascular spasms caused by the lightning strike, so the staff uses a Doppler ultrasound to identify peripheral pulses. Mr. Dunn's blood pressure is 148/86 mm Hg, but he still isn't breathing spontaneously, so he's put on mechanical ventilation. The ED physician notes that the only burn injury is a superficial burn in a fernlike pattern on Mr. Dunn's right arm. He slows the I.V. infusion to prevent cerebral edema, which may accompany lightning strike. He examines Mr. Dunn's ears and finds blood

(continued)

> **MANAGING LIGHTNING STRIKE** (continued)

behind both tympanic membranes, which were ruptured by high-pressure shock waves from the thunderclap. The physician orders a computed tomography scan of the brain, which rules out basilar skull fractures and intracerebral bleeding.

Mr. Dunn is transferred to the surgical intensive care unit for ventilator support and ECG monitoring for delayed cardiac arrhythmias. Because eye injuries are common in lightning strike victims, the ED physician orders an ophthalmology consult.

What should be done later?

As Mr. Dunn regains consciousness, he begins to breathe spontaneously and to assist the ventilator. He's weaned from the ventilator, but the ECG monitoring continues: Conduction disturbances, such as a prolonged QT interval, may not be evident until the second day.

A neuropsychologist will evaluate Mr. Dunn for long-term neurologic damage, including peripheral injury and associated pain, and psychological dysfunction, which isn't related to the severity of the injury.

After 3 days, Mr. Dunn is discharged home. He'll be followed by the neuropsychologist for several months to watch for lightning-associated neurologic injuries.

Day, M.W. "Action Stat: Lightning Strike," *Nursing* 33(6):104, June 2003. Used with permission.

> Prepare the patient with severe burns for skin grafting or wound debridement, if necessary.
> Test for hearing impairment.

Preventive steps

> Teach the patient about safety measures in the home, such as placing safety caps in all electrical outlets and ensuring that all electrical cords and appliance parts are out of the reach of children.
> Advise the patient to read and follow the safety instructions included with electrical appliances.
> Caution the patient to keep electrical appliances away from water and not to use such appliances in the shower, when wet, or when touching water or water pipes.

Pathophysiology recap

> The human body conducts electricity well.
> Electric shock results from contact with exposed electrical wiring or parts of electrical appliances, contact with lightning or high-voltage power lines, or other exposures related to occupation. (See *Managing lightning strike*.)

➤ In young children, electric shock can result from chewing on electrical cords and placing metal objects into an electrical outlet.

➤ Electric current in the body can cause thermal burns, cardiac arrest, and muscle, nerve, and tissue damage.

➤ Electrical burns that appear minor can have serious related internal damage, especially to the heart, muscles, or brain.

➤ Prognosis depends on the voltage to which the patient was exposed, the route the current traveled through the body, the patient's baseline health status, and the promptness of treatment.

➤ Death can result from direct contact with an electrical current.

➤ Hyperthermia

Also known as *heat syndrome,* hyperthermia is an elevation in body temperature over 99° F (37.2° C). It may result from environmental or internal conditions that increase heat production or impair heat dissipation.

Rapid assessment

➤ Assess the rate, pattern, and depth of respirations.

➤ Obtain the patient's history; ask about prolonged activity in a very warm or hot environment without adequate salt and fluid intake. Ask about nausea and abdominal cramps.

➤ Observe the patient for mild agitation.

➤ Obtain the patient's vital signs, noting mild hypertension, tachycardia, and a temperature between 99° and 103° F (37.2° and 39.5° C); these signs indicate *mild* hyperthermia. Hypotension, a rapid thready pulse, and a temperature up to 104° F (40° C) indicate moderate hyperthermia. Temperature above 106° F (41.1° C) indicates *critical* hyperthermia.

➤ In mild hyperthermia, note moist, cool skin. Assess for muscle tenderness, twitching, and spasms and hard, lumpy muscles.

➤ In moderate hyperthermia, the patient may report dizziness, headache, syncope, and confusion. Ask about thirst, nausea, vomiting, and muscle cramping. Observe for weakness, oliguria and pale, moist skin.

➤ In critical hyperthermia, obtain an electrocardiogram and assess for supraventricular or ventricular tachycardia. Evaluate the patient for confusion, combativeness, delirium, loss of consciousness, and seizures. Observe him for tachypnea; fixed, dilated pupils; and hot, dry, reddened skin.

Immediate actions

➤ Provide supplemental oxygen and prepare the patient for endotracheal intubation and mechanical ventilation, if necessary.

➤ Institute continuous cardiac monitoring and evaluate for arrhythmias.

➤ Prepare the patient for pulmonary artery catheter insertion to monitor core temperature.

In mild and moderate hyperthermia:
- ➤ Provide a cool environment.
- ➤ Allow the patient to rest.
- ➤ Encourage oral intake and administer I.V. fluids.
- ➤ Replace electrolytes, as necessary.

In critical hyperthermia:
- ➤ Remove the patient's clothing.
- ➤ Apply cool water to the skin, and then fan the patient with cool air.
- ➤ Administer diazepam or chlorpromazine to control shivering.

 ALERT *Shivering needs to be treated because it increases metabolic demand and oxygen consumption.*

- ➤ Apply hypothermia blankets and ice packs to the groin and axillae, if necessary.

 ALERT *The goal is to reduce the patient's temperature, but not too rapidly. Too rapid a reduction can lead to vasoconstriction, which can cause shivering.*

Follow-up actions
- ➤ Continue treatment until the patient's temperature drops below 102.2° F (39° C).
- ➤ Monitor the patient's vital signs frequently, including central venous pressure and pulmonary artery wedge pressure.
- ➤ Monitor intake and output.
- ➤ Monitor blood urea nitrogen and serum creatinine levels, and assess the patient for signs and symptoms of rhabdomyolysis, such as muscle pain, weakness, tenderness, malaise, nausea, vomiting, tachycardia, and dark reddish-brown urine.
- ➤ Monitor serum electrolyte levels and treat abnormalities.
- ➤ Monitor arterial blood gas levels for respiratory alkalosis and hypoxemia.

Preventive steps
- ➤ Caution the patient to reduce activity—especially outdoor activity—in hot, humid weather.
- ➤ Advise the patient to wear light-colored, lightweight, loose-fitting clothing during hot weather and to wear a hat and sunglasses.
- ➤ Instruct the patient to drink sufficient fluids, especially water, in hot weather and after vigorous physical activity. Warn him to avoid caffeine and alcohol in hot weather.
- ➤ Advise the patient to use air conditioning or to open windows and use a fan to help circulate air indoors.

Pathophysiology recap
- Humans normally adjust to excessive temperatures by complex cardio-vascular and neurologic changes that are coordinated by the hypothalamus.
- Heat loss offsets heat production to regulate the body temperature. The body does this by evaporation or vasodilation, which cools its surface by radiation, conduction, and convection. When heat loss mechanisms fail to offset heat production, the body retains heat. If body temperature remains elevated, fluid loss becomes excessive and hypovolemic shock can occur.
- Mild hyperthermia *(heat cramps)* occurs with excessive perspiration and loss of salt from the body.
- Moderate hyperthermia *(heat exhaustion)* occurs in exposure to high temperatures; blood accumulates in the skin in an attempt to decrease the body's temperature, causing a decrease in circulating blood volume and cerebral blood flow and leading to syncope.
- Critical hyperthermia *(heatstroke)* occurs when the body's temperature continues to rise and internal organs are damaged. If untreated, heat-stroke can result in death.
- Conditions that increase heat production include excessive exercise, infection, and drugs.
- Impaired heat dissipation results from high temperature and humidity, lack of acclimatization, excess clothing, cardiovascular disease, obesity, dehydration, sweat gland dysfunction, and illicit drug use.

➤ *Hypothermia*

Hypothermia is a core body temperature below 95° F (35° C). Severe hypothermia can be fatal.

Rapid assessment
- Obtain the patient's history; ask about the cause of hypothermia, the temperature to which the patient was exposed, and the length of exposure.
- Assess the patient's vital signs, noting a temperature of 89.6° to 95° F (32° and 35° C); this indicates *mild* hypothermia. A temperature of 86° to 89.6° F (30° to 32° C) indicates *moderate* hypothermia. Absence of peripheral pulses and audible heart sounds with a body temperature of 77° to 86° F (25° to 30° C) indicates *severe* hypothermia.
- In mild hypothermia, observe the patient for shivering and assess for slurred speech. Test for amnesia.
- In moderate hypothermia, assess the patient's level of consciousness, noting unresponsiveness. Observe for peripheral cyanosis. Assess for muscle rigidity.

➤ In severe hypothermia, observe for dilated pupils. Assess for a rigor-mortis-like state. Obtain an electrocardiogram and observe for ventricular fibrillation. Assess for absent deep tendon reflexes.

Immediate actions
➤ Initiate cardiopulmonary resuscitation (CPR), if necessary.

ALERT *Hypothermia helps protect the brain from anoxia, which normally accompanies prolonged cardiopulmonary arrest. Therefore, even if the patient has been unresponsive for a long time, CPR may resuscitate him, especially after a cold-water near drowning.*

➤ Initiate continuous cardiac monitoring.
➤ Administer supplemental oxygen, and prepare the patient for endotracheal intubation and mechanical ventilation, if necessary.
➤ Institute rewarming measures:
 – In passive rewarming, the patient rewarms on his own.
 – Active external rewarming is performed with heating blankets; warm water immersion; heated objects, such as water bottles; and radiant heat.
 – Active core rewarming includes the use of heated I.V. fluids, genitourinary tract irrigation, extracorporeal rewarming, hemodialysis, and peritoneal, gastric, and mediastinal lavage.

Follow-up actions
➤ Prepare the patient for a pulmonary artery catheter insertion to monitor core temperatures.
➤ Monitor the patient's vital signs, including core temperatures, frequently.
➤ Continue warming until the core body temperature is within 1° to 2° F (0.6° to 1.1° C) of the desired body temperature.
➤ If the patient has been hypothermic for longer than 45 minutes, administer additional fluids, as ordered, to compensate for the expansion of the vascular space that occurs during vasodilation in warming.
➤ Monitor arterial blood gas values and treat abnormalities.
➤ Monitor intake and output.
➤ Monitor serum electrolyte levels and treat abnormalities.

ALERT *Stay alert for signs and symptoms of hyperkalemia. If hyperkalemia occurs, administer calcium chloride, sodium bicarbonate, glucose, and insulin, as ordered. Anticipate the need for sodium polystyrene sulfonate enemas.*

Preventive steps
➤ Advise the patient, especially if he's elderly, to maintain proper insulation in the home and keep the indoor temperature 70° F (21.1° C) or higher.

➤ Caution the patient to wear warm clothing and use warm bedding.
➤ Advise the patient to get adequate nutrition, rest, and exercise.
➤ When the patient is expected to be out in the cold, especially for prolonged periods, advise him to:
 – wear loose-fitting clothing in layers
 – cover the hands, feet, and head (30% to 50% of body heat is lost through the head)
 – wear dry clothes and footwear and wind- and water-resistant outer garments
 – avoid alcohol.

Pathophysiology recap
➤ In hypothermia, metabolic changes slow the functions of most major organ systems.
➤ Renal blood flow and glomerular filtration rate are decreased.
➤ Vital organs are physiologically affected.
➤ Severe hypothermia results in decreased cerebral blood flow, diminished oxygen requirements, reduced cardiac output, and decreased arterial pressure.
➤ Causes of hypothermia include near-drowning in cold water, prolonged exposure to cold temperatures, disease or debility that alters homeostasis, and administration of large amounts of cold blood or blood products.
➤ Risk factors include youth, old age, lack of insulating body fat, wet or inadequate clothing, drug abuse, cardiac disease, smoking, fatigue, malnutrition, depletion of calorie reserves, and excessive alcohol intake.

➤ Insect stings

When a bee or wasp punctures the skin, it can cause a local reaction or, to those who are hypersensitive or allergic, an anaphylactic reaction. For 1 in every 100 people, a bee or wasp sting can be fatal.

Rapid assessment
➤ Obtain the patient's history; ask about the type of sting that occurred and the onset of signs and symptoms.
➤ For a local reaction, assess the sting site for erythema, pain, swelling, and itching. The reaction will dissipate in a few hours.
➤ For a large local reaction, assess the sting site for pain, swelling, and itching at the sting site and in other areas.
　In a systemic reaction (anaphylaxis):
➤ Obtain the patient's vital signs, noting hypotension and his level of consciousness.
➤ Assess for spontaneous respirations and, if present, determine rate, depth, and pattern.

➤ Observe for dyspnea and ask about a choking feeling in the throat. Auscultate the lungs for wheezing.
➤ Observe the patient's entire body for hives or swelling, especially his hands and face, and note itching around the eyes and darkened skin.
➤ Ask about difficulty breathing or swallowing, dizziness, weakness, a warm feeling, nausea, vomiting, stomach cramps, and diarrhea. Listen for hoarse speech.

Immediate actions
➤ Provide supplemental oxygen, and prepare the patient for endotracheal intubation and mechanical ventilation, if necessary.
➤ Remove the stinger, if present.
➤ Use an extractor pump, if available, to remove the venom.
➤ Administer epinephrine, bronchodilators, antihistamines, topical hydrocortisone, prednisone, and a topical anesthetic.

Follow-up actions
➤ Monitor the patient's vital signs frequently.
➤ Prepare the patient for insertion of an arterial catheter and monitor arterial blood gas values frequently.
➤ Observe the sting site and sites that the patient scratched for signs and symptoms of infection.
➤ Provide skin or wound care to the sting site.
➤ Keep the skin clean and keep the patient's fingernails short to help prevent infection caused by scratching.

Preventive steps
➤ Advise the patient to spray patio, picnic, and garbage areas with bee and wasp formula insecticides and to destroy nests. Caution him, however, to have an exterminator perform these tasks in severe or persistent infestations. The patient who's allergic to insect stings should also have an exterminator perform insect control measures.
➤ Explain that nests shouldn't be disturbed, nor should nests be burned or flooded in an attempt at removal; doing so will cause the insects to become more aggressive.
➤ Teach the patient to cover food, especially fruit, sugary foods, and soft drinks, when eating outdoors.
➤ Instruct the patient to keep garbage tightly sealed and dispose of it frequently.
➤ Advise the patient to protect his face and neck areas with his hands if a bee or wasp is going to sting in one of those locations.
➤ Instruct the patient to avoid heavy-scented shampoos, lotions, soaps, and perfumes—all of which attract bees and wasps—and to wear light-colored clothing and closed shoes.
➤ Teach the patient with known hypersensitivity to bee and wasp stings not to go outdoors alone, to wear medical identification, and to carry an epinephrine pen. If necessary, instruct him on the use of such a pen.

Pathophysiology recap

➤ A bee or wasp injects a venomous fluid under the skin when it stings.
➤ The severity of the reaction generally (but not always) correlates with the abruptness of the onset of symptoms; the more abrupt the onset, the more severe the reaction.
➤ When a patient has a systemic reaction to a sting, the intensity may increase with each following sting (this varies individually). Some people produce excess amounts of antibodies in their immune systems after the initial sting to which there's no reaction or a mild reaction. If stung again, the venom combines with the antibody produced after the first sting. This combination triggers an allergic response.
➤ Honey bees have barbed stingers that remain in the skin of the victim after the sting. It takes 2 to 3 minutes for the sac containing the venom to empty into the body.
➤ Wasps have lancelike stingers and can sting repeatedly. A wasp sting injects venom directly under the skin.

➤ Mammal bites

Bites from mammals, primarily dogs and cats, occur when the animal's canine teeth break the skin. In the United States, dogs inflict the greatest number of bites on humans. Most are minor but require medical attention nonetheless. Cat bites are far less common than dog bites, but the infection rate from cat bites surpasses the infection rate from dog bites.

 ALERT *Cat bites may appear less serious than they are; they carry a high risk for infection.*

Rapid assessment

➤ Obtain the patient's history.
➤ Ask about the type of animal that inflicted the bite, the animal's behavior, and whether the attack was provoked.
➤ Assess the patient's vital signs, noting hypotension, tachycardia, fever, and the depth, rate, and pattern of respirations.
➤ Palpate peripheral pulses.
➤ Evaluate the patient's motor function and sensation.
➤ Carefully inspect wounds, noting tissue damage, exposed tendons or bones, and visible foreign bodies such as teeth.

Immediate actions

➤ Provide supplemental oxygen, and prepare the patient for endotracheal intubation and mechanical ventilation, if necessary (usually only necessary with severe face and neck bites).
➤ Thoroughly irrigate wounds with an isotonic sodium chloride solution under high pressure using a 16G or 18G angiocatheter.

➤ MANAGING TETANUS PROPHYLAXIS

History of tetanus immunization (number of doses)	Tetanus-prone wounds		Non-tetanus-prone wounds	
	Td*	TIG**	Td	TIG
UNCERTAIN	Yes	Yes	Yes	No
0 TO 1	Yes	Yes	Yes	No
2	Yes	No (yes if 24 hours since wound was inflicted)	Yes	No
3 OR MORE	No (yes if more than 10 years since last dose)	No	No (yes if more than 10 years since last dose)	No

*Td = Tetanus and diphtheria toxoids adsorbed (for adult use), 0.5 ml
**TIG = Tetanus immune globulin (human), 250 units
Note: When Td and TIG are given concurrently, separate syringes and separate sites should be used.
Note: For children younger than age 7, tetanus and diphtheria toxoids and pertussis vaccine, adsorbed are preferred over tetanus toxoid alone. If pertussis vaccine is contraindicated, administer tetanus and diphtheria toxoids, adsorbed.

➤ Attempt to control severe bleeding using pressure.
➤ Administer antibiotics, analgesics, and isotonic I.V. fluids.
➤ Administer tetanus prophylaxis. (See *Managing tetanus prophylaxis*.)
➤ Be prepared to administer rabies prophylaxis if the patient suffered an unprovoked attack by an unfamiliar animal. (See *Rabies*.)

Follow-up actions
➤ Monitor the patient's vital signs frequently.
➤ Assess the patient for signs and symptoms of rabies.
➤ Monitor hemoglobin level and hematocrit, and transfuse with packed red blood cells, if necessary.
➤ Monitor the patient's white blood cell count, and monitor him for signs and symptoms of infection and cellulitis.
➤ Provide wound care, as ordered, using strict aseptic technique.

COMPLICATIONS
➤ *RABIES*

A potentially fatal complication of mammal bites (usually wild animals), rabies occurs after being bitten by an infected animal. The bite wound introduces the virus into the victim through the saliva of the infected animal. Rabies is an acute central nervous system (CNS) infection that typically causes death if untreated before the onset of symptoms. Treatment soon after exposure, however, may prevent fatal CNS involvement.

Signs and symptoms
After an incubation period of 1 to 3 months, rabies typically produces:
➤ local or radiating pain or burning and a sensation of cold
➤ pruritus and tingling at the bite site
➤ prodromal signs and symptoms, including a slight fever (100° to 102° F [37.8° to 38.9° C]), malaise, headache, anorexia, nausea, sore throat, and cough
➤ nervousness, anxiety, and irritability
➤ hyperesthesia, photophobia, and sensitivity to loud noises
➤ pupillary dilation
➤ tachycardia and shallow respirations
➤ pain and paresthesia in the bitten area
➤ excessive salivation, lacrimation, and perspiration.
  About 2 to 10 days after the onset of prodromal symptoms, a phase of excitation produces:
➤ agitation, marked restlessness, anxiety, and apprehension
➤ cranial nerve dysfunction resulting in ocular palsies, strabismus, asymmetrical pupillary dilation or constriction, absence of corneal reflexes, weakness of facial muscles, and hoarseness
➤ severe systemic symptoms, including tachycardia or bradycardia, cyclic respirations, urine retention, and a temperature of about 103° F (39.4° C)
➤ hydrophobia (literally, "fear of water"), in about 50% of affected patients
➤ difficulty swallowing, causing frothy saliva to drip from the patient's mouth
➤ forceful, painful pharyngeal muscle spasms, expelling liquid from the mouth and causing dehydration and, possibly, apnea, cyanosis, and death.
  Eventually, even the sight, mention, or thought of water causes uncontrollable pharyngeal muscle spasms and excessive salivation; after about 3 days, excitation and hydrophobia subside and the progressively paralytic, terminal phase of this illness begins.

Treatment
Treatment includes:
➤ cleaning all bite wounds (If the wound requires suturing, special treatment and suturing techniques must be used to allow proper drainage.)
➤ tetanus prophylaxis, if indicated
➤ antibiotics, as ordered, to control bacterial infection from the bite.
  After rabies exposure, a patient who has never been immunized must receive passive immunization with rabies immune globulin (RIG) and active

(continued)

> **RABIES** (continued)

immunization with human diploid cell vaccine (HDCV). If the patient has received HDCV before and has an adequate rabies antibody titer, he'll require only an HDCV booster; RIG immunization isn't necessary.

Nursing considerations
➤ When injecting rabies vaccine, rotate injection sites on the upper arm or thigh. Watch for and symptomatically treat redness, itching, pain, and tenderness at the injection site. Half of the RIG should be infiltrated into and around the bite wound, with the remainder given I.M.
➤ Cooperate with public health authorities to determine the vaccination status of the animal. If the animal is proven rabid, help identify others at risk.
   If rabies develops:
➤ Monitor cardiac and pulmonary function continuously.
➤ Isolate the patient. Wear a gown, gloves, and protection for the eyes and mouth when handling saliva and articles contaminated with saliva. Take precautions to avoid being bitten by the patient during the excitation phase.
➤ Keep the patient's room dark and quiet.
➤ Establish communication with the patient and his family. Provide psychological support to help them cope with the patient's symptoms and probable death.
   To help prevent rabies:
➤ Stress the need for vaccination of household pets that may be exposed to rabid wild animals.
➤ Warn people not to try to touch wild animals, especially if they appear ill or overly docile, a possible sign of rabies.
➤ Assist in the prophylactic administration of rabies vaccine to high-risk people, such as farm workers, forest rangers, spelunkers (cave explorers), and veterinarians.

➤ Prepare the patient with bone involvement for an X-ray or bone scan to rule out osteomyelitis and joint aspiration to rule out septic arthritis.
➤ Prepare the patient with a bite to the head for a skull X-ray or computed tomography scan of the head. Also assess him for signs and symptoms of meningitis.
➤ Prepare the patient for X-rays of bones in the area of the bite to detect foreign bodies that aren't visible and to assess for fractures.
➤ If indicated, prepare the patient for surgical interventions, such as foreign body removal, thrombectomy, and wound inspection, debridement, excision, or wound closure. Rarely, amputation may be necessary.

Preventive steps
➤ If the patient is a pet owner, advise him to leash his pets, especially in the presence of children, and to monitor his pets closely when outdoors.

➤ Teach children to avoid approaching animals, especially unfamiliar animals or those that are eating.

Pathophysiology recap
➤ Dogs have wide canine teeth and can use great force while biting.

 ALERT *Younger children are at risk for wounds in the head, neck, and face areas because the mouths of larger breeds of dogs are level with that area of children's bodies. Dog teeth are capable of penetrating the skull.*

➤ Cats have thin canine teeth that puncture the skin and force bacteria into deep tissues.
➤ Cats and dogs have potentially infectious aerobic and anaerobic bacteria in their oral cavities, such as *Staphylococcus, Streptococcus,* and *Pasteurella.*

➤ Near drowning

In near drowning, the victim survives (at least temporarily) the physiologic effects of submersion in fluid.

Rapid assessment
➤ Obtain the patient's history; ask about the cause of near drowning. Ask about headache, substernal chest pain, and vomiting.
➤ Assess the patient's vital signs, noting fever or a low temperature, tachycardia, and hypotension. Assess his level of consciousness (LOC) and respiratory status, noting shallow, gasping, or absent respirations.
➤ Auscultate the lungs for crackles, rhonchi, or wheezing.
➤ Auscultate the apical heart rate and palpate for a peripheral pulse.
➤ Observe the patient for seizures, apprehensiveness, irritability, restlessness, and lethargy.
➤ Obtain an electrocardiogram (ECG) and assess for arrhythmias or asystole.
➤ Auscultate for bowel sounds.

 ALERT *Bowel ischemia and necrosis may result from prolonged periods of hypoxemia and hypotension secondary to shunting of blood to more vital organs.*

Immediate actions
➤ Stabilize the patient's neck in case he has a cervical injury.
➤ Provide supplemental oxygen, and prepare the patient for endotracheal intubation and mechanical ventilation, if necessary.
➤ Prepare the patient for a cervical spine X-ray to rule out cervical fracture.

➤ Perform cardiopulmonary resuscitation, if needed.
➤ Place the patient in semi-Fowler's position to maximize chest expansion after cervical X-rays have ruled out cervical injury.
➤ Institute continuous cardiac monitoring.
➤ Obtain a serum sample for arterial blood gas levels to show the degree of hypoxia and acid-base imbalance and to identify hypoxemia, hypercapnia, and combined respiratory and metabolic acidosis.

 ALERT *If the patient is hypothermic, be sure to use warm humidified oxygen to prevent additional cooling.*

 ALERT *Positive end-expiratory pressure (PEEP) is especially helpful for the patient who experienced freshwater near drowning because alveoli remain open due to the pressure even without adequate surfactant. The patient may experience low levels of surfactant for 2 to 3 days after aspirating freshwater; therefore, discontinue PEEP carefully and monitor the patient closely for deterioration in respiratory status during discontinuation.*

➤ Perform active external rewarming and passive rewarming measures for mild hypothermia (89.6° to 95° F [32° to 35° C]), active external rewarming of truncal areas only and passive rewarming measures for moderate hypothermia (86° to 89.6° F [30° to 32° C]), and active internal rewarming measures for severe hypothermia (less than 86° F). (See "Hypothermia," page 371.)
➤ Obtain a 12-lead ECG to reveal myocardial ischemia.
➤ Administer sodium bicarbonate, bronchodilators, I.V. fluid replacement, vasopressors, and diuretics, as indicated.

 ALERT *Because a hypothermic patient experiences a decrease in drug metabolism, intervals between dosing of I.V. medications should be longer than usual. As the patient is rewarmed, stay alert for a boluslike effect due to vasodilation.*

Follow-up actions

➤ Prepare the patient for central venous or pulmonary artery catheter insertion.
➤ Monitor the patient's vital signs frequently, including oxygen saturation, central venous pressure, pulmonary artery wedge pressure, and core temperature.
➤ Provide nasotracheal or endotracheal suction, as needed, to clear secretions.
➤ Watch for signs and symptoms of increased intracranial pressure—decreased LOC, irritability, nausea, vomiting, altered pupillary response, altered motor response, or a disconjugate gaze.
➤ Insert a nasogastric tube to prevent vomiting and reduce the risk of further aspiration.

➤ Monitor serum electrolyte levels, especially for hyperkalemia due to acidosis or hemolysis

➤ Monitor complete blood count for increased white blood cells (WBCs) with alveolar inflammation or decreased WBCs with hypothermia.

➤ Insert an indwelling urinary catheter.

➤ Monitor intake and output and serum blood urea nitrogen and creatinine levels to determine kidney function.

➤ Prepare the patient for serial chest X-rays to reveal inflammation, fluid accumulation, fractures, foreign objects, and pulmonary infiltrates, which suggest pulmonary edema.

➤ Watch the patient for signs of impeding coagulopathy (petechiae, bruising, and bleeding or oozing from gums or venipuncture sites), and monitor serum coagulation studies.

➤ Provide a calm, quiet environment.

Preventive steps

➤ Remind parents never to leave an infant or child unattended in a bathtub or near a body of water. A child can drown in a toilet bowl or a bucket of water.

➤ Teach pool and swimming safety practices:
  – Never swim alone.
  – Avoid alcohol and drug use when around water.
  – Use flotation devices.
  – Wear proper swim wear and footwear.
  – Observe children when swimming.
  – Obtain swimming lessons, if needed.
  – Swim near the lifeguard.
  – Don't enter the water when riptides or currents are present.
  – Don't dive in shallow or unknown water depths.

➤ Teach boating safety practices:
  – Obtain a boating license.
  – Wear a life vest and instruct all passengers to do likewise.
  – Perform regular boat maintenance.
  – Don't use alcohol and drugs while boating.
  – Don't dive from the deck of a boat or swim near a boat.
  – Stay seated while the boat is moving.

Pathophysiology recap

➤ Aspiration of such contaminants as chlorine, mud, algae, weeds, and other foreign material can occur in all types of near drowning. Contaminants may lead to obstruction, aspiration, pneumonia, and pulmonary fibrosis.

➤ Cold water (69.8° F [21° C]) submersion may offer a protective effect by causing cardiac arrest and decreased tissue oxygen demand.

➤ Water rapidly conducts heat away from the body, resulting in the possibility of hypothermia even after drowning in warm water. (See *Physiologic changes in near drowning,* page 382.)

➤ PHYSIOLOGIC CHANGES IN NEAR DROWNING

The flowchart below shows the primary cellular alterations that occur during near drowning. Separate pathways are shown for saltwater and freshwater incidents. Hypothermia presents a separate pathway that may preserve neurologic function by decreasing the metabolic rate. All pathways lead to diffuse pulmonary edema.

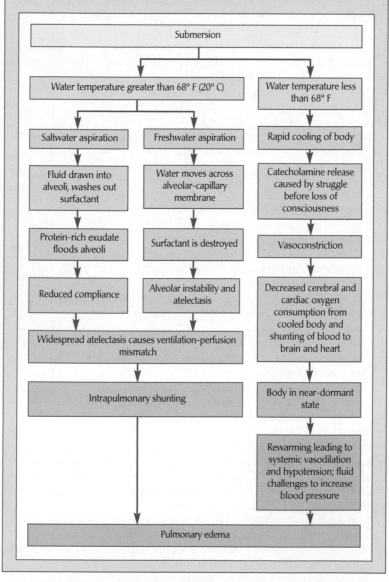

➤ In dry near drowning, the victim doesn't aspirate fluid but suffers respiratory obstruction or asphyxia.

➤ In wet near drowning, the victim aspirates fluid and suffers from asphyxia or secondary changes from fluid aspiration.

➤ In secondary near drowning, the victim suffers recurrence of respiratory distress (usually aspiration pneumonia or pulmonary edema) within minutes or 1 to 2 days after a near-drowning incident.

➤ In freshwater aspiration, water moves across the alveolar-capillary membrane and surfactant is destroyed. Alveolar instability and widespread atelectasis cause ventilation-perfusion mismatch. These changes, along with increased capillary permeability, lead to pulmonary edema and hypoxemia.

➤ In saltwater aspiration, the hypertonicity of seawater exerts an osmotic force, which pulls fluid from pulmonary capillaries into the alveoli. This results in an intrapulmonary shunt, which causes hypoxemia. Also, injury to the pulmonary capillary membrane causes pulmonary edema.

 ALERT *Saltwater aspiration is considered to be more dangerous than freshwater aspiration because it contains more types of bacteria.*

➤ *Organophosphate poisoning*

Organophosphates are toxic chemicals used in the home and in industry for such applications as insecticides and nerve gas. Poisoning can occur as a result of cutaneous contact, contact with mucous membranes, inhalation, or ingestion of the chemicals.

Rapid assessment
➤ Obtain the patient's history; ask about the route of contact — inhalation, cutaneous, or ingestion. Also ask about nausea, vomiting, diarrhea, abdominal pain, and muscle cramping.

➤ Listen for hoarseness, a sign of laryngospasm.

➤ Assess the patient's vital signs, noting bradycardia and hypotension (muscarinic effects) or tachycardia and hypertension (nicotinic effects).

➤ Observe the patient for anxiety, restlessness, confusion, seizures, insomnia, tremors, impaired memory, and coma.

➤ Auscultate the lungs for wheezing, indicating bronchospasm, or decreased breath sounds, indicating respiratory muscle paralysis.

➤ Obtain an electrocardiogram (ECG) and assess for arrhythmias.

➤ Observe the patient for rhinorrhea and cough and for increased salivation, lacrimation, and diaphoresis.

➤ Assess for urinary and fecal incontinence.

➤ Observe for muscle fasciculations and test for weakness, cogwheel rigidity, and paralysis.

Immediate actions

ALERT *Wear neoprene or nitrile gloves, gowns, and charcoal cartridge masks when treating the patient to avoid physical contact and inhalation of organophosphates.*

➤ Perform cardiopulmonary resuscitation, if necessary.
➤ Provide supplemental oxygen, and prepare the patient for endotracheal intubation and mechanical ventilation, if necessary.
➤ Remove the patient's clothing and discard it as hazardous waste.
➤ Clean the patient's skin with soap and water.
➤ Monitor erythrocyte and plasma cholinesterase levels.

ALERT *It takes 4 to 7 weeks for a laboratory to measure cholinesterase levels. A low level can only help diagnose the condition retrospectively. A diagnosis would be made if the serum cholinesterase was less than 50% of the normal level.*

➤ Administer sodium chloride for ocular irrigation in the patient with eye exposure, activated charcoal or sorbitol in the patient with GI contamination, and atropine in the patient with muscarinic symptoms.

ALERT *Initiate continuous cardiac monitoring and have a defibrillator and emergency cart at the bedside before administering atropine — it can cause arrhythmias.*

➤ Administer glycopyrrolate and pralidoxime.
➤ Give diazepam if seizures are present.

Follow-up actions

➤ Monitor the patient's vital signs frequently.
➤ Monitor arterial blood gas values and treat abnormalities.
➤ Monitor electrolyte levels and treat abnormalities.
➤ Obtain a 12-lead ECG and note arrhythmias.
➤ Monitor intake and output.
➤ Assess kidney function by monitoring serum blood urea nitrogen and creatinine levels.
➤ Monitor for a decreased white blood cell count consistent with a stress reaction, increased hematocrit due to fluid depletion, and acidosis secondary to poor tissue perfusion.
➤ Monitor bedside blood glucose levels for hyperglycemia due to catecholamine excess.

Preventive steps

➤ Advise all persons who come into contact with insecticides to practice such safety measures as the use of masks, gowns, gloves, goggles, respiratory filters, and hazardous material jumpsuits.

Pathophysiology recap

➤ Organophosphate poisoning occurs as a result of the compound's ability to inhibit acetylcholinesterase at cholinergic junctions of the nervous

system (postganglionic parasympathetic neuroeffector junctions, autonomic ganglia, and synapses in the central nervous system).
➤ Acetylcholinesterase breaks down acetylcholine after a nerve is stimulated.
➤ When acetylcholinesterase is inhibited, acetylcholine accumulates and there's an excessive stimulation followed by a depression.
➤ Organophosphates have an additive effect with repeated exposure causing progressive cholinesterase inhibition.
➤ Signs and symptoms of poisoning are due to an excessive amount of acetylcholine at the nerve endings (muscarinic and nicotinic receptors). This produces the same effect as hyperstimulation of the parasympathetic nervous system.

➤ Radiation exposure

Excessive exposure to radiation causes tissue damage.

Rapid assessment
➤ Assess the patient's vital signs, noting hypotension, tachycardia, and his level of consciousness.
➤ Assess the rate, depth, and pattern of respirations.
➤ If available, use a Geiger counter to help determine if radioactive material was ingested or inhaled and to evaluate the amount of radiation in open wounds.
➤ Assess the patient for signs of hypothyroidism, cataracts, alopecia, brittle nails, and dry, erythematous skin.
➤ Assess for malignant lesions.
➤ If acute hematopoietic radiation toxicity is suspected, assess the patient for pallor, weakness, oropharyngeal abscesses, nosebleeds, petechiae, hemorrhage, and bleeding from the skin, genitourinary tract, and GI tract.
➤ If GI radiation toxicity is suspected, assess for circulatory collapse, mouth and throat ulcers and infection, and intractable nausea, vomiting, and diarrhea.
➤ If cerebral radiation toxicity is suspected, assess the patient for lethargy, tremors, seizures, confusion, nausea, vomiting, diarrhea, and coma.
➤ If cardiovascular radiation toxicity is suspected, assess the patient for hypotension, shock, and cardiac arrhythmias. (See *Effects of whole body irradiation,* page 386.)

Immediate actions
➤ Initiate cardiopulmonary resuscitation, if necessary.
➤ Provide supplemental oxygen, and prepare the patient for endotracheal intubation and mechanical ventilation, if necessary.

➤ EFFECTS OF WHOLE BODY IRRADIATION

Symptoms resulting from whole body irradiation are dose-dependent. Below, you'll find the effects of radiation dosages ranging from 5 to 5,000 rads.

Radiation dosage (rads)	Clinical and laboratory findings
5 to 25	Patient asymptomatic; conventional blood studies normal; chromosome aberrations detectable
26 to 50	Patient asymptomatic; possible decrease in white blood cell (WBC) count
51 to 75	Patient asymptomatic; minor decreases in WBC and platelet counts in a few patients, especially if baseline values were established
76 to 125	Prodromal symptoms (anorexia, nausea, vomiting, fatigue) in 10% to 20% of patients within 2 days; mild decrease in WBC and platelet counts in some patients
126 to 200	Transient disability and clear hematologic changes in many patients; lymphocyte count decreased by about 50% within 48 hours
201 to 240	Probable radiation sickness and more than 50% decrease in lymphocyte count within 48 hours
241 to 400	Serious, disabling illness in most patients, with about 50% mortality if untreated; lymphocyte count decreased by 75% or more within 48 hours
401 to 4,999	Accelerated version of acute radiation syndrome with GI complications within 2 weeks; bleeding; death in most patients
5,000+	Fulminating course with cardiovascular, GI, and central nervous system complications, resulting in death within 24 to 72 hours

➤ For skin contamination, wash the patient's body thoroughly with mild soap and water.
➤ Debride and irrigate open wounds, as ordered.
➤ For ingested radioactive material, perform gastric lavage and whole-bowel irrigation, and administer activated charcoal, as ordered.
➤ Dispose of contaminated clothing properly.
➤ Dispose of contaminated excrement and body fluids according to facility policy.
➤ Use aseptic technique.

➤ Administer chelating agents, potassium iodide, aluminum phosphate gel, barium sulfate, I.V. fluids, and vasopressors, as indicated.

Follow-up actions
➤ Monitor the patient's vital signs frequently.
➤ Watch the patient for signs and symptoms of infection.
➤ Monitor for decreased hematocrit, hemoglobin level, and white blood cell, platelet, and lymphocyte counts.
➤ Monitor serum electrolyte levels, especially for decreased potassium and chloride, and treat abnormalities.
➤ Prepare the patient for X-rays to diagnose bone necrosis and bone marrow studies to identify dyscrasia.
➤ Provide a high-protein, high-calorie diet.
➤ Insert an indwelling urinary catheter.
➤ Monitor intake and output.
➤ Monitor thyroid function tests.
➤ If the patient was exposed to significant amounts of radiation, refer him to genetic counseling resources.

Preventive steps
➤ Advise the patient to avoid exposure to radiation when possible.
➤ Instruct the patient to use radiation shields over parts of the body that aren't being treated or studied during radiation or X-rays.
➤ Remind the patient to use occupational safety garments when working with radiation.

Pathophysiology recap
➤ The damage from radiation exposure varies with the amount of body area exposed, length of exposure, dosage absorbed, distance from the source, and presence of protective shielding.
➤ Charged atoms or ions form and react with other atoms to cause cell damage.
➤ Rapidly dividing cells are the most susceptible to radiation damage; highly differentiated cells are more resistant to radiation.
➤ Causes include exposure to radiation through inhalation, ingestion, or direct contact. Risk factors include cancer and employment in a radiation facility.

➤ Spider bites

In the United States, only two species of spider pose a life-threatening risk to humans—the black widow and the brown recluse. The black widow, which is found in all states except Alaska, generally stays in dark, dry places. A female will bite if she or her web is disturbed. Brown recluse spiders, which are found in the Midwest, also bite if disturbed, and are

> **IDENTIFYING BROWN RECLUSE AND BLACK WIDOW SPIDERS**

Brown recluse spider

The brown recluse spider is small and light brown, with three pairs of eyes. The hallmark is a violin-shaped darker area found on the cephalothorax. This spider is about 1" (2.5 cm) long, including the legs. Found in the south-central part of the United States, it favors dark areas, such as barns and woodsheds, and most commonly bites between April and October. The brown recluse spider injects a poison that causes its victim's blood to clot within 2 to 8 hours after the bite.

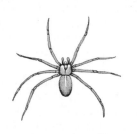

Black widow spider

The female black widow spider is glossy and coal-black with a red or orange hourglass mark on its underside; it's ½" (1.3 cm) in length, with legs 1½" (3.8 cm) long. Common throughout the United States, especially in warmer climates, the black widow spider is usually found in dark areas, such as outdoor privies and woodsheds. Its venom is toxic to the

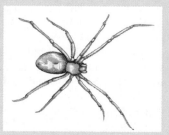

nerves and muscles of a human victim, causing muscle spasms in the arms and legs, rigidity of stomach muscles, and ascending paralysis that leads to difficulty swallowing and breathing; circulatory collapse may follow. The male black widow spider doesn't bite.

found in protected places, including clothing. (See *Identifying brown recluse and black widow spiders*.)

Rapid assessment

If it's confirmed that the patient was bitten by a brown recluse spider:

> Assess the patient's vital signs, noting fever, chills, malaise, and weakness.
> Determine the patient's level of consciousness (LOC), noting seizures.
> Obtain the patient's history; ask about nausea, vomiting, joint pain, itching at the site, and pain that increases in severity over time.
> Palpate the site to determine if it's hard.
> Inspect the site of the bite, noting a bluish ring around it, a bleb or blister, or necrotic arachnidism (several inches around the bite that become

necrotic and lead to an open sore that takes from months to years to heal).
➤ Look for petechiae.

If it's confirmed that the patient was bitten by a black widow spider:
➤ Assess the patient's vital signs, noting hypertension, tachycardia, and the respiratory rate, depth, and pattern.
➤ Determine the patient's LOC.
➤ Ask the patient if he's experiencing dizziness.
➤ Observe the bite site for swelling and two red puncture marks.
➤ Auscultate the apical pulse and palpate, noting a thready peripheral pulse.
➤ Assess for pinprick sensation followed by a dull pain and numbness.
➤ Watch the patient for extreme restlessness and seizures.
➤ Assess for hyperactive reflexes and, if the bite was in the leg, severe pain and muscle cramps.
➤ Assess for pain and rigidity in the chest, shoulders, and back if the patient sustained a bite on the arm.
➤ Assess for a painful and rigid abdomen.
➤ Observe the patient for pallor, chills, and sweats.

Immediate actions
➤ Perform cardiopulmonary resuscitation, if necessary.
➤ Provide supplemental oxygen, and prepare the patient for intubation and mechanical ventilation, if necessary.
➤ Immobilize the affected part of the body.
➤ Apply ice to the site.
➤ Administer I.V. fluids, corticosteroids, antibiotics, antihistamines, tranquilizers, tetanus prophylaxis (if indicated), and dapsone, as ordered.
➤ In the patient with a brown recluse spider bite, clean the lesion with a 1:20 Burow's aluminum acetate solution, apply antibiotic ointment, and elevate the affected part.
➤ In the patient with a black widow spider bite, remove jewelry and other constricting items before edema develops. Administer antivenin for severe black widow spider bites, I.V. calcium gluconate, and muscle relaxers.

 ALERT *Administer antivenin cautiously because it can result in anaphylactic shock and serum sickness.*

Follow-up actions
➤ Monitor the patient's vital signs frequently.
➤ Provide wound care, as ordered, using aseptic technique.
➤ Prepare the patient for debridement of necrotic skin and tissue and skin grafting, if necessary.
➤ Obtain a urinalysis, which will reveal hematuria after a black widow spider bite.

➤ Monitor the patient for signs and symptoms of infection.
➤ Monitor the white blood cell count as an indicator of infection (elevated after a black widow spider bite).
➤ Monitor the patient for hemolytic anemia and thrombocytopenia, especially after a brown recluse spider bite.

Preventive steps
➤ Advise the patient to keep garages and other dry, dark places that may harbor venomous spiders free from spider webs.
➤ Caution the patient to check clothing, shoes, sleeping areas, and other outdoor gear for spiders.

Pathophysiology recap
➤ The venom of the brown recluse spider is cytotoxic and hemolytic; it contains more than 8 components including enzymes and protein components.
➤ The venom of the black widow spider is a neurotoxin that causes systemic symptoms. Envenomation causes the release of large amounts of acetylcholine in neuromuscular junctions.

14
Emergencies due to drug toxicity and overdose

➤ Acetaminophen

Acetaminophen is the most widely used analgesic and antipyretic drug. In an acute acetaminophen overdose, plasma levels of 200 mcg/ml 4 hours after ingestion or 50 mcg/ml 12 hours after ingestion are associated with hepatotoxicity.

Rapid assessment
➤ Obtain the patient's history; ask about the drug ingested, the amount taken, and the time of ingestion.
➤ Assess the patient's vital signs, noting fever and hypotension.
➤ Assess the patient's level of consciousness, noting malaise, delirium, lethargy, coma, and seizures.
➤ Assess the rate, depth, and pattern of breathing and observe for cyanosis.
➤ Assess for abdominal pain, especially right upper quadrant tenderness.
➤ Ask the patient whether he has experienced anorexia and nausea and observe for vomiting.
➤ Observe for diaphoresis, jaundice, skin eruptions, and pallor.
➤ Watch the patient for signs and symptoms of bleeding.
➤ Assess for edema and ascites.

Immediate actions
➤ Perform cardiopulmonary resuscitation, if necessary.
➤ Administer supplemental oxygen, and prepare the patient for endotracheal intubation and mechanical ventilation, if necessary.
➤ Initiate suicide precautions, if necessary.
➤ Administer activated charcoal within 30 to 60 minutes of ingestion, if possible. Give acetylcysteine—the antidote for acetaminophen poisoning—within the first 24 hours of ingestion, if possible. Avoid giving acetylcysteine with activated charcoal because activated charcoal may absorb acetylcysteine and possibly reduce effectiveness. (See *Managing poisoning or overdose*, pages 392 to 394.)

(Text continues on page 395.)

➤ MANAGING POISONING OR OVERDOSE

Antidote and indications	Nursing considerations

ACETYLCYSTEINE (MUCOMYST, MUCOSIL, PARVOLEX)

➤ Treatment of acetaminophen toxicity	➤ Use cautiously in elderly or debilitated patients and in patients with asthma or severe respiratory insufficiency. ➤ Avoid use with activated charcoal. ➤ Don't combine with amphotericin B, ampicillin, chymotrypsin, erythromycin lactobionate, hydrogen peroxide, oxytetracycline, tetracycline, iodized oil, or trypsin. Administer separately. ➤ Don't give to semiconscious or unconscious patients.

ACTIVATED CHARCOAL (ACTIDOSE-AQUA, CHARCOAID, CHARCOCAPS, LIQUI-CHAR)

➤ Treatment of poisoning or overdose with most orally administered drugs, except caustic agents and hydrocarbons	➤ If possible, administer within 30 to 60 minutes of poisoning. Administer larger dose if patient has food in his stomach. ➤ Don't give with syrup of ipecac because charcoal inactivates ipecac. If a patient needs syrup of ipecac, give charcoal after he has finished vomiting. ➤ Don't give ice cream, milk, or sherbet because they reduce adsorption capacities of charcoal. ➤ Powdered form is most effective. Mix with tap water to form a thick syrup. You may add a small amount of fruit juice or flavoring to make the syrup more palatable. ➤ You may need to repeat the dose if the patient vomits shortly after administration.

AMYL NITRITE

➤ Antidote for cyanide poisoning	➤ Amyl nitrite is effective within 30 seconds, but its effects last only 3 to 5 minutes. ➤ To administer, wrap ampule in cloth and crush. Hold near the patient's nose and mouth so that he can inhale vapor. ➤ Monitor the patient for orthostatic hypotension. ➤ The patient may experience headache after administration.

DIGOXIN IMMUNE FAB (OVINE) (DIGIBIND)

➤ Treatment of potentially life-threatening digoxin intoxication	➤ Use cautiously in patients allergic to ovine proteins because the drug is derived from digoxin-specific antibody fragments obtained from immunized sheep. Perform skin test before administering. ➤ Use only in patients in shock or cardiac arrest with ventricular arrhythmias, such as ventricular tachycardia or fibrillation; with progressive bradycardia, such as severe sinus bradycardia; or with second- or third-degree atrioventricular block unresponsive to atropine.

➤ MANAGING POISONING OR OVERDOSE (continued)

Antidote and indications	Nursing considerations

DIGOXIN IMMUNE FAB (continued)

➤ Infuse through a 0.22-micron membrane filter, if possible.
➤ Refrigerate powder for reconstitution. If possible, use reconstituted drug immediately, although it may be refrigerated for up to 4 hours.
➤ Drug interferes with digoxin immunoassay measurements, resulting in misleading standard serum digoxin levels until the drug is cleared from the body (about 2 days).
➤ Total serum digoxin levels may rise after administration of this drug, reflecting fat-bound (inactive) digoxin.
➤ Monitor potassium levels closely.

METHYLENE BLUE

➤ Treatment of cyanide poisoning

➤ Don't give to patients with severe renal impairment or hypersensitivity to drug.
➤ Use with caution in glucose-6-phosphate dehydrogenase deficiency; may cause hemolysis.
➤ Avoid extravasation; subcutaneous injection may cause necrotic abscesses.
➤ Warn the patient that methylene blue will discolor his urine and stools and stain his skin. Hypochlorite solution rubbed on skin will remove stains.

NALOXONE (NARCAN)

➤ Treatment of respiratory depression caused by opioids
➤ Treatment of postoperative opioid depression
➤ Treatment of asphyxia neonatorum caused by administration of opioid analgesics to the mother in late labor

➤ Use cautiously in patients with cardiac irritability or opioid addiction.
➤ Monitor the patient's respiratory depth and rate. Be prepared to provide oxygen, ventilation, and other resuscitative measures.
➤ Duration of opioid may exceed that of naloxone, causing the patient to relapse into respiratory depression and requiring repeated administration.
➤ You may administer drug by continuous I.V. infusion to control adverse effects of epidurally administered morphine.
➤ You may see "overshoot" effect – the patient's respiratory rate after receiving drug exceeds his rate before respiratory depression occurred.
➤ Naloxone is the safest drug to use when the cause of respiratory depression is uncertain.
➤ Naloxone doesn't reverse respiratory depression caused by diazepam. The reversal agent for benzodiazepines is flumazenil.
➤ Although generally believed ineffective in treating respiratory depression caused by nonopioids, naloxone may reverse coma induced by alcohol intoxication.

(continued)

> **MANAGING POISONING OR OVERDOSE** *(continued)*

| Antidote and indications | Nursing considerations |

PRALIDOXIME (PROTOPAM CHLORIDE)

➤ Antidote for organophosphate poisoning and cholinergic drug overdose

➤ Don't give to patients poisoned with carbaryl (Sevin), a carbamate insecticide, because it increases Sevin's toxicity.
➤ Use with caution in patients with renal insufficiency, myasthenia gravis, asthma, or peptic ulcer.
➤ Use in hospitalized patients only; have respiratory and other supportive equipment available.
➤ Administer antidote as soon as possible after poisoning. Treatment is most effective if started within 24 hours of exposure.
➤ Before administering, suction secretions and make sure airway is patent.
➤ Dilute drug with sterile water without preservatives. Give atropine along with pralidoxime.
➤ If the patient's skin was exposed, remove his clothing and wash his skin and hair with sodium bicarbonate, soap, water, and alcohol as soon as possible. He may need a second washing. When washing the patient, wear protective gloves and clothes to avoid exposure.
➤ Observe the patient for 48 to 72 hours after he ingested the poison. Delayed absorption may occur. Watch for signs of rapid weakening in the patient with myasthenia gravis being treated for a cholinergic drug overdose. He may pass quickly from a cholinergic to a myasthenic crisis and require more cholinergic drugs to treat myasthenia. Keep edrophonium available.

SYRUP OF IPECAC (IPECAC SYRUP)

➤ Induction of vomiting in poisoning

➤ Syrup of ipecac is contraindicated for semicomatose, unconscious, and severely inebriated patients and for those with seizures, shock, or absent gag reflex.
➤ Don't give after ingestion of petroleum distillates or volatile oils because of the risk of aspiration pneumonitis. Don't give after ingestion of caustic substances, such as lye, because further injury can result.
➤ Before giving, make sure you have ipecac syrup, not ipecac fluid extract (14 times more concentrated, and deadly).
➤ If two doses don't induce vomiting, consider gastric lavage.
➤ If the patient also needs activated charcoal, give charcoal after he has vomited, or charcoal will neutralize the emetic effect.
➤ The American Academy of Pediatrics (AAP) no longer recommends using syrup of ipecac at home because it can be improperly administered and has been abused by persons with eating disorders such as bulimia. The AAP recommends that parents keep the universal poison control telephone number (1-800-222-1222) posted by their telephone.

ALERT *Start treatment immediately; don't wait for acetaminophen level results. Acetylcysteine must be administered as follows: give an oral loading dose followed by 17 oral maintenance doses, administered every 4 hours, for a total of 18 doses. Doses vomited within 1 hour of administration must be repeated. Remove charcoal by lavage before administering acetylcysteine because it may interfere with this agent's absorption. Dilute oral doses in cola or fruit before administering. If administering via nasogastric tube, mix the dose with water.*

➤ Administer vasopressors, dopamine, diuretics, and lactulose, as ordered.

Follow-up actions
➤ Monitor the patient's vital signs closely.
➤ Prepare the patient for hemodialysis to remove acetaminophen from the body.
➤ Monitor serum acetaminophen levels and liver function tests.
➤ Insert an indwelling urinary catheter.
➤ Assess renal function by monitoring intake and output and blood urea nitrogen and creatinine levels.
➤ Monitor serum electrolyte levels and treat abnormalities.
➤ Monitor coagulation studies.
➤ Administer fresh frozen plasma, platelets, and packed red blood cells to stop, prevent, and treat bleeding.
➤ Keep the head of the bed higher than 30 degrees to prevent hemorrhagic stroke and cerebral edema.
➤ Implement bleeding precautions.
➤ Provide a low-sodium, low-protein diet.

Preventive steps
➤ Advise the patient's families and friends to take all suicide threats seriously and provide referrals to a suicide support system.
➤ Instruct the patient to keep acetaminophen in its original, labeled container and to make sure that it and all medicine containers have childproof caps.
➤ Advise the patient to take acetaminophen only as directed.
➤ Warn the patient to avoid using nonsteroidal anti-inflammatory drugs and alcohol while taking acetaminophen.

Pathophysiology recap
➤ The maximum dose of acetaminophen over 24 hours is 4 g in adults and 10 to 15 mg/kg with a maximum of five doses a day in children. Toxicity occurs after ingestion of 150 mg/kg (or 7 g) at one time in adults.
➤ Acetaminophen is absorbed rapidly from the stomach and small intestine. The liver breaks it down into nontoxic components that are excreted in urine.

➤ When a toxic dose of acetaminophen is ingested, the metabolic pathways become overworked, and it's broken down into toxic components. These toxic components alter vital proteins and hepatocytes, resulting in liver tissue death.

Acetaminophen poisoning develops in stages:

➤ Stage 1 (12 to 24 hours after ingestion): nausea, vomiting, diaphoresis, and anorexia

➤ Stage 2 (24 to 48 hours after ingestion): clinically improved but elevated liver function test results

➤ Stage 3 (72 to 96 hours after ingestion): peak hepatotoxicity

➤ Stage 4 (7 to 8 days after ingestion): recovery or progression to complete liver failure.

➤ Barbiturates

Barbiturates are generally taken for seizure disorders or for pain. Although problems with barbiturate addiction have been replaced by addictions to more frequently prescribed depressant medications, such as benzodiazepines, barbiturate overdose remains a critical problem.

Rapid assessment

➤ Obtain the patient's history; ask about the drug ingested, the amount taken, and the time of ingestion.

➤ Obtain the patient's vital signs, noting hypotension and hypothermia followed by fever.

➤ Assess the patient's level of consciousness, noting lethargy, lack of coordination, slow speech, drowsiness, difficulty thinking and functioning, memory loss, and coma.

➤ Assess for shallow respirations.

➤ Observe for nystagmus, irritability, and a staggering gait.

➤ Assess the patient for decreased deep tendon reflexes.

Immediate actions

➤ Perform cardiopulmonary resuscitation, if needed.

➤ Provide supplemental oxygen, and prepare the patient for endotracheal (ET) intubation and mechanical ventilation, if necessary.

➤ Implement suicide precautions, if necessary.

➤ Send urine and serum samples for barbiturate levels (barbiturates will be detectable for up to 5 days after ingestion).

➤ If vomiting is contraindicated, perform gastric lavage while a cuffed ET tube is in place to prevent aspiration.

➤ Follow gastric lavage with administration of activated charcoal and saline cathartic.

➤ Administer vasopressors and I.V. fluids. If ingestion was recent, the patient is conscious, and the gag reflex is present, give syrup of ipecac.

➤ Be prepared to administer naloxone to treat an overdose of a barbiturate and an opiate.

Follow-up actions
➤ Monitor the patient's vital signs frequently.
➤ Monitor arterial blood gas values and treat abnormalities.
➤ Monitor intake and output.
➤ Reorient the patient as needed.
➤ Prepare the patient for hemodialysis if the drug level is persistent or if the overdose is severe.
➤ Provide emotional support to the patient and his family.

Preventive steps
➤ Instruct the patient to take barbiturates according to the physician's and pharmacist's instructions, and remind him not to take more than the maximum daily dose.
➤ Advise the patient to avoid illicit drugs, alcohol, and other depressants while taking barbiturates.
➤ Caution the patient to keep barbiturates in appropriately labeled containers and out of the reach of children.

Pathophysiology recap
➤ Barbiturates are depressant drugs. They suppress excitable tissue in the central and peripheral nervous system and in the cardiovascular and GI system by acting on gamma-aminobutyric acid receptors to suppress neurotransmission.

➤ Cocaine

Cocaine is a potent stimulant extracted from the leaves of the coca plant *(Erythroxylon coca)*. It has great potential for abuse and overdose, which can be fatal.

Rapid assessment
➤ Obtain the patient's history; ask about the drug ingested, the route of administration (I.V. or nasal), the amount taken, and the time of ingestion. Ask if any other drugs or alcohol were also taken.
➤ Obtain the patient's vital signs, noting hypertension, tachycardia, and fever.
➤ Assess the patient's level of consciousness and neurologic status, noting agitation, confusion, delirium, irritability, and seizures.
➤ Assess for diaphoresis, tachypnea, and shallow respirations.
➤ Ask the patient whether he has experienced chest pain.
➤ Obtain an electrocardiogram (ECG) and assess for arrhythmias.

Immediate actions

➤ Perform cardiopulmonary resuscitation, if necessary.
➤ Provide supplemental oxygen, and prepare the patient for endotracheal intubation and mechanical ventilation, if necessary.
➤ Initiate continuous cardiac monitoring.
➤ Provide cooling methods, such as cool baths and hypothermia blankets, if hyperthermia is present.
➤ Administer sedatives, antipyretics and, if the overdose resulted in a heart attack, thrombolytics.

Follow-up actions

➤ Monitor the patient's vital signs frequently.
➤ Obtain a 12-lead ECG to detect ischemic changes.
➤ Prepare the patient for cardiac catheterization and balloon angioplasty, if necessary.
➤ Monitor the patient for signs and symptoms of withdrawal.
➤ Refer the patient for drug rehabilitation.

Preventive steps

➤ Refer the patient's families and friends to an addiction support system.
➤ Advise parents to talk with their children about the effects of drugs and urge them to avoid drug use.

Pathophysiology recap

➤ Cocaine is a very addictive drug due to its euphoric effects. The euphoria occurs because cocaine causes an accumulation of dopamine in the brain and a continuous stimulation of neurons.
➤ A tolerance develops as the user increases the dose to prolong the euphoria after ingestion.
➤ The effects of cocaine are usually felt immediately after ingestion and last for a few minutes or a few hours.
➤ Effects of short-term use include vasoconstriction, dilated pupils, hyperthermia, tachycardia, hypertension, and myocardial infarction.
➤ Effects of long-term use include strange and violent behavior.

➤ Digoxin

Digoxin increases the strength of myocardial contractions, slows heart rate, and controls arrhythmias. While it works effectively to improve cardiac function, even a mild degree of toxicity can be dangerous—even fatal.

Rapid assessment

➤ Obtain the patient's history; ask about the drug ingested, the amount taken, and the time of ingestion.

➤ Assess the patient's level of consciousness, noting confusion, agitation, delirium, and seizures.

➤ Obtain the patient's vital signs, noting bradycardia.

➤ Ask about nausea, vomiting, anorexia, diarrhea, weakness, fatigue, headaches, hallucinations, paresthesia, and dizziness. Also ask about dyspnea, palpitations, and syncope.

➤ Ask about decreased general color vision with increased perception of yellow-green colors; also ask about halos and scotomas.

➤ Assess for diplopia, blurred vision, and photophobia.

➤ Obtain an electrocardiogram (ECG) and assess for arrhythmias — especially bradyarrhythmias, premature ventricular contractions, atrioventricular block, ventricular tachycardia, torsade de pointes, and asystole.

Immediate actions

➤ Initiate cardiopulmonary resuscitation, if necessary.

➤ Provide supplemental oxygen, and prepare the patient for endotracheal intubation and mechanical ventilation, if necessary.

➤ Institute continuous cardiac monitoring and obtain a 12-lead ECG.

➤ Initiate suicide precautions, if necessary.

➤ Obtain a serum sample to measure digoxin, serum electrolyte, blood urea nitrogen, and creatinine levels.

 ALERT *A patient with suspected digoxin toxicity should be treated according to his signs and symptoms, not according to the digoxin level.*

➤ Administer atropine, lidocaine, activated charcoal, I.V. fluids, and supplemental electrolytes, especially potassium and magnesium, as ordered.

➤ Administer digoxin immune fab (antidote to digoxin) for severe life-threatening digoxin toxicity.

Follow-up actions

➤ Monitor the patient's vital signs frequently.

➤ Discontinue digoxin.

➤ Prepare the patient for hemodialysis, if necessary.

➤ Prepare the patient for pacemaker insertion, if indicated.

➤ Monitor serum digoxin and electrolyte levels.

➤ Assess renal function by monitoring intake and output and blood urea nitrogen and creatinine levels.

➤ Encourage oral intake to maintain hydration.

Preventive steps

➤ Advise the patient to store digoxin in a labeled container with a safety cap and to keep it out of the reach of children.

➤ Instruct the patient to take digoxin according to the physician's and pharmacist's directions.

➤ Remind the patient to attend scheduled appointments for laboratory studies to monitor serum digoxin levels.
➤ Teach the patient about food and drug interactions.

Pathophysiology recap
➤ Digoxin inhibits the sodium-potassium adenosine triphosphatase pump. It enhances myocardial contraction by causing a rise in intracellular calcium.
➤ The automaticity of the Purkinje fibers is increased and the conduction through the atrioventricular node is decreased. Toxicity occurs with an increase in the automaticity and a decrease in the speed of conduction.
➤ Causes of digoxin toxicity include impaired renal function, dehydration, acidosis, myocardial ischemia, drug interactions, and electrolyte imbalances (especially hypokalemia, hypernatremia, and hypomagnesemia).

➤ Opioids

Opioids, also known as *narcotics,* are prescribed to relieve pain and facilitate sleep. The primary effect of opioid toxicity is respiratory depression.

Rapid assessment
➤ Assess the patient's vital signs, noting orthostatic hypotension, a decreased level of consciousness, drowsiness, euphoria, mental status changes, seizures, and pupillary changes (miosis).

 ALERT *Persistent or severe hypotension suggests the possibility of co-toxicity.*

➤ Obtain the patient's history; ask about the specific opioid ingested, amount taken, and time the ingestion occurred. Also ask about nausea and vomiting.
➤ Observe for respiratory depression, bradypnea (as slow as 4 to 6 breaths/minute), and hypopnea.
➤ Obtain an electrocardiogram (ECG) and assess for ventricular arrhythmias.
➤ Observe for needle tracks on the skin (with subcutaneous administration).
➤ Auscultate for decreased bowel sounds because opioids decrease GI motility.

Immediate actions
➤ Initiate cardiopulmonary resuscitation, if necessary.
➤ Provide supplemental oxygen, and prepare the patient for endotracheal intubation and mechanical ventilation, if necessary.

- Obtain a serum sample for arterial blood gas (ABG) analysis.
- Initiate suicide precautions, if necessary.
- Obtain a urine specimen for a baseline drug level (positive results occur 36 to 48 hours after ingestion).
- Administer I.V. naloxone (or naltrexone, which has a longer half-life) and activated charcoal.

 ALERT *If the patient is a long-term opioid user, adjust the dose of naloxone so that it's sufficient to reverse respiratory depression but not high enough to cause opioid withdrawal. Because the duration of action of the opioid is longer than that of naloxone, the respiratory depressant effects of the opioid may return as the effects of naloxone wear off. Additional I.V. push doses of naloxone and, possibly, a continuous infusion of naloxone may be necessary.*

After administering the medication, continuously assess the patient's respiratory status and continue oxygen therapy or mechanical ventilation, as needed.

Follow-up actions
- Monitor the patient's vital signs frequently.
- Monitor ABG levels.
- Monitor the patient's respiratory status and rate as well as the depth and pattern of respirations frequently.
- Monitor complete blood count and electrolyte and creatinine levels.
- Watch the patient for signs and symptoms of noncardiogenic pulmonary edema, a complication of overdose.
- Watch the patient for signs and symptoms of withdrawal as treatment continues.
- Obtain a 12-lead ECG.

Preventive steps
- Advise the patient to keep opioids in the original labeled container and out of the reach of children.
- Refer the patient with suspected or known suicidal ideation to a support group.
- Advise parents to teach children the ramifications of opioid toxicity and urge them to avoid drug use.
- Instruct the patient to take opioids according to the physician's and pharmacist's directions.

Pathophysiology recap
- Opioids activate opiate receptors and inhibit neurotransmission in the central and peripheral nervous systems. They decrease the perception of pain and reduce the response to the stimuli causing the pain. (See *Opioid types and mechanisms,* page 402.)
- Opioids are generally absorbed through the GI (especially the small intestine) and respiratory tracts.

➤ **OPIOID TYPES AND MECHANISMS**

Opioids block the release of neurotransmitters that send pain signals to the brain. The three categories of opioids are opioid agonists (narcotic analgesics), opioid antagonists (narcotic reversal agents), and mixed agonist-antagonists.

Opioid agonists
Opioid agonists relieve pain by binding to pain receptors, which, in effect, produces pain relief. Examples of opioid agonists are:
➤ codeine
➤ fentanyl
➤ hydromorphone
➤ morphine
➤ oxycodone.

Opioid antagonists
Opioid antagonists attach to opiate receptors without producing agonistic effects. They work by displacing the opioid at the receptor site and reversing the analgesic and respiratory depressant effects of the opioid.
    Examples of opioid antagonists are:
➤ naloxone
➤ naltrexone.

Mixed opioid agonist-antagonists
Mixed opioid agonist-antagonists relieve pain by binding to opiate receptors to effect varying degrees of agonistic and antagonistic activity.
    Examples of mixed opioid agonist-antagonists are:
➤ buprenorphine
➤ butorphanol
➤ pentazocine.

➤ The liver metabolizes most opioids, and the breakdown products are excreted in urine.
➤ Conditions that may potentiate opioid toxicity include liver failure and renal failure.

➤ *Salicylates*

Salicylates have analgesic, antipyretic, and anti-inflammatory properties. They can be taken orally or topically. Aspirin is the most common salicylate taken in overdose. Less commonly, overdose is after the topical use of salicylic acid in keratolytics or ingestion of methyl salicylate.

Rapid assessment
➤ Obtain the patient's history; ask about the drug ingested, the amount taken, and the time of ingestion. Also ask about nausea and vomiting.

➤ Assess the patient's vital signs, noting tachycardia and hypotension.

 ALERT *When obtaining the patient's history, remember to ask about aspirin and other over-the-counter (OTC) aspirin-related drugs; these drugs don't typically come to mind when patients are asked to list medications they're taking.*

➤ Assess the patient's level of consciousness, noting agitation, delirium, anxiety, difficulty concentrating, somnolence, lethargy, seizures, and coma.
➤ Observe for tachypnea and hyperventilation or respiratory arrest and apnea.
➤ Obtain an electrocardiogram (ECG) and assess for arrhythmias and asystole.
➤ Evaluate for GI bleeding; if not observed, perform a rectal examination to test for occult blood.
➤ Observe the patient for diaphoresis and signs and symptoms of dehydration.
➤ Test for decreased hearing due to ototoxicity and tinnitus (common if the salicylate level is greater than 30 mg/dl).

Immediate actions
➤ Provide supplemental oxygen, and prepare the patient for endotracheal intubation and mechanical ventilation, if necessary.
➤ Initiate suicide precautions, if indicated.
➤ Obtain a serum salicylate level and repeat every 2 hours until the level decreases.
➤ Obtain a serum sample for arterial blood gas analysis and evaluate for metabolic acidosis.
➤ Prepare the patient for gastric lavage, if necessary.

 ALERT *Protect the airway before performing gastric lavage to prevent aspiration.*

➤ Administer activated charcoal, a cathartic (one-time dose to prevent electrolyte imbalances), I.V. fluids, and sodium bicarbonate.

Follow-up actions
➤ Monitor the patient's vital signs frequently.
➤ Watch the patient for signs and symptoms of noncardiogenic pulmonary edema.
➤ Monitor serum electrolyte levels, especially for hypokalemia, and urine pH while performing urine alkalinization.
➤ Obtain serum samples for liver function tests and amylase and lipase as indicators of hepatitis and pancreatitis, respectively (more common in chronic toxicity).
➤ Monitor the patient for signs and symptoms of disseminated intravascular coagulation, especially in chronic toxicity.

➤ Obtain serum samples to monitor for elevated prothrombin time and International Normalized Ratio.
➤ Obtain a 12-lead ECG, noting abnormalities, especially if caused by hypokalemia.
➤ Prepare the patient for hemodialysis, if necessary.

Preventive steps
➤ Advise the patient to store salicylates in the original, labeled container and out of the reach of children.
➤ Inform the patient that salicylates can be dangerous even though they're dispensed OTC.
➤ Refer the patient with suspected or known suicidal ideation to a support group.

Pathophysiology recap
➤ Salicylates act on adenosine triphosphate and hinder reactions dependent on it, causing catabolism. This causes an increase in oxygen consumption, carbon dioxide production, glycolysis, and multiple organ failure.
➤ Ingestion amounts and toxicity vary; the following ranges are estimates:
  – Less than 150 mg/kg causes no to mild toxicity.
  – 150 to 300 mg/kg causes mild to moderate toxicity.
  – 301 to 500 mg/kg causes serious toxicity.
  – Greater than 500mg/kg causes potentially fatal toxicity.

➤ Warfarin

Warfarin, also known as *coumadin,* is the most common oral anticoagulant. It's used to prevent and treat blood clots in blood vessels and lungs. It's also used to treat blood clots due to heart attack or prosthetic heart valves, and it decreases the risk of a heart attack or embolic stroke. Toxicity can occur as a result of accidental or intentional overdose.

Rapid assessment
➤ Obtain the patient's history; ask about the drug ingested, the amount taken, and the time of ingestion.
➤ Assess the patient's level of consciousness, noting confusion, stupor, or unconsciousness.
➤ Obtain the patient's vital signs, noting hypotension and tachycardia due to decreased intravascular volume.
➤ Observe for bleeding—blood in stool or urine, black stools, melena, excessive menstrual bleeding, petechiae, excessive or easy bruising, excessive oozing from superficial injuries, nosebleeds, and bleeding mucous membranes.

Immediate actions
> Control active bleeding by applying pressure and assisting with cauterization.
> If hemorrhagic stroke is suspected, keep the head of the bed at 30 degrees to help decrease intracranial pressure (ICP).
> If a GI bleed is suspected, prepare the patient for nasogastric tube insertion and lavage.
> Discontinue therapy.
> Administer vitamin K (antidote to warfarin), and fresh frozen plasma and packed red blood cells, as needed.
> Administer activated charcoal.

Follow-up actions
> Implement suicide precautions, if necessary.
> Monitor the patient's vital signs frequently.
> Monitor for prolonged prothrombin time (PT) (may not be elevated until 2 days after ingestion), International Normalized Ratio (INR), decreased hemoglobin level, and hematocrit.
> Prepare the patient for a GI scope or surgery to control GI bleeding, if necessary.
> Prepare the patient for cystoscopy, if necessary.
> Restart warfarin treatment when appropriate; administer heparin if rapid anticoagulation is indicated.

Preventive steps
> Advise the patient to store warfarin in the original labeled container and out of the reach of children.
> Remind the patient to attend regularly scheduled appointments to monitor PT and INR while taking warfarin.
> Caution the patient to take warfarin according to the physician's and pharmacist's instructions and to report signs of bleeding.
> Teach the patient dietary and drug interactions that may alter the effect of warfarin.

Pathophysiology recap
> Warfarin hinders vitamin K synthesis by the liver. Coagulation factors dependent on vitamin K (factors II, VII, IX, and X, and anticoagulant proteins C and S) are also affected.
> A lack of functioning clotting factors and proteins leads to bleeding.
> After a dose of warfarin, the anticoagulant effect lasts 5 to 7 days.
> Warfarin binds to plasma protein, mostly albumin, which is why it interacts with many other drugs, such as antibacterials, antifungals, antiarrhythmics, anticonvulsants, nonsteroidal anti-inflammatory drugs, histamine-2 receptor antagonists, and immunosuppressants.
> Warfarin is distributed to the liver, lungs, spleen, and kidneys.
> Warfarin metabolism is affected by hepatic disease or failure but not by renal disease or failure.

15

Psychiatric emergencies

➤ *Anorexia nervosa*

The key feature of anorexia nervosa, an eating disorder, is self-imposed starvation due to a distorted body image and an intense, irrational fear of gaining weight, even when the patient is obviously emaciated.

Rapid assessment
- ➤ Assess the patient's vital signs, noting hypotension and bradycardia.
- ➤ Weigh the patient, noting a 25% or greater weight loss without a known illness.
- ➤ Interview the patient and assess for a morbid dread of being fat, an obsession with exercise and food, and a compulsion to be thin. Ask about laxative, enema, and diuretic abuse.
- ➤ Assess the patient for feelings of despair, hopelessness, and worthlessness as well as suicidal thoughts.
- ➤ Ask about amenorrhea, loss of libido, fatigue, sleep alterations alternating with hyperactivity and vigor, day-to-day food intake, and daily exercise.
- ➤ Ask about fertility issues.
- ➤ Observe the patient for angry and ritualistic behavior.
- ➤ Observe the patient for cold intolerance.
- ➤ Assess the patient for an emaciated appearance, with skeletal muscle atrophy, loss of fatty tissue, atrophy of breast tissue, blotchy or sallow skin, lanugo on the face and body, and dryness or loss of scalp hair.
- ➤ Observe the patient for dental caries and oral or pharyngeal abrasions that indicate vomiting.
- ➤ Palpate for painless salivary gland enlargement.
- ➤ Observe for bowel distention.
- ➤ Assess for hypoactive deep tendon reflexes. (See *Criteria for hospitalizing a patient with anorexia nervosa.*)

Immediate actions
- ➤ Initiate suicide precautions, if necessary.
- ➤ Administer hyperalimentation.
- ➤ Obtain laboratory tests, such as complete blood count, serum electrolytes, blood urea nitrogen, creatinine, liver function studies, and

> ## ➤ CRITERIA FOR HOSPITALIZING A PATIENT WITH ANOREXIA NERVOSA
>
> A patient with anorexia nervosa can be successfully treated on an outpatient basis. However, if the patient displays any of the following signs, hospitalization is mandatory:
> ➤ Rapid weight loss equal to 15% or more of normal body mass
> ➤ Persistent bradycardia (50 beats/minute or less)
> ➤ Hypotension with a systolic reading less than or equal to 90 mm Hg
> ➤ Hypothermia (core body temperature less than or equal to 97° F (36.1° C)
> ➤ Presence of medical complications or suicidal ideation
> ➤ Persistent sabotage or disruption of outpatient treatment—resolute denial of condition and the need for treatment

serum protein, to determine the degree of malnutrition and electrolyte imbalance.
➤ Obtain a 12-lead electrocardiogram (changes may include a prolonged QT interval and nonspecific ST and T wave changes), and monitor for cardiac arrhythmias.

Follow-up actions
➤ Monitor the patient's vital signs regularly.
➤ Monitor intake and output.
➤ Weigh the patient daily.
➤ Prepare the patient for behavior modification therapy and psychotherapy.
➤ Assist the patient in complying with treatment regimens.
➤ Make sure that the patient curtails physical activity.
➤ Administer vitamin and mineral supplements.
➤ Provide a reasonable diet (with or without liquid supplements) in the form of small, frequent meals with one-on-one supervision.
➤ Give the patient control over food choices, if possible.
➤ Provide emotional support.
➤ Refer the patient and her family to the Anorexia Nervosa and Related Eating Disorders national information and support organization.
➤ Advise family members to avoid discussing food with the patient.

Preventive steps
➤ Advise the patient's family and friends that early detection is the best way to treat the eating disorder. Encourage them to help the patient maintain a healthy self image and assist her in finding a healthy balance between a good diet and exercise.

Pathophysiology recap
➤ The causes of anorexia nervosa are unknown, however, social attitudes that equate slimness with beauty play some role in provoking this disorder; family factors are also implicated.
➤ Most researchers believe that refusing to eat is a subconscious effort to exert personal control over one's life.

➤ Bipolar disorder

Bipolar disorder is marked by severe pathologic mood swings from hyperactivity and euphoria to sadness and depression. It involves various symptom combinations and has manic and depressive phases.

Rapid assessment
For the manic patient:
➤ Interview him; note whether he appears grandiose, euphoric, expansive, or irritable. Determine the degree of his ability to exercise control over his activities and responses. Ask him about decreased need for sleep, increased physical activity, and excessive risk-taking behaviors.
➤ Note whether he describes hyperactive or excessive behavior or has plans to start projects for which he has little aptitude. Assess for an inflated sense of self-esteem, which may be delusional.
➤ Observe for bizarre activities, such as dressing in colorful or strange garments or wearing excessive makeup. Note accelerated speech, frequent changes of topic, flight of ideas, easy distraction, and sensitivity to external stimulation.
➤ Assess for signs of malnutrition and poor personal hygiene.
   For the hypomanic patient:
➤ Assess for a euphoric but unstable mood, pressured speech, and increased motor activity.
   For the depressed patient:
➤ Interview him and note a loss of self-esteem, overwhelming inertia, social withdrawal, and feelings of hopelessness, apathy, self-reproach, sadness, guilt, negativity, and fatigue. Ask about sleep disturbances, sexual dysfunction, headaches, chest pains, and heaviness in the limbs (these symptoms are usually worse in the morning).
➤ Assess for slow speech, delayed responses, and difficulty concentrating or thinking clearly without obvious disorientation. Evaluate him for reduced psychomotor activity, low muscle tone, weight loss, slowed gait, and constipation. Assess for hypochondria.
➤ Evaluate him for suicidal and homicidal ideation.

Immediate actions

➤ Initiate suicide precautions and ensure the safety of the patient and others (remove harmful objects from the patient's environment, observe him closely, and strictly supervise his medications).
➤ Administer lithium to relieve and prevent manic episodes.

ALERT *Lithium has a narrow therapeutic range. Treatment must be initiated cautiously and the dosage should be adjusted slowly. Therapeutic blood levels must be maintained for 7 to 10 days before the drug's beneficial effects appear.*

➤ Administer antipsychotic medications to reduce acute symptoms, such as delusions and hallucinations.
➤ Administer anticonvulsants to treat mood disorders and antidepressants to treat depressive symptoms.

ALERT *Be aware that the use of antidepressants during a depressive episode may trigger a manic episode.*

Follow-up actions

In episodes of mania:
➤ Encourage a high-calorie, high-carbohydrate diet with plenty of liquids.
➤ Encourage responsibility for personal care.
➤ Help set realistic goals.
➤ Provide emotional support.
➤ Provide structured diversionary activities.
➤ Reduce or eliminate group activities.
➤ Reorient the patient to time, place, and person, as needed.
➤ Set limits in a clear, calm, and self-confident manner.
➤ Listen to requests attentively, with a neutral attitude. Avoid power struggles.
➤ Watch the patient for signs of frustration; help him control his behavior.
➤ Watch the patient for signs and symptoms of lithium toxicity, such as diarrhea, abdominal cramps, vomiting, unsteadiness, and drowsiness.
➤ Monitor blood urea nitrogen and creatinine levels and intake and output as indicators of renal impairment.

ALERT *Lithium is excreted by the kidneys; renal impairment necessitates termination of the drug.*

In depressive episodes:
➤ Provide positive reinforcement.
➤ Provide a structured routine that includes activities to boost self-confidence and self-esteem.
➤ Encourage the patient to talk about or write down his feelings if he's having trouble expressing them.
➤ Listen attentively and respectfully.
➤ Assist with personal hygiene and feed the patient, if necessary.

➤ CYCLOTHYMIC DISORDER

A chronic mood disturbance of at least 2 years' duration, cyclothymic disorder involves numerous episodes of hypomania or depression that aren't of sufficient severity or duration to qualify as a major depressive episode or bipolar disorder.

Cyclothymia commonly starts in adolescence or early adulthood. Beginning insidiously, this disorder leads to persistent social and occupational dysfunction.

Signs and symptoms
In the hypomanic phase, the patient may experience insomnia, hyperactivity, inflated self-esteem, increased productivity and creativity, physical restlessness, rapid speech, and over-involvement in pleasurable activities, including an increased sexual drive. Depressive symptoms may include insomnia, feelings of inadequacy, decreased productivity, social withdrawal, loss of libido, loss of interest in pleasurable activities, lethargy, slow speech, and crying.

Diagnosis
Several medical disorders (for example, endocrinopathies, such as Cushing's syndrome, stroke, brain tumors, and head trauma) and drug overdose can produce a similar pattern of mood alteration. These organic causes must be ruled out before making a diagnosis of cyclothymic disorder.

➤ Offer small, frequent, high-fiber meals.
➤ Encourage physical activity and adequate rest periods.
➤ Watch for signs of mania in patients taking antidepressants.

Preventive steps
➤ Bipolar disorder can't be prevented; however, compliance with the treatment regimen can decrease the number and intensity of manic and depressive episodes.

Pathophysiology recap
➤ The cause of bipolar disorder is unclear, but hereditary, biological, and psychological factors may each play a role.
➤ Type I bipolar disorder is characterized by alternating episodes of mania and depression.
➤ Type II bipolar disorder is characterized by recurrent depressive episodes and occasional hypomanic episodes.
➤ Some patients experience a seasonal pattern, marked by a cyclic relation between the onset of the mood episode and a particular 60-day period of the year.
➤ Biochemical changes accompany mood swings, but it isn't clear whether the changes cause the mood swings or result from them.
➤ Intracellular sodium concentration increases during periods of mania and depression and returns to normal with recovery.

➤ Patients with mood disorders have a defect in the way the brain responds to certain neurotransmitters.
➤ Circadian rhythms that control hormone secretion, body temperature, and appetite may contribute to the disorder.
➤ Emotional or physical trauma and stressful events may precede the onset of bipolar disorder. (See *Cyclothymic disorder.*)

➤ *Delusional disorders*

Delusional disorders are marked by false beliefs with a plausible basis in reality. These beliefs involve erotomanic, grandiose, jealous, somatic, or persecutory themes. (See *Delusional themes,* page 412.)

Rapid assessment
➤ Obtain the patient's history; ask about social and marital relationships and problems, such as depression or sexual dysfunction. Also ask about social isolation or hostility. Note a denial of feelings of loneliness and relentless criticism or unreasonable demands on others.
➤ Observe the patient for evasiveness or reluctance to answer questions along with excessive talkativeness and detail in explanations. Assess for contradictory, jumbled, or irrational answers and statements.
➤ Observe the patient for expressions of denial, projection, and rationalization. Note accusatory statements.
➤ Observe the patient for nonverbal cues, such as excessive vigilance and obvious apprehension upon entering a room, sitting at the edge of the seat, folded arms, and clutching belongings.
➤ Because the patient may deny his feelings, disregard the circumstances that led to his hospitalization. Remember that he may refuse treatment. Ask family members to confirm assessment observations.

Immediate actions
➤ Ensure the safety of the patient and others.
➤ Administer antipsychotics to reduce hallucinations and delusions and relieve anxiety and agitation.

Follow-up actions
➤ Prepare the patient for counseling.
➤ Be direct, straightforward, and dependable.
➤ Respect the patient's privacy and personal space.
➤ Gradually increase social contacts after the patient is comfortable with the staff.
➤ Watch for refusal of mediations and food due to an irrational fear of poisoning.
➤ Monitor for adverse effects of antipsychotics — drug-induced parkinsonism, acute dystonia, akathisia, tardive dyskinesia, and malignant neuroleptic syndrome.

➤ DELUSIONAL THEMES

The delusions experienced by a patient with a delusional disorder are usually well systematized and follow a predominant theme. Common delusional themes are discussed here.

Erotomanic delusions

Erotomanic delusions are prevalent delusional themes that concern romantic or spiritual love. The patient believes that he shares an idealized (rather than sexual) relationship with someone of higher status – a superior at work, a celebrity, or an anonymous stranger.

The patient may keep this delusion secret, but more commonly will try to contact the object of his delusion by phone calls, letters (including e-mail), gifts, or even spying. He may attempt to rescue his beloved from imagined danger. Many patients with erotomanic delusions harass public figures and come to the attention of the police.

Grandiose delusions

The patient with grandiose delusions believes that he has great, unrecognized talent, special insights, prophetic power, or has made an important discovery. To achieve recognition, he may contact government agencies such as the Federal Bureau of Investigation. The patient with a religion-oriented delusion of grandeur may become a cult leader. Less commonly, he believes that he shares a special relationship with some well-known personality, such as a rock star or world leader. He may believe himself to be a famous person whose identity has been usurped by an imposter.

Jealous delusions

Jealous delusions focus on infidelity. For example, a patient may insist that his spouse or lover has been unfaithful and may search for evidence, such as spots on bed sheets, to justify the delusion. He may confront his partner, try to control her movements, follow her, or try to track down her suspected lover. He may physically assault her or, less likely, his perceived rival.

Persecutory delusions

The patient suffering from persecutory delusions, the most common type of delusion, believes that he's being followed, harassed, plotted against, poisoned, mocked, or deliberately prevented from achieving his long-term goals. These delusions may evolve into a simple or complex persecution scheme, in which even the slightest injustice is interpreted as part of the scheme.

Such a patient may file numerous lawsuits or seek redress from government agencies (querulous paranoia). A patient who becomes resentful and angry may lash out violently against the alleged offender.

Somatic delusions

Somatic delusions center on an imagined physical defect or deformity. The patient may perceive a foul odor coming from his skin, mouth, rectum, or another body part. Other delusions involve skin-crawling insects, internal parasites, or physical illness.

➤ Involve the patient's family in treatment.
➤ Administer clozapine, which differs chemically from other antipsychotic drugs, for patients who fail to respond to standard treatment.

 ALERT *The patient being treated with clozapine will require weekly blood monitoring.*

Preventive steps
➤ Delusional disorder can't be prevented, but the number of episodes can be decreased by counseling to help deal with childhood experiences, personality traits, and relationship management. Stress management, avoidance of alcohol, visual and hearing aids, and meaningful group interaction are also useful.

Pathophysiology recap
Although the exact mechanism of delusional disorders hasn't been identified, factors that may contribute to its development include:
➤ heredity
➤ feelings of inferiority in the family
➤ specific early childhood experiences with authoritarian family structure
➤ sensitive personality
➤ medical conditions, such as chronic alcoholism, head injury, and deafness
➤ aging—isolation, lack of stimulating interpersonal relationships, physical illness, and impaired hearing and vision
➤ severe stress.

➤ Major depression

Major depression is a syndrome of a persistently sad, dysphoric mood accompanied by lethargy, sleep and appetite disturbances, and an inability to experience pleasure (anhedonia).

Rapid assessment
➤ Obtain the patient's history; ask about life problems or losses, insomnia, and lack of interest in sexual activity. If present, note anhedonia, anger, anxiety, difficulty in concentrating or thinking clearly, distractibility, and indecisiveness.
➤ Ask about anorexia, constipation, or diarrhea; loss of appetite; or weight gain. Note any physical disorder or the use of prescription, over-the-counter, or illicit drugs. Ask about suicidal ideation and plans.
➤ Listen for expressions of doubt of self-worth or the ability to cope, and of unhappiness or apathy.
➤ Observe the patient for anergia and fatigue, restlessness, and reduced psychomotor activity.

Immediate actions

➤ Initiate suicide precautions and ensure the patient's safety.
➤ Obtain urine and serum specimens for toxicology screening.
➤ Administer selective serotonin reuptake inhibitors (SSRIs), such as flu-oxetine, paroxetine, or sertraline. (See *Managing attempted suicide.*) SSRIs are the first-choice treatment for most patients.
➤ Administer a serotonin and norepinephrine reuptake inhibitor (SNRI) such as venlafaxine. (SNRIs are generally used as second-line therapy.)
➤ Administer a tricyclic antidepressant (TCA) such as amitriptyline, as or-dered.
➤ If the patient doesn't respond to TCAs, be prepared to give a mono-amine oxidase (MAO) inhibitor such as isocarboxazid.
➤ Be prepared to administer other agents, such as maprotiline, trazodone, or bupropion, as ordered.

Follow-up actions

➤ Prepare the patient for psychological evaluation to determine the onset, severity, duration, and progression of depressive symptoms.
➤ Prepare the patient for electroconvulsive therapy if he's incapacitated, suicidal, or psychotically depressed or if antidepressants are contraindi-cated or ineffective.
➤ Prepare the patient for short-term psychotherapy — individual, family, and group.
➤ Share your observations of the patient's behavior with him.
➤ Avoid feigned cheerfulness but don't hesitate to laugh with the patient and point out the value of humor.
➤ Listen attentively and respectfully, preventing interruptions and avoid-ing judgmental responses.
➤ Provide a structured routine with noncompetitive activities.
➤ Urge the patient to join group activities and to socialize.
➤ Encourage the patient to express his feelings.
➤ Assist the patient with personal hygiene and encourage him to eat and feed himself. Offer small, frequent, high-fiber meals.
➤ Remind the patient that antidepressants may take several weeks to pro-duce an effect.
➤ Help the patient to recognize distorted perceptions that may contribute to his depression.
➤ Suggest that the patient chew sugarless gum or hard candy to combat the anticholinergic effects of many antidepressants.
➤ Because many antidepressants have a sedating effect, warn the patient to avoid activities that require alertness, including driving and operat-ing mechanical equipment, until the central nervous system (CNS) ef-fects of the drug are known.
➤ Instruct the patient taking TCAs to avoid drinking alcoholic beverages or taking other CNS depressants during therapy.

IN ACTION

➤ *MANAGING ATTEMPTED SUICIDE*

You're making end-of-shift rounds when you discover that one of your patients, Morton Long, 40, isn't in his bed. You find him with a sheet around his neck, hanging from the shower curtain rod. You call a code and rush to support him.

What's the situation?

Mr. Long was admitted to your medical-surgical unit for ascites and cirrhosis of the liver. On admission he was alert and cooperative, although his speech was slow, his tone low, and he avoided eye contact. He reported a history of alcohol and substance abuse and a family history of depression. He said he was feeling down because he'd recently lost his job and his wife had left him, moving his children to another state.

Mr. Long's admission vital signs were blood pressure, 110/60 mm Hg; temperature, 98.6° F (37° C); pulse, 100; and respirations, 22. His skin was warm and dry, his abdomen was distended, and you noted +1 edema of his legs.

What's your assessment?

Mr. Long gave several clues that he was depressed and might attempt suicide. During his admission interview he talked about his substance abuse history (frequently a precursor to suicide attempts), family history of depression, job loss, and recent separation from his family. Any one of these can be a red flag to alert you to serious depression.

What must you do immediately?

After calling a code, you attempt to get Mr. Long's weight off his neck by lifting his body. When the code team arrives, one person stabilizes Mr. Long's head and neck while you and another person support his body and a fourth person removes the sheet from his neck. You lower him onto a backboard and open his airway, using a jaw-thrust maneuver.

He's unresponsive and isn't breathing, but you palpate a carotid pulse. You begin rescue breathing, and he starts to breathe on his own.

The team members complete their evaluation and interventions and state that Mr. Long is clinically stable.

What should be done later?

Mr. Long is transferred to a monitored bed and watched for cardiac arrhythmias and delayed pulmonary complications related to edema of laryngeal structures. He'll have X-rays of his cervical spine taken before cervical spine stabilization is removed, and he'll need a computed tomography scan of the head if he isn't awake, alert, and oriented. Laboratory studies will be done to rule out physiologic causes of Mr. Long's depression. Mr. Long may need to be seen by an ear, nose, and throat specialist or trauma surgeon to check for laryngeal or carotid artery injuries.

(continued)

> **MANAGING ATTEMPTED SUICIDE** (continued)

Mr. Long will be placed under constant one-on-one observation until a psychiatric consultation can be arranged. He'll be encouraged then to discuss what led to the suicide attempt. (If you work in a hospital that has an inpatient psychiatric unit, suggest transferring Mr. Long there after he's stable.)

Stay alert for signs that a patient may be depressed and contemplating suicide. Screening tools, such as the Beck Depression Inventory, can be used at admission to screen the patient at risk. Follow your facility's procedures for suicide precautions and for referring the patient to mental health professionals who can determine his suicide risk and the appropriate level of suicide precautions.

McGlotten, S. "Action Stat: Attempted Suicide," *Nursing* 33(4):96, April 2003. Used with permission.

➤ Emphasize to the patient taking MAO inhibitors that he must avoid foods that contain tyramine, caffeine, or tryptophan.

ALERT *MAO inhibitors are associated with a high risk of toxicity, particularly when these agents interact with certain substances commonly found in many foods. Patients being treated with these drugs must comply with dietary restrictions because ingestion of tyramine can cause a hypertensive crisis, ingestion of tryptophan can cause severe neurologic symptoms, and ingestion of caffeine can cause cardiac problems. Instruct patients taking MAO inhibitors to avoid cheese, sour cream, beer, chianti or sherry, pickled herring, liver, canned figs, raisins, bananas, avocados, chocolate, soy sauce, fava beans, yeast extracts, meat tenderizers, coffee, and cola-flavored soft drinks.*

Preventive steps
➤ Major depression can't be prevented, but relapses can be reduced by following the treatment regimen. Some depressive episodes can be prevented by effective stress management, regular exercise, adequate sleep, and avoiding the use of drugs, alcohol, caffeine, and over-the-counter medications and supplements.

Pathophysiology recap
➤ Depression can be caused by:
  – genetic causes (depression is two to three times more common in people with a first-degree relative with the disorder)
  – psychological causes, such as feelings of helplessness and vulnerability, anger, hopelessness and pessimism, low self-esteem, and personal loss or severe stressor
  – medical conditions, such as metabolic disturbances (hypoxia and hypercalcemia), endocrine disorders (diabetes and Cushing's syndrome), neurologic disorders (Parkinson's and Alzheimer's), cancer, viral and bacterial infections (influenza and pneumonia), cardiovascular

COMPLICATIONS
➤ *SUICIDE*

Suicide is the act of intentionally taking one's life.

Signs and symptoms
A suicidal person will:
- ➤ have feelings of overwhelming anxiety (common trigger for suicide attempt)
- ➤ talk about feeling suicidal or wanting to die
- ➤ express feelings of hopelessness and helplessness
- ➤ become withdrawn (social isolation)
- ➤ claim that he's a burden to his family and friends
- ➤ use or abuse alcohol and drugs
- ➤ begin to put all his personal affairs in order
- ➤ give away prized possessions
- ➤ begin drafting a suicide note
- ➤ seek harm or danger.

Treatment
Treatment includes:
- ➤ admitting the patient to a psychiatric facility
- ➤ one-on-one observation
- ➤ safety precautions, such as removing all sharp objects, drugs and poisonous substances, cordlike items, and potentially dangerous appliances from the patient's surroundings
- ➤ antidepressant medications and antianxiety medications, as indicated.

Nursing considerations
- ➤ Provide emotional support.
- ➤ Establish trust.
- ➤ Allow the patient to express his feelings, and keep communication lines open.
- ➤ Assist the patient to participate in therapy and practice the suggestions of the therapist.
- ➤ Provide positive reinforcement.
- ➤ Provide distraction.
- ➤ Encourage the patient to comply with the treatment regimen.
- ➤ Involve family members in treatment.

disorders (heart failure), pulmonary disorders (chronic obstructive pulmonary disease), musculoskeletal disorders (degenerative arthritis), GI disorders (irritable bowel syndrome), GU problems (incontinence), collagen vascular diseases (lupus), and anemias
– drugs, such as antihypertensives, psychotropics, opioid and nonopioid analgesics, antiparkinsonian drugs, many cardiovascular medications, oral antidiabetics, antimicrobials, steroids, chemotherapeutic agents, cimetidine, and alcohol.
➤ Suicide is the most serious consequence of major depression. (See *Suicide*.)

➤ Panic disorder

Panic disorder is characterized by recurrent episodes of intense apprehension, terror, and feelings of impending doom. It represents anxiety in its most severe form.

Rapid assessment
- ➤ Obtain the patient's history, noting complaints of repeated spontaneous episodes of unexpected apprehension, fear or, rarely, intense discomfort that may last for minutes or hours and leave the patient shaken, fearful, and exhausted. These episodes occur several times per week—or daily—without exposure to a known anxiety-producing situation.
- ➤ Ask the patient about dyspnea, digestive disturbances, chest pain, and use of alcohol or illicit drugs.
- ➤ Assess the patient for signs and symptoms of intense anxiety, such as hyperventilation, tachycardia, trembling, and profuse sweating.

Immediate actions
- ➤ Initiate measures to ensure the patient's safety.
- ➤ If an attack occurs while you are with the patient, remain with him until it subsides.
- ➤ Maintain a calm, serene approach and avoid giving him insincere expressions of reassurance.
- ➤ Prevent excessive stimuli.
- ➤ Speak in short, simple sentences, and give one direction at a time.
- ➤ Allow the patient to pace around the room to expend energy; show him how to take slow, deep breaths.
- ➤ Encourage the patient to express his feelings.
- ➤ Obtain serum and urine samples to screen for abnormal levels of barbiturates, caffeine, and amphetamines, which can precipitate panic attacks.
- ➤ Administer antianxiety drugs, such as diazepam, alprazolam, and clonazepam. Give beta-adrenergic blockers, such as propranolol, and an antidepressants such as a selective serotonin reuptake inhibitor.

Follow-up actions
- ➤ Prepare the patient for behavioral therapy, especially when agoraphobia accompanies a panic disorder.
- ➤ Prepare the patient for psychotherapy.
- ➤ Teach relaxation techniques.
- ➤ Review all medications.
- ➤ Refer the patient to community resources such as the Anxiety Disorders Association of America.

Preventive steps
- ➤ Panic disorder can't be prevented, but some episodes can be reduced by avoiding stimulants, such as caffeine, cocaine, and alcohol.

Pathophysiology recap
➤ Initially unpredictable, panic disorder may become associated with specific situations or tasks. It commonly exists concurrently with agoraphobia.
➤ Panic disorder typically has an onset in late adolescence or early adulthood.
➤ Without treatment, it can persist for years, with alternating exacerbations and remissions.
➤ Patients with panic disorder are at high risk for psychoactive substance abuse disorder; these patients may resort to alcohol or anxiolytics in an attempt to relieve extreme anxiety.
➤ Potential physical causes of panic disorder may include alterations in brain biochemistry, especially in norepinephrine, serotonin, and gamma-aminobutyric acid activity, and a stressful or scary event, such as severe aspiration or choking during childhood.
➤ Psychological causes may include sudden loss and separation anxiety.

➤ Posttraumatic stress disorder
Characteristic psychological consequences that persist for at least 1 month after a traumatic event outside the range of typical human experience are classified as posttraumatic stress disorder (PTSD).

Rapid assessment
➤ Obtain the patient's psychosocial history; ask about early life experiences, interpersonal factors, military experiences, or other incidents that suggest the precipitating event.
➤ Ask the patient to determine the time of symptom onset—typically, immediately or soon after the trauma, although it may be months or years later.
➤ Ask about pangs of painful emotion, unwelcome thoughts, intrusive memories, dissociative episodes (flashbacks), difficulty sleeping, nightmares about the traumatic event, aggressive outbursts on awakening, chronic anxiety, or panic attacks.
➤ Assess the patient for rage and survivor guilt. Observe him for the use of violence to solve problems.
➤ Assess the patient for depression and suicidal ideation, phobic avoidance of situations that arouse memories of the traumatic event, memory impairment or difficulty concentrating, and feelings of detachment or estrangement that destroy interpersonal relationships.
➤ Ask about substance abuse.

Immediate actions
➤ Initiate suicide precautions and ensure the safety of the patient and others.

➤ Provide treatment for depression, alcohol or drug abuse, and medical conditions.
➤ Administer antianxiety medications and antidepressants, as ordered.

Follow-up actions
➤ Encourage the patient to express his grief, complete the mourning process, and develop coping skills to relieve anxiety and desensitize him to the memories of the traumatic event.
➤ Establish trust.
➤ Provide encouragement.
➤ Encourage joint assessment of angry outbursts.
➤ Encourage the patient to express his anger verbally, not physically.
➤ Prepare the patient for behavioral therapy, including relaxation techniques and psychotherapy.
➤ Encourage the patient to join a support group for persons with PTSD.

Preventive steps
➤ Counseling and crisis intervention immediately after the traumatizing event may help reduce long-term effects of PTSD.

Pathophysiology recap
➤ PTSD occurs in response to an extremely distressing event—a serious threat of harm to the patient or his family, such as war, abuse, or violent crime; a disaster, such as a destruction of a home or community by a bombing, fire, flood, tornado, or earthquake; or witnessing a death or serious injury of another person by torture, natural disaster, or by some type of accident.
➤ Preexisting psychopathology can predispose the patient to this disorder.

➤ *Rape trauma syndrome*

Rape is illicit sexual intercourse without consent. It's a violent assault in which sex is used as a weapon. It inflicts varying degrees of physical and psychological trauma. Rape trauma syndrome occurs during the period following the rape and encompasses the victim's short-term and long-term reactions and the methods she uses to cope with the assault.

Rapid assessment
➤ Assess the patient's vital signs.
➤ Evaluate for physical injuries.
➤ Obtain the patient's history; ask her to describe the events surrounding the rape.

 ALERT *Remember, health care notes may be used as evidence if the rapist is tried. Obtain an accurate and detailed history and record the victim's statements in first person, using quotation*

➤ IF THE RAPE VICTIM IS A CHILD

Carefully interview the child to assess how well she can deal with the situation after going home. Interview her alone, away from the parents. Tell the parents that this is being done for the child's comfort, not to keep secrets from them. Ask them what words the child is comfortable with when referring to parts of the anatomy.

History and examination

A young child will place only as much importance on an experience as others do unless there's physical pain. A good question to ask is, "Did someone touch you when you didn't want to be touched?" As with other rape victims, record information in the child's own words. A complete pelvic examination is necessary only if penetration has occurred; such an examination requires parental consent and administration of an analgesic or a local anesthetic.

Need for counseling

The child and her parents will need counseling to minimize possible emotional disturbances. Encourage the child to talk about the experience and try to alleviate confusion. After a rape, a young child may regress; an older child may become fearful about being left alone. The child's behavior may change at school or at home.

Help the parents understand that it's normal for them to feel angry and guilty, but warn them not to displace or project such feelings onto the child. Instruct them to assure the child that they aren't angry with her, that she's good, and that she didn't cause the incident. They should explain to her that they're sorry it happened but glad she's okay, and that the family will help her overcome her fears and confusion.

---

marks. Also document objective information provided by others. Never speculate or record subjective impressions or thoughts.

➤ Ask the patient about allergies, recent illnesses and history of sexually transmitted diseases, current pregnancy, details of her obstetric and gynecologic history, and date of her last menses.
➤ Ask whether the patient douched, bathed, or washed before coming to the hospital.

Immediate actions

➤ Take the patient to a private room where she can talk to a health professional or counselor before the physical examination. (See *If the rape victim is a child.*)
➤ Offer support and reassurance and assist the victim through the initial period and response after the rape.
➤ Help the victim explore her feelings.
➤ Listen, convey trust and respect, and remain nonjudgmental.
➤ Don't leave the patient alone unless she asks you to.
➤ Thoroughly explain to the patient the examination she'll have.

➤ Follow your facility's policy; make sure informed consent is obtained.
➤ Place clothing in a paper bag (plastic bags will cause secretions and seminal stains to mold, destroying their value as evidence).
➤ Carefully bag and label all possible evidence.
➤ Perform a physical examination, assist with a pelvic examination, obtain specimens for semen, and test for gonorrhea.
➤ Collect and label fingernail scrapings and foreign material obtained by combing pubic hair.
➤ For the male patient, obtain a pharyngeal specimen for gonorrhea culture and rectal aspirate for acid phosphatase or sperm antibodies.
➤ Clean and treat all lesions and injuries.
➤ Assist in photographing the patient (this may be delayed for a day or two until bruises and ecchymosis are more visible).
➤ Administer, as ordered, antibiotics to prevent sexually transmitted disease and norgestrel and ethinyl-estradiol to prevent pregnancy.

Follow-up actions
➤ Support and encourage the patient through the police interview.
➤ Help the patient verbalize anticipation of her family's response.
➤ Prepare the patient for X-rays to rule out fractures, if necessary.
➤ Schedule appointments for the patient to return for follow-up testing for pregnancy, as well as for human immunodeficiency virus and other sexually transmitted diseases.
➤ Provide ice packs to reduce vulvar edema.
➤ Refer the patient for psychological counseling to cope with the aftereffects of the attack.
➤ Refer the patient to support organizations, such as Women Organized Against Rape or a local rape crisis center, for empathy and advice.

Preventive steps
➤ Counseling and good support systems immediately after the event may help prevent rape trauma syndrome.

Pathophysiology recap
➤ In the United States, 1.3 adult females are raped every minute; most victims are between ages 10 to 19.
➤ One in seven reported rapes involves a prepubertal child.
➤ About 50% of rapes occur in the home.
➤ Most rapists are ages 15 to 24 and have planned the attack; in most cases, the victim is a female and the attacker is a male.
➤ Prognosis depends on physical and emotional support, counseling, and the victim's ability to cope with her fears and feelings.

➤ PHASES OF SCHIZOPHRENIA

Schizophrenia usually occurs in three phases: prodromal, active, and residual.

Prodromal phase

The *Diagnostic and Statistical Manual of Mental Disorders,* Fourth Edition, Text Revision *(DSM-IV-TR),* characterizes the prodromal phase as clear deterioration in functioning that occurs before the active phase of the disturbance, isn't due to a disturbance in mood or a psychoactive substance use disorder, and involves at least two of the following signs and symptoms:
- ➤ marked social isolation or withdrawal
- ➤ marked impairment in role functioning as wage-earner, student, or home-maker
- ➤ markedly peculiar behavior
- ➤ marked impairment in personal hygiene and grooming
- ➤ blunted or inappropriate affect
- ➤ digressive, vague, over-elaborate, or circumstantial speech, or poverty of speech, or poverty of content of speech
- ➤ odd beliefs or magical thinking that's inconsistent with cultural norms and influences the patient's behavior
- ➤ unusual perceptual experiences
- ➤ marked lack of initiative, interests, or energy.

Family members or friends may report personality changes. Typically insidious, this phase may extend over several months or years.

Active phase

During the active phase, the patient exhibits frankly psychotic symptoms. Psychiatric evaluation may reveal delusions, hallucinations, loosening of associations, incoherence, and catatonic behavior. The patient's psychosocial history may also disclose a particular stressor that occurred before the onset of this phase.

Residual phase

According to *DSM-IV-TR,* the residual phase follows the active phase and occurs when at least two of the symptoms noted in the prodromal phase persist. These symptoms don't result from a disturbance in mood or from a psychoactive substance use disorder.

The residual phase resembles the prodromal phase, except that disturbances in affect and role functioning usually are more severe. Delusions and hallucinations may persist.

➤ Schizophrenia

Schizophrenia is characterized by disturbances of at least 6 months' duration in thought content and form, perception, affect, sense of self, volition, interpersonal relationships, and psychomotor behavior. (See *Phases of schizophrenia.*)

Rapid assessment

Assess the patient for:

➤ ambivalence—coexisting strong positive and negative feelings, leading to emotional conflict
➤ apathy and other affective abnormalities
➤ clang associations—words that rhyme or sound alike used in an illogical, nonsensical manner
➤ concrete association—inability to form or understand abstract thoughts
➤ delusions—false ideas or beliefs accepted as real by the patient; delusions of grandeur, persecution, and reference (distorted belief regarding the relation between events and one's self); feelings of being controlled, somatic illness, and depersonalization
➤ echolalia—automatic and meaningless repetition of another's words or phrases
➤ echopraxia—involuntary repetition of movements observed in others
➤ flight of ideas—rapid succession of incomplete and loosely connected ideas
➤ hallucinations—false sensory perceptions with no basis in reality; usually visual or auditory, but may also be olfactory, gustatory, or tactile
➤ illusions—false sensory perceptions with some basis in reality
➤ loose associations—rapid shifts among unrelated ideas
➤ magical thinking—belief that thoughts or wishes can control others or events
➤ neologisms—bizarre words that have meaning only for the patient
➤ poor interpersonal relationships
➤ regression—return to an earlier developmental stage
➤ thought blocking—sudden interruption in the patient's train of thought
➤ withdrawal—disinterest in objects, people, or surroundings
➤ word salad—illogical word groupings.

Immediate actions

➤ Initiate suicide precautions and implement measures to ensure the safety of the patient and others.
➤ Apply physical restraints according to facility policy, if necessary.
➤ Administer antipsychotic drugs, antidepressants, and anxiolytics as indicated.
➤ Be prepared to administer clozapine in severely ill patients who fail to respond to standard treatment.

Follow-up actions

➤ Monitor the patient for adverse reactions to antipsychotic drugs. (See *Adverse effects of antipsychotic drugs.*)

 ALERT *Encourage the patient taking clozapine to return for follow-up blood studies to monitor for agranulocytosis, an adverse effect that occurs in 1% to 2% of patients taking this drug.*

➤ Prepare the patient for psychotherapy and family therapy.

➤ ADVERSE EFFECTS OF ANTIPSYCHOTIC DRUGS

The newer atypical agents, such as risperidone, olanzapine, quetiapine, sertindole, and ziprasidone, produce fewer extrapyramidal symptoms than the older class of antipsychotics. Risperidone is associated with increases in serum prolactin. Olanzapine, in moderate doses, induces little extrapyramidal symptoms, but has been associated with weight gain and blood glucose abnormalities. Quetiapine can cause weight gain, hypotension, and sedation.

Older classes of antipsychotic drugs (sometimes known as *neuroleptic drugs*) can cause sedative, anticholinergic, or extrapyramidal effects; orthostatic hypotension; and, rarely, neuroleptic malignant syndrome.

Sedative, anticholinergic, and extrapyramidal effects

High-potency drugs, such as haloperidol, are minimally sedative and anticholinergic but cause a high incidence of extrapyramidal adverse effects. Intermediate-potency agents, such as molindone, are associated with a moderate incidence of adverse effects, whereas low-potency drugs, such as chlorpromazine, are highly sedative and anticholinergic but produce few extrapyramidal adverse effects.

The most common extrapyramidal effects are dystonia, parkinsonism, and akathisia. Dystonia usually occurs in young male patients within the first few days of treatment. Characterized by severe tonic contractions of the muscles in the neck, mouth, and tongue, dystonia may be misdiagnosed as a psychotic symptom. Diphenhydramine or benztropine administered I.M. or I.V. provides rapid relief of this symptom.

Drug-induced parkinsonism results in bradykinesia, muscle rigidity, a shuffling or propulsive gait, a stooped posture, a flat facial affect, tremors, and drooling. Parkinsonism may occur from 1 week to several months after the initiation of drug treatment. Drugs prescribed to reverse or prevent this syndrome include benztropine, trihexyphenidyl, and amantadine.

Tardive dyskinesia can occur after only 6 months of continuous therapy and is usually irreversible. No effective treatment is available for this disorder, which is characterized by various involuntary movements of the mouth and jaw; flapping or writhing; purposeless, rapid, and jerky movements of the arms and legs; and dystonic posture of the neck and trunk.

Signs and symptoms of akathisia include restlessness, pacing, and an inability to rest or sit still. Propranolol relieves this adverse effect.

Orthostatic hypotension

Low-potency neuroleptics can cause orthostatic hypotension because they block alpha-adrenergic receptors. If hypotension is severe, the patient is placed in the supine position and given I.V. fluids for hypovolemia. If further treatment is necessary, an alpha-adrenergic agonist, such as norepinephrine, may be ordered to relieve hypotension. Mixed alpha- and beta-adrenergic drugs, such as epinephrine, or beta-adrenergic drugs, such as isoproterenol, shouldn't be given because they can further reduce blood pressure.

(continued)

> **ADVERSE EFFECTS OF ANTIPSYCHOTIC DRUGS** (continued)

Neuroleptic malignant syndrome

Neuroleptic malignant syndrome is a life-threatening syndrome that occurs in up to 1% of patients taking antipsychotic drugs. Signs and symptoms include fever, muscle rigidity, and an altered level of consciousness occurring hours to months after initiating drug therapy or increasing the dose. Treatment is symptomatic, largely consisting of dantrolene and other measures to counter muscle rigidity associated with hyperthermia. You'll need to monitor the patient's vital signs and mental status continuously.

➤ Encourage the patient to eat and monitor his nutritional intake and weight.

➤ Use an accepting, consistent approach and short, repeated contacts.

➤ Reward positive behavior to help promote independence.

➤ Engage the patient in reality-oriented activities involving human contact; explain that his private language, autistic inventions, or neologisms aren't understood.

➤ Explore hallucinations but don't argue about them; teach the patient techniques to interrupt his hallucinations.

➤ When talking with the patient, choose words and phrases that are clearly understood. Don't joke with him.

➤ Don't touch or crowd the patient without telling him first what you're going to do.

➤ Inform the patient about all medications and stress the importance of complying with the drug regimen.

Preventive steps

➤ Schizophrenia can't be prevented, but relapses can be prevented by strict compliance with the prescribed medication regimen.

Pathophysiology recap

➤ The onset of symptoms usually occurs during late adolescence or early adulthood and produces varying degrees of impairment.

➤ Causes of schizophrenia may be genetic, psychological (high stress levels), cultural (more common in lower socioeconomic groups), or biologic (excessive activity at dopaminergic synapses, increases in serotonin, structural abnormalities in the frontal and temporolimbic systems, and low birth weight).

➤ Somatization disorder

Somatization disorder is present when multiple recurrent signs and symptoms of several years' duration suggest that physical disorders exist without a verifiable disease or pathophysiologic condition to account for them.

Rapid assessment

➤ Obtain the patient's history; request his medical records to identify a pattern of multiple medical evaluations by different physicians at different facilities without significant findings.
➤ Observe the patient for anxiety and depression.
➤ Note the patient's report of physical complaints presented in a dramatic, vague, or exaggerated way, typically as part of a complicated medical history in which many medical diagnoses have been considered.
➤ Assess the patient for conversion or pseudoneurologic signs and symptoms, such as paralysis or blindness.
➤ Note GI discomfort, chronic pain, cardiopulmonary symptoms, reproductive difficulties (male or female), and psychosexual problems.
➤ Document extensive knowledge about tests, procedures, and medical jargon and disparaging comments about previous health care professionals and treatments.

Immediate actions

➤ Obtain a diagnostic evaluation to rule out organic causes for signs and symptoms.
➤ Inform the patient that he has no serious illness, but acknowledge his symptoms. Explain that he'll receive care to help him cope with them.
➤ Don't characterize his symptoms as imaginary.
➤ Explain all test results and their significance.

Follow-up actions

➤ Review the patient's complaints and the effectiveness of his coping strategies.
➤ Teach the patient to manage stress and point out the time relationship between stress and symptoms.
➤ Help the patient and his family understand his need for troublesome symptoms.
➤ Encourage psychiatric treatment but don't be surprised if the patient rejects the idea.

Preventive steps

➤ Somatization disorder can't be prevented, but the intensity of the symptoms may be reduced by counseling and stress management.

Pathophysiology recap

➤ Somatization disorder is usually chronic, with exacerbations during times of stress. It primarily affects females.
➤ Signs and symptoms, which are involuntary as the patient consciously wants to feel better, usually begin in adolescence; rarely, they may begin in the 20s.
➤ Genetic and environmental factors contribute to the development of the disorder.

Emergency cardiac drugs

Drug	Action	Indications
adenosine (Adenocard)	➤ Slows conduction through the atrioventricular (AV) node	Paroxysmal supraventricular tachycardia (PSVT)
amiodarone (Cordarone)	➤ Blocks sodium channels at rapid pacing frequencies	Life-threatening ventricular arrhythmias, such as recurrent ventricular fibrillation and recurrent, unstable ventricular tachycardia, atrial fibrillation, atrial flutter
atropine	➤ Blocks vagal effects on the sinoatrial (SA) and AV nodes and enhances conduction through the AV node and increases the heart rate.	Symptomatic sinus bradycardia, AV block, asystole and bradycardic pulseless electrical activity
digoxin	➤ Increases force and velocity of myocardial contraction; slows conduction through SA and AV nodes	Slows heart rate in sinus tachycardia from heart failure and controls rapid ventricular rate in patients with atrial fibrillation or flutter
diltiazem (Cardizem)	➤ Inhibits influx of calcium through the cell membrane, resulting in a depression of automaticity and conduction velocity in smooth and cardiac muscles	Atrial fibrillation, atrial flutter, atrial tachycardia

Adverse effects	Special considerations
➤ Chest pain ➤ Dyspnea ➤ Flushing ➤ Transient sinus bradycardia and ventricular ectopy	➤ Monitor cardiac rate and rhythm. ➤ A brief period of asystole (up to 15 seconds) may occur after rapid administration. ➤ Rapidly follow each dose with a 20-ml saline flush. ➤ Don't administer through a central line because a more prolonged asystole may result.
➤ Bradycardia ➤ Exacerbation of arrhythmia ➤ Fever ➤ Heart failure ➤ Hepatotoxicity ➤ Hyperthyroidism ➤ Hypotension ➤ Hypothyroidism ➤ Nausea and vomiting ➤ Ophthalmic abnormalities: Corneal microdeposits ➤ Photosensitivity and skin discoloration ➤ Pulmonary fibrosis	➤ Closely monitor the patient during loading phase. ➤ If the patient needs a dosage adjustment, monitor him for an extended time because of the drug's long and variable half-life and the difficulty in predicting the time needed to achieve new steady-state plasma drug level. ➤ Administer oral doses with meals. ➤ Monitor need to adjust dose of digoxin or warfarin. ➤ Monitor pulmonary, liver, and thyroid function tests.
➤ Blurred vision ➤ Dry mouth ➤ Palpitations ➤ Restlessness ➤ Tachycardia ➤ Urine retention	➤ Monitor cardiac rate and rhythm. ➤ Use with caution with myocardial ischemia. ➤ Not recommended for third-degree AV block and infranodal type II second-degree AV block. ➤ In adults, avoid doses less than 0.5 mg because of risk of paradoxical slowing. ➤ Isn't effective in denervated transplanted hearts.
➤ AV block ➤ Bradycardia ➤ Headaches ➤ Hypokalemia ➤ Nausea and vomiting ➤ Vision disturbances	➤ Digoxin is extremely toxic, with a narrow margin of safety between therapeutic range and toxicity. ➤ Vomiting is usually an early sign of drug toxicity. ➤ Check apical pulse before giving drug and discontinue digoxin, as ordered, if patient's pulse rate falls below 60 beats/minute.
➤ Abdominal discomfort ➤ Acute hepatic injury ➤ AV block ➤ Bradycardia ➤ Dizziness ➤ Edema ➤ Headache	➤ Closely monitor the patient when starting therapy and during dosage adjustments. ➤ Hypertensive patients treated with calcium channel blockers have a higher risk of heart attack than patients treated with diuretics or beta-adrenergic blockers. ➤ Abrupt withdrawal may result in increased frequency and duration of chest pain.

Drug	Action	Indications
diltiazem (*continued*)	➤ Different degrees of selectivity on vascular smooth muscle, myocardium, and conduction and pacemaker tissues	
disopyramide (Norpace)	➤ Decreases rate of diastolic depolarization and upstroke velocity; increases action potential duration; prolongs refractory period	Life-threatening ventricular arrhythmias such as sustained ventricular tachycardia
dofetilide (Tikosyn)	➤ Blocks cardiac potassium channels; increases duration of action potential by delaying repolarization	Maintains sinus rhythm in patients with chronic atrial fibrillation or atrial flutter
epinephrine	➤ Stimulates alpha and beta receptors in the sympathetic nervous system; relaxes bronchial smooth muscle by stimulating beta$_2$ receptors	Cardiac arrest (ventricular fibrillation [VF], pulseless ventricular tachycardia, asystole, pulseless electrical activity), symptomatic bradycardia, and for treatment of bronchospasm and anaphylaxis
flecainide (Tambocor)	➤ Decreases excitability, conduction velocity and automaticity due to slowed atrial, AV node, His-Purkinje system, and intraventricular conduction	Ventricular arrhythmias, supraventricular arrhythmias (patients without coronary artery disease), and atrial fibrillation and atrial flutter.
ibutilide (Corvert)	➤ Delays repolarization by activating slow, inward current (mostly sodium), which results in prolonged duration of atrial and ventricular action potential and refractoriness	Rapid conversion of recent-onset atrial fibrillation or atrial flutter
lidocaine (Xylocaine)	➤ Shortens the refractory period and suppresses the automaticity of ectopic foci without affecting conduction of impulses through cardiac tissue	Acute ventricular arrhythmias

Adverse effects	Special considerations
➤ Heart failure	➤ Monitor cardiac and respiratory function. ➤ Don't use for a patient with Wolff-Parkinson-White (WPW) syndrome or wide-QRS tachycardia of uncertain origin.
➤ Chest pain ➤ First-degree AV block ➤ Hypotension ➤ Long QT interval ➤ Nausea ➤ Widening of QRS	➤ Monitor for arrhythmias and electrocardiogram (ECG) changes; notify physician of widened QRS complex or prolonged QT interval. ➤ Disopyramide increases risk of death in patients with non–life-threatening ventricular arrhythmias. ➤ Use cautiously in patients with WPW syndrome or bundle-branch block.
➤ Chest pain ➤ Headache ➤ Torsades de pointes	➤ Don't use if baseline QTc is greater than 440 msec, if baseline heart rate is less than 50 beats/minute, or if severe renal impairment exists. ➤ Must be initiated by cardiologist, with continuous ECG monitoring for at least 3 days. ➤ Don't use with cimetidine, verapamil, ketoconazole, or trimethoprim.
➤ Angina ➤ Cerebral hemorrhage ➤ Hypertension ➤ Nervousness ➤ Palpitations ➤ Tachycardia	➤ Monitor cardiac rate and rhythm and blood pressure because increased heart rate and blood pressure may cause myocardial ischemia. ➤ Don't mix I.V. dose with alkaline solutions.
➤ Dizziness ➤ Dyspnea ➤ Headache ➤ Nausea ➤ Ventricular arrhythmias (new or worsened) ➤ Vision disturbances	➤ Contraindicated in patients with structural heart disease. ➤ Periodically monitor trough plasma levels because 40% is bound to plasma protein. ➤ Increase dosage as ordered at intervals of more than 4 days in patients with renal disease.
➤ Headache ➤ Hypotension ➤ Nausea ➤ Prolonged QT interval ➤ Torsades de pointes ➤ Worsening ventricular tachycardia	➤ Stop drug infusion as ordered when arrhythmia stops, if ventricular tachycardia occurs, or if QT interval becomes markedly prolonged. ➤ Perform continuous ECG monitoring for at least 4 hours after dose is completed because of proarrhythmic risk. ➤ Check potassium and magnesium levels and correct before giving drug.
➤ Dizziness ➤ Hallucinations ➤ Nervousness ➤ Seizures ➤ Tachycardia ➤ Tachypnea	➤ Monitor cardiac rhythm and notify physician of prolonged PR interval and widened QRS complex. ➤ Contraindicated in second- or third-degree AV block without pacing support, WPW syndrome, and Stokes-Adams syndrome. ➤ Reduce drug dosage as ordered in patients with heart failure or liver disease. ➤ Monitor patient closely for central nervous system changes.

Drug	Action	Indications
moricizine (Ethmozine)	➤ Shortens phase II and III repolarization, leading to decreased duration of the action potential and an effective refractory period	Life-threatening ventricular arrhythmias such as sustained ventricular tachycardia
procainamide (Procanbid, Pronestyl)	➤ Produces a direct cardiac effect to prolong the refractory period of the atria and (to a lesser extent) the His-Purkinje system and the ventricles	Potentially life-threatening ventricular arrhythmias; and atrial fibrillation with rapid rate in WPW syndrome
propafenone (Rythmol)	➤ Reduces upstroke velocity of monophasic action potential ➤ Reduces fast, inward current carried by sodium ions in Purkinje fibers ➤ Increases diastolic excitability threshold ➤ Prolongs effective refractory period	Life-threatening ventricular arrhythmias such as ventricular tachycardia when benefits of treatment outweigh risks
propranolol (Inderal)	➤ Antiarrhythmic action results from beta-adrenergic receptor blockade as well as a direct membrane stabilization action on cardiac cells	Ventricular tachycardias, supraventricular arrhythmias, and PVCs
sotalol (Betapace)	➤ Antiarrhythmic with beta-blocking effects and prolongation of the action potential ➤ Slows AV nodal conduction and increases AV nodal refractoriness	Life-threatening ventricular arrhythmias; maintains sinus rhythm in patients with history of symptomatic atrial fibrillation or atrial flutter
vasopressin	➤ Antidiuretic hormone acts at the cyclic adenosine monophosphate (cAMP) and increases permeability of renal tubular epithelium to water; at high doses, is a powerful vasoconstrictor of capillaries and small arterioles and may help maintain coronary perfusion pressure	Cardiac arrest with VF as an alternative to epinephrine

Adverse effects	Special considerations
➤ Bradycardia ➤ Dizziness ➤ Headache ➤ Nausea ➤ Sustained ventricular tachycardia	➤ Use cautiously in patients with sick sinus syndrome because of the possibility of sinus arrest. ➤ The patient should be hospitalized for initial dosing and monitored for heart failure. ➤ Give before meals because food delays rate of absorption.
➤ Agranulocytosis ➤ Diarrhea ➤ Dizziness ➤ Heart block ➤ Hypotension ➤ Liver failure ➤ Lupus erythematosus-like syndrome ➤ Nausea and vomiting	➤ Monitor for arrhythmias and notify physician of widened QRS complex or prolonged QT interval. ➤ Procainamide increases risk of death in patients with non–life-threatening arrhythmias. ➤ Use with caution in patients with liver or kidney dysfunction. ➤ Tell patient not to crush or break extended-release tablets.
➤ AV block ➤ Constipation ➤ Dizziness ➤ Headache ➤ Nausea and vomiting ➤ Unusual taste ➤ Ventricular tachycardia	➤ Monitor liver and renal function studies. ➤ Report significant widening of QRS complex and evidence of second- or third-degree AV block. ➤ Increase dosage more gradually, as ordered, in elderly patients and patients with previous myocardial damage.
➤ AV block ➤ Bradycardia ➤ Heart failure ➤ Hypotension ➤ Light-headedness ➤ Nausea and vomiting	➤ Propranolol is also used for treatment of hypertension, angina pectoris, and myocardial infarction (MI). ➤ Dosages may differ for hypertension, angina, or MI. ➤ Check apical pulse before giving drug. If extremes in pulse rate occur, stop drug and notify physician immediately. ➤ Report significant lengthening of PR interval and monitor for AV block. ➤ Drug masks common signs and symptoms of shock and hypoglycemia.
➤ Bradycardia ➤ Chest pain ➤ Dizziness ➤ Fatigue ➤ Palpitations ➤ QT prolongation	➤ Contraindicated in patients with bronchial asthma, sinus bradycardia, or second- or third-degree AV block without a pacemaker. ➤ Perform ECG monitoring for at least 3 days when therapy starts. ➤ Adjust dosage in renally impaired patients. ➤ Assess patient for QTc prolongation. ➤ Administer drug when patient has an empty stomach.
➤ Bronchoconstriction ➤ Chest pain ➤ Hypersensitivity ➤ Myocardial ischemia ➤ Water intoxication	➤ Monitor cardiac rhythm and blood pressure. ➤ Assess for hypersensitivity reactions, including urticaria, angioedema, bronchoconstriction and anaphylaxis.

Normal and abnormal serum drug levels

Drug name and therapeutic level for adults	Purpose of test	Significance of abnormal level
acetaminophen 10 to 20 mcg/ml (SI, 66.2 to 132.4 µmol/L)	Monitoring for overdose	➤ > 200 mcg/ml (SI, > 1,324 µmol/L) at 4 hours after ingestion or > 50 mcg/ml (SI, > 331 µmol/L) at 12 hours after ingestion signifies toxicity and potential for severe liver damage.
amikacin *Peak:* 20 to 30 mcg/ml (SI, 34.2 to 51.3 µmol/L) *Trough:* 1 to 8 mcg/ml (SI, 1.71 to 13.68 µmol/L)	Monitoring drug therapy	➤ Adjust time or amount of dose or both.
digoxin 0.8 to 2 ng/ml (SI, 1.024 to 2.56 nmol/L)	Monitoring drug therapy	➤ ≥ 3 ng/ml (SI, ≥ 3.8 nmol/L) may signify toxicity. ➤ Decreased level shows that drug may have decreased therapeutic effect.
ethosuximide 40 to 100 mcg/ml (SI, 283.2 to 708 µmol/L)	Monitoring drug therapy	➤ ≥ 100 mcg/ml (SI, ≥ 708 µmol/L) may signify toxicity. ➤ Decreased level shows that drug may have decreased therapeutic effect.
gentamicin *Peak:* 4 to 12 mcg/ml (SI, 8.36 to 25.08 µmol/L) *Trough:* < 2 mcg/ml (SI, < 4.18 µmol/L)	Monitoring drug therapy	➤ Adjust time or amount of dose or both.

Drug name and therapeutic level for adults	Purpose of test	Significance of abnormal level
lidocaine 2 to 5 mcg/ml (SI, 8.54 to 21.35 µmol/L)	Monitoring drug therapy and evaluating toxicity	➤ ≥ 6 mcg/ml (SI, ≥ 25.62 µmol/L) may signify toxicity. ➤ Decreased level shows that drug may have decreased therapeutic effect.
lithium *Therapeutic range:* 0.6 to 1.2 mEq/L (SI, 0.6 to 1.2 nmol/L)	Monitoring drug therapy and evaluating toxicity	➤ > 1.2 mEq/L (SI, > 1.2 nmol/L) may signify toxicity. ➤ Decreased level shows that drug may have decreased therapeutic effect.
nitroprusside (thiocyanate level) 4 to 20 mcg/ml	Evaluating toxicity	➤ > 100 mcg/ml may signify toxicity. ➤ Decreased level shows that drug may have decreased therapeutic effect.
phenobarbital 15 to 40 mcg/ml (SI, 64.65 to 172.4 µmol/L)	Monitoring drug therapy, evaluating toxicity, and evaluating for possible abuse	➤ Decreased level shows that drug may have decreased therapeutic effect
phenytoin *Plasma:* 10 to 20 mcg/ml (SI, 39.6 to 79.2 µmol/L)	Monitoring drug therapy and evaluating toxicity	➤ > 20 mcg/ml (SI, > 79.2 µmol/L) may signify toxicity. ➤ Decreased level shows that drug may have decreased therapeutic effect.
procainamide 3 to 10 mcg/ml (SI, 12.69 to 42.3 µmol/L)	Monitoring drug therapy and evaluating toxicity	➤ > 14 mcg/ml (SI, > 60 µmol/L) may signify toxicity. ➤ Decreased level shows that drug may have decreased therapeutic effect.
quinidine 2 to 6 mcg/ml (SI, 6.16 to 18.48 µmol/L)	Monitoring drug therapy and evaluating toxicity	➤ ≥ 7 mcg/ml (SI, ≥ 21.56 µmol/L) may signify toxicity. ➤ Decreased level shows that drug may have decreased therapeutic effect.

Drug name and therapeutic level for adults	Purpose of test	Significance of abnormal level
theophylline 10 to 20 mcg/ml (SI, 55.5 to 111 µmol/L)	Monitoring drug therapy and evaluating toxicity	➤ ≥20 mcg/ml (SI, ≥ 111 µmol/L) may signify toxicity. ➤ Decreased level shows that drug may have decreased therapeutic effect.
tobramycin *Peak:* 4 to 8 mcg/ml (SI, 4 to 16 µmol/L) *Trough:* < 2 mcg/ml (SI, < 4.28 µmol/L)	Monitoring drug therapy	➤ Adjust time or amount of dose or both.
valproic acid 50 to 100 mcg/ml (SI, 346.5 to 693 µmol/L)	Monitoring drug therapy	➤ Decreased level shows that drug may have decreased therapeutic effect.
vancomycin *Peak:* 20 to 40 mcg/ml (SI, 20 to 40 mg/L) *Trough:* 5 to 15 mcg/ml (SI, 5 to 15 mg/L)	Monitoring drug therapy	➤ Decreased level shows that drug may have decreased therapeutic effect.

Bioterrorism readiness

A terrorist attack that involves biological weapons, chemicals, or radiation can result in sudden or increased demand on facility services. Effective management of patients after such an attack can pose a multitude of challenges.

Biological agents

Follow a systematic approach when managing patients following a biological attack. Use standard precautions, including precautions for cleaning, disinfection, and sterilization of equipment and environment; follow additional precautions based on the biologic agent used and the degree of infection. Be sure to wear protective equipment, and wash your hands with antimicrobial soaps. Cohort patients with similar symptoms in a designated area of the facility when a large number of patients present at once. Also, limit transport of infected individuals, and don't discharge patients with bioterrorism-related infections until they're noninfectious. (See *Treatment for biological weapons exposure, page 440.*)

➤ TREATMENT FOR BIOLOGICAL WEAPONS EXPOSURE

Listed below are potentially threatening biological (bacterial and viral) agents as well as the treatments and vaccines that are currently available.

Implement standard precautions for all cases of suspected exposure. For smallpox, institute airborne precautions for the duration of the illness and until all scabs fall off. For pneumonic plague, institute droplet precautions for 72 hours after initiation of effective therapy.

Biological agent (condition)	Treatment
Bacillus anthracis (anthrax)	➤ Ciprofloxacin, doxycycline, or penicillin ➤ Vaccine: Limited supply available; recommended only for persons exposed to anthrax
Clostridium botulinum (botulism)	➤ Supportive: Endotracheal intubation and mechanical ventilation ➤ Passive immunization with equine antitoxin to lessen nerve damage ➤ Vaccine: Postexposure prophylaxis with equine botulinum antitoxin; botulinum toxoid available from Centers for Disease Control and Prevention; recombinant vaccine under development
Francisella tularensis (tularemia)	➤ Gentamicin or streptomycin; alternatively, doxycycline, chloramphenicol, or ciprofloxacin ➤ Vaccine: Live, attenuated vaccine currently under investigation and review by the Food and Drug Administration (FDA)
Variola major (smallpox)	➤ No FDA-approved antiviral available; cidofovir may be therapeutic if administered 1 to 2 days after exposure ➤ Vaccine: Prophylaxis within 3 to 4 days of exposure
Yersinia pestis (pneumonic plague)	➤ Streptomycin or gentamicin; alternatively, doxycycline, ciprofloxacin, or chloramphenicol ➤ Vaccine: No longer available

Chemical agents

As a nurse, you may be the first to recognize that a patient has been exposed to a chemical agent, and your rapid recognition will decrease the morbidity and mortality related to such a condition. However, keep in mind that the release of a chemical agent may not be easily identified because symptoms may mimic those of common diseases or may be delayed. In addition, you may be less familiar with the clinical presentation of chemical exposure. (See *Signs and symptoms of selected chemical agents.*)

➤ *SIGNS AND SYMPTOMS OF SELECTED CHEMICAL AGENTS*

Examples of signs and symptoms related to selected clinical agents are listed below.

Potential chemical agent	Signs and symptoms
Acrylamide	➤ Ataxia ➤ Delirium ➤ Depressed or absent deep tendon reflexes ➤ Encephalopathy ➤ "Glove and stocking" sensory loss ➤ Memory loss ➤ Muscle weakness and atrophy
Arsenic	➤ Abdominal pain ➤ Hypotension ➤ Profuse diarrhea (possibly bloody) ➤ Multisystem organ failure (possibly) ➤ Vomiting
Arsenic (inorganic)	➤ Ataxia ➤ Delirium ➤ Depressed or absent deep tendon reflexes ➤ Encephalopathy ➤ "Glove and stocking" sensory loss ➤ Memory loss ➤ Muscle weakness and atrophy
Barium	➤ Abdominal pain ➤ Hypokalemia ➤ Hypotension ➤ Profuse diarrhea (possibly bloody) ➤ Multisystem organ failure (possibly) ➤ Vomiting
Carbamate insecticides	➤ Altered mental status ➤ Bradycardia or tachycardia ➤ Bronchorrhea ➤ Diaphoresis ➤ Diarrhea ➤ Fasciculations ➤ Hypotension or hypertension ➤ Increased urination ➤ Lacrimation ➤ Miosis ➤ Salivation ➤ Seizures ➤ Weakness

(continued)

➤ **SIGNS AND SYMPTOMS OF SELECTED CHEMICAL AGENTS** (continued)

Potential chemical agent	Signs and symptoms
Carbamates (medicinal)	➤ Altered mental status ➤ Bradycardia or tachycardia ➤ Bronchorrhea ➤ Diaphoresis ➤ Diarrhea ➤ Fasciculations ➤ Hypotension or hypertension ➤ Increased urination ➤ Lacrimation ➤ Miosis ➤ Salivation ➤ Seizures ➤ Weakness
Carbon monoxide	➤ Altered mental status ➤ Dyspnea ➤ Headache ➤ Hypotension ➤ Metabolic acidosis ➤ Nausea ➤ Seizures ➤ Vomiting
Caustics (acids and alkalais)	➤ Lip, mouth, and pharyngeal ulcerations and burning pain
Colchicine	➤ Abdominal pain ➤ Hypotension ➤ Profuse diarrhea (possibly bloody) ➤ Multisystem organ failure (possibly) ➤ Vomiting
Cyanide	➤ Altered mental status ➤ Bitter almond odor ➤ Dyspnea ➤ Headache ➤ Hypotension ➤ Metabolic acidosis ➤ Nausea ➤ Seizures ➤ Vomiting
Diaquat	➤ Lip, mouth, and pharyngeal ulcerations and burning pain

➤ SIGNS AND SYMPTOMS OF SELECTED CHEMICAL AGENTS *(continued)*

Potential chemical agent	Signs and symptoms
Hydrogen sulfide	➤ Altered mental status ➤ Dyspnea ➤ Headache ➤ Hypotension ➤ Metabolic acidosis ➤ Nausea ➤ Seizures ➤ Vomiting
Inorganic mercuric salts	➤ Lip, mouth, and pharyngeal ulcerations and burning pain
Lead	➤ Ataxia ➤ Delirium ➤ Depressed or absent deep tendon reflexes ➤ Encephalopathy ➤ "Glove and stocking" sensory loss ➤ Memory loss ➤ Muscle weakness and atrophy
Mercury (organic)	➤ Ataxia ➤ Delirium ➤ Depressed or absent deep tendon reflexes ➤ Encephalopathy ➤ "Glove and stocking" sensory loss ➤ Memory loss ➤ Muscle weakness and atrophy ➤ Paresthesias ➤ Visual disturbances
Methemoglobin-causing agents	➤ Altered mental status ➤ Dyspnea ➤ Headache ➤ Hypotension ➤ Metabolic acidosis ➤ Nausea ➤ Seizures ➤ Vomiting
Mustards	➤ Lip, mouth, and pharyngeal ulcerations and burning

(continued)

➤ SIGNS AND SYMPTOMS OF SELECTED CHEMICAL AGENTS (continued)

Potential chemical agent	Signs and symptoms
Nicotine	➤ Altered mental status ➤ Bradycardia or tachycardia ➤ Bronchorrhea ➤ Diaphoresis ➤ Diarrhea ➤ Fasciculations ➤ Hypotension or hypertension ➤ Increased urination ➤ Lacrimation ➤ Miosis ➤ Salivation ➤ Seizures ➤ Weakness
Organophosphate insecticides	➤ Altered mental status ➤ Bradycardia or tachycardia ➤ Bronchorrhea ➤ Decreased acetylcholinesterase activity ➤ Diaphoresis ➤ Diarrhea ➤ Fasciculations ➤ Hypotension or hypertension ➤ Increased urination ➤ Lacrimation ➤ Miosis ➤ Salivation ➤ Seizures ➤ Weakness
Paraquat	➤ Dyspnea and hemoptysis secondary to pulmonary edema or hemorrhage; can progress to pulmonary fibrosis over days to weeks ➤ Lip, mouth, and pharyngeal ulcerations and burning pain
Ricin	➤ Abdominal pain ➤ Hypotension ➤ Multisystem organ failure (possibly) ➤ Profuse diarrhea (possibly bloody) ➤ Severe respiratory illness (if inhaled) ➤ Vomiting
Sodium azide	➤ Altered mental status ➤ Dyspnea ➤ Headache ➤ Hypotension ➤ Metabolic acidosis ➤ Nausea ➤ Seizures ➤ Vomiting

➤ **SIGNS AND SYMPTOMS OF SELECTED CHEMICAL AGENTS** (continued)

Potential chemical agent	Signs and symptoms
Sodium monoflucroacetate	➤ Altered mental status ➤ Dyspnea ➤ Headache ➤ Hypocalcemia or hypokalemia ➤ Hypotension ➤ Metabolic acidosis ➤ Nausea ➤ Seizures ➤ Vomiting
Strychnine	➤ Hypertension ➤ Intact sensorium ➤ Seizure-like, generalized muscle contractions or painful spasms (neck and limbs) ➤ Tachycardia
Thallium	➤ Alaxia ➤ Delirium ➤ Depressed or absent deep tendon reflexes ➤ Encephalopathy ➤ "Glove and stocking" sensory loss ➤ Memory loss ➤ Muscle weakness and atrophy

Adapted from the Centers for Disease Control and Prevention.
Available at: *http://www.cdc.gov/mmwr/preview/mmwrhtml/mm5239a3.htm.*

Clues that might suggest a covert release of a chemical agent include:
➤ sudden and unusual increase in number of patients with potential chemical-release-related illness
➤ unexplained deaths among young and otherwise healthy persons
➤ unexplained odor emissions by patients
➤ clusters of illness in persons who have common characteristics, such as drinking water from the same source
➤ rapid onset of symptoms after exposure to a potentially contaminated medium
➤ unexplained death of plants or wildlife
➤ syndrome suggesting a disease associated with a known chemical exposure.

Immediately report the release of chemicals, whether intentional or accidental, to your state health department and the Centers for Disease Control and Prevention.

Secondary contamination

Patients exposed only to gas or vapor and who have no gross deposition of the chemical on their clothing or skin are not likely to pose a secondary contamination risk. However, patients covered with liquid or solid chemical or those with condensed vapor may contaminate facility personnel by direct contact or off-gassing vapor. These patients should undergo a decontamination process that involves the removal of any clothing, flushing of the skin with plain water and mild soap, irrigation of irritated eyes with saline, or in the case of ingestion, administration of 4 to 8 ounces of water to dilute stomach contents.

Until the identity of the chemical agent is determined, consider the potential for secondary infection of facility personnel. Prior to the arrival of the patient, be sure that personal protective equipment has been distributed and donned and that areas which could become contaminated are cleared and secured. Most patients are transferred and treated in a critical care unit.

Treatment

➤ At all times, attention must be given to the patient's respiratory and cardiovascular status. Ensure a patent airway, intubate and ventilate as necessary and, if needed, support breathing and circulation through the use of cardiopulmonary resuscitation.

➤ Treat patients who are comatose, hypotensive, or have seizures or ventricular arrhythmias in the usual medical manner.

Radiologic agents

Radiation is a form of energy that exists in different forms. Individuals are exposed to small quantities of radiation daily from natural and man-made sources. Exposure to radiation can affect the body in a number of ways, but it may take several years to witness the adverse effects of exposure. Exposure to large doses of radiation because of an accidental or terrorist event is considered a medical emergency; death can occur in a few days or in a matter of months.

Secondary exposure

When treating patients with radiation exposure, facility personnel should institute standard precautions, wear two pairs of gloves for added protection and change them frequently, and establish multiple receptacles for contaminated waste. Obtain radiation survey meters in order to locate contamination areas and measure exposure rate.

Treatment

The first course of action is to medically stabilize the patient, if necessary, prior to initiating any significant decontamination procedures. Immediately remove and bag contaminated clothing, then decontaminate wounds and intact skin. (Recommended cleaning solutions include soap and water, hexachlorophene 3% detergent and water, or povidone iodine and water.) Wash the patient's hair with shampoo without conditioner. Use a radiation survey meter to monitor the progress of the decontamination.

Immediate care should focus on preventing internal contamination. Obtain nasal swabs as early as possible, as well as urine and feces specimens. Assist in the treatment of internal contamination to reduce the radiation dose from absorbed radionuclides and reduce the risk of long-term effects. Immediate treatments include:
- gastric lavage for ingestion of radioactive material within 2 hours of exposure
- antacids for ingested radionuclides
- cathartics for large ingestions
- increased fluid intake for tritium contamination
- oral potassium iodide for radioiodine contamination
- Prussian blue for cesium contamination
- chelating agents, such as calcium or zinc diethylene-triaminepentaacetate for plutonium and transuranics contamination
- oral aluminum phosphate or barium sulfate for strontium ingestion.

Selected references

Bickley, L.S., and Szilagyi, P.G. *Bates' Guide to Physical Examination and History Taking,* 8th ed. Philadelphia: Lippincott Williams & Wilkins, 2003.

Cummins, R.O., ed. *ACLS Provider Manual.* Dallas: American Heart Association, 2004.

Deal, B., et al. *Pediatric ECG Interpretation: An Illustrated Guide.* Elmsford, N.Y.: Blackwell Futura, 2004

ECG Interpretation Made Incredibly Easy, 3rd ed. Philadelphia: Lippincott Williams & Wilkins, 2005.

Greenberg, M.I., et al. *Greenberg's Text-Atlas of Emergency Medicine.* Philadelphia: Lippincott Williams & Wilkins, 2005.

Habif, T.P. *Clinical Dermatology: A Color Guide to Diagnosis and Therapy,* 4th ed. St. Louis: Mosby–Year Book, Inc., 2003.

Henderson, D.A., et al. *Bioterrorism: Guidelines for Medical and Public Health Management.* Chicago: American Medical Association, 2002.

Hesselson, A.B. *Simplified Interpretation of Pacemaker ECGs.* Elmsford, N.Y.: Blackwell Futura, 2003.

Hickey, J.V. *The Clinical Practice of Neurological and Neurosurgical Nursing,* 5th ed. Philadelphia: Lippincott Williams & Wilkins, 2003.

Ignatavicius, D.D., and Workman, M.L. *Medical-Surgical Nursing: Critical Thinking for Collaborative Care,* 4th ed. Philadelphia: W.B. Saunders Co., 2002.

Khan, M.G. *Rapid ECG Interpretation.* Philadelphia: W.B. Saunders Co., 2003.

Mastering ACLS, 2nd ed. Philadelphia: Lippincott Williams & Wilkins, 2006.

McAlister, F.A. "Atrial fibrillation, Shared Decision Making, and the Prevention of Stroke," *Stroke* 33(1):243-44, January 2002.

Morton, P.G., et al. *Critical Care Nursing: A Holistic Approach,* 8th ed. Philadelphia: Lippincott Williams & Wilkins, 2005.

Myers, J.W., et al. *Principles of Pathophysiology and Emergency Medical Care.* Clifton Park, N.Y.: Delmar, 2002.

Nursing2005 Drug Handbook, 25th ed. Philadelphia: Lippincott Williams & Wilkins, 2005.

Rakel, R., and Bope, E.T. *Conn's Current Therapy, 2004.* Philadelphia: W.B. Saunders Co., 2004.

Sadock, B.J., and Sadock, V.A. *Kaplan and Sadock's Comprehensive Textbook of Psychiatry,* 8th ed. Philadelphia: Lippincott Williams & Wilkins, 2005.

Tierney, L.M., et al. *Current Medical Diagnosis and Treatment,* 43rd ed. New York: McGraw-Hill Book Co., 2004.

Wood, S.L., et al. *Cardiac Nursing,* 5th ed. Philadelphia: Lippincott Williams & Wilkins, 2005.

Art credits

These pieces of art were borrowed from Lippincott Williams & Wilkins sources:

page 140, Smeltzer, S.C., and Bare, B.G. *Textbook of Medical-Surgical Nursing,* 9th ed. Philadelphia: Lippincott Williams & Wilkins, 2000.

pages 170 and 171, Hickey, J.V., *The Clinical Practice of Neurological and Neurosurgical Nursing,* 5th ed. Philadelphia: Lippincott Williams & Wilkins, 2002.

page 327, Bickley, L.S., and Szilagyi, P. *Bates' Guide to Physical Examination and History Taking,* 8th ed. Philadelphia: Lippincott Williams & Wilkins, 2003.

page 327, Pillitteri, A., *Maternal and Child Nursing,* 4th ed. Philadelphia: Lippincott Williams & Wilkins, 2003.

page 345, Smeltzer, S.C., and Bare, B.G. *Textbook of Medical-Surgical Nursing,* 9th ed. Philadelphia: Lippincott Williams & Wilkins, 2000.

Index

A

ABCDE primary survey, 2, 3t, 4
ABCs, primary survey and, 2, 3t
Abdominal aortic aneurysm. *See* Dissecting aortic aneurysm.
Abdominal trauma, blunt, 110-112
  effects of, 112i
ABG. *See* Arterial blood gas analysis.
Abruptio placentae, 259-263
  degrees of placental separation in, 260i
  fetal distress as complication of, 263
  managing, 261-262
Absence seizures, 176
Acceleration-deceleration injuries, 146
Acetaminophen overdose, 391, 395-396
  acetylcysteine as antidote for, 105t, 392t, 395
Acetylcysteine as acetaminophen overdose antidote, 105t, 392t, 395
Achilles tendon rupture, 215
Acidic substances, chemical burns to eye and, 315, 317
Activated charcoal as drug overdose antidote, 392t
Acute coronary syndrome. *See* Myocardial infarction.
Acute dermal gangrene. *See* Necrotizing fasciitis.
Acute glomerulonephritis, 279-280

Acute hematopoietic radiation toxicity, 385. *See also* Radiation exposure.
Acute infective tubulointerstitial nephritis, 280-282
Acute peripheral arterial occlusion, 9-10
Acute poststreptococcal glomerulonephritis, 279-280
Acute pyelonephritis, 280-282
Acute renal failure, 282-285
  pathophysiology of, 284-285, 284i
Acute respiratory distress syndrome, 67-72
  hypoxemia as hallmark of, 67
  progression of, 71-72, 72i
  prone positioning for, 69
Acute respiratory failure, 73-74
Acute tubular necrosis, 285-287
  pathophysiology of, 286-287, 286i
Acute tubulointerstitial nephritis. *See* Acute tubular necrosis.
Acyclovir, administration guidelines for, 151
Addisonian crisis. *See* Adrenal crisis.
Adrenal crisis, 218-220
  pathophysiology of, 219i, 220
Adult patient, ear characteristics of, 334i
Advanced cardiac life support, protocols for, 7
Air embolism, 11-13
  delayed, 11
  managing, 12-13

i refers to an illustration; t refers to a table.

i refers to an illustration; t refers to a table.

i refers to an illustration; t refers to a table.

i refers to an illustration; t refers to a table.

i refers to an illustration; t refers to a table.

i refers to an illustration; t refers to a table.

i refers to an illustration; t refers to a table.

i refers to an illustration; t refers to a table.

i refers to an illustration; t refers to a table.

i refers to an illustration; t refers to a table.

NOTES

NOTES

NOTES

NOTES

NOTES

NOTES

River's
Edge

*Also by Terri Blackstock
in Large Print:*

Emerald Windows
Covenant Child
Cape Refuge
Southern Storm
Evidence of Mercy
Justifiable Means
Ulterior Motives
Presumption of Guilt
Never Again Good-bye
When Dreams Cross
Blind Trust
Broken Wings
Seaside

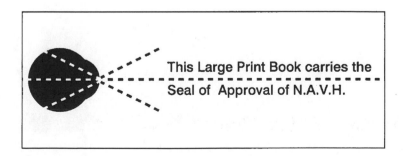
This Large Print Book carries the
Seal of Approval of N.A.V.H.

Cape Refuge Series
Book Three

River's
Edge

Terri Blackstock

Walker Large Print • Waterville, Maine

Published in 2005 by arrangement with
Zondervan Publishing House.

The text of this Large Print edition is unabridged.
Other aspects of the book may vary from the original edition.

Set in 16 pt. Plantin by Elena Picard.

Printed in the United States on permanent paper.

**The Library of Congress has cataloged the Thorndike
Press® edition as follows:**

Blackstock, Terri, 1957–
    River's edge / Terri Blackstock.
      p. cm. — (Cape Refuge series ; bk. 3)
    ISBN 0-7862-7182-5 (lg. print : hc : alk. paper)
    ISBN 1-59415-071-0 (lg. print : sc : alk. paper)
    1. Married women — Crimes against — Fiction.
2. Mayors — Election — Fiction. 3. Fertility clinics —
Fiction. 4. Georgia — Fiction. 5. Large type books.
I. Title.
PS3552.L34285R58 2005
  813'.54—dc22   2004062034

This book is lovingly
dedicated to the Nazarene

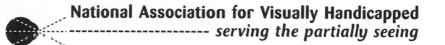

As the Founder/CEO of NAVH, the only national health agency solely devoted to those who, although not totally blind, have an eye disease which could lead to serious visual impairment, I am pleased to recognize Thorndike Press★ as one of the leading publishers in the large print field.

Founded in 1954 in San Francisco to prepare large print textbooks for partially seeing children, NAVH became the pioneer and standard setting agency in the preparation of large type.

Today, those publishers who meet our standards carry the prestigious "Seal of Approval" indicating high quality large print. We are delighted that Thorndike Press is one of the publishers whose titles meet these standards. We are also pleased to recognize the significant contribution Thorndike Press is making in this important and growing field.

Lorraine H. Marchi, L.H.D.
Founder/CEO
NAVH

★ Thorndike Press encompasses the following imprints: Thorndike, Wheeler, Walker and Large Print Press.

Preface

Cape Refuge is a fictitious island which I set just east of Savannah, Georgia, on the Atlantic Coast. To research it, I spent time on Tybee Island, a lovely little beachside community outside of Savannah. Many of my ideas for life in Cape Refuge came from there.

There's another island just south of Tybee called Little Tybee Island, an uninhabited marshland and wildlife refuge. For this novel, I turned Little Tybee into Cape Refuge, after a few alterations to the terrain and the coastline. I hope the kind people of Georgia's coast will forgive me.

I owe a big thanks to J. R. Roseberry, editor and publisher of the *Tybee News*, for his help in my research.

Acknowledgments

Each book I write requires a certain amount of research, and that research often forces me to seek out experts in particular fields. I couldn't write my novels without their help. For this book, I offer thanks to Dr. Steve Bigler and Dr. Tree James, for answering my random questions and brainstorming with me through plot scenarios. I owe a lot to Cissie Posey, who shared her struggles with infertility.

I'd also like to thank two groups of people who have helped my books reach more and more readers — booksellers and librarians. I consider my work a ministry, and I consider you to be my partners in that ministry. Thank you for all you do.

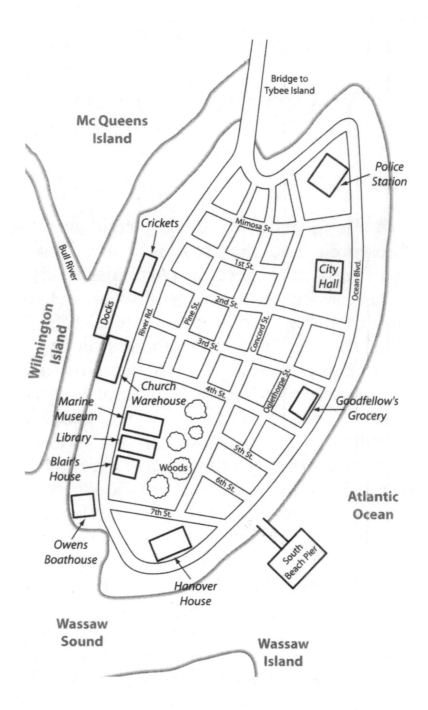

Mc Queens Island

Bridge to Tybee Island

Police Station

Crickets

Mimosa St.

City Hall

1st St.

Bull River

Ocean Blvd.

Docks

River Rd.

2nd St.

Pine St.

Wilmington Island

3rd St.

Concord St.

Church Warehouse

4th St.

Oglethorpe St.

Goodfellow's Grocery

Marine Museum

Library

Blair's House

Woods

5th St.

6th St.

Atlantic Ocean

7th St.

Owens Boathouse

Hanover House

South Beach Pier

Wassaw Sound

Wassaw Island

1

The cramps woke Morgan at 3:30 a.m., startling her out of a deep slumber. She'd been immersed in a dream about a little girl on a swing set, her long brown hair flowing on the breeze. She knew without a doubt that the child was the baby she was carrying.

The cramps offered a stark warning, as if her anxiety had shaped into a blunt instrument that bludgeoned her hope.

She sat up, her hand pressed over her flat stomach, and looked at Jonathan, who slept peacefully next to her. Should she wake him to tell him she was cramping, or just be still and wait for it to pass?

She had taken the home pregnancy test yesterday morning, then followed up with a blood test at her doctor's office that afternoon. Jonathan sat in the examining room with her, fidgeting and chattering to pass the time. When the nurse came back with the verdict, he sprang to his feet, muscles all tense, like a tiger tracking a gazelle.

"Before I tell you the results, I need to know if I'm bearing good or bad news."

Jonathan glanced at Morgan, and she knew he was way too close to calling the woman a smart aleck and warning her not to toy with them. "Come on, just tell us."

"But do you want to be pregnant? Is good news a yes or a no?"

Before he could grab the nurse by the shoulders and shake the playfulness out of her, Morgan blurted out, "Yes! More than anything!"

"Are we going to have a baby or not?" Jonathan asked.

"Congratulations!" The word burst out of the nurse's mouth, and Morgan came off the table, flinging herself into his arms, and they yelled like kids as he swung her around.

They agreed not to announce it until today, so they could share that first night of giddy excitement, crushing the secret between them.

They waited until Caleb, their eighteen-month-old foster child, was sound asleep, then went across the street to Hanover House's private stretch of beach. They giggled and danced under the May moonlight, to the music of the waves whooshing and frothing against the shore. When

12

they'd finally gone to bed, they lay awake until close to midnight, wondering if it would be a girl or a boy, and how soon they would be able to see their child on a sonogram. Jonathan held Morgan and whispered about soccer games and ballet, piano lessons and PTA.

Finally, they had both fallen asleep, and now she didn't want to wake him. It was probably nothing. Just something she ate last night. She would have to be more careful now.

But as the moments dragged on the cramping grew worse, and she couldn't ignore it. She folded her arms across her stomach and slid her feet out of bed. She sat up and realized it was worse, even, than she thought. There was blood.

"Oh, no." The words came out loud and unbidden, and Jonathan turned over and looked up at her in the night.

"Baby, what is it?"

She turned on the lamp. "Oh, Jonathan . . ."

He looked at her with an innocent, terrible dread, expecting something, though not clear what. Slowly, he sat up. "What?"

A sob rose in her throat as she pointed to the mattress.

For a moment they both just stared at it,

the blood-spot of a dream dying.

Their unformed, barely real, secret baby dying.

Then he jolted out of his stunned stupor and sprang out of bed. "Are you okay?"

"I'm losing it." The words bubbled up in her throat. "Jonathan, I'm losing the baby!"

"We're going to the hospital. Maybe it's not what you think. Maybe they can stop it." He pulled on the jeans hanging over a chair by the bed.

Maybe he was right. Maybe the baby was still there, nestled in its little sac, unscathed by whatever thing had broken loose in her. Or if not, maybe the medical staff could ward off danger, stop the impending doom, give her some magic pill to make it hang on.

She quickly got dressed while Jonathan woke Sadie — their seventeen-year-old foster daughter and Caleb's sister — to tell her of the emergency and ask her to listen for her little brother in case they weren't back when he awoke.

Then Jonathan helped Morgan out to the car as though she were a sick woman who couldn't walk on her own. She tried not to make sudden moves, not to walk too hard, not to cramp so tightly.

14

But it all seemed out of her control.

"It's okay, baby," Jonathan said as he drove at breakneck speed across the island. "We'll be in Savannah in no time."

Was it already too late? The drive from Cape Refuge to the closest hospital was too far. She cried quietly, staring out the windshield, praying that God would intervene.

"God's going to save her," he muttered as he drove. "He has to."

Morgan's face twisted. "Her . . . you said *her*." She looked over at him and saw the tears on his face. "You think it's a girl?"

He didn't answer. "God, please . . ."

She sobbed as he drove, her hand pressed against her stomach. *What kind of mother am I? I couldn't keep it safe for a day?* Her tears were cold against her face in the breeze of the air-conditioner.

Jonathan's lips moved in some silent monologue — a desperate preacher's prayer of faith and hope — or the angry railing of a seaman who saw terror coming and believed he could head it off with enough threats. His hands clutched the steering wheel, and occasionally he reached over to touch her with fearful reassurance.

Finally, they reached St. Joseph's, and

Jonathan pulled up to the emergency room door. He got out and ran to Morgan's side, helped her out. There was blood all over the back of her robe, and some of it had soaked into the seat.

"I need help here!" Jonathan helped her through the sliding glass door. "Please, someone help!"

But Morgan knew there was no help for her baby. It was already too late.

2

Two hours later, they rode home in silence, each mired in their own despair. As she'd known he would, the doctor confirmed her fears. She had miscarried her child.

Guilt and anguish ached through her body.

How would Jonathan ever forgive her?

They both wept quietly as the sun rose over the Atlantic, heralding a day that others would find beautiful and welcome. But she would do anything to turn the clock back to this time yesterday.

Jonathan pulled their car into the shade of the red cedars at the end of the gravel driveway. Their house loomed big in the morning light, the yellow paint glowing like the sun, the Victorian trim clean and white. Gus — one of the home's residents — had done some repairs on the house and coated it with fresh paint a couple of weeks ago. The full ferns on the porch overflowed their urns in bright, life-filled

green. Impatiens in yellow, red, and purple lined the front of the house, well cared for by the home's other residents. It was one of those chores that helped their charges integrate back into the world after time on the streets or in jail. Cause-and-effect lessons about working hard, taking care, cultivating and nurturing, and reaping good results. The testimony of a job well done.

She spoke that lesson to them so many times, reminding them that obedience to God, self-discipline, and love all added up to blessings too numerous to count.

Yet here she was, a poster child that the opposite was true.

The front door to the big yellow house was still closed. Maybe that meant that no one was up yet. If they were, the door would have been open, letting in light, along with the ocean sounds from just across the street, through the glass storm door.

Morgan hoped no one knew where she'd been. She didn't want to explain this to anyone but Sadie.

Jonathan helped her out of the car and walked her up the porch steps.

Sadie met them at the door, her eyes red-rimmed and worried. "I'm so glad to see you, Morgan!" She threw her arms

around her. "I thought you were dying or something."

"I'm sorry we worried you, honey." Morgan held her in a tight, reassuring embrace.

"Jonathan didn't say what was wrong. I saw the blood on your bed . . ."

"I'm fine, really."

"But what's wrong? What happened?"

Her effort not to cry twisted her face. "Honey, I found out yesterday that I was pregnant. And this morning . . . I miscarried."

At seventeen Sadie had seen the dark side of life, and she knew what it meant to grieve. Her expression bore the weight of Morgan's news, and she pulled her back into a hug. "Oh, Morgan. I'm so sorry."

Morgan didn't want the girl to suffer with her, so she tried to hold herself together. "I want you to keep this to yourself. I haven't even told Blair yet. And there's no need for anyone else to know, okay?"

Sadie wiped a tear. "Okay."

Jonathan stroked Morgan's hair. "Why don't you go get changed and lie down? I'll clean up the car."

She nodded and started toward the stairs.

"I changed the sheets," Sadie said. "The bed is clean."

"Thank you, sweetie."

Morgan went in, trudged up the stairs, and took a quick shower to clean up. She got dressed, and with her long, curly dark hair still wet, slipped into Caleb's room. He slept soundly in his crib, his thumb shoved into his mouth. Within the next hour, the eighteen-month-old would wake up and cry out for her. She wished she didn't have to wait.

She wanted to pick him up and hold him, crush him to herself, assuage those maternal hormones that hadn't gotten the news.

She didn't think she could have loved him more if he'd been her own son. But he wasn't.

Caleb Seth Caruso had a mother who was serving time in prison on drug charges. Morgan was merely a temporary caretaker until his mother was set free. She started to weep again, and left the room so she wouldn't wake him. He didn't deserve to see her like this.

She went back into the bedroom. Jonathan was sitting on the bed, his face white, expressionless. "I want you to lie down," he said. "When Caleb wakes up, I'll get him."

"Okay."

"Are you feeling all right? Physically, I mean?"

"Yeah, the cramping is getting better." She hated what that meant.

He sat down and looked at the wall, and she knew that he felt the loss as keenly as she. "We are going to be parents, sweetheart," he said. "I know it doesn't seem like it, but we are."

She nodded. They had been trying for over a year. In the scheme of things, she supposed it wasn't as bad as other couples who'd tried for seven, nine, twelve years. She thought of Ben Jackson — Jonathan's opponent in the mayoral race — and his wife, Lisa. They'd been trying for thirteen.

"Do you want to call Blair?" Jonathan's words cut into her thoughts.

Morgan thought of waking her sister up to tell her this news. It hardly seemed fair. Ever since Blair had bought the newspaper, she hadn't been getting adequate rest. "I'll tell her later."

She got into the bed, and Jonathan pulled the covers up over her and tucked her in. He bent over and kissed her cheek.

When he'd left her alone, she let her control slip away, and wept into her pillow.

Later that morning, the cramping stopped, and Morgan forced herself to get

21

out of bed. She went downstairs, and saw that the kitchen was spotless. Gus and Felicia had gone to work, and Sadie was at school. She saw Karen on the back porch feeding her own baby. There was no sign of Jonathan or Caleb. Maybe Jonathan had taken him with him to do some campaigning today.

His big debate with his two opponents in the mayoral race — Sam Sullivan and Ben Jackson — was tomorrow. Jonathan — who worked as a fishing tour guide, pastor of their small church, and director of Hanover House — had only come into the race a month ago, so he was way behind. The special election was scheduled for three weeks away, and he didn't have a moment to waste. If he won, he'd take office almost immediately, since the town had been without a mayor since the last one had been dethroned by scandal.

She went through the kitchen into the small office where she and Jonathan took care of the business of Hanover House. She sat down at the desk and moved a stack of donations out of her way. The home, a halfway house for people trying to change their lives, was supported by monthly contributions. She had yet to log them all this month, so much had been going on.

She picked up the telephone and dialed her sister's number. When there was no answer, she checked the clock. Ten o'clock. Of course Blair wasn't home. She dialed the newspaper office and got her voice-mail. She was probably out tracking down a story, trying to find an interesting angle to the mundane events of the island.

Discouraged, she hung up. She would try Blair again later. But would her sister understand her grief over a baby that she had only known for one day? How could she? No one could understand unless they had been there.

Then she remembered. Someone had.

She thought of the wife of Jonathan's fiercest opponent in the race. Lisa Jackson had been in Morgan's shoes four different times.

One would never have known of her struggle with infertility. It was a secret, closely held. Morgan wouldn't have known it herself, except that she had seen it on Lisa's face when they'd both wound up in the bathroom at a mutual friend's baby shower.

She had recognized those tears, and Lisa had recognized hers. Without saying a word, the two women, whose husbands were political archenemies, had embraced.

They'd sneaked out for coffee to comfort each other, and had poured out their hearts about their infertility and their desperate desire for children.

Maybe it would help to talk to her now.

You call me if you need to talk, honey. Day or night, I don't care. And if you don't mind, I'll do the same. These husbands of ours will just have to get used to it.

Morgan knew she'd meant it.

She knew Lisa probably wasn't home, since her real estate business kept her hopping. But she called and left a message on Lisa's voicemail, then tried her at her office. When her taped recording kicked in, Morgan decided to leave a message there too.

"Hey, Lisa," she said in a soft voice, "this is Morgan. Could you give me a call when you have a chance to talk? I really need to share something with you." She paused and tried to control the emotion wavering in her voice. "Something happened this morning. You're the only one I know who'll understand." She hung up and stared down at the phone. She hoped Lisa would return the call soon.

But hours later, Lisa had not called back, and neither had Blair. Jonathan came home with Caleb — he had only taken him

for a walk on the beach — and she busied herself with his care and the affairs of the house.

She longed for night and the sleep that would numb her pain, but when it finally came, she lay awake, thinking about the dream she'd had last night about the little girl on the swing.

She prayed that God would let her dream it again.

3

Police Chief Matthew Cade — simply Cade to everyone who knew him — came to Hanover House early the next morning. From the look on his face, Morgan knew he hadn't dropped in for breakfast. As Jonathan's closest friend and the love of her sister's life, he dropped in often — but not in full uniform.

He had bad news. She knew that look. It was the same tight expression he'd worn when he interrupted that City Council meeting last summer to tell her that her parents had been murdered.

"I hate to bother you this morning," he said. "I know you're all getting ready for the debate."

She felt like sinking against the wall, raising her arms to deflect the blow. "Something's wrong, Cade. What is it?"

"I'm here on police business. I need to ask you a few questions."

She shivered, and her mind raced with

possibilities. She still hadn't been able to get in touch with her sister. Had something happened to her? "Is it about Blair?"

He looked startled at the question. "No, why? What's wrong with Blair?"

"Nothing. I just haven't heard from her. I tried to call her yesterday but never got her."

His face relaxed. "I talked to her last night. She was working late, trying to cover a baseball game and an awards ceremony. She's fine. No, it's about Lisa Jackson."

"Lisa? What about her?"

"Morgan, Ben reported her missing last night."

"Missing? What do you mean, missing?"

"She didn't come home last night, and she missed several appointments yesterday. Important ones, apparently. She seems to have vanished sometime yesterday morning. We're talking to everyone who might have seen her yesterday. She had messages from you on her home and business voicemail. I wondered if you'd heard from her."

Morgan just gaped at him for a moment. "No. She never called me back."

"When's the last time you spoke to her?"

She shoved her long curls back from her face. "Uh . . . a few days ago."

"Did she give you any indication that she was upset about anything? Angry at Ben?"

"No, not at all. Cade, do you think something's happened to her?"

He seemed to consider whether or not to answer that. "Maybe not. I'm hoping she'll turn up today. Maybe she just left town for the night or something."

"But what does Ben think?"

"He seems to think that she's in trouble. He's pretty upset. He claims they hadn't had a fight, but with the stress of the mayoral race and the debate coming up, maybe she'd had enough and he didn't know it."

Morgan knew that was true. But it was more than that. The stress the Jacksons had been under with their fertility treatments was even more significant than the pressure of the race. But she didn't want to bring that up. "I'm sorry I can't help, Cade. All I know is that Lisa isn't the type to take off."

"I didn't think so either."

She walked him back to the door and looked into his eyes. He looked tired, as if he'd been up all night. His black hair looked a little disheveled, and his limp reminded her how recently his own life had been in jeopardy. "Are you okay, Cade? Taking care of yourself?"

"Yeah, I'm fine. Cane helps."

Morgan knew his transition from a crutch to a cane spoke well of his progress. He'd had surgery a month ago for multiple fractures in that leg. It had been set internally with steel rods, but his recovery was not yet behind him. She reached up to hug him. "If you see my sister, tell her to call me."

He smiled down at her. "Will do."

She watched him limp out to his squad car and get in, and she knew Blair would call her soon.

But what would she say when she called? *Hey, Blair. Whatcha been doing? Me? Oh, I found out I was pregnant, then miscarried the next day. Most people get nine months, then a bundle of joy. Not me. Nosirree, not me. My womb is like a tomb, rejecting life and creating death. My womb is a tomb . . . my womb is a tomb. I'm a poet and don't know it.*

Tears pushed to her throat again, and she told herself she would have to stop this. She wasn't this way. She didn't think bitter, cynical thoughts. But then, she obviously had a skewed picture of herself. She had pictured herself as a mother, raising a houseful of children — a big family, full of laughter and love . . .

But her body had kept secrets about its

29

malfunctions, as if it had other intentions entirely.

Was this anger normal? Had Lisa had these same thoughts of self-hatred, these raging thoughts that she had failed her child?

Morgan hoped Lisa was okay. Maybe she'd been plagued by the same kinds of self-recriminations, the need to escape herself and go somewhere alone to scream out and rail against the world and her body and all those busy, stressed-out moms who could never understand the broken and empty *longing* . . .

Maybe Lisa needed her, wherever she was.

Morgan blew her nose and dried her tears, then went to the phone. She dialed the Jackson's house. Ben answered on the first ring. "Hello?"

"Ben, this is Morgan Cleary. I just heard about Lisa."

"Who told you?"

"Cade came by to see if I'd seen or heard from her, since I'd left her some messages yesterday."

"And have you?"

"No. She never called back."

His voice cracked. "I haven't seen her since yesterday morning. She's just vanished. She's not answering her cell phone,

but that's nothing new since you can't get a signal on this godforsaken island. She missed several appointments yesterday. She even missed an important ultrasound she had scheduled. She would never do that. *Never*."

Morgan knew he was right. Lisa would never have missed an ultrasound, now that they'd decided to go through with another attempt at in vitro fertilization. Knowing when to harvest her egg was critical. "Ben, are you okay?"

"No, of course I'm not."

"Look, if you want to call off the debate this morning, I'm sure —"

"I don't care about the blasted debate! Let them declare Jonathan the winner, for all I care. *My wife is missing!*"

He slammed down the phone, and she felt shallow and silly for suggesting such a thing, as if he might have even considered showing up.

"Did I hear Cade?" Jonathan stood in the doorway, holding Caleb on his hip.

"Yes." She hung up the phone. "He said Lisa Jackson is missing. I just talked to Ben, and he's a basket case."

"Missing?"

"The police have been looking for her all night."

Jonathan stared at her for a moment, as if he didn't believe it. "You don't think this is a publicity stunt, do you? To get a few sympathy votes?"

She grunted. "Jonathan, I heard his voice. He's frantic. He doesn't even care about the debate right now. I think we should go over there."

He set Caleb down, and the child toddled over to his toy basket and took out a plastic train. "Morgan, of all people, he doesn't want me over there."

"Then I'll go by myself. He's there all alone, Jonathan. Someone needs to wait with him. And I'm worried about Lisa. She's my friend."

He sighed, as if he couldn't believe she was asking him to do this now. "All right, I guess we can go over for a little while."

She knew he was worried about the debate, which was scheduled for eleven. They still had three hours.

He got that sober, concerned look on his face and touched her chin. "Are you okay? Sure you're up to this?"

"I'm fine," she lied. "Really, I am."

He clearly had no choice but to take her word for it.

4

Ben Jackson's house was one of the more elegant ones on the island, situated near the northeastern point with a backyard view of the Atlantic. Beach property came at a premium on Cape Refuge, but it was well known that the Jacksons had money. That was why he was pulling ahead in the mayoral race.

He'd invested more money than either of the other two candidates. He'd had television commercials running on Savannah stations for the last month, as well as a billboard just off the bridge onto Tybee Island, and another one on the island expressway into Savannah. He had also taken out full-page ads in the *Savannah Morning News* and the *Cape Refuge Journal*. Even Blair had been forced to sell him the ad space that helped create his image as "The Man for the People."

The porch light was on, though the sun shone hot and bright. Ben had prob-

ably had it on all night.

She knocked. Jonathan stood behind her, his hands in his pockets. "I can't believe I'm here."

"Jonathan, take off your candidate's hat and put on your pastor's hat. We're here as Christians who care, not competitors."

Jonathan swallowed. "You're right."

Ben opened the door. His face was pale and his eyes were red, with dark circles shadowing them. He hadn't shaved, and his hair was tousled and dirty. "What are you doing here?"

"I wanted to come and sit with you," Morgan said. "You don't need to go through this alone."

He abandoned the door and headed back inside, and Morgan wondered if that was his invitation for them to come on in. She nudged Jonathan and they stepped inside, closing the door behind them.

They followed him into a great room decorated with rich silk draperies and faux-finished walls, with an adjoining kitchen that had a tin ceiling and shiny stainless steel appliances. Ben slumped over the amber granite counter. "What do you want?" He looked up at Jonathan. "Did you want to come over here and gloat that I'm finally getting mine?"

Morgan shot Jonathan a look that pleaded for him to answer gently.

"I would never do that. I came because Morgan said you were upset and you were alone. I thought maybe there was something we could do."

"You could go out and find her!" He ran a shaking hand through his hair. "You could tell me where she is. *That's* what you could do."

"Ben, are you sure she didn't just leave town for the night?" Morgan asked. "Maybe all the stress —"

"Absolutely no way. We were in the process of doing in vitro. It's a huge daily commitment. I have to give her shots the same time every day, pumping her body full of drugs and hormones. She would never go through all that for nothing. Never."

Jonathan sat down and rubbed his hands on his knees. "Those hormones, don't they cause mood swings, maybe even some irrational behavior? Maybe the pressure got to her —"

"She can take the stress," Ben cut in. "She always has. We've tried this three other times, and she was fine. This is a way of life for us. Has been for thirteen years. Yeah, the hormones make her moody. She

cries more often than she should. She's irritable and cranky, and sometimes she's
angry. Anyone would be when they've had
four miscarriages and nothing seems to
work. But she's not angry at *me*, and she
wouldn't have just taken off when we still
had some hope."

He went to the huge window with an
ocean view and peered out as if expecting
her to swim up with the waves and come
dripping across the beach.

"She was in a good mood yesterday
morning." His voice lowered. "She made
me breakfast, and I took the day off to go
fishing. I thought a day of relaxation would
help me to get my mind straight before the
debate. I got back midafternoon and showered and went to the doctor's office to
meet her there for the ultrasound we had
scheduled. She was supposed to ovulate
yesterday or today. It was critical that we
knew when she did. But she didn't show
up. And it wasn't until then I started to realize something must have happened to
her."

"Doesn't she have a business partner?"
Jonathan asked.

"Yeah, Rani Nixon."

Morgan thought of the beautiful African-
American woman who had once been a

successful New York model. When she'd gotten out of the business, she had moved here to open a real estate office with Lisa, her college roommate.

"I talked to her," he said. "At first she wasn't too concerned. Said that Lisa was probably out showing property, that she'd had several appointments and a couple of closings. But a little while later she called back and said that Lisa hadn't shown up for any of them. She'd heard from several clients who were upset."

"Is that when you called the police?"

"That's right. Chief Cade was here with some of the uniformed cops. Technically, he couldn't file a missing person's report for twenty-four hours, but I filled one out anyway. He probably took it back to the station and sat on it all night."

"No, that's not true," Jonathan said. "He told Morgan he'd been working on it."

Ben rubbed his neck. "He ought to be on leave. He practically just got out of the hospital. He can hardly walk, for Pete's sake, and he's trying to run a police force?"

Morgan saw Jonathan bristle. Revamping the police force had become one of the mayoral race's biggest issues. She hoped they wouldn't start debating now.

"He's as capable of running it now as he

ever was," Jonathan said.

Ben went to the window and looked out again. "That's exactly what I'm saying. He never was capable. Our illustrious former mayor was his uncle. Nepotism, pure and simple. The whole family is corrupt. He's not qualified to do that job, and it's time somebody else was appointed."

"When he finds Lisa, you'll change your opinion," Jonathan said. "Meanwhile, I'm calling off the debate."

Ben threw up his hands. "I don't care."

Jonathan looked at Morgan, and she knew he realized the urgency of the situation. This was no publicity hoax.

Ben Jackson was scared to death.

5

Blair Owens's morning walk always provided the last bits of peace in her day, before she started chasing down stories for the newspaper that came out three times a week. The newspaper business was new to her. For the past several years she had worked as a librarian, and only bought the paper a month ago. While she was widely known as a research whiz who could chase down facts like a greyhound after a rabbit, being a librarian had suited her specific paranoias. The burn scars that covered the right side of her face made her uncomfortable in public, but when she'd bought the paper, she'd been forced outside her walls. It took some getting used to, but she was finding that her new duties suited her personality even better.

She trudged through the sand and grass on the river side of the island to Cricket's, the little hole-in-the-wall diner on the dock where she had breakfast each morning. Often her walk had a payoff at the end,

when she found Cade sitting at the counter, sipping his coffee as if waiting for her to come in.

She hoped he would be there today. It had been a month since that first kiss between them, and ever since she'd walked around with butterflies in her stomach, wondering if it had meant as much to him as it had to her. Though he'd been spending a lot more time with her since then, she didn't want to assume anything. Word had gotten around that she and Cade were a couple, and people on the island were beginning to treat them as one. But in truth, she wasn't sure *what* they were. They had never expressed their feelings in words, but Cade's treatment of her had changed from intense friendship to flirtation. Not having that much experience with that type of relationship, she found herself feeling like a bumbling kid who had a crush on someone out of her league.

She got to the screen door of the small diner and pushed inside. Cade sat at the counter, wearing his khaki uniform. He swiveled on his stool at the sound of the door and smiled at her. She couldn't explain the thrill that went through her.

"Hey there," she said in a voice that she

hoped sounded friendly and cool. She fought the urge to lean over and kiss him, to touch his freshly shaven jaw or run her finger over his ear.

"I was hoping you'd come in before I had to leave."

"Where you going?"

"Work." He turned back to the counter as she sat down. "Colonel, get Blair a cup of coffee, will you?"

She studied Cade as the Colonel got her a cup. He looked as if he hadn't gotten much sleep last night. Had the pain kept him awake? She'd seen the struggle he encountered going from crutches to that cane, forcing himself to walk on the surgically repaired fractures, his bones held together only by the steel rods the surgeons had inserted. "You look tired."

"Yeah, I didn't get much sleep last night." He sipped his coffee. "Been working on a missing person case."

"Who's missing?"

"Lisa Jackson," the Colonel said over the bar.

Blair looked up and caught her breath. "Ben Jackson's wife? She's *missing*?"

Cade sipped his coffee and nodded. "Yeah. It's pretty much common knowledge now, since we've been questioning

people all over the island."

"Ben too," the proprietor said. "He was in here drilling everybody who came in last night. I'm thinking they probably had a fight and she ran off for the night. She'll turn up this morning, and they'll get it all worked out, I reckon. They have to. Neither one of them would want to jeopardize the mayoral debate."

Blair took her coffee and turned back to Cade. "How long's she been missing?"

"Not quite twenty-four hours, best we can tell. But I didn't see any point in waiting after Ben reported it. If she shows up today, so much the better."

She thought that over as she took a sip. "The stress of this debate probably got their tempers flaring. Ben can't be easy to live with right now."

"He's convinced something happened to her."

"Well, we both know that Ben's usually wrong. Does make for a more interesting story about the debate, though. I was picturing a big front-page article with a bunch of sound bites from their dogfight this morning, but now I can talk about missing wives and the stress this has put on the families. Heaven knows, it's been stressful for mine. Morgan has been so tense you

can hardly talk to her. You'd think Jonathan's been in politics for years."

"Don't exploit it, Blair. There's not a story there yet."

Blair tried not to look insulted. "Me? Hey, I just report the truth. You know I don't embellish."

"Every journalist embellishes, and your imagination is right up there with the best of them."

"You know I'm fair." At least, she hoped he knew. Before, when she had lived by her own set of rules, she might have exaggerated for the sake of subscriptions. But her life had changed. Just weeks ago, she had given her life to Christ, and everything had changed. Now, even in her work, she tried to live by the biblical principles of honesty and love. It wasn't always easy — sometimes she just didn't get it — but God was teaching her.

Cade slipped off the stool and got his cane. "I've got to go."

She tried to hide her disappointment. "You don't have time to eat?"

"I had a bowl of cereal at home." His voice dropped to a deep bass as he leaned in close to her ear. "I just came to see you."

She smiled up at him, knowing that her

feelings flashed like neon through the transparency of her eyes. He grinned as he limped out the door, letting the screen door bounce behind him.

When she turned back, she saw the Colonel grinning at her. "What?"

He started to chuckle. "You've got it as bad as he does."

Laughing softly, she brought the cup to her lips and hid behind it, hoping the Colonel hadn't read Cade wrong.

6

There was bad blood between Cade and Ben Jackson, but Cade knew he had to put it out of his mind during the course of this case. He couldn't dwell on rumors and stretched truths, on Ben's unfounded criticism of his department and Ben's promises to fire Cade if he was elected. If anything, Cade had over-compensated on Lisa's case to prove he wasn't holding anything against him. Most departments wouldn't even start a search until she'd been missing twenty-four hours, but Cade had a special interest in missing persons since he had so recently been one himself. It didn't matter that Lisa's husband was out to destroy him.

Cade knew Ben would have called him if he'd heard from Lisa, but he decided to go by his house after leaving Cricket's, just to update him on the search. He found Morgan and Jonathan there, and while it surprised him that Ben would have let Jonathan into his house, he was glad the man

wasn't alone. Morgan was known as one of the chief comforters on the island — one of the first to show up after any tragedy with a casserole and a hug.

Jonathan, who had grown more compassionate since becoming a pastor, would have a harder time comforting his political rival. But Cade knew his buddy was up to the task.

Ben looked even worse than he had last night. His eyes had a wild fear about them and his hands trembled, but he seemed grateful when he learned just how much the police department had already done to find Lisa.

He rubbed his stubbled jaw and looked up at Cade with misty eyes. "Listen, about all the stuff I've said about you during this campaign —"

"Don't worry about it, Ben. None of that matters. I'm just here to do my job."

Ben looked more humble than Cade had ever seen him. "I'm just saying that if I'd known I was going to need you like this, I sure would have been a little more careful what I said."

Morgan patted his shoulder. "Cade's not the type to hold grudges. You'll find her, won't you, Cade?"

"We're giving it everything we've got.

But I need to go over some more things with you, Ben."

Ben nodded, as if anxious to cooperate. "Of course. Anything."

Jonathan got up. "Look, we'll be leaving now so you guys can talk." He reached out to shake Ben's hand. "Let us know if you need anything, okay?"

Morgan gave Ben a hug. "Please, if she turns up, would you call us? We're going to get everybody to pray."

Ben rubbed his face. "I appreciate that."

"And we're not going to be debating without you," Jonathan said. "I'm calling it off."

"You don't have to do that. Sam will revolt."

"Of course I'm gonna do it. This is serious. He'll get over it."

Ben couldn't have looked less interested. He just fixed his eyes on Cade, clearly ready to begin. Cade got the feeling that the mayoral race was the farthest thing from Ben's mind.

7

Morgan was quiet as they drove home.

"You okay, babe?" Jonathan asked.

She leaned her head back on the head-rest. "Yeah."

"You were thinking about the baby, weren't you?"

She closed her eyes, hoping they'd look less haunted. "I was actually wondering if God still answers my prayers. Will he hear my prayers for Lisa, when he didn't hear my prayers for the baby?"

Silence fell between them. She was glad he didn't spout out some pat answer about how God heard but had a different plan. Even if it was true, she didn't want to hear it right now.

"Is it ever going to happen, Jonathan?"

"Of course it is." His voice sounded as weak and uncertain as hers.

She leaned her head against the window. "I'm not so sure. It took so long to get pregnant, and now this. There's got to be

something wrong." She looked back at him. "Jonathan, I think it's time for us to make an appointment at the fertility clinic."

He pulled into the driveway and cut off the engine but made no effort to get out of the car. "Don't you think it's too soon? It's only been a little over a year."

"If it's too soon, they'll tell us. Meanwhile, I just want some tests. I want to know if there's something wrong that can be fixed before much more time passes."

"You've got plenty of time left on your biological clock, Morgan. You're only twenty-nine."

"But I want a big family, and I don't understand why I can't get pregnant when teenagers do after one indiscretion. I need to know what's wrong with me."

He looked out the window for a long moment, staring at the wax myrtles along the driveway, their branches reaching up to the sky. Blair's car sat in the driveway. Was Sadie filling her in on the miscarriage? She hoped not.

"It could be me, honey." His words came out raspy, uncertain.

She shook her head. "You know that's not true. I was pregnant. I'm the one who lost the baby."

"But the bottom line is, something's going wrong with us. And if you feel like you need to go to the fertility clinic, I'm with you."

She had expected a fight. "Are you sure, Jonathan?"

"Of course I'm sure. Why wouldn't I be?"

"All the reasons you've said before. It seems like once we start on this cycle, it's hard to stop."

"It's worth a try, baby. Just one appointment. We can find out what our options are. Then we can decide if we want to go on." He squeezed her hand. "That okay?"

She wished the decision had made her feel better. It was simply a step, not the cure. "Yeah." She looked up at the porch. Her big ferns spilled over their hanging pots, cascading almost to the floor, in need of water. She suddenly felt too tired to tend to them. "Guess it's time to tell my sister what happened yesterday."

Jonathan looked as though he dreaded that as much as she did.

They went in and found Blair in the kitchen with Sadie and Caleb. The baby was in his high chair, shoving dry Cheerios into his mouth as he banged his spoon on the tray.

Blair was munching on a carrot and glanced at the Braves T-shirt Jonathan wore. "You're not wearing that to the debate, are you? Don't you realize this is the most important day of your political life, Jonathan?"

He headed for the phone. "There's not going to be a debate today, Blair."

She caught her breath and looked at her sister. "Because of Lisa Jackson?"

Morgan nodded. "How did you know?"

"I heard about it at Cricket's. Sadie said you'd gone over there. Is this for real?"

Morgan went to the coffee pot. It was still warm, so she poured a cup. "She's still missing. Ben's crazy with worry."

"You're sure it's not just some trumped up attempt to get attention?"

"Yes," Morgan said. "If you'd seen him, you wouldn't even ask. Besides, Lisa's not a publicity hound. She wouldn't have gone along with a scheme like that."

"She would if he tied her up and locked her in a room."

Morgan turned back to her sister and shot her a withering look. "That's not funny, Blair."

Blair looked as if she'd been unfairly judged. "Hey, I'm just saying people will do strange things for politics."

"This is not political," Morgan said.

Jonathan got off the phone and came out of the office. "Well, there's no way to completely call this off without going to the rally and making an announcement there. We're going to delay it a week, possibly two, depending on the availability of the Pier."

"Darn." Blair threw down her carrot. "I really hate that. I was all set for you to pull ahead in the race today." She looked at Sadie, who sat next to Caleb and was staring at Morgan as if she expected her to burst into tears. "Sadie, I guess you and I can chase down the Lisa story today. See if we can find out anything."

Sadie had worked briefly for the previous owner of the paper, so Blair had hired her to help out after school and on weekends. She had proved to be a valuable employee. But Sadie looked as if something was troubling her.

"I was thinking . . . since the rally's off, do you think I could go to Atlanta and see my mom? I haven't seen her in about a month. We've been so busy, and she doesn't get that many visitors. It always cheers her up when I come."

Blair shrugged. "I can do without you. The paper doesn't even come out until

Tuesday. I'm sure I can cover everything by myself today."

Morgan smiled at the girl. "You can take my car, honey. Give her a kiss from Caleb."

A grin broke out on Sadie's face, and Morgan realized how much the teen still missed her mother. Saturdays were the only days that Sadie could go visit. The fact that it was a six-hour round-trip made it prohibitive on any other day.

"Before you leave, Sadie, I need to talk to Blair upstairs. Can you watch Caleb for a few minutes?"

Sadie gave her a knowing look. "Sure. Come on, Caleb. Come with me while I get ready to go see Mommy." Caleb toddled off, holding Sadie's hand.

Blair got up and studied Morgan's face. "Everything okay?"

"Let's go talk." Morgan was quiet as she led her sister up the stairs. She could hear Karen — one of the home's residents — changing her baby's diaper in her room, talking to the seven-week-old infant in a soft, sweet voice. She had turned out to be a devoted mother to Emory — not something Morgan would have expected from a former crack addict.

Morgan led Blair into their parents' old room. Though they had died months ago,

Morgan had left their room just as it was. The scents in the pillows and the curtains had long ago faded, but the room still filled them both with comfort when the grief got a foothold.

Morgan sank onto the bed.

"Sis, are you all right?" Blair whispered.

Morgan pressed the corners of her eyes, trying hard not to cry. "I had a miscarriage yesterday."

It took a moment for the words to hit full force. "A miscarriage? You were pregnant?"

"I'd only found out the day before. We were going to announce it yesterday."

"Oh, honey." Blair sat down on the bed next to her and pulled her into her arms. "I am so sorry."

Morgan laid her head on Blair's shoulder. "I tried to call you several times yesterday, but I never got you."

"Why didn't you leave a message? I would have called back."

"I don't know. I guess I couldn't decide whether I really wanted to talk or not. Oh, Blair, I really wanted to be pregnant."

"I know you did." Blair grabbed a Kleenex box from the nightstand and handed one to Morgan, then wadded one up for herself. "I don't even know what to say."

"There's nothing *to* say. It just is."

"At least you know you *can* get pregnant now."

Morgan wished Blair hadn't said that. "What good is it to be able to fertilize an egg and have it implant into your uterus if you can't make it hold on? Lisa's had *four* miscarriages. She's been trying for thirteen years. What if I'm going to be like that?"

"You're not, okay? It's nothing like that."

Morgan blew her nose. "I don't know, Blair. I have a bad feeling."

"Well, don't." Her voice held a determined certainty. "You're perfectly fine."

"I miss Mama." Morgan's voice broke off, and Blair pulled her back into her arms and let go of her own emotions. "I miss her so much."

"Me too," Blair whispered. "She would know what to say. She wouldn't spout off like I do, without a thought."

"Words aren't the answer," Morgan told her. "But she would pray. Mama was the world's best prayer warrior."

"Now, that I can do," Blair whispered.

8

Morgan recognized the angry voice at the front door as she and Blair came downstairs.

"I heard you're planning to call off the debate. Who do you think you are, making that decision without even asking me?"

Morgan looked at Blair.

"Sam Sullivan," they said at the same time.

Sam was the third candidate in the mayoral race — the one who wrote the book on cut-throat campaigning. Morgan might have known he wouldn't take the cancellation well.

She reached the bottom of the stairs and joined Jonathan at the door.

"Lisa Jackson is missing," he was saying. "Under the circumstances, we could hardly have gone on with it."

"You and me could have done it." The tips of Sam's ears turned pink. "If somebody can't show up, that's his tough luck. But this was supposed to go off. We have

advertisements up all over town — *paid* advertisements, I might add. It ain't right to call it off without consulting everybody involved."

Jonathan shook his head. "We can put it off, Sam. It won't hurt a thing."

Sam looked like a good-ole-boy version of Rodney Dangerfield, with his flattop and his don't-get-no-respect attitude. "You think you're pretty smart, don't you, Jonathan? Throwing us off guard like this when we were all prepared. You know darn well that Ben Jackson'll do anything for publicity, and this is the biggest stunt he's pulled yet."

"I thought of that," Jonathan said, "but I really don't believe that's what's happening here. I was with him this morning."

"I knew it!" Sam threw his hands up. "So you two are in cahoots then. I might have known. And if you don't think I'm gonna let this be known to every reporter in the area —"

"Milk it for all it's worth," Jonathan said. "Knock yourself out. If you want to look like a man who doesn't have an ounce of compassion, go for it."

"I have a good mind to hold that rally anyway. To stand up there by myself and take advantage of the opportunity."

"Like I said, knock yourself out." Jonathan swung the storm door open to let Sam out. "Nice of you to drop by, Sam. Sorry you have to leave so soon."

Sam spotted Morgan and Blair standing in the doorway. "Blair Owens, you better write about this in that paper of yours! Tell 'em how he talked to me. You can't play favorites."

Blair crossed her arms. "I'm on it, Sam."

He marched out the door, grumbling something about derailing this election and suing for the advertisement money. Jonathan let the door bounce shut behind him.

Blair chuckled. "That man is like a caricature of himself. Every reporter's dream."

Jonathan ground his teeth together. "Coming into my house and chewing *me* out. He can have at it. I hope he does prance down to the Pier and show his true colors."

"Are you going to show up and make the announcement?"

"You bet I am," Jonathan said. "And if Sam tries to stand in my way, the crowd will see what he's made of."

9

The drive to the prison, which was located one hour east of Atlanta, seemed farther every time Sadie made the trip. She passed the time listening to music, but by the time she got there she dreaded having to drive home again.

She went through the degrading hoops necessary for security — emptying her pockets, removing her shoes, enduring a search that left her feeling humiliated — then took her place at one of the visiting booths as she waited for them to get her mother. She hadn't been able to hug her mother in a year, since her arrest and felony conviction on drug charges. A panel of smudged glass separated them, and they had to talk via the telephones that hung on either side of the glass.

The atmosphere was not conducive to a relaxing visit. Every conversation in the room could be overheard. The glass partition didn't go to the ceiling, only high

59

enough to prevent contact. Angry voices and expletives flew around her. She sat with rigid muscles, as if ready to defend herself from sudden assault.

In the booth next to her, a man cursed into the phone, and she could hear the inmate's angry reaction as she hit the glass with her fists, causing Sadie's own booth to jerk. The woman shrieked at her visitor, and for a moment Sadie thought the inmate might come over the partition and latch onto his neck.

Sadie fought the urge to run out. If she did, her mother would be crushed.

She watched through the glass as two guards came to quiet the inmate. The woman swung at one of them, and in an instant, they had wrestled her to the door, no doubt escorting her to lockdown where she would feed her rage.

"Leave her alone!" Her visitor was on his feet, shouting. "She didn't do nothin'. I got the right to visit my wife!" He kicked his chair, and it fell against Sadie. She sprang up and tried to move away.

Another guard pushed her aside and escorted the rabid husband out. Sadie watched until he was gone, afraid he would run back in and wreak more havoc. She felt small and fragile — and close to

tears — as she sat back down to wait for her mother.

Other conversations around her were thankfully less heated. A baby cried at one of the booths, and a two-year-old had been set free to run around barefoot on the dirty floor.

There was no air-conditioning, and the room was approaching eighty degrees. The heat did nothing to help the smell of backed-up sewage in the bathroom or the heavy scent of body odor on the stagnant air.

The door opened, and Sadie saw Sheila step in and look from window to window. When she saw Sadie, her face lit up. That look made all of this worth it.

Sheila grabbed the phone and sat down. "Hey, baby —" she touched the glass — "I thought you couldn't come today."

Sadie put her hand against the glass. Her side was sticky. "My plans changed at the last minute. How are you?"

Her mother looked good, in spite of the brown jumpsuit she'd worn every day of her incarceration. Her hair was pulled up in a pony tail, making her look younger than thirty-two. Sadie knew most people thought they were sisters, rather than mother and daughter. Sadie was the result

of a teen pregnancy, and her upbringing bore that out.

"How's Caleb?" her mother asked.

Sadie pulled the current pictures out of her pocket and pressed them against the glass. "I took this one earlier this week. Look how curly his hair's gotten. He's always real busy and talks a lot. You should hear him. He's a real scream."

Her mother's head tilted at the sight of the pictures, and she got tears in her eyes. "I wish you could bring him to see me."

"It would be too hard, Mom. The ride is too long. He'd never be able to stay in his car seat that long. And when we got here, you wouldn't even be able to hold him."

Sheila wiped a tear. "Maybe we could get special permission. Some of the girls here have been able to do that. One of my cell mates had a baby right here in jail two months ago. They took it from her the next day, but they let her hold her baby sometimes when her mother brings her. I could get the chaplain to work it out for me. They listen to him."

Sadie sighed. She couldn't imagine subjecting her little brother to this place. "We'll see, Mom. Maybe we can work it out sometime. But I'll leave you these pictures."

"Did you get my letter yet? About my lawyer?"

Sadie shook her head. "When did you send it?"

"Two days ago. You probably would have gotten it today." That smile came back to Sheila's face. "Baby, I'm not getting my hopes up or anything, and I don't want you to either, but I found out that the legislature just passed a law to help overcrowding in the prisons. For nonviolent crimes, they're letting people out after serving only twenty percent of their sentence. I'm not sure whether my conviction falls within the right timeline. I may qualify and I may not. My public defender is looking into it."

Sadie almost jumped out of her seat. "You mean you could get out?"

"It's possible. I have four more years. If I fall under the twenty percent rule, I could get out now. But don't get your hopes up, baby. It may not work out. Hardly anything ever does."

Sadie's heart was pounding. "Mom, that's great! What if it *does* work out? You could be free."

Sheila leaned in to the window and giggled. "Wouldn't that be a miracle?"

"God's given us miracles before, Mom."

Sheila's eyes grew misty again. "Yeah, he has."

"Oh, Mom, you would love Cape Refuge. It's so beautiful. Probably the most beautiful place on earth. At least, it's the most beautiful place I've ever seen."

Sheila paused for a moment. "Baby, I don't know if I want to come to Cape Refuge."

Sadie's heart deflated. "Why not? You don't want to go back to where we were before."

"Tell you what. We'll just cross that bridge when we come to it."

Sadie thought about that statement as she drove back to Cape Refuge. She couldn't consider the thought that her mother might choose to go back to Atlanta if she was released early. Somehow, she had to talk her into coming to Cape Refuge and starting a new life.

There simply was no other option.

She prayed that God would have mercy on her mother and give her this second chance that no one had expected. Then she imagined Sheila walking along the beach with her, barefoot in the sand, swinging little Caleb between them, and splashing his feet in the water. She pictured her being serene and happy, like

Morgan, taking care of her family and watching over them.

It was a picture far removed from the reality she had known before her mother went to jail, but she hadn't given up on the hope that she could change.

"Please let it happen, Lord," she prayed as she drove. "Change Mom's heart, and give her a new start."

10

Detective Joe McCormick, the only detective on Cade's force, had not been with Cade last night when Ben reported Lisa missing. Since she still hadn't been found, and the possibility that she'd met with foul play increased with each passing hour, Cade decided to bring McCormick in. Maybe something in Ben's story would send up a red flag in the detective's mind.

McCormick took notes as Ben went over his story again. When Ben finished, McCormick studied his notes. "Where were you fishing yesterday, Ben?"

"I took my boat and went out to the reefs."

"Catch anything?"

"Yeah. Six black sea bass. They're in the freezer."

"Then you took the time to clean them before you went to meet Lisa?"

"Yeah. It didn't take that long. Then I showered and headed to the doctor's office."

"How long were you out there?"

"Until about two. Appointment was three-thirty."

"Did you communicate with her at all from the time you left Cape Refuge until you came back?" McCormick asked.

Ben shook his head. "Not at all. She had all these appointments scheduled. It was a big day for her. She was closing on some houses and looking forward to that appointment. And I don't have to tell you that our cell phones don't work on the island. When she's in Savannah I can usually get her, but not here."

"Was she worried about anything — upset at all?"

He shrugged. "Just the usual."

"What usual?" McCormick asked.

"Well, you know, we were both stressed about the debate, and she was worried about whether this in vitro would work. She had this big-deal Hollywood producer coming, and she was supposed to help him scout locations for his newest movie."

"I've got his name," Cade said. "We're questioning him today."

"She never made it to that appointment. Rani said she had to fill in for Lisa."

McCormick rubbed his chin as he studied Ben's face. Cade knew what he was

looking for. The husband always had to be considered a suspect when a wife met with foul play, but so far, Cade hadn't found any guile in Ben's body language or glitches in his story. They still weren't sure there had been any foul play.

"Had a lot on her plate, huh?" McCormick asked.

"Yeah, but she always does."

Does. Present tense was a good sign.

"I expected her at home when I got here because we were going to ride to the fertility clinic together, only she didn't show up. So I called her at the office. Rani hadn't seen her. Nobody'd seen her, but I didn't worry. I figured she'd meet me at the doctor's office. There was no way she was going to miss it." He stopped talking and rubbed his mouth hard. "It wasn't until I got there that I realized something must have happened to her. That's when I started getting worried."

Cade heard a car door slamming outside, and Ben sprang up and lunged for the window, as if expecting to see Lisa getting out of her car. But it wasn't Lisa. A television van from Savannah had parked in front of the house, and a camera crew was setting up. Cade saw the coiffed correspondent trudging across the lawn to the door.

"It's the press," Ben said. The disappointment hung over him like a lead cloak. He dropped back into the chair. "I thought it was her."

Cade watched him cover his face and fight tears. He didn't know how to comfort the man, but he felt sure this wasn't an act. The worry and dread seemed genuine.

The bell rang. "Do you want to talk to them?" Cade asked softly.

Ben slid his hands down his face and looked toward the front door. "I guess it might help. Get the word out."

It wasn't the answer Cade expected, but he saw the wisdom behind it. Maybe it was a good idea.

Ben went to the door and told the reporter that he'd be out in a minute to give a statement, then he turned back to Cade and McCormick. "I need to figure out what I'm going to say."

"Find a picture of her to give them," Cade said. "Describe her car and when she was last seen. That kind of thing."

Ben grabbed a framed picture off of an end table. "This one should do." His hands trembled as he took it out of the gilded frame. He looked scattered, as if his mind raced with pleas for his wife. "Are we finished here?"

Cade looked at McCormick. He nodded. "Ben, last night we checked all the hotels on the island, to see if she might have checked in. She didn't. Today we're checking the hotels in nearby towns. Are there any other towns we should check? Any family members she might have gone to stay with?"

"No. I talked to her parents in Cordele last night, and they haven't heard from her. She's an only child. There's no place I can think of where she would have gone."

"We're putting a statewide APB out on her car, and I'm going to ask South Carolina and Florida to do the same. Maybe someone will spot it." Cade got up and reached for his cane. McCormick followed him to the door.

Ben stopped them at the door and grabbed Cade's arm, his desperate gaze locking into Cade's. "Find her, Cade. She has to be all right."

Cade knew better than to give him meaningless assurances. "We'll do everything we can, Ben."

Ben's face sagged with the heaviness of his fear. "Look, would you two mind going out and standing with me while I make my statement? They might want to ask you a few questions."

70

"I'm not going to give a statement," Cade said, "but our presence will let them know that we're looking."

The three of them stepped out into the front yard, and the television camera started rolling. Cade saw Blair's car pulling up, and she hurried up the yard, as if she didn't want to miss a thing.

He hoped the publicity would bring Lisa home and that later they would all feel like idiots for making so much out of nothing. Yet he had no intention of resting on that assumption. If he had anything to say about it, Lisa would be found today.

11

Her friend's disappearance haunted Morgan all morning, and she finally decided to drive to Lisa's real estate office to talk to her partner. Rani Nixon's Mercedes Roadster was the only car in the parking lot, and Morgan supposed that the staff must be off on Saturday.

The sun blazed on the black asphalt, its heat radiating upward. She was glad the debate wasn't going to be today. She still felt weak from the miscarriage and had dreaded standing out at the South Beach Pier, trying to look perky in ninety-five-degree heat.

The cool air from the air-conditioner blasted her as she went into the building. She stepped into the quiet waiting area and looked around. Morgan had never been in here before, so she wasn't sure where Rani's office was, but she could hear the woman's low voice from one of the offices at the back. She went to the doorway

and saw the woman talking on the phone. Rani saw her and lifted a hand in a wave, then held it there as if telling her she'd be right with her.

"Yeah, look, if she does come by, would you please have her call? We're all very worried about her." Rani sniffed and wiped her nose with a wadded ball of tissue.

Morgan looked away, feeling as if she'd stepped in on an intimate moment.

"We hope not too. Yeah, I know."

Morgan looked up at her again, a sense of awe falling over her at the strikingly attractive woman. Rani Nixon still looked like a cover model. With her Halle Berry features and short-cropped black hair, she looked as if she should have a mob of paparazzi following her around. When she'd given up her career five years ago and moved to Cape Refuge to work with Lisa, she had been an instant success. Everyone wanted to do business with the celebrity. Her reputation, her money, and her aggressive nature had all added up to skyrocketing success for their real estate business.

Rani got off the phone. "Morgan, isn't it?" She stood up, her five-feet-ten-inches making Morgan feel dwarfed.

"Yes." The woman had a Wall Street handshake, and Morgan was intimidated.

"It's good to see you. I just wanted to come by and talk to you about Lisa. I'm really worried about her."

"You and the rest of us. I haven't slept all night. I've been worried sick." She motioned for Morgan to sit down, and Rani took her chair again. "So how did you come to hear about it?"

"I left some messages for Lisa yesterday, so Cade came to question me this morning about whether I'd talked with her. I hadn't. She never called back."

Rani shook her head and leaned forward. "I have a bad feeling, Morgan. A real bad feeling."

That wasn't what Morgan wanted to hear. "Why?"

"Because she had a million things going on yesterday. Trust me, she wouldn't have just bagged them. I spent the whole day trying to do spin control and cover for her, and that never happens. And the kicker is she missed her doctor's appointment."

"At the fertility clinic." Morgan wanted Rani to know that Lisa hadn't kept that secret from her.

"Yeah, she's practically psycho about those things. Her body's pumped so full of hormones that if Ben's one minute late for one of those appointments, she just about

74

goes ballistic. No way did she just decide to skip town and not go."

"Well, that's the thing. Don't you think those hormones just may have pushed her over the edge?"

"Hey, she's moody, but she's not crazy. I meant she was psycho about the appointments, the fertility, the whole baby thing. It's an obsession with her, you know? I didn't mean that her hormones were really making her crazy. A little irritable maybe. A little moody. And come on, she missed half a million worth of commissions yesterday. No way that would happen."

"Was there any place she went where her car might have broken down or something?"

"There's no telling. Her car hasn't turned up, so we don't know." She dug into her drawer and came up with a cigarette and lighter. "You don't mind, do you?" she asked as she lit it. She took a drag and blew the smoke out in a stream, then tossed the lighter back into the drawer. "Lisa hates when I smoke in the office. I've been trying to quit, but it's impossible with this stuff going on."

Morgan tried not to cough.

"Anyway, if the cops know what they're doing — and frankly, I'm not so sure —

they're interviewing everyone she was supposed to meet with yesterday."

Morgan ignored the comment about Cade's police force. "They'll find her. I know Cade real well. He's very good at what he does."

"Let's hope you're right. But with one detective and a half-crippled chief, I'm skeptical. If Lisa's all right, she would have called by now. If she could get to a phone, that is. If this blasted place could just get a cell phone signal — I've never heard of anything so primitive. It almost kept me from moving here. And it hurts with selling real estate, I can tell you. People prefer to go somewhere else if they can't even make a call."

Morgan didn't bother to mention that they always had Ma Bell. "Did she have a cell phone with her?"

"Yes, and I've tried to call it a million times. She's not answering. If she were off the island somewhere, she'd at least check her voicemail." She brought the cigarette to her lips again. "I swear, I think he had something to do with it."

"What? Who?"

"That Ben." She blew the smoke toward the ceiling. "I wouldn't put it past him."

Morgan just gaped at her. "Are you sug-

gesting he would hurt Lisa?"

Rani gave Morgan a conspiratorial look. "I'm not accusing him of anything, okay? I'm just saying, there's been trouble in paradise for a long time."

Morgan didn't know whether to be relieved or concerned. If it really had been a fight, then maybe Lisa was off nursing her anger. Maybe she'd be back.

Rani tapped her cigarette on an ashtray shaped like a manicured hand. "Lisa comes in here a few weeks ago with tears in her eyes. She'd just collected the mail in her office, and you'll never guess what she found."

Morgan couldn't imagine. "What?"

"A letter from a woman who claimed to be Ben's lover."

Morgan's mouth fell open. "You're kidding."

"The woman told her that she'd been having an affair with Ben for months and that he'd been promising that he was going to leave Lisa."

"Who was it from?"

"That's just it." Rani leaned on her desk, her gaze locking into Morgan's. "There was no signature and no return address. The letter was postmarked Cape Refuge. No clue who sent it."

"Did Lisa confront Ben?"

"Of course she did." Rani stubbed out her cigarette. "That jerk just told her he had no idea where the letter had come from, that it was a bunch of lies. He told her that if she didn't believe him, she could hire a detective to follow him around. She bought it."

"Did she hire the detective?"

"No. She convinced herself he was telling the truth. She figured he wouldn't be working so hard at trying to have a baby with her if he planned to leave her. And besides that, he seemed to be available at a moment's notice. Not like he was hiding anything." She waved her hand in the air. "They were doing this temperature thing, checking her body for ovulation, all this stuff, and whenever she'd call him, he'd drop whatever he was doing and meet her — at home, at the doctor's office, wherever she needed him. He also convinced her he'd never do such a stupid thing when he was trying to run for mayor. It would ruin his chances in a town like this."

"Well, that does sound reasonable," Morgan said. "Ben is always worried about image. You'd think he wouldn't be so stupid as to have an affair when so much was at stake."

"You would think." She set her chin on her hand and let out a long sigh. "But I wasn't believing it. I've seen this kind of thing before. People *are* stupid when they're cheating. And then she got more letters."

Morgan frowned. "How many?"

"Three or four more. And every time, he denied it, but I think Lisa was starting to get wise. The last one really concerned her, though, and I could see on her face that her faith in him was starting to falter. I tried to convince her to call his bluff and hire a detective just like he'd suggested, but I don't think she ever did."

Morgan felt sick. Maybe the pain she'd seen on Lisa's face so many times hadn't just been mourning over her infertility. Maybe there was something much deeper.

"Rani, have you told the police about this?"

Rani lit another cigarette. "I've been going around and around about it. I didn't know if I should, because it opens a whole new can of worms. And if Lisa hasn't just run off, they might assume she has and stop looking."

"Cade wouldn't do that. You have to tell them. This is relevant information."

"If Ben has any decency, he'll tell them himself."

"Not if he's hiding something." Morgan thought back over Ben's countenance this morning. Did he look like a guilty man, someone who'd been having an affair, cheating on his wife, lying to her all along? No. The truth was, he had been beside himself, panicked over the disappearance of his wife. It couldn't have been an act.

Or could it?

"The thing is, even if he was having an affair," Rani said, "I don't think he would have killed her."

Morgan shivered. "*Killed* her?"

"Well, yeah. I mean, to get her out of the way so he could be with his lover or whatever."

Morgan had considered that Lisa could be dead, but only as a fleeting thought. Now, the idea that Ben might have done it disturbed her more than she could explain. "Rani, you have to tell the police."

Rani stared at her for a long moment, turning the idea over in her mind. "I guess you're right. I wonder if she kept those letters in her desk. They came here, after all. Maybe I can find them." She slid her chair back and walked out, her perfume trailing in the air behind her, mingling with the smoke.

Morgan followed her into Lisa's office.

The walls looked like polished marble, and the carpet was a deep wine color. Tiffany lamps accented the antique desk and the sitting area. Morgan could just imagine Lisa making deals in an office like this.

Rani pulled out the drawers and searched through them until she came to the bottom drawer and found a box of letters.

"Bingo. Pay dirt." She pulled the letters out, then tossed them onto the desk. "Take a look if you don't believe me."

"Uh . . . no. I don't feel comfortable doing that. Let's just take them to Cade. Let him read them."

Rani shrugged. "Okay, maybe they do have some relevance. Let me get my purse."

When Rani had locked the office, Morgan looked at her. "Do you want me to follow you there and talk to Cade with you?" She felt foolish for asking. Rani was tough, assertive. She didn't need anyone to hold her hand.

But the woman surprised her. "Yeah, it might not hurt to have a little moral support, if you don't mind."

Morgan followed the Roadster to the police station, thinking about those letters and praying that they didn't mean some-

thing terrible had really happened to Lisa. Was Ben Jackson grieving over his wife's disappearance — or his own guilt? Was he covering for a lover who might have taken matters into her own hands?

The questions filled her with nauseating urgency. She only hoped Cade could answer them.

12

The stage on the beach next to the South Beach Pier had been built for the rally, decorated with the American and Georgia state flags. It was wired to blast the debate for hundreds of yards. The crowd had already assembled when Jonathan pulled up in his car and found a parking place in the spot reserved for the candidates. Sam Sullivan was already there, working the crowd, wearing a light blue seersucker suit and a Panama hat that made him look like Rodney Dangerfield impersonating Harry Truman.

Art Russell — one of the City Council members — met Jonathan in the sand before he reached the crowd.

"Jonathan, are you really calling this off? We have vendors here selling food and drinks. A lot of people went to a lot of trouble. The square dancers are all here in full costume, ready to perform."

"We have to call it off, Art. It's not right

to hold a political rally without all the candidates."

"But Ben had the choice to show up."

Jonathan kept walking. "No, he didn't. His wife is missing. I'm not going to take advantage of it, and neither is Sam."

Art looked back at the crowd. "You know he's planning to take the stage himself."

"Not if I can stop him."

Jonathan didn't bother to shake any hands as he walked through the crowd and right up onto the platform. Sarah Williford, the council member who was going to introduce them, was already sitting in her spot as if afraid that someone else might get it. The woman, looking as though she'd stepped out of a sixties commune, had dressed for the occasion in a flowing dress, which looked like it was made of cheesecloth, and a pair of flat sandals.

Jonathan didn't bother to speak to her. He went straight to the microphone and tapped it. "Excuse me, could I have your attention, please? Everybody, could I have your attention?"

Sam Sullivan cried out, then made a beeline through the crowd. In his hurry, he almost stumbled up the stairs.

Jonathan ignored him and kept talking. "Ladies and gentlemen, I'm afraid we're going to have to call off the debate. Ben Jackson won't be able to make it. It seems that his wife, Lisa, has been missing since yesterday." A wave of surprise whispered over the crowd. "We'll reschedule the debate for two weeks from today, since it wouldn't be right to do it without him at a time like this."

By now, Sam was on the stage. He glared at Jonathan like he had hijacked the spotlight and grabbed the microphone out of his hand.

"We need your help and the help of anybody else on this island who's so inclined," Sam said. "Lisa — bless her heart — was last seen yesterday morning. If any of you have any information about any sightings of her yesterday at any time of the day, we would ask you to call the Cape Refuge police and report it. It's not a time for politics. It's a time for working together, to help a brother in need."

Cade stood back gaping at the man. Did anyone really buy this sudden concern? He hoped the people saw through Sam's self-sacrificing act.

Jonathan took the mike back. "I spoke to Cade before coming here, and he said

we're going to need a lot of volunteers to search the island. Since all of you are already assembled here, I'm going to open up a table over to the side here where people can sign up to help."

"When did she go missing?" Ronald Myers shouted from the crowd.

"Sometime yesterday," Jonathan said. "No one's sure yet."

"I saw her Wednesday," Fran Lincoln said. "She was in line at the bank, and we struck up a conversation. She was in a real big hurry to get away."

"Everybody's in a hurry when they talk to you," someone returned. Jonathan saw her ex-husband snickering at the back of the crowd.

"I'll bet Ben campaigned her right outta her mind," Bo Patterson suggested. "She's prob'ly curled up in fetal position on some shrink's couch."

Half the crowd laughed, and the rest expressed indignation.

"I hope it's something simple like that," Jonathan said. "But she needs earnest prayer right now. In fact, I'd like to lead us in that."

Most of the people bowed their heads, and a hush fell over the group. Jonathan made a petition for Lisa's safety and Ben's

comfort. When he'd said *amen,* he looked over at Sam. His opponent — an avowed atheist — looked as if he might grab Jonathan by the throat and wrestle him to the ground.

"So, Sam, do you have something you'd like to add?"

Jonathan could have sworn smoke was coming out of the man's ears. He wondered if he'd invoke the "separation of church and state," but Sam was too shrewd for that. Too many of his constituents believed in God.

"Just that I'll be helping at that table too. Maybe we can divide up and take groups out to search various areas."

Jonathan smiled and looked down at his feet. Sam wasn't going to give him the opportunity to show his leadership skills all alone. He figured it could only help.

He stepped off the stage and went to the table that had been set up to give out campaign flyers. He wasn't sure where Cade would want them to start looking, but from the number of people assembling to get in line at the table, he knew that they would have a good start on searching for Lisa today.

"Jonathan, a word with you, please."

Jonathan looked at the man who had

stepped to the front of the line. He looked familiar, but Jonathan wasn't sure where he'd seen him before.

"Vince Barr, of the *Observer*." The man reached across the table to shake his hand.

"Of course." Jonathan remembered the sleazy reporter for the tabloid based in Savannah. He'd been amused at some of his recent headlines. One claimed that George Bush had been kidnapped and replaced by an alien — complete with pictures of the offending space ship in the sky. Usually mayoral debates in small towns weren't up his alley.

"It's about Lisa Jackson's disappearance. I heard about it on the police scanner, and I've been trying to get information for our Tuesday issue. Have you spoken to Mr. Jackson?"

Jonathan wasn't about to tell this man a thing. "I thought you guys just made stuff up. You don't really do interviews, do you?"

He grinned. "Of course we do interviews. This is serious news."

"Yeah, but it's not national."

"They didn't think Laci Peterson's disappearance was national either, but you never know. It's always good to have a leg up on things just in case something comes

of it. So did you talk to him?"

"Yes, I talked to him. He's very upset."

"Do you think he'd grant an interview?"

"I really couldn't say." Jonathan turned to the line of volunteers forming and passed a legal pad across the table. "If you'd all just sign in, I'll try to get word to Cade that we're ready to start looking where he tells us."

"How well do you know Lisa and Ben Jackson?" the reporter cut in.

Jonathan shot him another look. "Well enough."

"Were they happy? Had there been any trouble in their marriage?"

"I don't know any of that. They seemed happy."

"What kind of man is Ben Jackson?"

Jonathan didn't like where Vince was going with this. "If you don't mind, I'm busy. But you can sign up as a volunteer, if you want. The search itself will be a story. Maybe there's even an alien or two involved."

Vince chuckled again and started to back away. "Thanks anyway. I'm sure I'll find someone who'll give me information."

13

Ben Jackson owned a fleet of shrimp trawlers and a shrimping warehouse on the Savannah dock, one of many operations in the industrialized area that serviced the marine commerce. Since adult white shrimp spawned near the shores in May, it was a busy time for his captains and crews.

Cade knew Ben oversaw the warehouse operations and the shipping of the shrimp to other states, but he wasn't here today. Cade had driven here in hopes of talking to his employees, to feel them out about the possibility that Ben had a mistress.

Rani's revelation about the letters had changed his thinking about the case. Sympathy for Ben had kept him from exploring the man's possible guilt in his wife's disappearance, but the letters forced his hand. If they had, indeed, been written by his mistress, then Ben could be hiding much more than infidelity. The letters provided motive for two different people to want Lisa out of

the way. If there truly was another woman, Cade was determined to find out who. The more he knew, the better equipped he'd be when he confronted Ben about the letters.

One of the rigs had just returned with its catch from a run up the South Carolina coast, so no one noticed right away when Cade came into the warehouse. The crews busied themselves with deheading, sorting, and packing the catch in ice. Though the place was clean and cool, the smell of shrimp filled his nostrils and attached itself to his hair and clothes. He looked around at the dockworkers on Ben's payroll. They were mostly tough, rugged men with foul mouths — which pretty much ruled out the possibility that Ben had a mistress here.

Cade identified the supervisor in charge of the shift and headed toward him. The man looked as if he hadn't showered in days. He wore an old charcoal gray T-shirt with big sweat rings under the armpits. Someone nudged him as Cade approached, and he met Cade halfway across the floor.

"Thought I might see the po-lice here today. I'm J. B. Hutchins, Ben's operations manager."

Cade introduced himself. "Why did you expect the police?"

"What with Lisa missin' and all. TV stations were here, snoopin' around about Ben. Only fittin' that the po-lice would show up, askin' questions." He could see that the man was excited by the day's events.

"What kind of questions did the press ask you today?"

"You know, stuff about their marriage and whatnot. Whether Lisa was depressed."

"And what did you tell them?"

"I told them they were a solid couple. Happily married, far as I could see. I didn't see Lisa all that much."

"J.B., was there anybody else in their lives, somebody who might have threatened Lisa or . . . might have come between them at any point?"

"Come between them?" J.B.'s voice echoed over the warehouse. "You mean like an affair or somethin'? Heck, no. Lisa would never do that."

His immediate assumption that Cade was talking about Lisa surprised him. "What about Ben?"

J.B. let a laugh echo over the room. "No way. Ben ain't the type to do that. He has a

one-track mind. Like with this mayor's race, it's all he thinks about. He's like that with his marriage. He'd never go with no other woman."

"Was there anybody who might have been angry at Ben or Lisa? Angry customers? Disgruntled crewmen?"

"Not that I know of."

"No threats? Nothing out of the ordinary?"

"Naw, none." He stuck his hands into his back pockets. "What do you think? She got kidnapped or somethin'?"

Cade evaded. "We're still investigating. Looking at every possibility." He saw J.B. look toward the door, and Cade glanced behind him.

Blair stood at the doorway. He wondered how much she'd heard.

"Grand Central Station," J.B. muttered. "People comin' and goin' all day today, askin' all sorts of questions. I'll be glad when she gets found."

"Listen, if you think of anything, give me a call at the station, will you?"

"Sure, I will." J.B. reached out to shake his hand and then headed back to the crew.

Cade limped over to Blair and grinned down at her. "What are you doing here?"

She grinned back. "Same thing you are. Snooping around. Digging up dirt."

Cade grunted. "That's what you think I'm doing?"

She didn't answer that. "So what's this about Ben having an affair?"

Cade's grin crashed. "Where did you hear that?" He had explicitly instructed Morgan and Rani to keep that to themselves.

"You were asking like you thought maybe it was a possibility. You must know something."

He wasn't sure he believed that was how she knew, but he tried to rally. "You misunderstood, Blair. I only came here to see if anyone knew anything about Lisa."

She turned her face up to him, that maddening determination sparkling in her eyes. "Come on, Cade. Ben's your first suspect. That's a no-brainer."

"We don't have any suspects yet, Blair. We don't know that a crime has been committed."

"Yeah, and that's what they said when *you* were missing."

She had a point. He dropped his voice to a near whisper. "That's precisely why I'm not taking this lightly."

Her eyes squinted, and he felt she could

see right into him and read his every thought. "So who is she?"

"Who is who?"

"The other woman. You obviously think Ben was having an affair."

He sighed. "Blair, your creative auditory skills amaze me. And that intuition of yours is sometimes wrong."

"Sometimes. But not often."

It was true. He knew it, but he wasn't about to encourage her. "I've got work to do." He started limping toward the crew.

"Have you found Lisa's car yet?"

"No, it hasn't turned up. Hopefully that's because she's driving it." Sighing, he turned back around.

"Are people out looking for it?"

"Of course they are. In fact, Jonathan's organizing a search party. We're going to comb the island this afternoon. I have men from the Sheriff's Department, the Highway Department, the State Police, and the Savannah and Tybee police departments on their way to help out."

She pulled out her notebook. "One more question."

He turned around and she stepped closer. She was a whole head shorter than he. He happened to know that her shoulder fit right under his. If he pulled her against

him, she would hear his heart beating.

But her personality seemed to put her at eye level. "What question, Blair?"

Her eyes lost that eye-of-the-tiger glint, and her face softened. "You're not over-doing it, are you? With the leg, I mean."

He was glad she *couldn't* hear his heart. "I'm chief of police. I'm doing what I have to do, injury notwithstanding."

"You didn't answer my question."

He looked toward the activity of Ben's workers. A gentle smile pulled at his lips. "I'm fine, Blair. Thanks. How about your skedaddling on out of here so I can inter-view some people? A woman's life could be at stake, and every delay could cost her."

"Are you running me off?"

"Yes, I am."

"All right, but I'm coming back when you leave. By the way, thanks for the lead."

He might have known. "I didn't give you a lead, Blair."

"If I find out her name, do you want me to tell you?"

He groaned. "What if she's just a fig-ment of your imagination?"

"I'll find that out too."

He tried to get serious. "Blair, a man's reputation is at stake, and he has enough problems right now."

"Not to worry. I'm not out to ruin anybody. But I'm still going to dig. I think I'll go talk to some of Lisa's friends, see what they know."

He knew Rani would be among them. Blair would know about the letters within the hour. "Guess I can't stop you."

"Got that right."

Sighing, he started back toward the crew.

"Take care of your leg, okay? Don't go tromping through the woods looking for her. There are plenty others who can do that."

"I'll call you later." He wouldn't let himself look back at her as he walked away. She clearly enjoyed driving him crazy.

And as aggravated as he was at her, he had to admit he enjoyed it a little, too.

14

Rani Nixon let the top down on her Roadster as she flew through town. Her bones felt weary from not having slept the night before. She'd spent too much time dialing and redialing Lisa's cell phone, yelling messages for her to call and put them all out of their misery. She'd gone to every property that Lisa might have shown the day she disappeared, searching every room and praying that she wouldn't come upon Lisa's body. But so far she had no clues as to where her best friend was. So this morning, when the telephone call came from the psychic, she agreed to meet him without hesitation.

His name was Carson Graham, and though she didn't know him, she had done a quick search on her computer and found a webpage that described the services he performed. He did palm readings, astrological charts, and tarot cards, and his bio claimed he had helped the police solve sev-

eral cases through doing psychic readings on victims.

"I just wanted to offer my services," he'd told her. "Perhaps you could bring me something of Mrs. Jackson's — something she wore that I could use to do a reading."

Rani had frowned and clutched the phone. "Why did you call me and not the police or her husband?"

"I tried calling her husband," he said. "I kept getting his voicemail, and I don't know how to get in touch with him. As for the police, I used to help the department all the time until Chief Cade was hired. Let's just say he hasn't needed my services, and I didn't think he would be open to my helping with the case, but I know I can at least generate some clues."

Rani liked the sound of that. One good clue and they could find Lisa. She was sure of it. "What do you need? I'll bring it to you."

"Just something of hers, something personal. Something she wore or used a lot. Whatever you have in your possession."

"I have a sweater," she said. "She left it in my car the day before when we were previewing properties."

"That would be perfect."

"Where can I meet you?"

"How about if you meet me at Winston's Restaurant? You can buy me lunch, and I won't charge you for my services."

She hadn't thought about a charge, but she figured it was worth it. She'd pay anything to know where Lisa was. "All right. I'll be there in twenty minutes."

"Just ask the hostess for me," he said. "She'll lead you to the table."

Rani got to the restaurant a little while later, holding Lisa's sweater folded over her arm.

The hostess led her to Carson Graham. He looked like he belonged on an infomercial for Ronco products. His goatee needed trimming and his hair needed to grow. She suspected he shaved his head as an offensive against his baldness.

She greeted him and handed him the sweater.

"I took the liberty of ordering you coffee," he said. "I didn't know how you take it."

"Black's good."

"What about lunch? Would you like to order before we get started?"

She really didn't want to be bothered with food right now. "You go ahead. I'm not hungry."

"From the looks of you, you could stand a good meal." His laughter was inappropriate and a bit too loud.

At five ten, Rani had always been bone thin. When she'd worked in New York, she had learned to eat high-protein and low-carb to stay lean. She'd kept the diet ever since. She preferred lean meats and salads over the breads and pastas that everyone else considered staples. "I'll pass, thanks."

"Gonna make me eat alone?"

She saw that her lack of appetite was distracting him. She was going to have to order. "Okay, I'll eat something."

He called the waitress over and placed an order big enough to feed a baseball team. When it was her turn, she ordered a salad.

The waitress hurried off, and Rani turned back to the man. "Tell me, can you see anything yet just from holding the sweater?"

He smiled and brought it to his face, taking in a deep breath. "Actually, I think I need to be alone so I can concentrate."

She wished he'd take a to-go box so he could get on with it. "When will you know something?"

"I think later today. I realize that time is of the essence."

"You don't have any impressions yet? Nothing?"

"I told you, I have to be alone."

She sank back into her chair. What if she was barking up the wrong tree? But what could it hurt, giving a psychic a chance to find Lisa? It was as good as any other leads they had.

"Tell me about your friend." He took a long sloppy drink, dribbling some on his chin. "Any information you give me might help me to get a better handle on her."

She dug into her purse. "I brought a picture of her. You've probably already seen it on the news."

"Yes. She's very pretty."

"You got that right." Rani handed him the photo. "She's my best friend. I've known her since college. We were roommates the whole four years. Then we each kind of went our separate ways, had our own careers for a while. She got into real estate, and I was in modeling. When I decided to leave New York, she asked me if I'd like to come here and go into business with her. I did, and we've been together ever since."

"Tell me, what kind of person was Lisa?"

Rani didn't appreciate the use of the past tense. She hoped he hadn't come up with that from some kind of psychic vibration.

"Lisa *is* a wonderful person. She's devoted to her husband. She's ambitious, efficient, diligent, vibrant, effusive . . . all the things that spell success. That's what Lisa *is*."

He leaned in, his eyes squinting. "Did she have any dark secrets she was hiding?"

That aggravated her. "Look, I don't have to tell you this stuff. Either you know it or you don't. You said you could find her based on something she owned. I'm hoping you can do that. If you can't, I want that sweater back."

"Of course. I didn't mean to step on any toes. I was just trying to get a feel for her."

"Yeah, well, it's not my job to fill in the blanks for you. Either you're for real or you're not."

"I assure you, I'm for real. You'll see."

The waitress delivered their food, and Rani watched him dive in. He wasn't even insulted by her doubt in him. Maybe that was a good sign.

With a mouthful of baked potato, he said, "Perhaps I should tell you a little bit about my background."

"Yes, that would be helpful."

He swallowed and took a long swig of iced tea. "I've known since I was a boy that I had some powers. ESP, some people call it. I seemed to always be able to find lost

things, and I knew things about people that no one had told me. When I got into college, I joined a parapsychology club and started to meet other people like myself. We sort of encouraged each other and helped each other develop our gifts."

Rani's anger started to fade. This was the kind of thing she wanted to hear. It sounded authentic.

"You claimed that you had helped the police solve crimes before. Which crimes?"

"Oh, there've been quite a few." He buttered his roll. "I gave the Atlanta police clues one time that helped them find a sniper who was terrorizing the citizens, and two or three times I've given Savannah police information that has led to convictions of bank robbers, kidnappers, drug dealers. Before Chief Cade was here, I used to help Chief Baxter from time to time. He wasn't one to give me a lot of credit, but I think I was helpful in a number of cases."

Rani smiled. *Perfect.*

"When Elizabeth Smart was missing, I had a vision that she was with a man and a woman. Saw her wearing a burka-type thing on her head, and I knew she was alive."

"Did you tell the police?"

"Yes, I called them, but that wasn't much to go on. Turns out I was right, though."

Rani was impressed. "Is that documented?"

"What? Who Elizabeth Smart was with? Of course it is."

"No, I mean your phone call to the police."

He breathed a laugh. "I doubt it. Like I said, it wasn't a lot to go on. I didn't have a location or a name. Since it wasn't a real physical siting, they didn't put much stock in it."

He went on about other cases he'd solved, and by the time he'd finished eating, she was a believer. She was glad she'd come.

As he took Lisa's sweater and went toward his van, which had "Palm Readings" in big letters on the side, Rani shook his hand. "You'll call me the moment you have something?"

"Of course I will."

"And don't worry about the police. If you have a lead, I'll make sure they follow it."

"Good deal."

She hurried back home to wait for his call.

15

The phone call Rani had been waiting for came an hour later. She saw Carson's name on her caller ID, and she snatched up the receiver. "Hello?"

"It's Carson," he said.

She'd gone back home and paced her living room a thousand times since lunch. "Have you got anything?"

"Yes, I'm afraid I do. But I'd rather not discuss it over the phone. Do you think we could talk in person?"

Rani hesitated. What could be so bad? She cleared her throat and swallowed hard. "Okay. Do you want me to come to your place?"

"Yes. Do you know where it is?"

"The palm reader's shop on Ocean Boulevard?"

"That's right."

"I'll be right over."

She drove too fast, her heart pounding. If the news was good, wouldn't he have

told her over the phone? Did guys like Carson ever deliver good news? Then she thought of Elizabeth Smart. He'd had good news then, if anyone had listened.

She pulled into the parking lot in front of his small eggplant-colored house. There was a painted sign out front that had been faded by the sun. It read, "Palm Reading and Tarot Cards — $20." She went up the steps and knocked on the door. He answered quickly.

His face was sober as he invited her in.

The front room looked as if it had been decorated by an elderly spinster. The walls were paneled in dark laminate, and the furnishings were old enough to need replacing, but not old enough to qualify as antiques.

She stepped into the front room. It smelled of strawberry candles and incense, and the lights were too dim. She turned to face him. "Tell me."

"Sit down." He pointed her to a plush easy chair. Her heart raced as she sat down, terror taking her breath away. He took the seat across from her. They were almost knee to knee.

She couldn't wait any longer. "So what did you find out?"

He picked up the sweater he had lying

107

on an end table and moved it around in his hands. "Rani, I'm really sorry. I hate to be the bearer of bad news."

Rani wilted back. She knew it. "Just spit it out. Come on."

"I'm afraid your friend is dead."

Rani had expected it — had even rehearsed it — but now she found that it hit her in the gut.

"That's what you saw? That she's dead?"

"I saw more than that. I'm sensing that there was foul play of some kind, though I can't say exactly what the nature of it was. When I hold the sweater, I just feel a lot of tension and fear."

Rani sat up straighter, blinking back the tears in her eyes. He could be wrong . . . He could be blowing smoke, conning her. He probably didn't know what he was talking about.

"I believe I know where she is. In a vision, I saw her car going into the water about half a mile east of Bull Bridge."

Fear rammed its fist into her chest again. This was more specific than she'd expected.

"I believe if you find that car, you're going to find her. Tell the police to search there first."

She got up, trying to think. Lisa wasn't

dead. The man was a fraud. Just an evil, conniving, con artist trying to get his name in the paper. She tried to believe it was a hoax, but her heart wasn't buying. She looked down at a statue of a Buddha on a table, trying to think.

"I tried to get more," he said. "But it just didn't come to me. It's hard to know how these visions work. Sometimes I get parts of things, sometimes wholes. I guess the important thing, though, is that we notify the police."

Rani nodded and started digging through her purse for her keys. Then she realized she already had them in her hand. "I'll go straight there from here."

"If you need me to talk to them, I will, but as I've told you before, Chief Cade doesn't like me very much."

Rani wanted out of there. She started for the door. "I'll handle it."

"And would you do me a favor? Let me know if and when you find her?"

Nodding absently, Rani headed back out to her car and closed herself in. She sat there for a moment, staring at the steering wheel.

Lisa wasn't dead. He was flat wrong.

She pulled out into traffic, wishing for numbness. It couldn't be true, yet what if

it was? What if her friend was dead at the bottom of the river?

She couldn't make herself go to that place for fear she would find her. Instead, she drove to the police station as fast as she could.

16

Cade had gone to the site where Lisa was supposed to have shown property yesterday — a plot of land on the edge of some forest land, on the eastern side of the island. Rani got the location and decided to go there and tell Cade herself what Carson Graham had said. If she gave the information to someone else, it might be ignored.

She found the site easily. Cars lined the street out in front of the land, and a table was set up near the road, where police officers were registering volunteers and giving them instructions. She tromped in her high heels through the grass, right up to the table.

"You'll need to change your shoes, ma'am," a young cop said. "It's rough treading in those woods."

"I'm not here to search. I need to speak to Chief Cade."

"He's busy right now."

She leaned on the table and glared into his face. "Go find him and tell him it's

Rani Nixon, and that I have information about where Lisa is!"

The cop sprang up. "Okay, just stay here for a minute."

She paced back and forth in front of the table, waiting for Cade to come out of the house. In a moment, he emerged, looking fatigued and distracted. His limp was more pronounced than it had been earlier.

"What is it, Rani?" he asked. "Have you heard from her?"

"No. Cade, I need to talk to you privately."

He looked concerned and motioned for her to walk with him. Taking her away from the crowd, he said, "Okay, Rani. What is it?"

Rani shoved her fingers through her cropped hair. "Cade, I know this is going to sound crazy, but this man named Carson Graham contacted me. He's a psychic and he told me —"

"Hold it." Cade raised a hand to stop her story. "I'm not buying anything Carson Graham told you. That guy is a complete fraud."

She hesitated, gaping at him. "He *told* me you didn't like him, but that doesn't matter. I just need you to listen to what he said."

"Rani, that guy tries to get in on every investigation. Trust me, he just gets in the way. Every now and then he hits on something that's vaguely close to the truth, and then he takes full credit for it when the crime is solved. You can't believe a thing he says."

"Okay, maybe he's just a lying jerk. But what if he's right?"

Cade looked down at his cane. "Okay, Rani, what did he tell you?"

"He told me she's dead." She burst into tears. "That she's in her car at the bottom of the Bull River, half a mile east of the Bull Bridge."

Cade sighed. "Rani, I can't send divers to a place based on some psychic's vision."

"Just go over there. Wouldn't you see something if a car had gone into the water? I mean, wouldn't there be tire tracks or something?"

He seemed to consider that. "All right, Rani. I'll go over there myself and have a look. That's all I can promise you. I'm not wasting a lot of my department's resources on one of Carson Graham's wild-goose chases."

"Good enough. I just want you to see. I don't want it to be true."

17

Cade drove to the Bull Bridge, clocked out a half mile to the east. The land along the river was largely protected by the state's Department of Resources, which had laid down strict rules about the homes built along the river. They hadn't approved many of them before the DOR decided no more could be built — much to the delight of the few property owners, who knew their property values would shoot higher because of the rarity of riverfront homes.

The homes were widely spaced, with hundreds of yards between them. They were secluded and built among the trees, maintaining the integrity of the land along Bull River.

He left his car and walked through the trees until he reached a place where he used to come fishing as a boy. It reminded him of the place where Andy and Opie fished during the whistling theme song of *Andy Griffith*. He walked along the dirt

patches and grass, looking down toward the meandering river and scanning the ground for any signs of Lisa.

He didn't even know why he was wasting his time. Some people on the island bought Carson Graham's lies hook, line, and sinker. He had a nightclub psychic act that wasn't doing so well. When tourist season was hopping, business picked up, but rumor had it that the proprietor was thinking about bringing in a magician to replace Graham.

As long as his lies were just part of a nightclub act or a palm reading business, Cade had decided the man wasn't all that harmful, but this took the cake. Exploiting a woman's disappearance by preying on the people who loved her beat everything.

He kept walking, leaning on his cane, wishing he could go home and put ice on his leg. Each step made it ache more, and he felt it swelling against his pant leg. He had a two-bit psychic to blame for this. A psychic who had sent him on a wild-goose chase. He was probably hiding and watching, laughing it up that Cade had followed up on his tip.

He started to turn back, then stopped as something caught his eye. Tire tracks dug into the bank, going right into the river.

He stood there a moment, staring. Was it possible Carson Graham had gotten it right this time? Was it just a coincidence? Was there really a car at the bottom of that river?

He studied the tracks and saw footprints mashed in next to them. This wasn't a place to put a boat in — the launch ramp was only a mile down. The half shoe prints looked as if someone had pushed hard against a heavy weight.

He had no choice now. He was going to have to find out.

He went back to his car and radioed the Department of Resources to ask if they could send divers over with sonar equipment. They would be at Cape Refuge within the hour.

He then set about to cordon off the tire tracks and footprints until they could study them for evidence, in the event that a car . . . and Lisa . . . were found on the bottom of that river.

18

Blair knew they must have found something when she heard Cade's voice on the police radio, ordering all units to a place a half mile east of the Bull Bridge. She'd been on her way to photograph the search on the eastern side of the island, but now she turned her car around and headed to Bull River.

Squad cars from Cade's department and the Chatham County Sheriff's Department blocked off the road in front of a cluster of trees. She couldn't see what was going on behind them, but there was clearly a lot of activity. She saw Rani arguing with an officer at the edge of the crime scene tape, so she got out and crossed the grass.

"Rani, has there been news on Lisa?"

Rani turned around. She was frantic, almost hysterical. "You bet there has! But they won't let me in. I can't see anything."

"What happened?"

"I got a tip that Lisa's Lexus had gone

117

into the river right here. I gave the tip to Cade, but he didn't believe me until he came over here to check out the place. He must have found something!"

Blair scanned the landscape. Maybe she could find a place with a view of the water . . . It was forest land for as far as she could see right now, with no houses in sight. But Blair knew there was a house a couple hundred feet away on the other side of the trees. The house had a view of a portion of the river directly behind it. She knew it had a pier, and it might give her a view of what was going on upriver.

"Who gave you the tip, Rani?"

"Carson Graham, that's who."

Blair turned back to her. "The palm reader?"

"He's a *psychic*, Blair, and he did a reading on Lisa today."

"Come on. You're kidding me."

"Hey, I was a skeptic at first too. And I'm praying he's wrong. But look at all this!"

Blair dropped her notepad. This was going to be a wash. She didn't even know why Cade would entertain anything that guy said. She heard a helicopter overhead. Shading her eyes, she looked up and saw the chopper with the word *Observer* on the side. The tabloid hadn't missed a beat to

get the best seat in the house.

"I heard someone say they're using sonar equipment to look for the car," Rani said.

Blair couldn't believe they would go to all this trouble for a hoax. "Wow, they must really think she's there."

"She is! I just know it!"

Blair looked around. "I've got to get a vantage point, even if I have to go across the river."

"I'm coming with you," Rani said.

"There's a house down the way," Blair said. "Do you happen to know who owns it?"

"Oh, yeah. It belongs to Melanie and Andy Adams. I sold it to them."

Blair knew the couple. "Great. Let's go ask them if we can use their pier."

They went back out to the street, where a crowd of other reporters and onlookers had formed. No one was getting past the police line.

Blair led Rani toward the house, hoping no one else had already thought of this. She went to the door and knocked. Melanie, a nervous-looking blonde, answered quickly. "Hi."

"Melanie, I don't know if you remember me . . ."

"Of course I do. Nobody ever forgets you, Blair."

Blair thought that was a reference to her scars, but she tried not to dwell on it. "Melanie, would you mind if we go out on your pier to see if we can tell what the police are doing?"

"The police?" Melanie's face changed, and she looked out past them.

"Yes. They're looking for Lisa Jackson, and apparently they think she's in the water. We don't know for sure what they've found, if anything."

"Lisa Jackson? Here?" Her face drained of its color as she peered at the police. "Well . . . sure. Yes, you can use it. I'll come too." She came out with Blair and followed her and Rani around the house to the pier.

As they walked around Melanie's yard, Blair bit her lip. Maybe this wasn't going to help after all. Privacy hedges lined the sides of the property, and forest separated Melanie's yard from where the police worked. Their part of the river was on a narrow bend that restricted their view to the right or the left.

Blair saw a few people with television cameras across the river, trying to get pictures of the search. She hurried out onto the pier, looked to the left, and saw one of the search boats on the water. "Yes! We'll

see some of it, anyway."

Rani came and stood beside Blair. "They haven't found her. They wouldn't still be looking if they'd found her."

Melanie stood behind Blair, gazing off toward the activity. "I hate this. It's freaky. My husband is going to die when he hears about this."

The heat was intense, steaming off of the water. Blair slowly sat down on the boards. "This could take a while. We might as well get comfortable."

"I don't want to be comfortable," Rani said. "My best friend might be in that water."

19

"We got something!"

The yell came out over the water, and Cade went as close to the bank as he could without getting wet. The call came from one of the boats in the middle of the river, a little to his right.

"What is it?" he asked into his radio.

The response crackled. "Sonar's showing a big object, straight down. We're getting the divers down there. Might be a car."

He prayed that it wouldn't be. From here, he could see Blair sitting on the Adamses' pier, her hand shading her eyes as she watched the activity. Rani towered behind her, standing next to Melanie.

Then the call came. "It's a car, Chief. A Lexus XL330, and there's a woman's body in it."

Lisa. His heart slammed against his ribcage, and he stood there a moment, trying to process the reality.

Ben . . . how was he going to tell him?

Should he get him over here or tell him later? Would someone else get to him first?

He went to Alex Johnson, who was holding back the crowd. "Alex, do me a favor and go get Ben. Pick him up and bring him here."

The young cop looked as if he'd rather be beaten. "Really, Chief? You want him to see this? What do I tell him?"

"Just tell him we may have found her car. Nothing else."

Alex rushed away, and Cade called the medical examiner's office and told him to hurry.

He went back to the bank and waited.

The radio crackled. "Chief, what do you want the divers to do?"

"Just hold tight. We need to leave the body in the car so we won't disturb the evidence. The ME is on his way, and the Georgia DOR will have to pull it out."

It looked as if the search for Lisa was over.

But this wasn't the way he'd expected it to end.

20

By the time the DOR tugboat was in position to pull the car up, a huge crowd had gathered. The media, trying to get a better shot, had collected on the opposite side of the river with cameras, and a news helicopter circled overhead. Cade saw Jonathan and Morgan with baby Caleb, tearfully arriving on the scene. Alex brought Ben back with him, and he stood, pale, face full of dread, as he watched the DOR working to pull the car up.

Cade had roped off the area around the crime scene to keep the evidence from being disturbed. Finally, the cable began to creak and squeal as the tail of the vehicle came up out of the water. It was Lisa's burgundy Lexus.

And then he saw her as the front end was lifted out — Lisa Jackson, still strapped in by her seat belt, her hair floating in the murky water-filled car . . . exactly where Carson Graham had said she would be.

The boat moved the car to the bank, then lowered it hard onto the grassy area a hundred feet from where it went in, so as not to disturb the tracks and footprints. They opened the door, and the water gushed out.

The sight of Lisa in that car hit Cade in the gut. For a moment he stood there, staring at her through the wet windshield as if there were some possibility she would begin to cough. He told himself to move, to look for blood or a gunshot wound or evidence of suicide or foul play — to do *something* befitting of a police chief who'd just discovered a body — but he couldn't catch his breath.

The medical examiner moved into action, checking for any sign of life. "No pulse," he said.

"She's not dead!" Ben's words cracked out over the area. "Help her, you idiots!" Ben broke through the barricade of officers keeping him back and wrestled his way to the car. Cade tried to hold him back, but he fought to get to her door.

"She's not dead! *Do* something!"

"Ben, you can't touch anything! You'll compromise the evidence."

"Lisa!" He began to shake, and the anguish on his face cut through to Cade's

125

soul. "Dear God, who did this to her?" Ben started to sob, and Cade felt torn between offering comfort to the man and dragging him away. "Please . . . maybe there's a pulse."

Cade pulled him away. "Ben, she's dead."

The words seemed to drag the strength right out of the grieving husband, and Ben covered his face and wailed out his pain.

Cade turned away. He had work to do; he didn't have time to fall apart.

"You can't just leave her like that," Ben cried. "Get her out of there!"

"We will as soon as we can, Ben. Just stay back, okay?"

There was too much that had to be done before they could move her. The detectives had to take pictures of the car from every angle, with her exactly as she'd been found. Everything was critical, from the fact that she wore her seat belt, which didn't sound like something a suicidal person would do, to the angle of any gunshot wound or injury that might explain how she died. If she was killed and then pushed into the river, the killer might have left some clue behind. They couldn't risk losing that by moving her.

Ben was led back to the shade, where

Cade could hear the anguished sounds of his grief.

McCormick came to stand beside him. "You think his grief is for real, Cade?"

"Looks real to me. My gut tells me he's not responsible."

But his gut couldn't dictate his conclusions. The evidence would have to do that. He looked at the body, still in the car. There would be many questions answered there, and many new questions raised.

He hated investigating homicides, but someone was going to have to do it. There was a killer out there somewhere, and Cade wouldn't rest until he found him.

Blair couldn't see what was happening, but she heard yelling, and the one boat she could see drifted out of sight around the bend. She decided to try to get a little closer.

The three of them followed the river line at the back of Melanie's property. There was a small path between the trees and the riverbank, cutting right to the place where the police worked.

They got around the bend, and finally had a clear view of them pulling the Lexus out.

Rani cried out. "Lisa's car!"

Then Blair heard Ben's wailing and watched as he tried to get to the car.

She knew Lisa was there.

Rani screamed out her despair and denial, then bolted out of the trees toward the car too, but she was wrestled back.

Ben was weeping in a crowd of police, standing back from the scene.

Blair didn't know what to do. They needed pictures for the paper, but somehow, it seemed cruel and opportunistic to snap them now.

She saw that Morgan and Jonathan had been allowed past the crime scene tape and were trying to comfort Ben. He staggered toward them and fell into Morgan's arms, and she held him for a long time.

Blair blinked back her tears. No . . . she wouldn't take pictures now.

Others found no problem with photographing the scene. Vince Barr of the *Observer* had gotten through the barricade somehow and was using his telescopic lens to get pictures of Lisa inside the car. Where was his helicopter? Had he parachuted out or just taken a leap into the water? She wouldn't put either past him.

She sidled up beside him. "Don't you think you've gotten enough, Vince? You're not really going to publish pictures of her

dead body, are you?"

"What do you think?" he asked with a smirk.

She thought of the JonBenet Ramsey case and the pictures his rag had published of the murdered child. Yes, he would indeed publish them. "Don't you have the slightest bit of integrity, Vince?"

He lowered the camera long enough to shoot her a smarmy grin. "Don't be such an amateur, Blair. Integrity doesn't pay the bills. Graphic pictures do."

21

"I didn't think she was dead. She was somewhere in trouble, but not dead. Not Lisa." Ben's words seemed to echo in the large great room of his home. Jonathan and Morgan had managed to convince him to let them bring him home, and now they wondered what comfort they could give the man in his shock.

"She would never have killed herself. *Never.* She had no reason . . ."

Morgan wondered if he was right. Could her despair over her marriage have driven her to suicide? Had the hormones and the stress over the IVF procedure and the mayoral race pushed her over the edge?

"I can prove it!" he said suddenly. "Have you seen the nursery?"

She wiped her face. "No."

"Let me show you." He started through the house, his gait angry and determined, his breathing hard. She and Jonathan followed.

Ben led them into a sage-colored room, with a junglelike mural painted on the wall and characters from Disney's *Jungle Book* hidden among the trees. A custom crib with legs that looked like little tree trunks sat in the center of the room, and a green rocker and chaise lounge sat at angles across from it.

"Lisa did all this herself." His voice was raspy and trembling. "She wouldn't take her life when we were right on the verge . . ." He sat down in the rocker. "Having a baby was what she lived for. It was her goal . . . and we were close to reaching it. If I'd known that she wouldn't live to see it, I wouldn't have let her waste all those years."

"But you didn't know," Morgan whispered. "How could you know?"

He reached out for the bed, touched the sheets, then crumbled again. "Who did that to her? I can't even imagine."

The assault of those words surprised Morgan, reviving her own helpless, rabid, broken questions in the aftermath of her parents' murders. Jonathan seemed to sense her memory and set a gentle hand on her shoulder.

Morgan shook herself out of her own stroll down murder lane, and drew on her

store of tried and true helps in tragedy. "Ben, is there anyone you want me to call?"

Ben looked up, his face stricken. "Oh, God help me, I have to call our families."

"I could do it, Ben."

He shook his head. "No, I have to. They have to hear it from me."

As he picked up the phone, Morgan went back into the kitchen, and she and Jonathan prayed quietly for those poor family members he called.

22

Lisa Jackson hadn't killed herself. Cade was certain of that. The medical examiner had ruled out suicide almost immediately. The marks on her neck indicated that she'd died of strangulation with a telephone cord they'd found on the floor of the car. Because there was no water in her lungs, it was clear she died before entering the water. The lividity on her skin — the purplish pooling of blood at the lowest points of a corpse — indicated that she was killed before being placed in the car.

Cade tried to puzzle the pieces together. Had someone come into her home after Ben left, murdered her, loaded her body into her own car, and driven her into a river in broad daylight? Granted, it had gone in at a secluded part of the river, in a place where no one was likely to see. Still, it seemed like a tremendous risk . . .

Unless the driver of the car had been its other owner. If Ben killed her and drove

her across town, no one would have noticed anything out of the ordinary. He would simply have driven through the trees to the quiet fishing hole, strapped her into the driver's seat, put the car in neutral, and given it a shove into the water.

But why would he kill her? Could it have anything to do with those letters?

And what about Carson Graham? How had he known where Lisa could be found?

Could *he* have committed the murder?

The shoe prints were a clue, but they hadn't gotten a match just yet. They'd determined the prints came from a size eleven men's shoe — the same size Ben wore.

Cade put Ben's house under surveillance until he could get over there to question him further. If Ben was guilty, he didn't want him making a run for it.

While the forensics team from the State Police worked the crime scene, Cade went to pay Carson Graham a visit. He pulled up on the dirt parking lot in front of the peeling blue house, and before he could knock, Graham opened the door. He grinned as if he'd been expecting him. "You found her body, didn't you?"

Cade hadn't expected him to be quite so delighted with the find. "I want to talk to you, Graham."

"Certainly. I'm always eager to help. You know that."

Cade walked into the dark house, which smelled of incense, and looked at the lit candles clustered around the room. A few fake Tiffany lamps provided a little more lighting, but the place had a carefully created air of dusty mystery.

The man lowered himself into a Chippendale chair and gestured for Cade to take the one facing him across a small round table. "Want me to do a reading for you, Cade? Perhaps I could aid in finding the killer."

"No, thanks." Cade took the seat, studying the man's face. "How did you know, Graham? The truth."

"I saw it in a vision. That's a fact. I wish I'd seen the identity of the killer, but I'm afraid I didn't."

Cade cleared his throat and leaned forward. "Where were you yesterday morning, Carson?"

"I was right here, sleeping late. I didn't have any appointments, and I'd had a late show over at the Frankfurt Inn the night before."

"Do you have any witnesses who could vouch for that?"

"Well, I didn't have anyone in bed with

135

me, if that's what you mean. My wife worked a double shift at the hospital that night and didn't get in until almost noon yesterday. But I can guarantee that you won't find anyone who saw me anywhere else. Ask the neighbors. My van was here all day." The arrogance on his face faded somewhat. "I know it's hard for you to believe, Cade, but psychic phenomena are real. I've never met Lisa Jackson in my life. All I know of her is what I've seen on the news — and the vision I got when I held her sweater."

Cade stared at the man for a moment, knowing in his gut that Carson was somehow involved in Lisa's death. He might not have killed her, but he felt certain he knew who had. How else would he have directed them to her body? "Graham, what size shoe do you wear?"

The man looked surprised at the question. "Size nine. Why?"

Cade studied his feet. He wore a size ten himself, and Graham's feet did look smaller. He figured he was telling the truth.

Graham seemed to sense Cade's thoughts and he almost looked amused. "You're not going to pin this on me, Chief. I'm a bona fide psychic, whether you can

deal with that or not. My advice to you is to embrace that knowledge and use it to your advantage. I'm more than happy to work with you on future cases. Of course, we both know that after the election, you may not even have a job."

He had guts. Cade would give him that much — though he didn't think much of his intellect. Provoking the police chief wasn't wise when one was tied up with a murder case and had no alibi. Cade got up. "Don't leave town, Graham. We might want to question you again."

"I have no place to go. Don't worry about it."

Cade couldn't help worrying as he limped through the door.

"You take care of that leg now," Carson called out behind him.

Cade got into his car and glanced back up as he drove away. Carson Graham stood outside his front door, arms crossed, chuckling like a man who'd just won the lottery.

23

Despite his suspicions about Graham, Cade had no choice but to center his investigation on the other main suspect — Ben Jackson. The grieving husband was inconsolable when Cade and McCormick showed up at his house with the news that strangulation had been Lisa's cause of death.

Morgan and Jonathan tried to comfort Ben, but anger, rage, and grief all booked time on his face, glazing his eyes with tortured visions. "My Lisa, she didn't have any enemies. Everyone who knew her loved her. Who could do this? *Why?*"

Cade didn't even try to answer those questions. "Ben, Lisa was killed before she was put into her car. It may have happened here."

Ben's face changed, and he looked around him, his eyes rapidly darting around the room, as if looking for some sign that a killer had been here. "In my

house? You think he came in here and murdered my wife?"

"We can't say for sure. But we'll need to search your house."

"Of course, yes. That's fine. If the killer was here, maybe some evidence was left." He walked to the back door and looked down at the lock. "Nothing was stolen. I would have noticed. And there wasn't any sign of a break-in." He swung around and settled his wild eyes on Cade. "Do you think it was someone she knew? Someone she let in willingly?"

"Those are questions we're asking, too. We'll know more after we've had time to go through the house."

"Go ahead. The sooner the better. I want you to find him, Cade. I want to know what happened . . ." His face twisted in his anguish.

Cade looked at the floor. McCormick gave him a quiet moment, then said, "Ben, we need to sit down with you and go over a few things."

"Anything," Ben said. "Anything you want to know."

Jonathan got up. "We'll go, Ben, so you can talk to them."

Morgan's face mirrored Ben's pain as she gave him another hug. "Ben, call us

when they're finished. We don't want you to be alone."

Ben was unresponsive as Morgan and Jonathan whispered goodbyes and left. Instead, Ben kept his eyes on McCormick, seemingly anxious to talk. "Okay, go ahead. What do you want to ask me?"

McCormick pulled out a stool at the counter, but Ben kept standing. In a quiet voice, McCormick asked him the question that had plagued Cade all day. "Ben, is there something you failed to tell us about your marriage?"

Ben clearly looked perplexed. "Like what?"

"Like the letters Lisa got from someone claiming to be your mistress?"

Ben groaned and pulled out a stool. Dropping into it, he rubbed his face. "I might have known. Who told you that? Rani? Had to be Rani."

McCormick didn't answer.

"Ben, who is she?" Cade asked.

"Nobody! I'm telling you, I was not having an affair. There *is* no other woman."

"Then how do you explain the letters?"

"Exactly the way I explained them to Lisa. Some crackpot was trying to cause problems for me before the election."

"You realize that if you were seeing someone, we'll find out." McCormick's tone was still soft, steady. "It wouldn't be wise to withhold that kind of information, Ben."

Ben leaned forward and locked his eyes into McCormick's. "I told you, I'm not lying. There is no woman! Trace those letters. I'd *love* to see where they're from. Maybe it was a way of luring Lisa somewhere. Maybe the killer sent them."

Cade just stared at him for a long moment, studying his face and his body language for some sign of guile, but he saw none. "Ben, was there anyone who might have had designs on you? Anyone who may have harbored some secret fantasy? Anyone you'd gotten to be close friends with, even if it was platonic?"

"No. I'm a busy man. I don't have time for stuff like that."

"Did Lisa believe that?"

"Of course she did. She knows how I am. She had no reason to suspect that I was having an affair until those letters started coming."

"And then she did suspect it?" McCormick asked.

"Well, yeah, she suspected it when she first got them. She came home all upset,

141

crying her eyes out, accusing me of all sorts of things. It took some doing to convince her that they weren't true. And then they kept coming. Every week I had to mount a new defense, but ultimately I always convinced her."

Ben leaned back in his chair. "The last letter came a few days ago. I think by the time that one came Lisa resolved herself to the fact that it was a pack of lies. It wasn't an issue. We had other things to think about."

Cade could see that Ben wasn't going to change his story. They'd know more when they sent the letters out for a handwriting analysis and tested them for fibers and prints.

"You know, you should search her office, too," Ben said. "If he didn't do it here, maybe it was there. Or some other clue . . . Last night I went there and checked her desk for a note or anything, or a notation on her calendar. I didn't find anything, but maybe I missed something. I don't even know what to look for."

"We plan to do that," Cade said. "But for now, we'll need you to leave the house. Where will you be in case we need to contact you?"

Ben breathed in a ragged breath. "At the

office, I guess. Do I need to stay overnight?"

"Probably," Cade said. "We're going to be a while."

"All right. I'll pack a bag."

Cade felt a surge of pity for the man. If he was innocent, he was being run from his home even as he struggled to absorb his shock. On a night when he would need to curl up with Lisa's things, he was exiled to a cold warehouse that smelled of shrimp. "You could probably stay at Hanover House if you wanted. Morgan and Jonathan wouldn't want you sleeping on a cot somewhere."

"I'll be fine. I have a lot of phone calls to make. I have to make arrangements . . ." He looked around as he spoke, as if trying to decide what to take with him. "I think I need to be alone. I need to think . . ."

Thinking was just what Ben didn't need to be doing. Cade walked with Ben to his bedroom and watched as he packed a few things into a small suitcase.

As he watched Ben pull away in his car, Cade turned all of the man's reactions and behaviors over in his mind. There was nothing there to indicate that he was lying. At least, nothing apparent.

"What do you think?" McCormick asked him.

Cade looked back at his detective. "I don't know. He's acting like a man who's just lost his wife."

"Yeah, seems genuine to me, too. But you know things aren't always the way they seem."

Cade knew that better than anyone, so he pressed past his own gut feelings and called for the detectives the State Police had loaned him to help with the search of the house.

24

"I know the timing is bad, mon, but you'll be seein' why I don't want to wait to say what I got to say."

Gus and Karen had been waiting on the porch for Morgan and Jonathan when they'd gotten home, and had followed them into the kitchen with solemn looks on their faces.

Jonathan shot Morgan a look, and she wondered what to brace herself for now.

"Sure, Gus. Is something wrong?"

The Jamaican fidgeted with a button on his shirt as he sat down at the table. Karen took the seat next to him. He cleared his throat, as if preparing to make a speech.

Gus had lived there for over a year since getting out of prison, and in that time he'd grown into a man of integrity and character with a good job and a future, ready to stand on his own. He planned to move into his own apartment within the next couple of weeks, and Morgan knew she was going

to miss him terribly. But it was time. It was clear that something romantic was developing between him and Karen, and dating among the residents was forbidden.

"Nothing wrong." He grinned at Karen, and she grinned back, and suddenly Morgan knew.

"Don't tell me —" Jonathan smiled — "let me guess. When you move out, you want permission to date Karen."

Gus took Karen's hand in his. "Not exactly, mon. I don't want your permission to date her. I want your permission to *marry* her."

Morgan caught her breath so hard that she almost choked. Jonathan touched her back as she coughed her way through the shock. She got up and grabbed a glass from the cabinet, filled it with water, and threw it back. Able to breathe again, she turned back to them.

"You all right, babe?" Jonathan asked.

"Yes. I'm sorry, I just . . . Wow. I didn't expect that." Gus and Karen were beaming. She forced herself to smile.

Now it was Jonathan's turn to clear his throat. "Well, I have to say . . . This is uncharted territory for Hanover House."

"I know it is, mon. It's uncharted for us, too."

Morgan searched her mind for the right response. Just a few weeks ago, Karen had come to them nine months pregnant, fearful that her baby's abusive father would endanger her child. She had a history of drug addiction and had served time in prison. Though she had done well in their program so far, it was no guarantee that she was strong enough for marriage.

"Gus, we appreciate you coming to us," Jonathan said, "and we're happy that the two of you want to commit to each other. But Karen, you've only been here a few weeks. I'm not sure you're ready for this kind of thing. You thought you were ready to stand on your own when you got out of prison, but you've said yourself that you backslid and went back to your old ways."

"Not the drugs," Karen said. "I didn't go back to the crack. I been clean of drugs for three years now, so it's not like I have that calling to me. I did get weak and wound up pregnant with Emory. I know all that, Jonathan, but this is different. Gus is the kind of man I been dreaming of. He's a good man, who can take care of us. And he loves Emory."

"Emory needs a daddy, mon," Gus told Jonathan. "You know he does."

Jonathan couldn't argue with that. "The

thing is, I don't want Karen to always turn to a man for her security. I want her to learn to lean on Christ."

Karen took Jonathan's hand and made him look at her. "I am leaning on Christ. I really am, Jonathan. And Gus will help me. You told me a husband is s'pose to be a spiritual leader. Gus is a strong man who loves the Lord. He'll help me grow, like you help Morgan."

"But you haven't known each other but a few weeks," Morgan said. "Wouldn't it be better to take some time to date and get to know each other better?"

Karen let Jonathan's hand go and put her hands over her face.

But Gus wouldn't give up. He put his arm around her shoulders. "We do know each other, Morgan. We been spendin' lots of time getting to know each other. Nothin's happened, so you don't have to worry, but we been around each other a lot. I seen what kind of mama she is to Emory. She's a good woman. I know all I need to know."

Karen slid her fingers down her face and met Morgan's eyes.

Silence passed between them, and Morgan just stared at both of them. "We need to pray about this."

"We been praying already, Morgan, ever since we knew we were in love." Gus took Karen's hand in both of his. "And what we came to is that we need your blessing. If we don't get it, we'll wait until we can."

That surprised Morgan even more. She looked at Jonathan and saw that he was equally moved. "You would do that? Wait, just because we wanted you to?"

Karen nodded. "If we knew you'd been praying about it and still felt we should wait, then we would. If we're s'pose to do this now, like we think God is telling us, then he'll tell you, too. I know I still need what I can get at Hanover House. I need the Bible study and the structure. It makes me strong. I like being part of your family."

"We thought of two ways to go about this," Gus said. "We could get married and I could stay at Hanover House. I could just give up my room and move in with Karen, so's she could stay in the program. Or she could move in with me in my new apartment and come back here for the Bible studies every day."

They heard the front door open, and Morgan knew that Sadie was home. "Let us pray about it, okay? We want what's best for you. We really do."

"We know you do, Morgan," Gus said.

"And I want what's best for Karen and Emory, whatever that is, but I want to start thinking of her as my wife, and him as my son. The apostle Paul said it's better to marry than to burn with lust."

Morgan thought she might choke again, so she grabbed her glass and went for more water.

"But lust is not a good reason for marriage," Jonathan said. "That's not what Paul meant."

"That ain't all, mon," Gus said. "I love this woman. I want to spend my life with her."

Morgan gulped the water down and turned back to them. When Jonathan met her eyes again, he was grinning. She couldn't help answering that smile.

"Well, I have to say that it's good to have some happy news," she said, "after all that's happened today."

Sadie stepped into the kitchen, looking haggard from her long drive. Morgan went to kiss her on the cheek. "Hey, sweetie. Come in and I'll fix you something to eat."

"No, I got something on the way." Sadie looked around. "Am I interrupting something?"

"No," Gus said. "We just be talking, Sadie. We're done. How was your trip?"

"Long." Sadie went to the refrigerator and got out a drink. "How was your day? Did anything happen with Lisa?"

Morgan's fragile joy for Gus and Karen faded. "They found her body at the bottom of the river."

Sadie spun around. "Oh, Morgan. I'm so sorry . . . Are you okay?"

"Yeah, I'm fine."

"Her poor husband. How is he?"

"Not well. He's taking it hard." She didn't want to talk about it now, so she changed the subject. "Sit down and tell us about your visit. Was your mom okay?"

"She was great, and she had some good news. Well, *maybe* some good news. She may be getting out early."

Morgan wasn't sure she'd heard her right. "What? How?"

"Some new law that says nonviolent of-fenders only have to serve twenty percent of their sentence because of overcrowding in the prison. She's not sure if she quali-fies, but her lawyer is looking into it."

A fifth of her sentence? Morgan looked at Jonathan, quietly passing her concern to him. If that was the case, her time served would be all that was required of her.

Jonathan leaned on the table. "Sadie, I don't want you to get your hopes up about

this. Morgan and I have been working in prison ministry for a while. It happens all the time — the inmates hear rumors about new laws and think they're getting out early. Mostly, they're disappointed. They want to be released so bad that they cling to every remote hope that comes along."

Karen agreed. "It's true. Whole time I was in jail, I just knew that I was gon' get out the very next week. First I thought somebody would post my bond. Then when they didn't, I thought I could get my public defender to file for a motion to reconsider. Then I tried to figure out ways to work off my sentence, get house arrest, whatever. Never did happen. Half the time I couldn't even get the lawyer to come see me."

"Me too," Gus added. "You turn into a mathematician when you're in the can. You get your time, minus time served, and then you get a day's credit for every day you work, time off for good behavior, and then the sixty percent law or the forty percent law, or the possibility of parole, or a mistake in the DOC office . . ."

"And it never added up the way we thought."

Morgan thought Sadie might cry. "Honey, it's something to pray about."

"But it could work out." Sadie's pleading

152

expression broke Morgan's heart. "Maybe it will. Maybe God's just giving her a second chance. He does that. I know he does."

Morgan took her hand. "Of course he does. He's the author of second chances."

Morgan could see from the girl's face that they had ruined her hopes. She wished she had just kept her reservations to herself.

"I'm tired," Sadie said. "I think I'll go on up to bed and read for a while."

Morgan hoped she wasn't going upstairs to cry. "Honey, I'm sorry we brought you down."

"Yeah, Sadie, we didn't mean to do that," Karen said.

Gus's face softened. "We hope your mama does get out. It happened to my cell mates sometimes, just never to me."

"It's okay." Sadie looked back at Morgan. "I'm sorry about Lisa. I know she was your friend."

"Thank you, sweetie."

"Good night, everybody." Sadie left the room, and silence fell over them all.

"She's right," Karen said quietly. "God does give lots of second chances." She reached for Gus's hand again.

Morgan knew they had an awful lot to pray about that night.

25

"Well, there's no blood," McCormick said after five hours of searching the house, "but that's no surprise since there weren't any open wounds. But the telephone doesn't bode well."

Cade had to agree. They had found a phone without a cord in the living room, suggesting that the murder weapon had come from the house. If Ben had removed the cord to kill her, wouldn't he have thought to replace it? Even if he'd forgotten, he would have been reminded each time the other phones in the house rang.

As they'd searched the premises, they'd found a good deal of evidence suggesting that these two people had a future together. They hadn't found a thing suggesting marital discord or even a struggle of any kind.

They bagged a truckload of things that might later prove to be evidence, vacuumed the floor for fibers, and dusted for

fingerprints. They confiscated her computer and canvassed the neighborhood for anyone who might have information.

And then they found the shoes.

They were the same size as the shoes that made the prints at the crime scene, with the same Nike design on the bottom. But it was a common running shoe, so the find didn't mean that Ben had been the one to push his wife into the river.

Unless the lab could prove that the dirt on the bottom was the same dirt that had been on the riverbank.

The officers also sealed off Lisa's office and confiscated Ben's boat and car. He handed everything over freely and got a rental car to drive.

By ten-thirty, Cade put night-shift officers outside the real estate office and the Jackson home to stand guard so he and McCormick could call it a night. They would all need some sleep if they were to make any sense of the evidence they'd gathered.

It was after eleven when he got into his truck, wincing as he pulled his swollen leg in. He sat behind the wheel for a moment and stared out the window into the night.

He was bone-tired and drained, yet he

didn't want to go home. His day felt unfinished. He needed to see Blair.

She was probably in bed already, sleeping soundly, but it wouldn't hurt to drive by and see if the lights were on.

He drove down Ocean Boulevard, his eyes scanning the moonlit beach and the businesses along the road. Did a killer lurk there somewhere? Was he laid up in one of the condos along the beach, or watching the local coverage of his murder on a hotel room TV?

Anger surged through Cade. He loved this town and the people who lived here and he wanted to protect them from evil, but sometimes evil slipped through anyway.

He rounded the island, where the road was darker along Wassaw Sound. Some of the houses were dark for the night, with lone porchlights the only security other than a locked door.

But Blair's house was still lit up, and relief flooded through him as he pulled onto the gravel parking lot she shared with the library. Maybe she'd waited up, hoping he'd come by. Warmth flooded through him at the thought.

He went to the door and tapped lightly on it. He saw her pull the curtains up from

the window. She opened the door and smiled out at him.

"Hey." The word was soft, drawn out, packing more punch than a simple greeting. It said she was glad to see him, that she'd been hoping he would come.

"Sorry it's so late." He leaned against the casing.

She looked sleepy and disheveled in a pair of sweat pants and a wrinkled T-shirt. "It's not too late. It's exactly the right time." She took his hand and pulled him in, and he felt the stress of the day melting away as he entered the warm glow of her living room.

"Sit down," she said. "Your leg is killing you."

He hadn't realized how badly he was limping, but he didn't argue. He sat down, and she got a cushion to put his leg on. "Here, prop it up. You want some aspirin?"

"No, I'll live." He slid down, resting his head on the back of the couch. It was the most comfortable he'd been all day.

She sat down next to him, pulling her feet beneath her. "Rough day, huh? Did you find anything in the house?"

"Blair, you know I can't talk about it."

"I know. But I've been doing a little searching on my own. You might be inter-

ested in a few things I came up with. But if you don't want to talk about it . . ."

He grinned. This was her way. She played that game of *you-scratch-my-back-and-I'll-scratch-yours* whenever there was an important investigation going on. The truth was, she usually had better information than he did. She had a gift, one that law enforcement officers would kill to have, and he didn't discount it.

"Okay, Blair. Tell me."

Clearly delighted that he'd taken the bait, she shifted to face him fully. "Okay, so I'm looking around town and interviewing people to find out who might have seen Lisa Jackson last. Lo and behold, Alan Freeman told me that maybe Lisa went looking for Ben's girlfriend."

"That guy? Alan Freeman is a well of misinformation," Cade said. "You know that. He thinks he's an expert on everything."

"I realize that, but I wanted to know where he heard it, so I drilled him as hard as I could, and I found out that he heard it from some of the women in the ladies' book club. Well, I don't have to tell you, I know every one of them, so I got on the phone and started calling around. Every single one of them had heard rumors of Ben Jackson's affair. No one had a name.

No one knew anything except that there was some mystery mistress."

Cade sat up straighter. "Yeah?"

"Finally, I traced the rumor back to Sarah Grady, and she refused to tell me who told her."

Cade's hopes crashed. "Blair, you're starting to sound like one of those high school girls on the telephone."

"I know, but don't you see, Cade? It's not just the rumor that's important." Her eyes widened. "It's where the rumor *started*. Tracing this rumor back to its roots is going to take us either to the mistress or to the person who started the rumor, who ultimately may have written the letters."

Cade closed his eyes and sighed. "I didn't tell you about any letters."

She waved the comment off. "My sister let it slip out when I called her this afternoon."

Cade might have known. "Morgan knew better than that."

"Don't worry. She was horrified after she did it, but I'm pretty good at prying information out of people. She hardly had a chance."

"She still shouldn't have given you that kind of information. You're the media, for heaven's sake."

"Well, don't blame her. Her defenses

were low. She's really depressed today and she was hoping I'd find the killer."

"You? I'm the one leading this investigation!"

"Yeah, but she knows I'm just like you. I don't give up until I have answers that make sense."

He rubbed his eyes, realizing he was more tired than he thought. "So did you follow the rumor mill any further?"

"Not quite, but tomorrow I'm going to get to the end of it, I can promise you that. Either there's a mistress or there's a liar trying to stir up trouble. Either one could be our killer."

Cade chuckled softly and stroked her hair. "I'm glad you're on my side."

"I'll keep you updated, even if you don't return the favor. And Cade, go easy on Morgan. She's not herself today."

Cade relaxed his head back again. "I guess the murder rocked us all."

"It's not just that. It's something else. Just between you and me, Morgan had a miscarriage yesterday."

"What?" He dropped his leg and sat up straight. "Jonathan didn't tell me she was pregnant!"

"They had just found out. Hadn't even told *me* yet."

"Oh, no." He thought of the blow that must have been to his best friend and his wife. "That's awful. I need to call him."

"Not tonight. They're exhausted. But see, that's why she called Lisa, because Lisa's been infertile all these years, and they'd gotten to be friends through that common bond. Morgan wants a baby so bad."

Cade knew Jonathan yearned for a child too. His poor friends. They must be heartbroken. "I wonder what went wrong."

"They don't know. They're making an appointment with the fertility doctor Monday. The same one Lisa was seeing."

"Sims?" Cade had heard plenty about the doctor from Ben today. He got comfortable again and propped his leg back up. "I've heard he's pretty good." He reached up and pushed Blair's hair back from her face. He knew she didn't like it when he did that. Her self-consciousness about her scars made her hide behind that hair, but he liked having a clear view of her eyes. "Do you ever think about having children?"

Those scars turned pink, and she looked away. "Sometimes. It's hard to picture — me, as a mom. I'm probably better aunt material."

"I can picture it," he whispered. "You'd be a terrific mom."

She studied his face — a million thoughts and twice as many emotions flashing across her features, but for once, she didn't voice them. Instead, she got up. "You want something to drink?"

She was changing the subject, so he let her off the hook. "Yeah, I'll take some water."

He watched her retreat into the kitchen, wondering why the thought of motherhood would seem so foreign to her. She'd had a wonderful mother of her own, and while she didn't have the "earth mother" traits Morgan had, she was devoted and nurturing to those she cared about.

After a moment, he got up and followed her into the kitchen. Leaning against the counter, he watched her fuss over putting ice in the glass. He met her eyes and saw her swallow. Then she looked away and let her hair fall back along her face.

If only she understood how beautiful she was.

"Come here." He took her hand and pulled her toward him. She came, looking up at him with those wide eyes that seemed so uncertain — even a little afraid — as if she might be misreading his

interest and making a fool of herself.

Slowly, he bent down and slid his fingers through her hair, against her soft neck. Her pulse raced against his fingertips as she melted in the kiss. She caused a longing deep inside him, a sweet homesick pull for some home he'd never had. It made him ache.

When the kiss broke, he kept his forehead against hers and let that ache linger.

It wasn't safe, the two of them here . . . alone like this, with these feelings that seemed bigger than the strength he had.

"I'd better go."

"Why?" Her question was a breath against his lips.

"Because I really want to stay." He kissed her forehead. "You know?"

She breathed a soft laugh. "Yeah, I know."

He pulled himself away, got his cane, and went to the front door. Blair followed him, her hands in the pockets of her sweatpants, as if she couldn't trust them at her sides. He opened the door, looked down at her, but couldn't think of a thing to say. Finally, he drew in a deep breath, then let it out in a rough sigh. Then with a soft grin, he said, "Good night, Blair."

"Good night," she whispered.

He didn't kiss her again — didn't dare — for fear he'd never get out that door. But his heart hammered as if he had.

He hoped he would be able to sleep tonight.

Blair lay in bed, staring up at the ceiling, a soft smile on her lips. She'd had sleepless nights thinking about Cade before, but usually her thoughts were dismal and hopeless. This time they held a giddiness that she'd rarely experienced in her life.

Cade made her feel so pretty. She would never have believed that anyone would think such a thing, yet every time he looked at her with that soft grin in his eyes, she saw herself as a beautiful woman. Was it possible that someday her scars wouldn't even be an issue, that she would go through an entire day without thinking about them?

Or was she just setting herself up for a humiliating heartbreak?

Almost frantic at the thought, she slid out of bed to her knees and sent a plea up to heaven that the Lord wouldn't let her overestimate Cade's feelings for her. She didn't think she could stand his rejection.

She had loved Cade far longer than she'd been willing to admit to herself, and while

he'd shown signs that he'd been interested as well, he'd never made a single gesture toward her until after she'd embraced Christ. He had cried at her baptism four weeks ago when Jonathan immersed her at the beach across the street from Hanover House, with the congregation of their church gathered around for the occasion. She came up out of the water feeling clean and triumphant, and the crowd burst into cheers. Cade was the first to hug her as she came dripping onto the shore.

She sensed he'd been praying for her for a very long time.

Her salvation was like the dawning of day to her, moving from a life of dull gray to one of bursting yellows. She understood the term *born again*. As a babe in Christ, she felt the new life God had spoken of in his Word.

Cade was an extra blessing, one that she would have to take as God decided to give. She couldn't rush this, anymore than others could have rushed her salvation.

Yet waiting was hard, and it made for lots of restless nights, especially when possibilities loomed like dormant dreams stirring themselves awake.

Could Cade really feel the same about her?

She decided to hope just this once, and that hope turned into another prayer. Maybe God would smile on her and give her this desire of her heart.

26

Blair got to Cricket's an hour before church the next morning and took a booth in case Cade joined her. After breakfast, she would walk across to the Church on the Dock that met in the old warehouse. Her parents had planted the church years ago, and after they died, Jonathan stepped into the role of pastor. Blair had only returned to its pews last month after staying away for years. Now the act of worship was something she looked forward to.

She wondered if Cade would even have time to come by this morning, much less worship, with the investigation still in its infant stages. She hoped he'd rested his leg and gotten some sleep last night.

She was on her second cup of coffee when he came in. He looked exhausted, but his eyes lit up with that contagious light that made her see herself in a new way.

"I can't stay," he told her as he slipped in across from her.

"I know. You look tired. Did your leg keep you up?"

"Among other things." His grin brought the heat rushing to her face. "Listen, I wanted to talk to you about what you're writing."

"Okay."

"Paper comes out Tuesday, right? I want you to mention that the police department has a tip line and that we're waiting to hear from anyone who may have seen Lisa's car Friday. We especially want to know if someone else was driving it."

"You got it. I'll put it on the front page."

He pulled an index card out of his pocket. It had the number on it.

She took her notepad out of her bag. "So, where's the car?"

"We moved it to the crime lab in Savannah. Forensics is going through it."

"And the autopsy?"

"They'll be doing it tomorrow. I plan to be there when they do."

"You'll update me, won't you? I don't want to put the paper to bed tomorrow night until I've got the latest info."

"You know I'll tell you what I can."

"Coffee, Cade?" the Colonel called from the bar.

"Yeah, a tall one to go, Colonel."

Blair leaned on the table, fixing her eyes on Cade. "So, tell me about Carson Graham."

Cade laced his fingers in front of his face. "That's the other thing I wanted to talk to you about. I meant to bring it up last night, but . . . I got sidetracked."

She looked down at her coffee and moved her stirring stick around. Should she joke about last night or pretend it hadn't happened? Feeling awkward, she chose the latter. "Weird, huh? How do you think he knew?"

"Good question."

"He told Rani he'd helped the police before. Is that true?"

"The guy's a pest," Cade said. "Apparently he gave Chief Baxter some no-brainer tips before I was here and claimed credit for solving those crimes. We're talking vague stuff, nothing specific. Anybody could have come up with the same tips if you just gave it a little thought."

The Colonel brought Cade's coffee, and Cade busied himself adding sugar and cream. "He tries to get involved on every major crime. Even when your parents were killed, he had some cockamamy story about who he thought did it based on some vision he'd had. None of it panned out."

"But he was right on the money this time. I mean, don't you find that bizarre? You can't seriously attribute that to luck."

Cade sipped his coffee. "What *can* you attribute it to, Blair?"

Blair thought it over for a moment. "Maybe God? Maybe God's speaking to him. Or even through him."

"God doesn't use psychics."

"But what about the spiritual gift of prophesy? Isn't that the same thing?"

"Not at all." He sipped through the plastic top. "The Bible forbids us to go to psychics. Psychics and sorcerers and those who do what the Bible calls *divination* are an abomination to God."

Blair didn't remember seeing that in the Bible. "Are you sure?"

"Of course I'm sure. Pull up that Bible program of yours and do a search. You'll see."

"So you're saying that if a psychic can't be of God, then he must be of Satan?"

Cade shook his head. "I'm not even sure it's that spiritual. I mean, think about it. Half of what they predict is based on common sense and probable outcome. When a woman says that her husband all of a sudden wants a divorce, that he's been staying out all night, it's kind of a no-

170

brainer to suggest that he might be having an affair. Based on that probable outcome, the so-called psychic makes a prediction. And *voilà,* it turns out to be true. That doesn't mean he has any special powers."

Blair leaned back, processing that. "But what about the cases where they are specific and turn out to be right?"

"Well, even if they did have *some* power, if the Bible forbids it, then it can't be of God."

Blair wasn't sure she could attribute it to Satan, either. Carson Graham didn't seem evil. She would have to look that up on her own and see what the Bible really said.

"Just do me a favor, Blair. When you write about him, please don't make it sound like he cracked the case. Every desperate person in town will be lining up for a reading from him. We both know that's not where they're going to find answers."

"I'll only report what happened, Cade. Just the facts."

27

Blair didn't hear from Cade again that day, and by Monday, she knew he was probably working on the investigation around the clock. She spent the day interviewing people about the murder, trying to find out if Ben indeed had a mistress. She continued to trace the rumor back to its origin, but hadn't reached it yet.

Sadie came after school to help her lay out the paper. When she had to go home to study for exams, Blair stayed at the office, proofing every article one more time.

Finally satisfied that it was ready, she kicked her shoes off and padded in her sock feet back to the printing room to start the presses. The person who had owned the newspaper before her only had a weekly edition. Ever since Blair took over, there was too much news to settle on once a week, so she'd put out an edition each Tuesday and Friday. That meant that Monday and Thursday nights she got little

sleep. In the past few weeks, as more subscriptions had sold, she'd been able to draw more from the wire services and news syndicates. She'd also occasionally paid a few stringers, who brought in stories that interested them, and Sadie, who was gifted in both journalism and photography.

The mayoral race kept things going strong. Blair even got a lot of comments from islanders that they'd canceled their subscriptions to the *Savannah Morning News* since her paper seemed to have everything they needed to keep them up-to-date.

She got the printer started. Maybe she should sell the equipment and start hiring an outside printing company to do this part of her job. But then she couldn't make changes at the last moment, and she needed that flexibility.

It would be several hours before the newspaper would be printed, and then she'd have to bundle the stacks and have them ready for the paperboys who would report at 5:00 a.m.

She pulled one of the front pages off the printer. She hoped Cade wasn't upset by the headline: "Psychic Leads Police to Body." There were two pictures on the front, one of Lisa Jackson and the other a

photo of Carson Graham that Blair had pulled from his website. She had tried re-wording the headline, but she couldn't tell the story of police finding the body until she told how they knew it was there. It was headline material, and all the other papers were reporting it as such.

She had to keep the integrity of her paper by giving the readers all of the facts. They expected it of her, after all. Surely Cade wouldn't find fault with that.

28

"Lisa Jackson Found Dead — Husband's Footprint Found at Crime Scene."

Cade stared at the headline of the *Observer*, the national tabloid whose weekly issue had come out that morning. How had Vince Barr known about the shoe print?

He grabbed his cane, got up, and, waving the paper, went into the squad room. "I want to know who leaked this, and I want to know *now!*"

Billy Caldwell rose from his desk. "What, Chief?"

" *'Husband's Footprint Found at Crime Scene'*! Who told this reporter that?"

Alex Johnson and McCormick emerged from the interview room, and Sarah, the dispatcher, looked up at him with wide eyes. "I didn't even know about it, Chief."

Cade swung around to Johnson and McCormick. "I want to know who did it so I can personally end his career in law en-

forcement and arrest him for interfering with an investigation."

"Whoa, Chief." McCormick held out his hands, as if calming a bucking horse. "You don't know it was one of us. It could have been one of the borrowed investigators. There were enough people working the scene."

Cade flung the paper across the room. "We don't even know for sure that it was Ben's shoes that made those prints! And here they are publishing it in a national tabloid!" He grabbed the paper back up and saw the articles further down the front page. *"Local Psychic Helps Police Find Body."* Carson Graham's picture had a place almost as prominent as Ben's or Lisa's.

When he turned to page two, his heart felt as if it would slam right through his chest, alien-style. Pictures of Lisa's dead, wet body, slumped in that car dripping with seaweed, filled half the page. He ripped the page in two and flung both halves down. "This is all we need. A media circus making Lisa Jackson into a freak show and Ben into a homicidal maniac." He pointed to the cops in front of him. "No one talks to the media about this case, do you hear me?" His staff nodded, and he

turned to Sarah. "Get on the radio and tell every one of my men that. No one talks to the media — or they lose their job. No second chances. Tell them I'm not playing."

He went back into his office and sank back into his chair. The phone was ringing, and no one out there was answering it. It was probably a reporter. He felt like ripping the cord out of the wall and throwing it across the room.

He leaned his elbows up on the desk and looked down at today's copy of the *Cape Refuge Journal*, which had also come out this morning. Its headline was almost as bad as the Observer's.

"Psychic Leads Police to Body."

As if on cue, Alex stuck his head around the door. "Uh, Chief, Blair's here to see you."

Great. He'd been wanting to talk to her, too. "Send her in."

Blair bolted in, looking like she hadn't yet been to bed. "Cade, I just saw Vince Barr's article. Why didn't you tell me about the footprint?"

"Because it's not public information, Blair! I don't know who told him, but when I find out, somebody's gonna lose their job! Barr's reporting of it was irresponsible."

Blair sank into a chair. "And that surprises you? That a tabloid would be irresponsible?"

"Speaking of irresponsible . . ." Cade got up, came around his desk, and closed his door. He picked up the *Cape Refuge Journal*. "What do you call this?"

She grunted. "The edition I stayed up all night to get out. What's wrong?"

"It's the headline that's wrong!" He flung the paper back down. "You gave this psychic undue credence, Blair. I asked you not to!"

"Cade, you asked me not to make him a hero, and I didn't. Did you even read the article?"

"I didn't have to. The headline says it all."

"No, it doesn't. The article explains what happened. Cade, if I didn't report it, I'd be the only one. The *Savannah Morning News* reported it Sunday."

"But our residents expect more from you. They expect accuracy. For you to back up what they said just makes it look true. You could have found another angle. *'Police Find Body in River'* would have been fine, but that's not sensational enough."

Blair got up and faced him squarely. "Okay, is that it? That you didn't get credit?"

That did it. He felt as if his body was going to implode right there. "It's not about credit, Blair," he said through his teeth. "It's about the fact that my job is already pretty much on the line. If anybody but Jonathan makes mayor, I'm out of here. How do you think it makes me look to be taking advice from some two-bit con artist?"

"You didn't take his advice. You followed up on a lead. You were doing your job, and that's what I wrote!" She picked up the paper and shook it out. "Here —" she poked her finger at a paragraph — "right here, I said that you were skeptical about the lead, but when you followed up you saw evidence that a car may have gone in the river. The fact is that you would not have seen the tire tracks if it hadn't been for Carson Graham. That's all I said. I have to do my job, Cade, just like you have to do yours. You can't expect me to hedge on the facts. I put your tip line on the front page. I quoted you and told how you'd gotten others in from different departments to help with the search. You're the real hero here."

"I'm not trying to be the hero!" He grabbed the paper out of her hands and stuffed it into the trash can. "I'm trying to solve a murder! It's not about me. It's

about an innocent woman who was strangled to death in our town. But you and Vince Barr and all those other reporters have made it a freak show, with Carson Graham as the star. Giving away key bits of evidence that no one but the police were supposed to know —"

"Then it's true about the footprints?"

"I don't believe this." She was still playing reporter, using their argument as another chance to get a scoop. Chewing his lip, he went back to his desk, trying to calm his anger. Slowly, he lowered back into his chair. "This interview is over, Blair. I have nothing more to say."

The anger on her face matched his as she bent over his desk. "It's not an interview, Cade, and you know it. I just asked you a question. I'm not Vince Barr. I'm not the one who printed pictures of her corpse, so you can stop taking it out on me."

"I'm not taking it out on you."

"I bought that paper so that I could report the news in this community with integrity and intelligence. I use my Christian principles in deciding what goes into that paper, and you know it. I don't appreciate your implications that I'm irresponsible or opportunistic."

He wondered if his own face was as red

as her scars. "Christian principles, huh? Then tell me why you would help that fly-by-night fortune-teller elevate his name. I'm absolutely amazed that you spent so many years dissecting Christianity because it didn't make sense to you, but you're accepting that guy's claims without a second thought. Did you read what the Bible says about guys like him, Blair, or did you just blow that off?"

She straightened. "I've been busy, just like you have. Are you questioning my Christianity?"

"I'm questioning your knowledge of the Bible. If you knew what it said about psychics, you wouldn't be giving this guy a standing ovation."

The words hit dead-on. "You act like I've joined a cult or something. I just wrote an article. And it's not a big surprise that I'm not as well versed in the Bible as you are when I've only been a Christian for a month! But none of that has anything to do with my reporting the facts. He told you where she was. That's all there is."

"How did he *know?*" Cade wanted to hit something, but he knew the raised voices were already giving his men enough to talk about. Blasted paper-thin walls. They'd probably heard every single word. Whose

idea was it to turn a laundromat into a police station, anyway? "Did you ever question that, Blair? How did this so-called psychic know where she was?"

Her face changed. "So you think he was involved in her death?"

He couldn't believe that had come out of his mouth. He needed some sleep, some Advil for his aching leg . . . and while he was at it, a resolution to this murder case. He took in a long, deep breath and lowered his voice. "I don't know, Blair. All I know is that God didn't give him a vision. But when his show packs in more people this week than the churches packed in Sunday, you can pat yourself on the back for advancing the cause of the crackpots."

He got up, came around the desk, and opened the door. "Now I've got work to do."

He stormed past the officers at their desks, pretending to be busy as if they hadn't heard the exchange. Pushing out the front door, he went to his truck and got in.

Blair was coming out as he backed up and pulled out of the parking lot. He was more determined than ever to find the killer and solve the puzzle of Carson Graham's involvement before this whole thing got out of hand.

29

As tired as Blair was from her all-nighter, she found herself unable to sleep when she went home. Anger seethed through her at the things Cade had said, but more than that, she felt stark disappointment that he'd walked out on her.

They'd argued before, but not in the last month, since the two of them had gotten closer. She'd wondered if they still had that kind of fight in them. His accusations made her livid. Did he doubt her faith because of a headline? Did he consider her a superficial Christian because she hadn't had time to study what the Bible said about psychics?

She tried to swallow back her anger and, taking his challenge, went to get her father's Bible. She took it to her laptop, sat at the kitchen table, and pulled up her Bible program. She keyed in a few words and began flipping through the Scriptures that spoke on the subject of psychics.

Deuteronomy 18 had much to say on the subject. She turned to that place in her father's Bible, and read aloud.

"There shall not be found among you anyone who makes his son or his daughter pass through the fire, one who uses divination, one who practices witchcraft, or one who interprets omens, or a sorcerer, or one who casts a spell, or a medium, or a spiritist, or one who calls up the dead. For whoever does these things is detestable to the LORD; and because of these detestable things the LORD your God will drive them out before you. You shall be blameless before the LORD your God. For those nations, which you shall dispossess, listen to those who practice witchcraft and to diviners, but as for you, the LORD your God has not allowed you to do so."

She sat back and stared down at the page. It was clear what God thought about the practices of people like Carson Graham.

But did that mean that he was a fake? If he didn't get his vision from God, where *had* he gotten it? What had given him the power to see where Lisa's body lay?

She closed her Bible and stared at a spot on the table. Maybe Cade's suspicions were right. Maybe Carson had inside knowledge that had nothing to do with psychic powers. Maybe he *had* been involved.

She checked more of the passages that came up on her computer screen. In 1 Samuel 28 Saul had consulted a medium, and the woman brought up the dead Samuel, who prophesied Saul's death. If that woman had the power to bring someone back from the dead, was it just a one-time fluke for God's purposes? Had she been a fraud up until that point, then been stunned when Samuel appeared? God had used a donkey before to speak his truth. Was it so far-fetched that he might use a woman he considered wicked to speak Samuel's prophecy?

Or did she really have special powers apart from God, who would never have gifted her with something he considered detestable?

She read about the spiritists and magicians who couldn't recite Nebuchadnezzer's dreams, and how Daniel did so through the spirit of prophecy. Had those spiritists been able to do so before?

Finally, she found the passage in Acts 16

in which a fortune-teller followed Paul around for days, yelling out that he was a "bond servant of the Most High God." She had spoken the truth, yet Paul had turned around and cast a demon out of her. Immediately, she'd lost her power to tell fortunes.

So what did that tell her? She got up and walked around the kitchen, trying to think it through. Apparently some psychics really did have demonic power to do the things they did, though it sounded like they could not see the future. Deuteronomy 18:21–22 said, "You may say in your heart, 'How will we know the word which the LORD has not spoken?' When a prophet speaks in the name of the LORD, if the thing does not come about or come true, that is the thing which the LORD has not spoken."

If they really had power to see the future, then they wouldn't ever get it wrong.

But did they have the power to see visions of things that had already happened? Did demons, who knew the evil that had already happened to Lisa, put that vision into Carson's head?

She went back to the Bible, determined to mold her anger at Cade into something productive. She would study until she got to the bottom of this, and then she would

show Cade that his implications about her faith were unjust and untrue.

Knowledge could only help.

30

Lisa's fertility doctor, Alan Sims, the one who had worked with her and Ben through their long, arduous struggle to have a child, wasn't at his clinic. His receptionist told Cade that Sims had taken the day off to attend Lisa's funeral that afternoon.

Cade found the man's home on Cape Refuge — a three-story Tudor-style house situated on an acre in one of the more upscale neighborhoods in town. Since he'd been personally interviewing everyone who'd been scheduled to see Lisa on the day of her murder, he needed to talk to the doctor to see if he had any insights to give him about her death. It was the kind of thing McCormick might have done better, but he was tied up reviewing the evidence that had been taken from Lisa's car and body, so Cade had come himself. It was welcome work since he couldn't stand the thought of sitting in his office, stewing about Blair's article and dealing with

phone calls from the press.

He rang the front bell and waited. After a moment, the doctor himself answered. "Chief Cade?"

"Dr. Sims, I'm sorry to bother you at home, but your office told me you'd taken the day off. Do you mind if I come in and talk to you for a minute?"

"Sure, come on in." Sims was unshaven and smelled of whiskey. Barefoot and wearing a wrinkled T-shirt and a pair of jeans, he led Cade into his living room. A shirt lay wadded on the couch, and several pairs of shoes and socks lay on the floor. A plate, several glasses, and some wadded napkins cluttered the coffee table.

"Excuse the mess." He grabbed some newspapers off of a chair so Cade could sit down. "My maid is AWOL, and my wife has been in Europe for the past week. It doesn't usually look like this. This thing with Lisa really shook me up. I haven't even been able to think clearly." He sat down on the couch, and Cade took the chair. "You build a relationship, you know? She wasn't just a patient. She was a friend."

"I can imagine," Cade said. "I'm afraid I didn't know her very well myself. Dr. Sims, could you tell me about the last time you saw her?"

He set his elbows on his knees and raked his hands through his hair. "That was the day before she disappeared. I saw her every day last week. We were doing daily sonograms so we'd know exactly when she ovulated. We had to know when we could harvest her egg. Timing is critical."

"Did she ever mention any problems or turmoil in her life? Or anyone she might be afraid of?"

"Not really. Fighting infertility is a very long road and it's not always pleasant. The Jacksons had a lot of disappointments and were under quite a bit of stress, not to mention all the drugs that she was on and the pressure that Ben was under with the election."

Cade thought of those letters again. "Did Lisa ever express concerns about her marriage?"

"Not really. I know he had asked her to wait until after the election to do the last IVF. But she felt panicked, like her time was running out. Every month counted. I had noticed a little more tension between them lately." He stopped, ran his hands down his face, and looked at Cade over his fingertips. "Chief, do you think he killed her?"

Cade wasn't going to answer that. "Was

there anything in Ben's character that would make you think he was capable of that?"

His hands went back through his hair. Cade noticed they were shaking. "You never know what anyone's really capable of, do you?"

31

"And now to comment on this bizarre murder case in Cape Refuge, Georgia, Vince Barr of the *Observer* joins us via satellite. Welcome, Vince."

Blair caught her breath and turned up the television. Had FOX News really asked the sleazy tabloid reporter to talk about Lisa's case?

"This morning your paper called this case to the attention of the national media," Shepherd Smith said. "It seems that this woman named Lisa Jackson turned up missing just days ago, and then her car was found in the river."

"That's right, Shep," Vince said, as if he was a regular on their show instead of some two-bit paparazzi looking for an alien behind every bush. "And the interesting thing about this case is that a psychic is the one who led the police to her body. He apparently was given a sweater that belonged to Lisa, and from that he got a vision. He

told her closest friend where her body could be found."

As he spoke, FOX flashed pictures of Lisa Jackson on the screen.

"And the sheriff listened to him, and indeed, her body was found there, in her car."

"He's not a sheriff!" Blair bit out to the television.

"Tell us about Lisa Jackson," Smith said. "I understand she was a real estate maven in the area."

"She was, and a very popular one, at that. Her business partner is former model Rani Nixon —"

"Rani Nixon? One of the highest paid models in Manhattan just a few years ago. So that's where she wound up."

"That's right. She went into business with Lisa when she retired from modeling."

Blair couldn't imagine what he thought Rani had to do with anything, but she supposed that had probably been a part of his pitch to FOX when he'd tried to sell them the story.

The photos of Lisa stopped flashing, and the camera went back to Vince. He looked like he'd dyed his hair overnight. He'd been decidedly grayer yesterday.

"Lisa and her husband had been married for twenty years," he went on, "and by all accounts, seemed happy. They had gone through years of infertility treatments and were, in fact, about to do their third in vitro procedure when Lisa disappeared."

"Vince, in your article this morning, you said that the husband's footprints were found at the scene where her car went into the river."

The helicopter footage of the search for Lisa's body came on, then the tape from across the river, and then closer up of when he'd taken pictures of the body. Blair thought of grabbing a vase and slamming it into the screen, but she decided to wait until she saw him face-to-face.

"Yes. They found shoes in his house that matched the prints."

"Is this confirmed?"

"Anonymously. I got this tip from a very reliable source."

"And they're putting her time of death at midmorning, isn't that right? So do they think he just drove her car there with her dead body in it and pushed it into the river in broad daylight?"

"The site where she went in is a pretty isolated area on the river. He could have easily done it without anyone seeing him.

And apparently did."

"Have any arrests been made yet?"

"Not yet, Shep. Understand, this is a very small sheriff's department, used to dealing with car thefts and parking violations. If it weren't for Carson Graham's psychic reading, they'd probably still be searching for her."

"Thefts and parking violations!" Blair threw the remote across the room, then went to the set and punched the power button to turn it off. Hadn't Cade solved four murders in the past few months? She couldn't watch another moment. She hoped Cade hadn't seen that. He would be more enraged than he already was, and she didn't blame him.

Suddenly she realized that she wasn't angry at him anymore. Her feelings of defensiveness over him spoke volumes.

How dare that man minimize Cade's competence?

She thought of what Cade had said about her making Carson Graham out to be a hero. He was even more of a hero now, and he would probably be invited onto every news show in the country after this.

Could Cade be right about his involvement being more than just a psychic vi-

sion? Could the psychic have had something to do with Lisa's death?

She decided her first interview of the day would be with Graham himself. She called him, and he answered on the first ring.

"Carson Graham. How can I help you today?"

She swallowed. "Carson, this is Blair Owens. I was wondering if I could come by and talk to you this morning."

"Would you like a personal reading or is this newspaper business?"

She rolled her eyes. "Newspaper. I'd like an interview."

"Well, certainly." His syrupy, soft voice was reminiscent of a funeral director. "I have some time right now if you could come on over, but I can only spare a few minutes. I'm getting quite a large number of media requests today."

She hurried over and pulled up into the gravel parking lot of the old house, situated on Ocean Boulevard just off of the Tybee Bridge, one of the busiest roads on Cape Refuge, where every gullible soul who came in or out of town would see his sign. She shivered as she looked up at the place, wondering if she should be afraid. She could be walking into danger on several levels. If Carson was a fraud, and really

196

was involved in Lisa's death, he could be dangerous. And if he wasn't a fraud but a real psychic, were there demons hovering around him? She wished she knew more about the spiritual aspects of his "gift."

Carson Graham met her at the door. "Blair, so good to see you." He took her hand in both of his. "Come in, dear. Would you like coffee? Coke?"

"No, thanks. I'm good."

Withdrawing her hand, she looked around at the candles clustered around the room, their light flickering eerily against the wall. The smell of incense almost made her sneeze.

"You sure keep it dark in here."

"That's for privacy and concentration. I'll open the drapes if you'd like."

She shrugged, as if she didn't care one way or another, but she was glad when he did. As light filled the room, she realized it didn't look nearly as elegant as she'd thought. Dust particles danced on the sun rays, revealing the scratches and age in most of the cheap furniture. Shabby without the chic.

He sat down across from her. "Thank you for the headline today, Blair. It was such a pleasant surprise. My work is usually done behind the scenes. I don't expect

that kind of credit."

She cleared her throat. So Cade was right. "I just reported the facts. But today I was thinking about doing a piece on the process behind being a psychic. Where you got your gift, how you've developed it, what exactly you see . . . that kind of thing."

"Of course. And I'm glad you used the word *gift*. It really is that, you know. A gift from God."

Blair hadn't expected that. Her eyebrows came up. "God, huh? So you believe God is the one who gave you this power?"

"Of course he did. He's the one who opens my eyes to see, if you will."

Blair jotted that down. *Eyes to see.* Bible lingo. "So tell me about your average vision. How does it work?"

He shifted in his seat. "Well, to tell you the truth, it comes in different ways. Usually, I'll take my subject's hand, and impressions just begin flooding my brain." He reached out for her hand. "May I?"

"Maybe some other time."

He laughed softly. "Oh, a skeptic, huh? Well, you know, I don't always *have* to touch that person to get those impressions. Sometimes they come without it. Like now, for instance. I'm sensing that you're in love."

She tapped her pencil on her pad and

hoped her scars weren't flaming. "Is that right?"

"Yes. I sense that it's a strange feeling to you, because in the past you haven't let yourself be that vulnerable. And you never thought romance was in your cards. But let me tell you, Blair. It is."

Part of her wanted to follow this lure — see if he could tell her where her relationship with Cade would lead. But wasn't it becoming common knowledge? After their first kiss, which happened in front of dozens of police officers, hadn't word spread all over the island?

"You've been hurt in the past. You've suffered intense grief."

She sighed and propped her chin on her hand. "Come on, Carson. Everybody in town knows I lost my parents."

"But your scars have caused you no end of grief, haven't they? You put on the air of a tough broad, but the truth is that all you've ever really wanted was someone of your own to love you."

Now she knew her scars were flaming. She felt her chest tightening, her heart ramming against it. "Could we get back to the interview?"

"This *is* part of the interview, Blair. I'm showing you how this works."

"I didn't come here for a reading. I'm here as a reporter."

"Don't worry, I won't charge you. He is going to marry you, you know."

Her heart jolted. "Who is?"

"This person you're in love with."

She stared down at her notepad as an unexpected wave of anger surged up inside her. Why Graham's words angered her so, she wasn't sure. Tapping her pencil on her paper, she gritted her teeth. "On the day after Lisa's disappearance, Rani Nixon came to see you. Is that right?"

"Yes," he said with a condescending smile. "She gave me Lisa's sweater. I took it home and sat alone, right here in this room, holding that sweater. And that's when I saw where she was."

"So, did you go into a trance or something? An out-of-body experience?"

"No trance. I just saw impressions of her in her Lexus, going into the water. Very similar to the one I see of you in a wedding dress."

She stared down at her notes and forced herself to go on. "How did you know exactly where on the river she was?"

"I just knew. It's very hard to explain, Blair. I saw her dead in the water, and I just knew exactly where it was. Half a mile

east of the Bull River Bridge. I know it sounds crazy. But that's the way it is."

She thought back over those Scripture passages she'd read this morning. "Carson, you mentioned that your power came from God. What religion are you?"

He seemed to stiffen. "I'm not really into religion, Blair. Not organized religion, anyway. I worship God in my mind. My body is his temple. And I like to think that the people who come to me for readings, whether it's here or at my show, feel that their experiences are very close to religious experiences."

That was telling. So his belief in God was ethereal. "Do you believe in heaven?"

"Yes, of course."

"What about hell?"

"I believe in a hell on earth. How else can you describe poverty, death, depression?"

"No hell," she jotted down. "Okay, so how about Satan?"

He chuckled as if he knew exactly what she was getting at. "Are you trying to figure out if I'm demon possessed?" He seemed genuinely delighted. "Look at me, Blair. Do I look evil?"

She had to admit he didn't. A little silly, maybe, but not evil.

"My power does not come from the Devil or demons, Blair. I'm gifted by God. It's as simple as that. God wanted Lisa to be found, and so he used me to do that."

Blair jotted that down verbatim, but didn't know if she would use it in her article. Cade was right. There would be readers who would conclude that Carson was a prophet from God.

"Blair, I think that God wants you to be happy, and he's going to use me to help you with that, too."

Again, anger pulsed through her. How dare he try to hit her vulnerability — and in the name of God!

"He's already thinking about marriage, Blair. This man you love can't imagine a life without you. I see a proposal in your very near future."

Her heart began to swell with hope, but then she remembered the Scripture. She wasn't supposed to listen to a psychic or believe in his prophecies. Besides, if he could really read Cade's feelings right now, he would see only anger . . . not romance.

"I have to go." She got up and shoved her pad back into her bag. "I think I have all I need."

"You work too hard, Blair. Yet you have the potential to turn the *Journal* into a

202

daily paper of great import. I advise you to hire a staff to help you and shoot high. I can already see the *Cape Refuge Journal* in a four-story building with dozens of employees. You're familiar with the old South Farm Insurance Building, aren't you? I see the *Journal* occupying that building, Blair."

She paused for a moment and looked up at him. She had never thought of using that building. It was too big. It seemed too soon to think that big.

"You must not be hindered by your logic."

It was as if he could read her thoughts.

"I see your circulation being far greater than the population of this island. You must be bold, fearless in your expansion. You must make daring decisions without looking back."

She felt the pull of his vision, the hope of his promise . . .

. . . and suddenly realized how seductive his words could be. No wonder millions of dollars a year were spent on psychic hotlines.

She started to the door, and he followed her. "You should come to my show one night. Then you could really see me in action. You could be my guest."

"Maybe sometime I will. Thanks for the

interview, Carson."

"So will this be in Friday's issue?"

"Maybe. I don't know for sure."

She got to her car and pulled out of the parking lot as fast as she could. As she drove away, she understood how easily people could be taken in by him.

He told them exactly what they wanted to hear.

32

The funeral was held in Savannah at an old, opulent church that Ben and Lisa had rarely attended. Seated in the pews was a Who's Who of the wealthiest people in the area. Morgan almost felt out of place.

The priest clearly didn't know Lisa. He talked about her in generic terms, read Scripture that had little to do with her, and gave a sermon on the battle between good and evil. She supposed that was his vague reference to Lisa's killer, and that the good was a veiled reference to God. How sad that at a time like this, the man of the cloth could give them nothing more than that.

Rani Nixon had been asked to give Lisa's eulogy, since she was her oldest friend. Rani had on a sleek black dress like something she would have worn on the cover of *Vogue*, with a sheer black sari thrown around her shoulders. Despite her sophistication and prideful carriage, she looked as fragile as blown glass.

Morgan prayed that the woman could get through it without tears.

Rani strode to the pulpit and stood there looking out at them, as if waiting for the camera to snap. Finally, she spoke. "Lisa Jackson was my best friend." Her mouth quivered at the corners. "I met her in college, when we were assigned together as roommates. I was this tall, lanky, skinny black kid who expected someone of my race as a roommate. Lisa came in, and the first thing she said was, 'You're black.'" Rani smiled weakly. "She always did have remarkable insight."

The crowd laughed softly, and Morgan's tension melted away. Rani could do this.

"I told her that if she had a problem sharing a dorm room with someone of a different race, I would be glad to go to the housing director and ask him to move me. She looked at me for a minute and said, 'It's not your race that worries me. It's your size. I was really hoping we could share our wardrobes.'"

Morgan smiled. That sounded like Lisa.

"She hugged me then, and we began to unpack, and before the day was over, she'd found four or five of my blouses that she could wear." She paused. "I don't think I ever saw those again."

More laughter. This was perfect. Since the murder, she'd only been able to dwell on the negatives in Lisa's life. It was good to remember the things that brought smiles.

Rani's smile faded, and her mouth trembled as she tried to hold back her tears. "We continued to live together for the next four years. We told each other every secret, concocted schemes together, and suffered through the ups and downs of romance. I remember the night she met Ben."

She stopped then, staring down at her notes, her nostrils flaring because of the struggle going on within her. "She said it was love at first sight. That he was her knight in shining armor. That she knew . . . nothing bad could ever happen to her if he was in her life."

She lost the battle with her tears then, and her face twisted with pain. Wetting her lips, she looked out at Ben, sitting in the front row. "Did you know that, Ben? Did you know she trusted you that much?"

Morgan touched Jonathan's hand, and he squeezed. She glanced at Ben in the front row and saw that his shoulders were shaking as he wept into his hands.

Blair, who sat on the other side of Jonathan, leaned up to meet Morgan's eyes.

What is she doing? her eyes asked.

"Lisa will be deeply missed." Rani went back to her notes. "My life will never be the same without her. No one's will, not if they knew her well."

She went back to her seat, wiping the tears off her face.

Morgan breathed a sigh of relief. For a moment there, she had expected something more. A confrontation, perhaps, given Rani's feelings about Ben and the letters.

Unfortunately, the danger was not over. As they all got into their cars for the funeral procession to the grave site, Morgan stopped Rani. "Do you want to ride with us, Rani?"

Rani's eyes followed Ben into the limo at the front of the line. He was weeping again and hugging a mourner. Rani's face tightened at the sight. Morgan wondered if she'd heard her.

"Rani?"

"What? Oh, no, I think I need to ride alone."

"Are you sure?"

"Yeah." She clipped off to her Roadster and slipped behind the wheel.

"She's right on the edge of losing it," Jonathan said.

"And she's sure he did it." Morgan realized she could hardly blame her. The letters didn't make Ben look good.

Yet Ben's grief seemed authentic. He was clearly broken, just as he'd been the day Lisa had been found.

They drove in the silent procession to a new memorial garden that wasn't yet sprinkled with graves.

Ben had chosen a lovely spot for Lisa's burial — on a hill beneath the shade of a sprawling oak tree and near a summer garden of marigolds, periwinkles, and brightly colored pansies. It was a soft reminder that life flourished, even where death was planted.

The graveside service was brief and somber, and after the priest had given his final words, Ben got up and hugged Lisa's weeping parents. They clung to each other before the casket, sobbing openly.

Morgan looked at Rani, saw that her eyes were dry. She sat with her hard eyes fixed on Ben, her lips tight across her teeth. She was a powder keg about to explode . . .

"Stop it!"

Everyone turned to look at Rani, as she came out of her chair. Tears stained her

dark face. "You're not fooling anyone!"

Ben let go of his in-laws and turned his wet face to Rani. "What?"

"Everyone here knows you're the one who put her in that car and shoved her into the river!"

Morgan gasped and reached for Rani. "Honey, don't —"

Rani jerked out of her grasp and strode toward Lisa's parents, who looked at her as if they'd just plunged into a new dimension of their grief. "He killed your daughter, Mr. and Mrs. Hinton. I know he did!"

Ben stepped toward her. "Rani, I know you're upset. We all are. But you can't go accusing me like that. I loved her."

Rani slapped him.

Morgan gasped as he stumbled back, almost falling.

"Are you crazy?" he shouted.

"You were having an affair!" She grabbed his shirt and shook him. "Who was she, Ben? Is she here? Did *she* make you do it?"

"Rani!" Lisa's mother said.

"That's a lie!" Ben cried. "It's not true!"

"Did Lisa finally get wise and threaten to leave you before the election?" Rani railed. "Did you kill her for the votes, Ben? Is that why Lisa's dead?"

Someone tried to restrain her, but she jerked away. Throwing her hands over her mouth, she ran back to her car.

Everyone stood frozen as Rani screeched away.

Morgan turned back to Ben. He stood there alone, sobbing as he looked around. "I didn't do it," he said softly. "I would never kill her. She was my bride. The letters were a lie." He broke down, and several friends came to hold him up.

Morgan couldn't escape that image of Rani's active rage, and she couldn't help wondering if she was right.

33

Blair rode back to Cape Refuge with Morgan and Jonathan. "That was unbelievable. Dramatic, but unbelievable. And I saw Vince Barr there. I'm sure he was taking notes."

Morgan looked back at her. "Don't be flip, Blair. It was very sad."

It was a day for reprimands, Blair thought. She was getting tired of it. She decided to switch gears. "Someone needs to tell Cade what happened. Jonathan, I nominate you."

Jonathan looked at her in the rearview mirror. "Me? Why not you?"

She sighed. "Because I don't think we're speaking."

Morgan twisted in her seat and looked back at her. "What happened?"

She sighed. "Today's paper happened. He went ballistic over the headline."

Morgan sent Jonathan a knowing look.

"Oh, don't tell me. You two are hot about it, too?"

"Not hot," Jonathan said. "But we wondered what you were thinking."

Blair leaned up on the seat. "Okay, so the headline rubbed you all the wrong way. It's no reason to question my Christianity."

"He did that?" Morgan asked. "Oh, Blair."

Blair leaned back and looked out the window. "He was furious at the *Observer* for telling about the shoes and printing those pictures, so he took it all out on me."

"He was probably just frustrated," Jonathan said. "His job's in jeopardy, you know. He doesn't need more fodder for his critics. But that's no reason for him to question your faith."

She thought of the things Cade had said that morning, and the pain came back again. "He did," she said softly. "Made me wonder if he's doubted it all along. I guess all this time he's been thinking that I faked a religious experience just to get his attention."

"Honey, he knows better than that."

"No, he doesn't, Morgan. I mean, if I was gonna do that, I'd have done it long before now. And can't he see that I've changed?"

213

Jonathan considered her words. "Of course he does. He just got his feathers ruffled. He's probably just tired and cranky."

"I'm the one who hasn't slept." Blair was quiet for the rest of the ride home. She wondered if Cade had nursed his anger for her all day.

When they reached Hanover House, a Mercedes Roadster sat in the driveway.

"Uh-oh," Morgan said. "Rani's here."

Blair perked up and got her notepad out of her bag. This could be interesting.

As they pulled up next to her, Rani got out of her car. Her eyes were red and puffy, but she had managed to pull herself together. "I need to talk to Blair," she announced as they opened the car doors.

Blair got out of the car, bracing herself. "What is it, Rani?"

Rani faced off with her, towering above her. "Don't write about what I did at the funeral, Blair. Please. It wouldn't serve any purpose."

"Rani, you did it in public, right out in front of everybody."

"But I just lost it! I don't want that in the papers. The gossip will be bad enough without you confirming it."

"I wasn't even the only media there,

Rani. This is a case of national interest now. Vince Barr from the *Observer* was there."

"I'll deal with him. But right now I'm asking you. Blair, please. If you have any decorum at all . . ."

Morgan and Jonathan turned to her, their eyes echoing Rani's pleading. So many critics, she thought. So many self-proclaimed editors.

"Okay, I won't write it. But this is the last time you or anyone else is going to tell me what to print."

Rani let out a breath.

"Are you okay?" Morgan asked her.

Rani shook her head. "No, I'm not. He killed her, Morgan. I know he did." She glanced back at Blair. "Off the record."

"Off the record, off the record," Blair mocked under her breath as Morgan led Rani to the porch. Why did people think *off the record* absolved them of any responsibility for the things they blurted? Didn't she have to agree that it was off the record? Weren't they supposed to say it *before* they spouted out revelations? Maybe she hadn't been in journalism long enough, but she knew manipulation when she saw it.

Rani sat down on the swing, and Morgan took the seat beside her, patting her hand

like the proverbial earth mother.

"They should have arrested him by now," Rani said. "Or at the very least, identified the other woman. They have the shoes. The letters. They should test them for fibers, fingerprints, handwriting. I watch *CSI*. I know what they can do. What are they waiting for?"

"They're going through all the evidence," Blair said. "They're not equipped to do this without outside help. The force is too small and their budget isn't adequate, which is why we need a new mayor. One who'll give enough money to the police force so they can do their jobs better."

"So what have you found out, Blair? Sometimes reporters can get to the heart of things faster than the police can."

Blair shook her head. "I haven't gotten any closer than the police have. And if I did, I wouldn't tell you two, because you'd try to talk me out of reporting it."

"Rani, I know how things look. But I really don't think it's Ben," Morgan said weakly. "I'm a good judge of those things, and I've been around him a lot in the last few days."

Blair almost laughed as she came up the porch. "No, you're not! You're a terrible

judge. You think with your heart. You let people convince you that they're good when they're really not. And do I need to remind you that just a week ago you thought Ben Jackson was the scum of the earth? You remember, Morgan. When he was putting up all those signs and running those ads, throwing hundred dollar bills around like they were M&Ms, while you and Jonathan could barely get fliers into the hands of the voters?"

"So we were competitive with him. It wasn't like we thought he was a killer!"

"And speaking of the election," Blair said, "I don't think Jonathan should stop campaigning just because of this. It's too important. He's got to win this race. He should get back to work this very after-noon. Door-to-door, shaking hands, person-to-person."

Morgan bristled. "It doesn't hurt to take a few days off of campaigning to honor someone who's just lost his wife."

"You don't see Sam Sullivan taking time off."

Morgan threw up her hands. "Fine. Let him move ahead. I'm tired of this whole mess."

"Me, too." Rani sat there a moment as if trying to hold herself together. "I really

miss her. I keep wanting to pick up the phone and tell her stuff. Who am I gonna talk to now?"

Blair looked down at her feet. She knew that feeling. There were still times when she picked up the phone to dial her mother. She wondered how long that would last.

She looked back at Rani. Was she just seeking friendship and someone to talk to, or had she really come by to shut Blair up?

Maybe Blair would get to know Rani better, when all of this died down. They had a few things in common now, after all. By the time it was all behind them, they each might need a friend.

34

Cade found that the lab report on Ben's shoes answered the questions the media had already answered. The dirt on the shoes *was* the same dirt found at the scene where Lisa's car had been pushed in. That, added to the phone cord that had come from Ben's home — the same cord that had been used to strangle Lisa — as well as the alibi that couldn't be confirmed, gave Cade probable cause for an arrest, and the DA had insisted that he go ahead and bring Ben in.

He'd hoped to make the arrest quietly, but there were already dozens of media standing outside Ben's place, taking pictures of every person who came or went. They shouted questions at Cade and his officers as they went to the door.

Ben opened it before they could ring the bell. He took one look at Cade, then threw up his hands. "What do you want?"

Cade stepped inside, out of the sight of the reporters. Johnson and Caldwell came

in behind him. "Ben, we have a warrant to arrest you for Lisa's murder —"

"Cade, I can explain the shoes. They were in her car. I left them in there the day before when we went for our appointment. She picked me up at work, and I changed my shoes because I didn't want to wear dirty tennis shoes to the doctor. The killer must have gotten them out and used them to set me up."

"Ben, we found them in your bedroom, under your bed."

"I didn't put them there! Don't you understand?"

Cade nodded for Johnson to cuff him. "I'm sorry, Ben."

"Cade, don't do this! You know I didn't kill my wife!"

Cade didn't like doing it, especially when he still had such deep reservations about Ben being the killer, but he couldn't go by his gut. He had to go by the evidence, and the DA had given him orders.

He hated parading Ben through the reporters, allowing them to get pictures of the grieving husband whose life had been twisted into pieces. If Ben turned out to be innocent, Cade wasn't sure he would ever forgive himself.

"Is this about the shoes, Sheriff?" Vince

Barr called out through the cameras.

Cade turned back to him. "I'm not the sheriff. I'm the police chief. At least get your facts straight before you go on national television with your wild tabloid stories, Barr."

As he got Ben into the squad car and drove him away from the circus, Cade vowed he wouldn't rest on this arrest.

Until he was absolutely convinced that Ben was guilty, he would keep looking for Lisa's killer.

35

The fertility clinic had a cancellation for Wednesday afternoon. Morgan had been thrilled to get in so soon, but then it hit her that the cancellation might well have been Lisa's daily appointment.

Jonathan seemed as nervous as she as they stepped into the clinic that they hoped would change their lives. Women and men of various ages sat around the room, paging through magazines or talking softly. One woman with a baby sat in the corner, a testimony to the success of the clinic.

Morgan felt a surge of hope. Maybe one day she would come in here with her own baby in her arms. She checked in and filled out the paperwork, and then they waited.

She grew more tense as the moments ticked by, and when her name was finally called, she almost jumped out of her seat.

The nurse led them to the doctor's office. He wasn't there yet, so she looked

around at all his medical degrees. A bulletin board with baby pictures hung on the wall behind their chairs. "Look, Jonathan."

He turned and looked up at the pictures, some of them of multiple births. "I think we're in the right place," he said.

Dr. Sims came in after a few minutes. He bore a strong resemblance to Mark Harmon, the actor, and he had kind eyes. He greeted them both warmly, then took his seat behind the desk. "I saw you at Lisa's funeral yesterday," he said in a quiet voice. "Were you good friends?"

"Yes, we'd gotten to be over the last few weeks. She's the one who wanted me to come see you."

He adjusted himself in his seat, then looked down at Morgan's file. After a moment, she realized he was struggling with his emotion.

"It's terrible what happened to her." He rubbed his eyes and cleared his throat. "It's such a tragedy. And what happened at the funeral yesterday . . ." He brought his troubled eyes to Morgan's. "You don't think he actually killed her, do you?"

The question surprised Morgan. "We've been with him since before she was found. He's a wreck. I can't imagine that he did."

He stared at the file again, unseeing. "I

considered them both friends. When you see somebody as often as I see some of my patients, for years at a time, and you know their deepest longings and you're trying to help them fulfill them . . . you get close to them." His voice broke, and he clasped his hands in front of his mouth. "It's very hard."

"We feel the same way, Doctor," Jonathan said.

He sat up straighter, took a deep breath, then scanned her records. "Well, you certainly have reason to come here. Anytime you've been trying over a year to get pregnant and it hasn't happened, one has to wonder why."

"We're not sure that we're ready to go the whole infertility route, Doc," Jonathan said. "We just want to know what's wrong. Then we'll decide if we want to pursue it."

"Of course. That's what I recommend to all my patients. You have to know what your options are. The first thing I'd like to do is to test Jonathan to see if his readings are normal."

"Me?" Jonathan asked. "But Morgan's already been pregnant. Wouldn't that mean that things are all right with me?"

"It's routine, Jonathan. It's an easy test, just to make sure you don't have a problem

that, combined with Morgan's, is making it harder for her to get pregnant. If nothing's wrong with you, then we'll do what's called a hysterosalpingogram for you, Morgan."

Morgan had never heard of that. "A what?"

He smiled. "We call it a hysterogram for short. It's when we shoot dye into your uterus and fallopian tubes to check for blockages. That'll tell us if the problem is with you. Then we'll know how to proceed."

"So when can we get started?" Jonathan asked.

"Well, we can test you today, Jonathan, if that's all right."

"Of course." Morgan laughed. "I didn't expect to jump in so soon."

"Why wait?" Sims' voice softened. "I'm very hopeful that you're going to have a baby soon, and this time, you'll carry it to term. In fact, I feel this is a personal goal. Lisa died before she could ever hold a baby in her arms. Let's make sure that we get it right with you."

36

"So you think this is going to work, huh?"

Blair had come over to Hanover House to hear about the doctor visit, but her question was heavy with skepticism.

Morgan sat at the table, Caleb in her lap. The child was finger painting with chocolate pudding and working on a picture that Morgan held still. It looked like mocha chaos, but Caleb was thrilled with the effort.

"I don't know. We'll see what the test results show."

"Is he going to put you through the hormonal wringer, like he does all those other women?"

"I hope not."

"See?" Caleb cried out, indicating that he was finished.

She kissed Caleb's chubby cheek and picked up his picture. "Look how beautiful this is. Caleb, this is the best picture you've done! Blair, isn't this wonderful?"

Blair grinned and ruffled the child's hair.

"Caleb, that's beautiful," she said in a delighted voice. "It looks like the inner workings of a headache."

"Blair!" Morgan grinned. Caleb thought it was high praise. "We have to let it dry now."

"More," he said.

"All right. I think you've got enough pudding for five more on your hands." She got another piece of manila paper and set it in front of them. As Caleb began slapping it with his chocolate-blobbed hands, Blair set her chin on her palm.

"So is this doctor going to make you jump through hoops?"

"I hope it won't come to that. We won't know anything until he sees the test results, and maybe they'll tell us everything. Maybe it's just a mild case of something that they can fix. A blocked tube or something. He'll find it. I know he will."

"Morgan, maybe you just haven't given it enough time. Maybe you're jumping ahead of God."

"I don't think so. I think he's given me this doctor to help me with the process. He does work through doctors, sometimes."

"Of course he does, but I don't want to see you get as caught up in this as Ben and Lisa were."

Caleb finished his picture again and began licking his hands. His face looked as if he'd been bobbing for apples in a bucketful of cocoa.

"I'm serious, Morgan. You're not going to make this an obsession, are you?"

Morgan took the baby to the sink. "Lisa and Ben were desperate to have a baby. They were doing whatever it took. What's wrong with that?"

"I'm not sure, but there needs to be balance."

"Well, let's see if you feel the same way if you ever have trouble getting pregnant."

Blair almost laughed. "Me? I can't even keep a relationship, much less do the family thing."

"What do you mean, you can't keep a relationship? Hasn't he called?"

"Nope. I haven't talked to him since he chewed me out yesterday."

Morgan cleaned Caleb up, then set him down. He toddled to his toy basket. She regarded her sister. "Are you okay?" But she could see that Blair wasn't.

"I could have sworn we were getting closer. He was over Monday night, and we had a real tender moment there . . . But now I think he's lost interest. I can't believe he questioned my faith."

Morgan wiped the pudding off the table, then rinsed her rag out over the sink. "He didn't mean it."

"Yes, he did. All these years he's known me as a proud unbeliever, and I guess that's a tough image to shake, but I would never fake my conversion. I don't do that kind of thing, and he knows it."

"Maybe you've blown his silence way out of proportion. Maybe he's just busy. He knows what you're like, and he knows you've changed." She dried her hands. "Besides, I think he's secretly been in love with you since before you believed."

"In love?" Blair uttered the words with astonishment. "He's never told me he loved me, and there's not one thing to indicate that he had feelings for me then."

"No, not one thing. More like a dozen things. I could see it in his eyes. It was pretty clear, even though he never would have made a move. He takes the Bible very seriously when it says not to yoke yourself with unbelievers."

"Well, I'm not an unbeliever now. It's maddening, this feeling of being at his mercy. All these years I was content knowing that I was going to be alone, that no man would have me because of these hideous scars."

"They're not hideous."

"And finally, now I've had a taste of what it's like to be in love. I don't much like being that vulnerable."

Morgan just smiled. "He'll call you, Blair. You know he will."

"When?"

"I don't know when, but he will. Just give him a little credit, okay? He's not the type to just dump somebody without telling them."

"But we never had an understanding or anything. Can you dump someone that you've never had any kind of commitment to?"

"Cade would never lead you on if he didn't intend to follow through."

"Well, he's not leading me on now. I'm just sitting here like an idiot, waiting for a phone call. I hate that."

"I know you do, but you do it very well." She laughed. "He's going to call eventually, but right now he's just stressed out. You'll hear from him soon enough."

The telephone rang, and Morgan laughed. "Maybe that's him now."

Blair grunted. "Fat chance. Maybe the results of your tests?"

"Too soon." Morgan picked up the phone. "Hello?"

"May I speak to Morgan or Jonathan Cleary?" It was a man's voice, crisp and rapid.

"This is Morgan."

"Morgan, this is Anthony Hammond. I'm the attorney for Sheila Caruso."

Morgan caught her breath. "Yes, what can I do for you, Mr. Hammond?"

Caleb started pounding a wooden spoon on his toy piano. Morgan motioned for Blair to distract him.

"I wanted to let you know that Sheila's going to be released in a little over a week."

Morgan froze. *"What?"*

Blair picked Caleb up and looked at her. "What is it?"

Morgan held her hand up to quiet her. "How can she be released in a week? She was supposed to be in for four more years."

"The legislature issued a new law a couple of weeks ago that nonviolent offenders only have to serve twenty percent of their sentence. She's already served that."

"Yes, I heard that might be a possibility, but I didn't think —" His words ricocheted through her head, making her dizzy. She groped for a chair. "What are her plans, Mr. Hammond? Regarding her children, I mean."

"I'm not sure yet, but she plans to contact her daughter soon. I just felt you should be notified, as the foster parent of her children."

When he hung up, Morgan set the phone back in its cradle. Her mind raced with images of her foster children being dragged away. She took Caleb from Blair and held him tight.

"Sheila's getting out?" Blair asked in a whisper.

"That's right." Her voice sounded as if it came from someone else. "Next week."

"No way! Morgan, what are her plans?"

"I don't know." She choked the words out. "But she's going to want her kids."

Caleb touched her face. She took his hand and kissed it. "She can't take him back, Blair. She's not ready to be a mother."

"Oh, Sis." She reached out to Morgan, pulling her into a hug. "What are you gonna do?"

Morgan tried to think. She couldn't let it happen. Sheila was not equipped to care for Caleb. Her irresponsibility had almost gotten both of her children killed.

"There's only one answer. She'll have to come here. We'll just have to convince her to do that, and then she can mother Caleb

as much as she wants to, right here in our home. And so can I."

"Do you think she will?"

"We'll just have to convince her." Fear took hold of Morgan's heart, for she knew Sheila might have other plans.

37

The test was the hardest and most important one Sadie had taken all year. She had studied her brains out, and she had a headache and a cramp in her hand from writing the essay questions.

Already half the class had turned their exam papers in. All she had to do was take the test up to her teacher and tenth grade would finally be behind her. Then she could work full-time for Blair for the summer and stop worrying about the stress and dread of being a seventeen-year-old sophomore.

She finally realized she had done her absolute best and couldn't improve on any of her answers, so she got her books and turned the test in.

"Thank you, Sadie." Mrs. Whitlow smiled at her. "Have a good summer."

She walked out into the hall. Lockers were slamming in celebration as students came out of their exams, exhila-

rated that school was over.

But no one was happier than she. She walked up the corridor, wishing she'd never have to see this place again. She had begged Morgan to let her homeschool next year so she could work more hours for Blair. Neither Morgan nor Jonathan liked the idea.

But she hadn't given up. If being a seventeen-year-old sophomore was bad, being an eighteen-year-old junior was sure to be worse. She had come to Cape Refuge a sixteen-year-old ninth-grade dropout, running for her life from her mother's drug-addicted, violent boyfriend. Everyone in the school knew of her checkered past, and her few attempts at fitting in had been disastrous. Her hours at school were among the loneliest of her life.

When she got home, she heard the sounds of Caleb laughing in the kitchen and baby Emory crying upstairs. She loved those sounds. It sounded like a family, a warm contrast to the social chills she got at school.

"I'm home!" she cried out.

"Hey, sweetie." Morgan came out of the kitchen. She still didn't look good since her miscarriage — her face was pale, and she'd lost a few pounds. Sadie knew she

wasn't eating or sleeping much. She hoped Morgan was really all right. "How was your exam?"

"Not bad. Now I'm free." Sadie set her backpack near the bottom of the stairs so she could take it up when she went.

"I have some good news for you."

Sadie examined her face. Morgan didn't look like she had good news. She seemed to be balancing on the edge of tears. "What?"

"It's about your mother." She planted a smile on her face. It was a valiant effort, but it didn't reach to her eyes. "You were right. God is giving her a second chance."

"She's getting out?" The words burst out of her.

"Next week," Morgan said.

Sadie let out a scream and began jumping up and down. She hugged Morgan. "Did you talk to her?"

"No, her lawyer called."

Sadie squealed. "Oh, my gosh! I bet she's just freaking out." She ran into the kitchen and found Caleb sitting among several pots and pans that he banged on with his favorite wooden spoon. She grabbed him up and kissed him. "Caleb, Mom's coming home!"

He giggled, though he didn't have a clue

what she was talking about.

"Mom's coming home!" She swung around to Morgan. "She's coming here, right?"

Morgan's smile faltered. "I don't know, honey."

"But she has to. We can't leave." Only then did Sadie understand the reason for the tension on Morgan's face.

"She's welcome here," Morgan said.

"Oh, Morgan, do you think she'll come?"

Tears came to Morgan's eyes, and she took Caleb out of Sadie's arms. "I hope so."

Any other possibility seemed too far-fetched to consider. Sadie thought of her mother coming here, seeing the beautiful house, and soaking up the love and warmth of the family. She had never really had that before. "She will. I'll convince her. Don't worry, Morgan. It's going to be all right. I'll go visit her Saturday and talk her into it. Where else would she go?"

With that, she ran up the stairs and began to clean up her room, to prepare for her mother.

38

"How do you people work in this place? Can you at least turn up the air-conditioner?"

Cade looked at the cocky detective at the back of the group. He'd had to cram all of the crime scene investigators — three from the State Police, plus McCormick and himself — into the small interview room at the police department. It wasn't big enough for this many people.

"Yeah," someone else complained. "Place feels like a boiler room."

"Or maybe a laundromat." The three guest detectives laughed.

Cade didn't find it amusing. "We're trying to cool it down. I'll make this fast." He stood in front of the dry-erase boards he had temporarily hung on the wall and pointed to the column with "BODY" at the top. "Strangle marks on her neck. No other bruises or cuts, no signs of a struggle. The medical examiner put her death at ten-thirty Friday morning. She was dead be-

fore she went into the water."

"So the husband is in custody?" one of the detectives asked.

"That's right. The DA wanted me to bring him in, but the truth is, he doesn't have enough of a case to convict. And I'm not entirely convinced the husband's the killer. The letters, shoes, and telephone cord do seem to implicate him, but he claims that the shoes were in her car at the time of the murder and that the killer must have brought them back to his house and put them under the bed where we'd find them."

"That's a stretch."

"Yeah, it is," Cade admitted. "And then there's the phone cord that came from their house. And we have the letters. Don't yet know where they came from, but we have handwriting analysts working on that. Either there was another woman, which certainly could be the motive, or someone was trying to sabotage Ben Jackson's marriage . . ."

"Or his campaign," McCormick added.

"Have you considered one of his opponents?" someone asked.

"Could be," Cade said. "Alibi's iffy. And he's been pretty cut-throat during this campaign."

"What about the other one?"

"Jonathan Cleary?" Cade knew Jonathan hadn't done it, but he didn't want to appear biased. "Has a strong alibi. His wife had a miscarriage that morning. They were at the hospital, then he didn't leave her until later in the day. The residents of their house are witnesses."

A knock sounded on the door, and he opened it. Alex Johnson stood there with an uncomfortable look on his face. "Uh . . . Chief. You may want to take a look at this. That *Observer* guy is on FOX News again."

Cade groaned and stepped into the squad room. The television was on in the corner, with the volume turned down low. Video was playing of Ben's arrest, of Cade walking him through the crowd to the squad car, and of Cade's comments about not being the sheriff.

Vince had made him look like a jerk. Cade turned it up and heard Vince talking over the video. ". . . rumors that Ben Jackson was having an affair. It seems that the other woman had been writing letters to Lisa, telling her about the affair. According to her friend Rani Nixon, Lisa had confronted her husband about the affair, but he convinced her it was a hoax."

Cade just stood there, frozen, trying to stay calm. In the reflection of the television screen, he saw that all of the detectives in the meeting had come out and were watching it, too.

He brought his hand up and raked his fingers through his hair. He was glad Vince Barr wasn't within his reach. He might have actually given the national media a new story to cover.

Cade turned back to the men. "I guess the meeting's over. McCormick, tell them what we need from them."

His jaw flexed as he went into his office and put his foot up on the desk. If he could keep the media out of his way long enough to conduct this investigation, they might actually figure out who the killer was.

The media would try Ben in the court of public opinion, before they even had a case that could convict him. Meanwhile, if Ben wasn't their guy, the real killer was getting a good laugh out of the whole blasted thing.

39

The test results cleared Jonathan of blame for their fertility problems, which laid it squarely at Morgan's feet. Dr. Sims scheduled a hysterogram for the next day and assured her they would know more after that.

Morgan knew she should be grateful that the first test had shown no problems, but a heaviness lay over her heart at the thought of the road they were headed down.

When she saw Sam Sullivan's car pulling into the driveway, she thought of meeting him at the door and warning him that Jonathan was on his boat, trying to earn a living, and that she wasn't in the mood for his harassment today.

Instead, she met him out on the porch and forced herself to greet him like she would any other visitor.

He looked as if he'd just won the lottery. "Did you hear that Ben has been taken off the ballot?"

Morgan crossed her arms. "Where did you hear that?"

"Down at City Hall. There was a question on whether he qualified to run, given his arrest, but apparently he told them to pull him out of the race. Looks like it's just Jonathan and me now. We've officially rescheduled the debate for a week from Saturday."

"That's fine, Sam. That'll be three days before the election."

He chuckled and rubbed his hands together as if he couldn't wait to take Jonathan on. "Sure he's up to a one-on-one?"

Morgan tried to smile. "I'm sure he's ready, Sam."

He started back to his car, but stopped before getting in. "Oh, by the way, did you hear about the deal I just made for a cell phone tower on the island?"

Her smile faltered. "No, I didn't."

"I sold them some of my land. Prime real estate. We'll have cell service out here before we know it."

He winked like a car salesman and got into his Mercedes.

Morgan watched him drive away. So that was his ace in the hole. He would become the island hero by giving the people something they wanted.

It would be hard to compete with that. She only hoped the people had sense enough to see past it.

40

Cade hadn't planned to come to the City Council meeting tonight. He had enough to do and didn't relish wasting time with this group of gabbing, self-important council members, but they had demanded his presence and an update on the investigation.

He asked them to put him first on the agenda so he could get in and out quickly, but as was always the case, they ignored his wishes, bickering about when the next meeting was going to be and who would be introducing the candidates at the upcoming debate.

He looked at his watch and wished they would hurry.

Finally, they came to an agreement, and Art Russell banged his gavel.

"Next on the agenda tonight we'd like to address some questions to Chief Cade. Cade, would you mind stepping up to the microphone, please?"

Cade looked around. Other than council

members, there were only six people in attendance tonight. "What do I need a microphone for, Art? There's nobody here."

"Very well. Stay where you are. We wanted to talk to you about this investigation and how much it's costing Cape Refuge."

Sarah Williford had a Tootsie Pop in her mouth. She took it out to address him. "Cade, you're way over your department's budget on this."

"That's right," Cade said. "I never budgeted in a murder. Since I only have one detective in the department, I had to go to outside departments to do the crime scene investigations. And yes, they do have to be paid for the overtime hours. Some of that money will come from the state, and some of it will come from their own departments, but we are going to have to come up with some of it."

"How long are you going to need those folks?" George O'Neal asked from the end of the table. He must have been out fishing today, for his skin was ridiculously red. "You've made an arrest. Looks like you could send them on their way."

"Come on, George. We're going to use the help as long as we need it. There's more to an investigation than making an

arrest. I can't short-circuit this investigation just to save the city a few bucks."

Sarah piped in. "I'm just saying that you don't have to drag it out if you already know who did it."

Cade cleared his throat and tried to stay calm. "Sarah, I'm not going to try and explain to you the finer points of investigating a homicide. You're just going to have to trust me to do my job."

"We're just saying you don't need an outside group to help you solve a murder that's already been solved."

"This is why your days as chief are numbered," Art Russell muttered.

Cade ground his teeth, the muscles in his jaw popping, and considered handing them his resignation right then and there, but he couldn't let pride and emotion guide him. "I have no intention of discussing the details of this case in front of this body. And I will not close an investigation just for your convenience or your budget. Now, if you'll excuse me, I have work to do."

Cade turned and limped back to the door he'd come in and prayed again that Jonathan would be elected mayor, before the business of this town got further out of hand.

41

Cade sat at his desk, staring down at the paperwork he had to deal with before he could get back to the investigation. Anger still beat through him at the City Council's audacity.

What did they expect him to do? With a force of fourteen people, including himself, it was impossible to evaluate the evidence from the car, the body, the bank of the river, the Jackson house, Lisa's business, Ben's boat, and all the other possible crime scenes, without outside help.

"Hey, Chief. Somebody here to see you."

Cade looked up at Alex. "I'm kind of busy."

"It's Lisa Jackson's parents."

Cade sat back hard and rubbed his eyes. He couldn't send them away. They were probably crazy with grief over their daughter. He looked around. He had reports stacked up on the chair in front of his desk and three feet of files on his desk.

If he moved anything, he'd lose his whole train of thought.

He could meet them in the interview room, but first he'd have to remove the dry erase boards he'd been charting the investigation on. He couldn't let them see them.

"Alex, do me a favor. Go in the interview room and turn those boards to face the wall. I'll take them in there."

"Will do, Chief."

Cade got his cane and limped out of the office. The couple stood at the door, looking awkwardly around. The woman, who appeared to be just over sixty, had a vacant expression in her eyes as she stared at the air. Her fingers rubbed her white collar nervously. Lisa's father wore an expression that hovered between despair and indignation.

"Mr. and Mrs. Hinton, I'm Chief Matthew Cade," he said in a soft voice. "Sorry to keep you waiting."

Lisa's father shook his hand. "Al Hinton. My wife, Marge."

Cade led them into the interview room and gestured for them to sit down. He closed the door and took his seat at the table. "Mr. and Mrs. Hinton, first let me say how sorry I am about your loss."

Mr. Hinton cleared his throat. "We need to know if . . . we need to understand . . ."

"Why would Ben kill our daughter?" Marge blurted.

Cade knew that Ben's arrest had to make their tragedy double-edged. "Mrs. Hinton, your son-in-law is innocent until proven guilty. I can't really discuss the details of the investigation."

"Just tell us, is it true about the shoes and the letters?" Al asked in a raspy voice. "That's all they're talking about on the news."

Cade thought of Vince Barr and all the damage he was doing to this case. "There were some shoes found in Ben and Lisa's house, and they matched the footprints at the scene of the crime."

"And there were letters from some girl-friend?"

"We don't yet know who those letters were from or even that they were true."

Mrs. Hinton got up and stared down at him through raw, swollen eyes. "Chief Cade, we've loved Ben all these years. He's like a son to us. We can't imagine he would do such a thing, that he would hurt our daughter when he seemed to love her so much."

"Has he said why?" Al asked. "Has he

given any indication of what might have caused this?"

Cade wanted very much to tell them that he wasn't convinced that Ben was the killer, that he may indeed be the devoted husband they believed, but doing so would undermine the district attorney and make things even worse than they were already.

"Would you like to see him and ask him yourself?"

Al looked like he might seize the opportunity, but Marge began to cry harder. "I can't look him in the eye, knowing he might have hurt Lisa. I can't sit there and listen to him lie."

Cade got up and went around the table to Mrs. Hinton. He bent down to her and touched her shoulder. "Ma'am, I can tell you that the investigation is not over. We're still gathering evidence, still getting tips. All the pieces of this puzzle aren't in place yet. It could be that things will change. When's the last time you spoke to your daughter?"

"The night before she disappeared." She dug into her purse for a tissue and dabbed at her nose. "She called and was anxious over the IVF. She felt it had to work, that it was her last chance to get pregnant."

"Did she mention anything else she was

upset or worried about?"

"No, not at all. We talked about my arthritis. I dominated the conversation." She stopped and tried to rein her emotions in. "I wouldn't have, if I'd known it was the last time I'd ever talk to her. I would have told her I loved her. I would have listened more."

Cade wished he could take off his chief-of-police hat, and just hold her hand to comfort her. "Don't you think she knew you loved her?"

Al put his arm around her, and she laid her head on his shoulder and wept. "She knows, Mother. Lisa knows."

Marge looked up at Cade, her eyes pleading. "Do you think she suffered, Chief Cade? Do you think it was a horrible death?"

"No ma'am," he whispered. "It looks like her death was quick." He didn't know that for sure, but it was the only thing kind enough to say. "Mr. and Mrs. Hinton, whoever did this to your daughter will be brought to justice. I'll see to it here, and God is going to see to it in the next life."

But it didn't satisfy the mourning couple. He supposed nothing ever would.

42

"He met her on the Internet, and next thing we knew he had run off to South America to marry the girl. Brought her back with her four kids, both parents, and a bedridden grandmother who we've been supporting ever since. If that ain't bad enough, her ex-husband comes high-tailin' it after 'em, threatenin' to kill my boy."

Morgan lay on the hospital bed, watching the IV drip into her arm, grateful for the conversation going on just beyond the curtain. The unsuspecting nurse had gone to prep the woman for surgery and been treated to the saga of her family. Morgan had to admit it was fascinating and got her mind off of the hysterogram. She hadn't slept last night, fearing the procedure and what it might reveal.

When it was time, they wheeled her into a sterile room and sedated her with an amnesiac drug. The next thing she knew, the procedure was over, and she had no

memory of it. Jonathan was with her. He helped her get dressed, then they waited for the results.

When Dr. Sims came in, he looked cheerful. Hope fluttered to life in her heart.

"How are you feeling?"

"Okay," she said. "Do you have my results?"

"I sure do." He took the rolling chair and sat down in it, crossing his legs. "I think it's good news again. There were no blockages, no endometriosis, nothing evident to keep you from getting pregnant."

"Yes!" Jonathan punched the air.

Morgan knew she should be happy, but she couldn't muster any joy. "Nothing? Nothing at all?" She tried to swallow the constriction in her throat and turned her troubled eyes to Jonathan. His excitement deflated visibly. "I was hoping you'd find something you could fix. But if you didn't, do we just go on like this? Unable to get pregnant, then when I do, losing the baby?"

"I understand your feelings, Morgan." The doctor smiled and patted her knee. "We're not finished yet. We're going to take some blood from you before you go home. We'll do an FSH test and see what

your follicle-stimulating hormone level is. We'll see if that could be the problem."

Jonathan squeezed her hand. "And what if it is that?"

"Well, that would mean that you're having trouble producing enough eggs. We can put you on a hormone called Pergonal, which may help you with that, and there are a number of options." He looked into her face. "Morgan, I'm not going to give up until we see a baby in your arms. You got that?"

Morgan tried to smile. "Thank you, Doctor." She glanced at Jonathan. "But I'm also worried about the cost of all this. Being self-employed, we don't have very good health insurance. We're not even sure it'll pay for the hysterogram. If we don't find something soon, I'm not sure we can afford to go further."

"We'll go further," Jonathan said. "We'll go as far as we need to. We may just have to take time between tests to save up."

"I'm sure we can work something out," Sims said. "Just get with my bookkeeper, and she'll give you some options." He grinned and winked at Jonathan. "Of course, if you're elected mayor, you'll be on the city's health insurance. Some policies even provide for one or two IVF procedures."

Morgan hadn't thought of that. She looked hopefully at Jonathan.

"Guess it would be one of the perks of the job."

"Now all you have to do is get elected." Sims started from the room. "You've got my vote." He looked back at them before closing the door. "I'll send someone in to take your blood, Morgan. We'll call you with the results sometime Monday. Chin up, okay? You're going to be a mommy before you know it."

43

"I'm comin' home, baby!" Sheila Caruso stood on the other side of the prison's visitation glass the next day, her arms raised in a victory celebration.

Laughing, Sadie slapped her hands against the glass.

Morgan smiled at the exchange. Though Sheila was being released in just a few days, Morgan had decided to come with Sadie to visit her today, hoping she could help her talk her mother into coming to Hanover House.

Sheila was still a pretty woman, even with the lines of years of drug abuse etched onto her face. Her hair was a golden blonde and shone as if she'd used some fifty-bucks-a-bottle conditioner on it. Her eyes were as blue and round as Sadie's. When Sheila grabbed up the phone, Sadie put her receiver between her ear and Morgan's, so they could both hear her.

"I'm getting out!" Sheila yelled. "Can you believe it?"

"Mom, I'm so excited!"

"I was sitting in my cell feeling sorry for myself, and my lawyer comes to visit me. So I come down here and he tells me and I just went, like, nuts, jumping up and down and hollering. They threatened me with lockdown if I didn't shut up."

Morgan tried to jump in. "We're really excited for you, Sheila."

"Mom, you remember Morgan."

"Of course I do. Hey, Morgan."

Morgan took the phone. "Sheila, I wanted to come with Sadie today because I wanted to let you know that we would love for you to come and stay with us when you get out. Sadie and Caleb are doing very well at Hanover House, and we were really hoping you would join them there. That would give you time to get on your feet, get a job, and save some money."

"Yeah, Mom. It's a beautiful place. You'd really like it."

The zeal in Sheila's eyes seemed to go dull as she clutched the phone. "Are you sure you want me to?"

"Yes," Morgan said. "We have a vacant room. And it's a great answer because you could be with Caleb and Sadie

without uprooting them."

Sheila began to jitter. "I've thought about it some. But I don't know if it's the right thing." She looked at Morgan through the glass. "Don't get me wrong, now. I'm so grateful to you and your husband for all you've done for my kids. I really am. I'm just not sure what I want to do."

Morgan's heart sank. *Please God . . .*

"Caleb's really happy there, Mom." Sadie's voice was tight and louder than normal. "It would really hurt him if you moved him now."

Sheila shook her head. "But he's my son. He needs to get to know me again."

"He will!" Morgan's words burst out on a rush of fear. She swallowed and tried to steady her voice. "He is your son, Sheila. I just thought we could make it a little easier for him —"

Sheila sighed. "I didn't even think you would take somebody like me without making me fill out an application, get a bunch of references . . . or something like that. Hanover House doesn't take just anybody."

Morgan's chest had locked tight and her breathing was shallow. She tried to stay calm. "It's true, we do have an application

process, but since we already have your children, we're going to make it easy for you. You'll still have to abide by our rules and follow our structured program. We are a Christian home, Sheila, and we try very hard to give the people who come to live with us a new way of life. We give them a foundation in the Bible so that when they're on their own, they can live by those principles. And best of all, it's free. You can stay there without charge until you start working, and then we have a sliding fee for room and board until you're able to live on your own."

"Abiding by the rules," Sheila repeated. "See, that's the thing. I've been abiding by rules for the last year now. I don't think I'd like it too much to have somebody telling me what I can and can't do."

Morgan kicked herself for choosing the wrong words. If she hadn't mentioned rules, maybe it would have gone down easier. "So often people who get out of jail wind up in desperate situations, unable to pay their rent or buy food, and the stress of life outside causes them to go back to drugs. We've had a really high success rate with people standing on their own and never going back to jail after they get out of our program."

"It's a really good program, Mom," Sadie said. "The house is beautiful, and it's in the greatest town in the world, and the people in the house are like a real family."

"But I *have* a family."

Panic hit Morgan like a tidal wave. Sheila was going to take Caleb and Sadie away. That little boy would be ripped out of his home, away from the people he loved.

For the second time, she would lose a child.

"Mom, what's wrong?" Sadie asked. "Don't you understand how great this is? Where else do you have to go?"

"I have friends who can help me get started. Until I get on my feet."

Sadie's look broke Morgan's heart. "But you know what those friends do to you! Mom, I don't want you to go back down to that again. Being dependent on those people who call themselves your friends. Getting involved with some guy who treats you awful and ruins your life. And ours, too."

Morgan put her arm around Sadie to calm her, but then she saw the possessive, bitter look on Sheila's face. She let her go.

"I won't do that again, baby. I've learned my lesson."

Morgan thought of telling her that she wouldn't have to follow the rules if that was what was dissuading her. She could come and go as she pleased, do anything she wanted, if she would just let her keep Caleb.

But she knew better.

Her mouth trembled, and she knew she couldn't hold back the tears any longer. She didn't want Sheila to know how desperately she wanted this. She sensed that would play against her.

"Tell you what," she said. "I'll leave you and Sadie to talk about this alone. If you have any questions, I'll come back and talk to you before we leave."

Sheila put her face in her palm, and Morgan knew Sadie's expression had hurt her, too. "I'll just be out in the front room if you need me, Sadie."

She hurried out of the room before the tears assaulted her. By the time she reached the waiting room, she was sobbing. She found a chair at the back of the room and sat down facing the wall. Covering her face, she wept quietly. No one around her seemed to notice or care.

In the visitation room, Sadie tried not to cry. "It would be cruel to take Caleb away

from Hanover House." Her voice was soft, careful. "He's really bonded with Morgan and Jonathan."

Sheila's face hardened. "He's mine, not theirs."

"I know, but it's going to take time for him to warm up to you again. You said yourself that he doesn't know you."

Sheila looked wounded. "And how will he *get* to know me if they're around all the time?"

"He will, Mom. He takes to people. He loves everybody in the home. He'll warm right up to you."

"I want him to know that I'm his mother, and she's not."

"Mom, he will know that eventually. But he's been with them longer than he's been with you."

"That's not my fault!"

Isn't it? Sadie wanted to say. Wasn't it all her fault for putting her drugs and her men above her children?

Sheila leaned forward, clutching the phone to her ear. "Baby, listen to me. Just think about if we went back to Atlanta. We could be a family again, just the three of us. If you came with him, Sadie, he'd be fine."

"Me? To Atlanta?" She finally lost her

battle with her emotions. Tears came to her eyes. "Mom, I have a life in Cape Refuge. I love my job, and I don't want to leave Hanover House. It's the only safe place I've ever lived."

Sadie's tears seemed to push Sheila over the edge. "If they're around, he's *never* going to turn to me. I'll never really have him back!"

Sadie saw the desperation in her mother's eyes, and suddenly her anger melted away. "Mom, we didn't expect you to be out for four more years. It's a God thing that you're getting out early. Morgan and Jonathan taught me that the Lord restores the years that the locusts ate."

"Locusts? What do *locusts* have to do with anything?"

"It means that all the years that were lost to prison or abuse or addiction can be given back. He can help you start over. But you need to do it his way."

Sheila wiped the tears from her face. She was still so pretty, Sadie thought, even in prison browns.

"Baby, I know you don't have a lot of faith in me, but I'm different now. I've been clean from drugs for almost a year."

"You couldn't help being clean, Mom. You've been locked up. You don't know

what it's going to be like when you're back in Atlanta and all your old friends start coming out of the woodwork, and you have the stress of trying to hold down a job and raise a baby."

"But I'll have you to help me, Sadie."

Sadie sat back in her chair and stared at her mother. She wanted to be with her more than anything, but setting up housekeeping with her in their old neighborhood was like moving back into the garbage dump after sitting at the king's table. Going back would be suicide.

"Mom, if it weren't for Morgan and Jonathan, we both might be dead right now. Please, just say you'll try it. What could it hurt?"

Sheila crumpled then and began to cry, and Sadie wished she could go through the glass and hold her. She had always been her mother's caretaker, the one who comforted, the one who let her off the hook.

She prayed she wouldn't do it this time. "Caleb will love you, just like he did before. But make yourself a *part* of his life. Don't just snatch him out of it."

Sheila sat there crying like a teenager with a broken heart. "I love you, Sadie," she said finally. "But you're putting me between a rock and a hard place."

Good, Sadie thought. "Maybe that's the only place where we'll all be safe, Mom. Between that rock and that hard place."

44

Cade was still angry at Blair, but the truth was, he missed her.

He had run into Jonathan campaigning in town, and he'd mentioned that Blair was babysitting at Hanover House. "Why don't you go by and give her a hand?"

Did his best friend know about their fight? "I'm kind of busy, buddy."

"Come on, man. You can take five minutes."

Now he found himself driving by Hanover House, looking to see if Blair's car was still there. She'd been as busy as he had for the last few days. Several times he'd driven by her house, but she never seemed to be home. Did she miss him? Was she nursing her anger at his reaction to her article . . . ?

Or did she even notice he hadn't been by?

He started to pass the house, like some teenage kid on a drive-by. Then he kicked

himself and pulled into the driveway.

He went up the porch and heard chaos through the storm door. Caleb was crying at the top of his lungs, the telephone was ringing, and the buzzer on the oven was shrieking out. Worried, he didn't bother to knock. As he stepped inside, something shattered on the kitchen floor.

He bolted into the kitchen.

Blair stood there with her back to him, dancing screaming Caleb on her hip and staring down at the shattered glass. The phone kept ringing. "It's okay, kiddo," she was saying. "Come on, calm down. You're dealing with an amateur here."

"Is everything all right?" he yelled over the noise.

She swung around at Cade's voice. The glass crunched under her shoes. "Oh, thank goodness you're here!" The phone kept ringing and the buzzer shrilled out over Caleb's screams. "Here. Please, can you hold him for a second? Watch the chocolate on his face."

Cade leaned his cane against the wall and started to take the child.

"Watch out, there's glass on the floor." She thrust the filthy baby into Cade's arms and ran to the buzzer. The phone kept shrilling as she took a pan of smoking

brownies out of the oven and dropped the pan into the sink with a clank. Smoke filled the kitchen.

She crunched to the phone. "Hello?"

The baby kicked and screamed in Cade's arms, crying to be put down, but there was no way he could set him down with the glass on the floor. He slid toward the back door and opened it to air the room out, then slid through the glass to the sink. He turned on the water and grabbed a paper towel. With his arm around Caleb's waist, he turned the child face out and swiped the wet paper towel over his face. His cries rose an octave.

"No, I need to get someone over there right away," Blair said into the phone. "It's the first cell phone service on the island. I can't. I've got to babysit. Please, can you cover it for me? No, Sadie can't go. She's out of town today. You've been wanting me to hire you, Jeff. Just do this story and we'll talk."

Caleb kept crying, so Cade lifted him over his head and wiggled him, trying to make him laugh. The baby looked tortured.

Blair propped the phone between her ear and shoulder, and crunched to the refrigerator. She grabbed out his little cup and

handed it to him. Caleb knocked it out of her hand.

"Oh, brother," she whispered. "No, I wasn't talking to you, Jeff. Would you? Oh, thank you! You're a lifesaver." She grabbed the broom and started sweeping the glass.

Cade lifted the baby again, trying to make him catch his breath. The smell that wafted past his face made Cade catch his, instead. "So *that's* it, huh?"

Blair put her hand over the phone. "What's it?"

He held the baby out in front of him. "Dirty diaper."

"Great. Morgan keeps them upstairs."

Cade glared at her. "Surely you don't expect me to —"

She held out a hand to stop him. "Yes, Jeff. Drop the film by here when you're done, all right? And make sure you get statements from the cell phone company. I suppose you'll have to get one from Sam Sullivan, too, and also some of the citizens who are there."

He'd have to go for it. Holding the baby out in front of him, he left the kitchen and carefully started up the stairs. Without his cane, it was slow going. The child kicked and screamed, his face as red as the chocolate-covered shirt he wore.

He found Caleb's room and laid the baby on the changing table. His crying covered the scales as Cade took his dirty diaper off. He found the covered garbage pail and dropped it in.

The smell was lethal. How did people do this? He looked around, and saw nothing with which to clean the baby up.

Caleb kicked and cried, and Cade tried to keep him on the table while he looked on the shelves beneath him, searching for toilet paper. There was none.

What was he going to do now?

He was the chief of police, for Pete's sake. He had averted disasters, chased criminals, solved murders. Changing a diaper couldn't be that hard.

But why didn't Morgan have toilet paper nearby?

He would have to go get it from the bathroom, he decided. Instead of taking Caleb with him, he picked him back up and put him in the crib, hoping he wouldn't sit his dirty bottom down. "Just stand there, bud. Don't touch anything. I'll be right back."

Caleb began rattling the side of the crib like a psychotic prisoner.

"Come on, Caleb," he called from the hallway. "Can't you just cooperate a little?

I don't know what to do here."

He limped to the bathroom and grabbed the roll of toilet paper off its holder, then hurried back into the nursery, trailing tissue behind him. He grabbed the baby back up and took him back to the table. He tried to wipe his bottom, but it wasn't easy.

"Give a guy a break," he said in a soft voice. "Come on, bud, I just want to clean you up."

"I'm so sorry, Cade!"

He turned to see Blair at the doorway, looking as frantic as he felt. She'd brought his cane.

"He needs a bath," he said. "I can't get him clean."

"Did you try the baby wipes?"

Baby wipes. Of course. He'd seen the commercials. She grabbed out the box that was conveniently placed on the shelf below the changing table, and took over.

"I'm so sorry I left you with him! He's really been pretty good most of the morning, then the universe kind of exploded. About the same time as his bowels, apparently." She got him clean, then grabbed a fresh diaper. Caleb finally stopped crying.

"Why isn't he potty trained?"

Blair grinned. "Because he's only eigh-

teen months old. They don't potty train them until at least four or five."

"You're insane. They start school at four or five, and I don't know any teachers who have to change diapers."

"*I'm* insane? You're the one who tried to clean him up with toilet paper!"

Cade started to laugh, softly at first, but then the laughter bent him over. It was contagious, and Blair caught it. She set Caleb down before she dropped him.

The two screamed out their laughter, and Caleb stood there smiling up at them. Cade tried to stop laughing, but it had wound itself within him, sapping his strength. He saw that Blair had the same problem. Tears rolled down her face as she fell against him.

It was the most beautiful sight he'd seen in days.

Blair wiped her face. "You didn't say why you came by," she said as her laughter played down. "Did someone call 911? Report us for disturbing the peace?"

He drew in a deep breath. "Jonathan told me you were here."

Her laughter settled, and her eyes grew wide. "And you came anyway?"

"Yeah —" he grinned — "I came anyway."

He wanted to kiss her, squeeze the breath out of her, and beg her to update him on every minute of her days since he'd seen her last.

But Caleb made a run for it.

"Oh, no, you don't, kiddo!" Blair started after him and grabbed him up.

Caleb screamed with glee as she hoisted him on her hip again. She started down the stairs. "Come on, let's go outside where we can't destroy anything."

Cade followed her down and out to the backyard. She set the boy down, and he ran to his big plastic gym. Sighing, she dropped into one of the lawn chairs. Cade dropped into one next to her.

"So, how are you?"

"Okay," she said. "You?"

"Better now."

She smiled at him, and he realized how much he'd missed those bright eyes. "Jonathan told me Caleb's mother's getting out of jail."

"Yeah," Blair said. "Morgan's really depressed. If she doesn't talk Sheila into coming here, I don't know what she'll do."

Cade looked at the boy, who chattered to himself as he climbed the three-step slide. "I'm praying for her."

"Me too," she said. "I do that now, you

know. Pray, I mean. Now that I'm a Christian and all. A real one."

Cade hated himself for ever suggesting she wasn't. "I know you are, Blair. I didn't mean what I said. I was just mad."

"No kidding."

He smirked. "I'm still ticked that you gave credence to Carson Graham, but I'm man enough to forgive you."

"And I'm woman enough to accept your apology."

"Apology?" he said. "I'm not apologizing."

"And I'm not admitting wrong."

He couldn't help smiling. "You make me crazy, you know that?"

"You've mentioned it before."

He watched Caleb try to go up the slide the wrong way. "So, what're you doing tonight?"

"What have you got in mind?"

"I wanted to drop by Carson Graham's show, just to see how he operates. Want to come?"

"I don't know. The Bible calls that stuff detestable. You should look it up."

Touché. "I'm not going for entertainment, but I want it to look like I am."

"So is he a suspect?"

"Let's just say he's a person of interest.

I'm not entirely sure Ben's the right man. And that's off the record."

Blair locked her eyes on him as she considered his offer. "What time will you pick me up?"

45

Caleb was sleeping when Morgan and Sadie got back. Morgan went upstairs to check on him. The child lay face down, his cheek mashed against the mattress, his thumb in his mouth. Did his mother know he was a thumb sucker? Would she let him do it or slap his hand away?

She leaned over the crib rail and picked the boy up. He stirred awake, his face warm against her neck. She carried him into her room and laid him gently down on the bed. He put his thumb back in his mouth and began sucking again as she curled up next to him.

Stroking his little head, she began to cry. *Please, Lord. Don't take this baby away from me.*

Even if Sheila did come to live with them, Morgan's days of mothering the baby would end.

Did she even have a choice?

What if he's the only baby I ever have?

She touched her stomach and wondered how it would be to feel the swell of a baby, the flutter of his movement, the kick from a little foot. Even the morning sickness would be welcome.

She cried into the pillow and prayed that the results of her hormone test would be good news, and not further deplete her hope.

Monday morning, when Morgan and Jonathan went to learn the results of her FSH test, she knew the news was not good. Dr. Sims met them in his office, a grim expression on his usually pleasant face.

"As I told you before I did the test, the follicle-stimulating hormone enables your ovaries to produce eggs. Whenever the FSH level is over twenty, it tells us that your ovaries may not be working like they should."

"What was my level, Doctor?"

"Forty-two."

She felt as if he'd thrust a fist into the middle of her stomach, knocking the breath out of her.

Jonathan took her hand. "So, what does that mean? Will we be able to have children?"

The doctor sighed. "I never say never."

Morgan's heart plunged.

"At this point, I usually put a patient on Pergonal, which helps stimulate follicle growth. In your case, with such high numbers, I think a more aggressive approach might be in order."

"Aggressive?" Jonathan asked.

Morgan tried not to cry. "But I don't understand. My miscarriage didn't have anything to do with my eggs, did it?"

Dr. Sims got up and came around the desk, and sat on the edge of it, facing them like a friend instead of a doctor. "Morgan, we don't know for sure what caused your miscarriage, but it may have had to do with the maturity of the egg. My goal in treating you would be to stimulate the follicle production with Pergonal, harvest the egg at the right time, and then fertilize it in our lab."

Morgan couldn't believe she was hearing him right. "Are you suggesting in vitro fertilization?"

"That's exactly what I'm suggesting. We've had a tremendous success rate with this procedure."

"Wait a minute." Jonathan looked as if he'd been threatened. "I thought IVF was a last resort, for people who had no other hope. I thought you were supposed to try everything else first."

The doctor shrugged. "Some do, but I realize how much the two of you want a family. While you're trying other things, Morgan's biological clock is ticking."

"Dr. Sims, she's only twenty-nine. It's not like her time is running out."

"Can I be honest with you?" Sims asked in a soft voice.

"That's what we want, Doc."

"Lisa tried everything else first. By the time she and Ben decided to try IVF the first time, she was pushing forty."

It made sense. Morgan looked up at Jonathan, wishing he wouldn't reject the idea outright. They needed to listen, at least.

"How much money are we talking about for a procedure like that, Doctor?"

He went back around the desk and sat down. "It varies. Insurance usually doesn't cover the retrieval of the egg, the embryology lab, or the transfer of the embryo. The cost in my office usually averages ten thousand dollars, depending on several factors."

Jonathan looked sick.

"What if it's not successful?" Morgan asked. "Would other attempts be included in that price?"

"No, that cost is per treatment. It's a very high-tech procedure, and it's expen-

280

sive. Most people think it's worth it when they're holding that baby in their arms."

Morgan couldn't imagine coming up with ten thousand dollars for something that might not even work. She met Jonathan's eyes and saw the helplessness there.

"We could never afford that," he said. "No way."

"Some of my patients take out loans. Mortgage their houses, that kind of thing. There are ways to make it work. I haven't known a single couple to regret the sacrifice."

Tears were coming, and Morgan couldn't stop them. "I never thought it would be this way. I thought I'd get married and have a baby, then another baby, and another . . . Infertility never crossed my mind."

Dr. Sims looked as if he hurt with her. "Morgan, I know this is difficult. I can tell from the short times I've spent with you that you would be a wonderful mother. We're going to make it happen, okay?"

Later, as they drove home, Morgan wept quietly.

Jonathan took her hand. "Honey, it's going to be all right. If God wants us to have a baby, we will."

That was just it. What if he *didn't* want them to? "I feel kind of like Sarah," she said, "working it all out in my own way. Is Pergonal my Hagar? Is IVF my Ishmael?"

"What if it's God's provision?"

"Why would he need to provide that way, when he could just touch me and make me conceive? He's the one who creates life. Why can't he create it in me?" She looked over at Jonathan and saw the tears brimming in his eyes.

"Are you saying we just need to trust?" Jonathan asked. "To wait for God's timing?"

"I don't know! What if we do that and never have a baby and realize that we missed the opportunities he gave us?"

"We could adopt, if it came to that."

"That takes years, too. I want to be pregnant, Jonathan. I want to have a baby that looks like us. I want to be able to say, 'You're just like your father.' And I don't want any biological mother coming to take him back."

"It wouldn't be the same as having a foster child. An adopted child would really be ours."

Silence fell over them as Morgan thought of little Caleb. She knew she had it in her to love a baby that wasn't biologi-

cally hers, but she wasn't ready to give up the idea of having her own child. "Caleb's not ours, and we're going to lose him."

"No, we're not," Jonathan insisted. "Sheila will come. You'll see."

"But I wanted to be his mother."

He reached over and pulled her into his arms, and he held her for a long time.

"I have to surrender," she said finally. "I have to just surrender to whatever God is doing. I have to believe it's the best thing."

"Honey, if God wants us to do the whole infertility thing, he'll show us. We'll have peace about it. We have to be open to seeing the signs when he gives them. But in my heart, I see you as a mother, Morgan, and I see myself as a father. It's going to happen, honey, one way or another. If we have to do these treatments, we will. If we have to go to some foreign country to adopt, we'll do it. We'll do whatever is necessary to have the family that I know God has planned for us. We're going to go through this together, whatever we decide."

Morgan looked out the window, her heart sending up pleading prayers for help.

Even with all the best science had to offer, Morgan knew God was their only real hope.

46

Blair had trouble deciding what to wear on her pseudo-date to Carson Graham's show. She hated herself for being so self-conscious and vain, when she'd once had such contempt for women who spent too much time in front of the mirror.

She settled on a pair of white slacks and a pink blouse, one she'd bought on a whim when she'd been starry-eyed about Cade. Sitting in front of the mirror, she put on her makeup, paying careful attention to her eyes. She wanted to knock his socks off tonight, even if they were going for business.

But it was almost hopeless.

She put her hand over the right side of her face, imagining what she'd look like without the scars. She might have been print-ad pretty, like her sister. Pageant material. Drop-dead gorgeous.

She moved her hand and saw the whole picture, the same face Cade saw each time he looked at her.

She parted her hair on the side and brushed it to fall in front of her scars. If it hung just right and shone just enough, maybe he would be distracted from her scars.

The doorbell rang and Blair turned away from the mirror. She wouldn't look at her reflection again for the rest of the night. There was no use ruining a perfectly promising date.

The sight of Cade made her heart jolt. He wasn't in uniform tonight. He wore a pair of jeans and a pullover shirt — and a gentle smile on his face. "Hey there. You look nice."

She fought the urge to turn her face away. "Thanks. So do you."

He stepped inside and bent down to kiss her. Then slowly, he swept her hair back from her face, exposing it fully. His gaze swept over her face — all of it — and if she hadn't known better, she would have believed there was pure pleasure in his eyes.

Her heart beat like a jackhammer as he took her hand and escorted her to his truck.

He is going to marry you, you know. Carson Graham's prediction came back to her, fluttering like a hummingbird through her heart.

She tried to put it out of her mind, but it was there, a hope spoken aloud, stamped on her subconscious, always lingering in her mind.

No matter how often she told herself the man was a fake, she still hoped the psychic knew what he was talking about.

47

The club at the Frankfurt Inn was filling up fast, and Blair wished they had come earlier to get a decent table. She followed Cade through the crowd to a small table in the back corner of the room.

"Can you believe this crowd?" he muttered as they sat down.

"Yeah. Looks like Lisa's murder was a real boon to Carson."

"It's the big break he's been waiting for." Cade's eyes scanned the crowd at the many familiar faces. He saw George O'Neill and Harold Delaney, two of the town's city councilmen, sitting near the front with frosty mugs of beer.

"Is that Bruce over there?" Blair pointed through the people.

Cade looked and saw the newest member of his police force sitting at a table full of friends. He sighed. "Great. Even my own men are buying into this stuff."

Blair's eyes swept over the crowd. A

couple of church members sat at another table, watching them as if wondering what would bring them here. She supposed she couldn't blame them for their curiosity. "If this guy's a fake, he sure has a lot of people fooled."

"*If* he's a fake?" Cade breathed a laugh. "He is one, Blair. He's a con artist and a liar."

The lights flickered, indicating that the show would begin soon. Blair looked toward the stage as people hurried to find seats. Was Cade right, and so many others wrong? *He is going to marry you, you know.* Graham had been right before. The pianist sat down at the piano at the side of the stage and began a Broadway-type intro that quieted everyone.

Blair spotted Rani coming in, and when she saw them, Rani made a beeline toward them. She smelled of cigarette smoke and Obsession perfume. "Hey, guys. Mind if I share your table?"

"Sure," Cade said. "Pull up a chair."

She sat down and grinned at them both. "I'm so glad to see you two here. Finally, you'll see what Carson is all about. I've been to his show every night since I met him. It's fascinating. Tell the truth, Cade. You're starting to believe, aren't you?"

Cade bristled. "No, actually, I'm not. I'm just here to watch."

A spotlight came on as the music crescendoed. The manager of the Frankfurt Inn walked onto the stage and introduced Carson Graham as if he were a rock star.

The crowd applauded enthusiastically and the curtains parted. Carson stepped out, arrayed in a purple sequined coat with a red satin shirt. His head, freshly shaved, shone in the lights.

He clutched the mike like a nightclub singer. "Thank you, thank you everybody. Thank you for coming."

Rani clapped so hard she almost came out of her seat. Blair just looked at Cade, noting the tension on his face.

"Ladies and gentlemen, my beautiful assistant, Amber — who also happens to be my bride — is coming around the audience with a velvet bag right now. She'd like for you to throw in personal objects. If you have a cigarette lighter or a pen, a pair of glasses — anything — just throw it in. But beware! When I pull your object out of the bag, I might be inclined to tell some of your deepest, darkest secrets."

A nervous chuckle went across the room, and then Graham's wife — who Blair knew

held a job as a nurse at a Savannah hospital — came into the audience with a velvet bag. A spotlight followed her around the room as people dropped in their objects.

"Wanna put anything in to test him?" Blair asked Cade on a whisper.

"No, I don't."

"I have something." Rani dug through her purse as the wife headed in her direction. She pulled out a big tortoise-shell barrette. "It's Lisa's."

Cade stiffened even more. "Do me a favor, and don't let them know it's hers."

"Okay, but he'll know. You'll see."

Amber came to their table, and Rani dropped the barrette in. After accepting a few more items, she pranced back up to the stage and handed the bag to Carson.

Carson sat on a stool, which had been spray-painted gold, and reached in for the first object. He pulled out a handkerchief and held it by one corner with two fingers.

"I hope this isn't used." Laughter rippled over the crowd. He shook the cloth out, revealing a flower embroidered at the center of it. "I'm sensing that this handkerchief belongs to a woman." Again, laughter.

He laid it across his knee and stroked his

hand across it. "A very pretty woman. I'm seeing bright sunshine associated with this handkerchief. This could be a woman who works outside, maybe spends a lot of time at the beach."

A woman at one of the tables began to laugh, and the group around her began to whisper.

"Rocket science," Cade muttered. "We live on the ocean."

"Is this yours?" Carson asked the woman.

"Yes," she said as the spotlight sought her out.

His face sobered. "You've recently been to a wedding or a funeral. Am I right about that?"

She caught her breath. "Oh, my gosh. Yes, I've been to a wedding."

"How hard is that?" Cade muttered to Blair. "Everybody's been to a funeral or a wedding."

"You met a man there," Carson went on. "He might have been in the wedding party . . . or maybe just a guest. Is that right?"

"That would cover just about every man there," Blair whispered.

Rani shushed her.

"Yes. He was an usher."

291

"And some romance may have developed."

The woman hesitated, but he kept going. "Not really a romance, but just some interest . . . maybe a little chemistry?"

She smiled as if she'd been caught. "Maybe."

"I think that man that you met may actually be someone you need to get to know a little better."

Her eyebrows came up. "Really?"

"I see another wedding in your future. Only this time you're the one wearing white."

The group at her table began to laugh raucously. The crowd applauded.

Cade leaned over to Blair's ear. "And how can you refute anything he just said? All you can do is wait to see if it happens. Smoke and mirrors. And if she gets married, she'll think he got it right. He predicted her walking down the aisle in white."

Blair thought about his prediction about her own marriage. It had been specific, that Cade would propose. But was it such a stretch? Wasn't it what she'd hoped for? If it happened, did it mean that Carson Graham was gifted or that he was just a good guesser?

Or was he off-base altogether since there had been no mention of any kind of commitment between them, much less marriage?

Blair watched as Carson pulled out an unsmoked cigarette with lipstick stains on the filter. He held it up, took a sniff of it, and turned it around in his fingers. "This belongs to someone who is trying to quit smoking."

The crowd chuckled.

"But this person is also grieving over the death of someone she loved."

"Oh, he's right!" a woman said, and the spotlight quickly found her. "Yes, that's true."

"It was someone very close to you."

Blair thought that could apply to her. In fact, it could apply to almost everyone.

The woman paused, as if not sure whether to help him or not. "My mother," she blurted out.

"You've got to stop blaming yourself," he said suddenly.

The woman just stared at him, stricken.

Blair's mind raced critically ahead. Wasn't guilt a natural aspect of grief? Didn't everyone who'd lost a parent blame themselves for something they hadn't done?

"You have regrets over the way you treated her," Carson said. "You want to know if she's forgiven you. But she wants you to know that there's nothing to forgive."

Whether he'd hit the nail on the head or not, the audience sat spellbound, hanging on every word.

"What, is he a medium now too?" Cade whispered.

Carson came out into the audience and made his way to the woman. He handed the cigarette back to her. "You've also been sad that your mother won't be at your wedding."

The woman gasped. Blair looked at Cade.

"Engagement ring," Cade whispered. "Either that, or she's a plant."

Maybe . . . but maybe not.

"She wants you to know that she will be there. She's not going to miss it for anything."

The woman began to cry, and the man next to her pulled her against him.

Rani turned back to them with tears in her eyes. "Isn't he wonderful? He's given her so much comfort."

Blair didn't say anything.

Carson dug into Amber's bag again.

This time he came up with the barrette Rani had dropped in.

Cade shot Rani a look, reminding her not to react.

"How can you think he's not for real?" she whispered. "He told us where she was!"

"Please, Rani," Cade whispered. "Just sit tight. See what he says."

"All right, but only to prove it to you."

Carson stood among the tables, holding the barrette to his head. "This barrette belongs to a blonde woman. I'm picturing a pretty woman with blondish hair."

Blair looked at Cade. Lisa was a brunette.

Rani looked distressed.

"Kind of a sandy blonde, with a little brown. Highlights of auburn."

"He didn't mention gray," Cade muttered under his breath.

Carson looked around the room, as if reading the faces to see whom this might belong to. "I get the impression this barrette belongs to a very troubled person."

Cade glanced at Rani, saw that it was taking all her effort not to respond.

"Who put this in here?" he asked finally. "I need to see you. I'm getting some very vivid impressions . . ."

295

Rani looked back at Cade, but he slowly shook his head.

"Don't want to tell me?" Carson shrugged then and dropped the barrette back into the bag. "Let's move on to something else."

Rani shot Cade a condemning look. "I should have stood up."

"Why?" Cade whispered back. "If you had stood up, he would have known right away that it was something to do with Lisa. That's all that's been on your mind lately."

Blair leaned toward Rani. "If he was for real, Rani, wouldn't the object have told him something?"

"He said he got some vivid impressions! Maybe they were too vivid. Maybe he just had more scruples than to blurt them out."

"Or maybe he was drawing a blank," Blair said.

Rani sat there for a few moments longer, as Carson made more educated guesses about the people whose objects had been in that bag. Finally, she got up and strode out.

"Guess she's mad," Cade said, "but maybe she learned something."

They watched as Carson demonstrated his performance skills and his keen ability

to read body language. But it clearly wasn't magic.

When they were finally driving home, Blair looked over at Cade. "If the guy's a fraud, how did he know where Lisa's body was?"

"That is exactly what I intend to find out."

48

"She's coming!" Sadie's cry shook the walls of Hanover House the next day. "Mama's getting out tomorrow, and she's agreed to come here!" She bounced down the stairs and into the kitchen, and she grabbed Caleb off the floor. "Caleb Seth Caruso, your mommy's coming home!"

Morgan felt the staggering relief taking hold of her, but even as it did, a profound sadness followed. "Are you sure she's coming here?"

"Yes. She called collect and said that they're releasing her tomorrow! I can't believe it," she squealed. "I'll have my whole family back together. This is the new beginning that Mom needs."

It was the new beginning Sadie needed, too. Maybe there would be healing for her in Sheila's release, but Morgan couldn't imagine it being best for Caleb.

Or for her.

As soon as she was able to get away

without Sadie wondering why, she slipped out and drove to Blair's house. She needed for her sister to pray with her.

Blair saw the pain on her sister's face the moment she let her in. "Oh, no. Sheila refused to come?"

"No, she's coming tomorrow." Tears hung in Morgan's eyes, ready to shatter. "I know I should be happy, but I'm scared, Blair."

Blair was struck by the frantic expression on Morgan's face, the smear of mascara under her eyes as if she'd cried on the way over, the nervous way she kept wiping her hands on her jeans and sliding them into her pockets.

"Sit down," Blair said.

Morgan pulled out a chair at Blair's kitchen table and dropped into it. Blair wished she had some cookies to offer her, like their mother would have done. If not cookies, then wisdom. But she didn't have much of that, either.

Morgan was the wise one, the more mature Christian, the one who cast her cares before the Lord and left them there. Morgan had prayed so often for Blair, but it was only recently that she had been able to ask for prayer in return. Blair was glad

that pattern had been broken.

"What specifically do you want me to pray, Morgan?"

"That I'll love her." Morgan wiped the smear of mascara under her eyes. "That I'll be a bigger person. I'm so disappointed in myself, Blair. I should want what's best for Caleb, not myself. If I can give Caleb back his mother and teach her how to parent him, then I'd be glorifying God. But I have these selfish thoughts."

"How does Jonathan feel?"

Morgan shook her head. "He's worried, too. But I'm Caleb's primary caretaker. I do everything for him. How can I turn it all over to her?"

"Morgan, that's a natural response. You need to stop beating yourself up."

"Do I? Or am I just an ungrateful wimp?"

"No, Sis. You have a tender mother's heart that's just about broken in two. One side for your miscarried baby, and the other side for Caleb."

Morgan lost it then, and Blair pulled her into her arms and held her for a long time. She needed to pray. A fierce sense of responsibility gripped her, and she started to pray aloud. She felt the Holy Spirit directing her thoughts and words, adminis-

tering a healing balm over her sister's heart.

When they'd finished praying, Blair let her sister go. "Sis, you rescued Caleb and Sadie from pure evil. You've loved them and given them things that they've never had before. Even if the day comes when Sheila takes them away, I know you would do it all over again."

"Of course I would."

"It's going to be all right. You're just like Mama. You give and give, and every time it glorifies God. Sometimes it's going to hurt. Break your heart, even. But you'll keep doing it, because that's the way you are."

Morgan reached for her again, and they wept together until there were no more tears.

Later that day, Morgan lay on the bed, curled up next to Jonathan.

"It's gonna be okay, baby," he said. "I know it is. We'll make it work. God is looking out for Caleb. He's going to take care of him."

"But I want to take care of him."

"You will. Sheila will need your help. She'll be grateful for it."

Morgan wondered if that was true. The

woman she'd seen in jail a few days ago didn't seem grateful or even willing to let Morgan help.

"You know, we need to talk about where we're going to put her."

"I was thinking Mrs. Hern's room, since she's gone to the nursing home."

"Or Gus's room."

They hadn't had the chance to really consider Gus's request. "I guess we need to talk about that, don't we?"

"Yeah," Jonathan said. "I've been praying about him and Karen a lot."

"So have I. What do you think?"

Jonathan sat up and leaned back against the post at the foot of the bed. "Ordinarily, I would say that it's way too soon for Karen, that she needs to finish our program, that she doesn't need to take on the responsibility of being a wife."

"But this isn't an ordinary situation."

"No, it isn't. Karen has the baby, and Emory needs a father."

"Gus would love to be his daddy," Morgan said. "He's been around since he was born. I have no doubt in my mind that Gus is ready to handle the responsibility of a family. If they stay here, then Karen can finish the program, and we can help her with her parenting skills and give her a

solid foundation to overcome her addictions once and for all."

"Besides," Jonathan said, "I hated to see Gus leave. He's like family."

Morgan smiled. "Then we're going to give them our blessing?"

Jonathan sighed. "Are we crazy?"

"I don't think so. I mean, I've been thinking that maybe this was all part of God's provision for Karen and Emory. Maybe he brought her here so that she'd meet Gus. Emory's father is a violent, abusive drug dealer who had no intention of marrying her, and even if he did, he'd put Emory in danger. Maybe God was taking care of her by making Gus fall in love with her."

Jonathan reached across the bed and kissed her. "As if we didn't have enough to do, now we've got a wedding to plan."

"Let's go tell them!"

They hurried downstairs and found Gus and Karen sitting on the sun porch with Emory.

"You guys don't have time for lounging around when you have so much to do," Jonathan said.

Gus got up. "You need help with something, mon?"

"You bet I do," Jonathan said. "I need

help figuring out where we're going to have your wedding."

Karen screamed and shot out of her seat, and they all threw themselves into joyful hugs.

49

The Tuesday issue of the *Observer* was even more sensational than the one the week before. McCormick had brought it to Cade in his office, and Cade had lost his appetite for breakfast. He scanned it now as his coffee slowly got cold. It was packed full of articles about Ben and Lisa's life together, about the journey their infertility had taken them on, about the rumored affair . . .

Vince Barr had more pictures of Lisa's wet, dead body in her car, pictures of her parents at the funeral, an article about Rani's outburst last week, and a lengthy interview with Lisa's best friend, in which she accused Ben of the murder again.

He chronicled the searches of Ben's home, car, boat, and business, complete with interviews with each of his employees, defending his character and denying that he'd ever had another woman.

He even profiled Ben's opponents in the election, with questions about whether

Jonathan or Sam might have had anything to do with the murder.

He was thorough, imaginative, and left no stone unturned.

Too bad one of those big networks who kept interviewing him about the case didn't just hire him so he could turn to the scandals of politicians and athletic stars — and get off Cade's back. Cade knew Barr wasn't about to let the case go until he'd milked it for everything it was worth.

When Cade finished scouring the tabloid, he turned to Blair's new issue, which had also come out today. She'd handled things tastefully and accurately, in contrast to Vince's fiction, though she hadn't sold nearly as many copies.

It wasn't fair, but it would be all right. Blair would build her circulation, and eventually she would give even the Tampa paper a run for its money. He knew her potential. She could do anything she set her mind to.

Blair perused the *Observer*, gritting her teeth at the things Vince Barr had reported. The man had gall.

She set the paper down and looked around at her cluttered office. She'd been up most of the night trying to get the paper

out. She was exhausted. She didn't know how much longer she could keep up this pace, and for all the work, she still put out a less-than-stellar little paper that few took seriously.

She'd been thinking about hiring a night staff — maybe two or three people to handle the printing — since she'd bought the paper. But ever since Carson Graham had made the prediction about her buying the South Farm Insurance Building, her imagination had been running wild. What if she really could expand that much, start putting the paper out every day, and grow her circulation to all of Georgia rather than just the island? She was good enough. Her investigative skills, coupled with her research and writing skills, could catapult her to the top echelon of the media in no time . . .

Not that she was listening to Carson. She knew better than that. The idea had already been in her mind somewhere, dormant. A dream planted by God. Carson simply awakened it.

Inspired by the vision, she decided to drive over to that vacant building, just to see. She crossed the island and found the building, which had been vacated when the insurance company had moved to bigger

facilities in Savannah. A "For Sale" sign sat on the front lawn. Rani and Lisa's real estate company had listed the property.

There was no way she could afford it, but it had been on the market for a long time. Maybe they would consider some sort of lease.

But even that would be out of her budget, wouldn't it?

Her heart began to pound, and her mind began to calculate. She had spent every penny she had in savings to buy the paper. It had been a good investment, but she had nothing left. Still . . . there might be a way if God was in this . . .

But that was the question, wasn't it? Was this a seed planted by God, or was it something else entirely?

She drove back home, muscles drawn tight by the anxiety of dreaming too big, the stress of wanting more than was in reach. It wasn't like her to be greedy, to take shortcuts to success. If she had to go into deep debt to expand, if she had to scheme against her own accounting, if she had to take such tremendous risks when she'd barely gotten the paper off the ground — then she was pretty sure this wasn't of God.

Until she was sure it was, she would put

the plans on the back burner. But keeping herself from thinking about them might not be all that easy. Her Pandora's box of dreams was open now. She didn't know if it was possible to close it again.

50

Morgan rose Saturday morning while it was still dark and went downstairs to gather herself before Caleb got up. Karen was already up, sitting out on the sun porch nursing Emory.

Morgan put a pot of coffee on, then stepped out to join her. "Good morning. You're up early."

Karen smiled up at her. "Emory woke me up. If I can get him to sleep till five I'm happy. Besides, I'm so excited about the wedding, and there's so much to do. I couldn't hardly sleep anyway."

Morgan hugged her. "You sure you can get it all together that quick? A week from Saturday is awfully soon."

"I'd do it today if I could. I can't believe how the good Lord has blessed me."

When the couple had chosen to have it so soon and asked to have it at Hanover House, Morgan and Jonathan pointed out that it was impossible to do much in prep-

aration. The debate was this Saturday; the election Tuesday. But Gus and Karen didn't want any flowers other than the ones already planted in the front garden. Melba Jefferson, a dear friend of the family, got the news and immediately volunteered to make Karen's wedding dress. They wanted it simple and sweet.

Church members offered to help with the food, the music, and the chairs on the front lawn, and Jonathan would conduct the ceremony. Morgan just hoped it wouldn't rain.

"So are you getting ready to go get Sadie's mama?"

"I am." Morgan sat down next to her. "It's a three-hour drive, so I hope to get off early. Jonathan's staying behind to do some campaigning."

"You want me to keep Caleb for you?"

Morgan thought about that for a moment. "I'm trying to decide whether to take him with us or not."

"It's a long trip. Three hours, one way."

"I know, but when I put myself in Sheila's place, I think how anxious she must be to spend time with him. She'll want to hold him the minute she's free. She could sit by him in the backseat and bond with him. I think he'll be okay if

311

we make frequent stops."

"That's sweet of you to think of her, Morgan. I know this is hard for you."

Morgan hated being so transparent. "I want her to be happy here. I want to give her every opportunity to be what her children need her to be."

"That's what you gave me," Karen said. "A chance to start over, get my life right. And watching you mother Caleb has taught me how to be a mama to Emory."

Ironic, Morgan thought. Here she was, not even a mother herself, modeling motherhood to the mothers who would live in the house. That heaviness fell over her heart again. "Well, I guess I'd better get Sadie up, and I need to go through the clothes we've had donated. Sheila may not have anything to wear."

"Guaranteed she's not the same size she was when she went in. I was two sizes bigger when I got out."

That had been the problem with virtually all of the women who came here from jail. They'd spent whatever money they'd earned working in jail on candy bars and junk food at the commissary. It helped anesthetize the grief, boredom, and loneliness. She went to the closet where they kept the donated clothing and

312

picked out a couple of outfits in different sizes close to what Sheila probably wore. She was still slim, but she'd been nothing but skin and bones when she'd been arrested.

Help me to think of her today, Lord. Not me.

If she could focus on her, maybe she would get through the day without falling apart.

Sheila was waiting in the holding room in the prison when Morgan, Sadie, and Caleb went in. She still wore her brown prison jumpsuit, dingy white socks, and the fluorescent orange flip-flops that were issued to all the inmates.

Sadie carried Caleb in, and the moment she saw her mother she let out a joyful yell. Sheila bolted out of her chair and threw her arms around them.

Morgan stood back, holding the clothes over her arm. Sheila took Caleb and covered his face with kisses.

It was as it should be.

"He's so big. Look at him. He's grown up. He's not a baby anymore."

The child stared up at his mother, as if he didn't quite know how to react. Morgan prayed he wouldn't cry.

"His hair has a curl. I didn't know he had curly hair."

"I sent you pictures, Mom," Sadie said. "Don't you remember seeing the curl?"

"It's not the same." She ruffled his hair and kissed him again. He smiled — miraculously . . . beautifully. "Look at you, smiling at your mama. Oh, you're so different in person, Caleb! Do you even remember me?"

Of course he didn't, Morgan thought. He'd only been a few months old when she'd been arrested.

She stepped up then. "Sheila, we're so glad you're coming home with us."

Sheila looked as if she could have floated out the door. "Well, I'm ready to get out of this place, only they won't let me go in the state-issued jumpsuit."

"I brought you some clothes. I wasn't sure of the size, but one of these should work."

Sheila took one of the pairs of jeans with her free hand and held it up to her. "You people are unbelievable, you know that? I'm just blown away."

"Go change, Mom," Sadie said. "I can't wait to get you out of here."

Reluctantly Sheila handed Caleb back to Sadie and, giddy with excitement, disap-

peared into a bathroom.

When she'd finished dressing and signed all of her paperwork, they left the depressing building. Morgan unlocked the car and opened the door to the backseat. "I thought you'd want to sit next to his car seat. Here, I'll put him in."

"I can do it. I remember how to put a kid into a car seat."

Morgan didn't like hearing Caleb referred to as a kid, but she knew loving parents did it all the time. She got into the driver's seat as all three Carusos lined up in the back.

They had scarcely gotten to the highway back to Savannah, when Caleb started to cry. Morgan listened helplessly as both Sadie and Sheila tried to calm him.

She glanced into the rearview mirror. "Maybe we should pull over. He might need to be changed. We need lunch, anyway."

"I can change him," Sheila said quickly, and before Morgan could stop her, she had unclipped his car seat and pulled him out. "He just wants his mama, don't you, Caleb?"

Alarms went off in Morgan's head. "He really needs to be in the car seat, Sheila. It's dangerous to have him out of it. It's

315

also against the law."

"Well, what are they gonna do, put me back in jail for holding my own baby?"

Morgan swallowed and decided to pull over at the next exit.

Caleb didn't like the new arrangement, so he cried louder, kicking and bucking to get out of her lap. He was just about to break free when Morgan pulled into a McDonald's. "We can eat and let him play for a little while. He'll probably be ready for a nap by the time we get back into the car."

She could see the frustration on Sheila's face, and she told herself to have compassion. Sheila was trying, after all, even if her methods were a little wrong.

Caleb got sleepy after lunch and fussed until Morgan finally took him. He laid his head down on Morgan's shoulder and began to suck his thumb. She saw the disappointment on Sheila's face, so she tried to distract her. "I'll go change him. If you guys need anything, there's a big convenience store next door." She pulled out a twenty dollar bill and handed it to Sheila. "I'm going to pull the car over there and get some gas."

Sheila's face changed, and mother and daughter hurried across to the store, like

best girlfriends on a shopping spree. It had been over a year since Sheila had been in a store. She would probably head straight for the Cokes, as the residents often did. Then she'd get some mascara, if they sold it, maybe some lip gloss. Things that made her feel human again.

Morgan tried to get her bearings. She changed Caleb and hooked him back into his car seat. "Go to sleep, sweetie," she said, kissing his forehead. "You're being such a good boy."

His eyelids began to close even as she got into the driver's seat and pulled over to the gas pumps. She looked toward the door and saw Sadie coming out. Her face was pale, and she looked as if she might burst into tears.

"What is it, honey? Is everything okay?"

Sheila came out then. A lit cigarette hung from her mouth. She held a brand new pack in her hand.

Morgan glanced back at Sadie.

"I told her, but she wouldn't listen. Morgan, please don't get mad."

Sadie got into the car. Morgan waited for Sheila to reach her. "Sheila, if you read the rules of the program at Hanover House, you know that smoking is forbidden."

"Well, we're not at the house yet. Don't worry. I won't smoke in the car."

"I'd rather you didn't smoke at all."

Sheila huffed and took the cigarette out, exhaled a long stream of smoke. She looked poised to argue, but then seemed to think better of it. Dropping the cigarette, she stomped it out.

"I don't want you bringing the pack home, Sheila."

Sheila sighed. "Well, you paid for it. You want me to just toss it?"

"I'd appreciate that."

Her face was tight as she dropped it ceremoniously into the trash can, then got back into the car.

"Thank you, Sheila." Morgan took the nozzle out and put the gas cap back on.

Sheila didn't answer. She just closed the door hard.

Morgan didn't know why she felt like crying as she got back into the car. This happened almost every time they got a new resident. They were always happy and grateful to be accepted, but as soon as the rules and the reality sank in, they began to resent Morgan and Jonathan. Usually, if they could just stick it out for the first month or so, the resentment would eventually fade, and the real work could begin.

But she wanted it to be different with Sheila. Her children were watching.

Sheila seemed to be sulking as she sat next to her sleeping child. Her arms were crossed, and she stared out the window as Morgan pulled back onto the interstate. Sadie was just as quiet.

As she drove, Morgan realized they were walking a tightrope between strict adherence to the rules and the knowledge that Sheila could leave, taking Caleb if Sheila felt provoked. Morgan couldn't let her love for the child temper her expectations. It wouldn't help Sheila change her life. It wouldn't do her any good at all. Since the other tenants had to follow the rules, it wouldn't be fair to bend them for Sheila.

If Morgan were still pregnant, everything would be different. Maybe it would be easier for her to let go. Or maybe not.

After a while, Sadie tried to get her mother's mind off of her anger. "Mom, there was a murder a couple of weeks ago in Cape Refuge. I've been helping Blair cover it for the paper. This woman, Lisa, was found in her car at the bottom of the river . . ."

This woman, Lisa, Morgan thought. Her friend, who had been barren. She wondered if this third treatment would have

helped Lisa conceive, if she had been close to seeing her dreams come true.

Maybe they could still come true for her. In vitro was a drastic approach so soon in her infertility struggle. But maybe the doctor was right. Maybe they needed the big guns first. She didn't want to wind up like Lisa, with an empty womb and an empty crib where Caleb used to be.

When she got home, she would tell Jonathan she wanted to try. Somehow, she would come up with the money. But Dr. Sims was right. She couldn't put a price on having a family.

Whatever it cost, she would figure out how to get the money. Even if it meant mortgaging Hanover House.

51

"Have you seen this autopsy report?"

McCormick's question cut into Cade's thoughts as he studied Carson Graham's phone records. "No. Anything we didn't know?"

McCormick came in and dropped the report on his desk. "You might want to take a look at it."

Cade glanced down at the long report. It would take him a while to read it.

"Look under General Health History. The part about her uterus."

Cade scanned the pages until he found that section. "What's a bicornuate uterus?"

McCormick sat down. "I looked it up. It's when the uterus is split in two parts, and there's a wall between them. It causes a woman to miscarry early in her pregnancies, which is obviously why Lisa was never able to have a baby. Read on."

Cade looked back down at the report. Keith Parker, the medical examiner, had

made a notation. "Subject's IVF procedures were misinformed and suggest malpractice."

Cade froze. "Malpractice? Why?"

"I don't know, but I thought it was worth following up on."

"I'll call Keith." He dialed the number and waited as the call was routed to the medical examiner. "Yeah, Keith, this is Cade from Cape Refuge."

The ME sounded rushed, busy. "Yeah, Cade. What can I do for you?"

"Listen, I was just looking over your report on Lisa Jackson, and I wanted to ask you about something. You mentioned that Lisa had a bicornuate uterus."

He was quiet for a moment, and Cade pictured him fumbling through her file. Finally, he spoke. "Yeah, that's right."

"Are you sure about that?"

"Absolutely. I saw it myself."

"You mentioned that her IVF procedures suggested malpractice. What did you mean by that?"

"I mean that any doctor who performed an in vitro procedure on a woman with a bicornuate uterus was either stupid or a fraud. Her problem was not in conceiving. She simply couldn't carry a baby for very long."

Cade tried to follow what this meant. "So is it possible her fertility doctor didn't know this?"

"Hardly. It's a birth defect. He would have seen it in a hysterogram, which is one of the earliest tests he would have done on her. He also would have seen it in any laparoscopy. And he would have done those in the first two IVF procedures when he harvested the eggs. No way he didn't see it."

Cade locked eyes with McCormick across his desk and changed the phone to his other ear. This couldn't be right. Had Sims lied to her?

"Keith, can this be corrected?"

"Sometimes it can."

"Then why wouldn't the doctor have done that?"

The ME hesitated. "The only reason I can think of is that there's more money in stringing her along. Three procedures would cost over thirty thousand dollars, and that doesn't even add in all the other treatments he'd tried on her over the years. He had a long-term money bag there, and much of it didn't have to go through insurance companies. It was cash out of pocket."

Cade felt sick. Could someone really be that manipulative? That evil? To drag

someone's hopes and dreams through such trials just for a buck?

When Cade hung up, he told Mc-Cormick what Keith had said. "I think it's time to interview Sims again."

McCormick agreed. "You think he had anything to do with her death?"

Cade drew in a long breath. "I wouldn't rule anything out. But even if he didn't, he could be lying to all his patients. He has no business practicing medicine. And because of Lisa's murder, he's going to be exposed."

"Looks like we have *two* major crimes to investigate," McCormick said.

Cade nodded. "I think I need to call the DA."

52

Sadie didn't like the distant, restless look she saw in her mother's eyes as night began to fall. So many times she had anticipated Sheila seeing Hanover House for the first time, with its garden of color lining the front of the house and the big, luscious ferns spilling onto the porch. It looked like something from one of those foggy dreams of heaven, a picture of hope. The reality of a home.

But Sheila didn't catch that vision. Even when they showed her the room Sadie had worked so hard to fix up for her, Sheila's gaze strayed to the window, as if she scoped out her escape.

"I know it's all really stressful to you, Mom. Being in a strange place and having so much expected of you. But it's going to be all right. You'll get comfortable in a few days. Caleb will get to know you."

"I don't see why he has to go to bed so early. He was down before dark."

"It gets dark pretty late this time of year.

He's little. He needs his sleep."

"You used to stay up till after midnight," Sheila said. "It never hurt you any."

Sadie didn't want to tell her that many of the choices Sheila had made about her childhood had hurt her. "He's got a routine. It's good for him."

Sheila turned to look at her. "What does he call her?"

"Who?"

"Morgan. Does he call her *Mama?*"

"Usually he calls her *Mo.* I guess it's his shortened version of Morgan. Sometimes *Mo-mo.*"

"It sounds awfully close to Mama." Sheila's voice sounded hollow, and in it Sadie heard the waver of fear.

"It doesn't matter what he calls her. It matters that he's happy. It's good that there are people like Morgan and Jonathan, Mom. They can love without expecting anything in return."

Sheila gave her a faint smile. "It's just that it makes the rest of us look bad. I don't need any help with that." She turned from the mirror and sat down on the bed. "I'm easily replaced, you know."

Sadie's heart broke at the words. "How can you say that? You haven't been replaced."

Sheila's eyes rimmed with tears. "I've always been a problem to the people around me. Even when I was a little kid, and my mama was going through her string of men, I was always in the way. They farmed me out to everybody they knew. Aunts and uncles and neighbors and foster homes. Nothing — nobody — was ever really mine."

Sadie sat down next to her. "I'm yours, Mom. I always will be. And so will Caleb."

"But can you see why I don't want to be here? I'm in the way again, in a place that's not mine, trying to fit back into my own family. The people here only know me as an ex-con, a drug addict, a terrible mother. How can they see me as anything else, when that's what I am?"

"Mom, Morgan and Jonathan think everyone is worthwhile. Take Gus Hampton, for instance. He's been in prison most of his adult life for everything from armed robbery to drug trafficking. They took him in here and helped him change his life. Now he has a good job, and next Saturday he's marrying Karen. You met her downstairs. The one with the baby. Karen has been in and out of prison, too. She came here pregnant, fearing for her baby's life if she stayed with her violent boyfriend. But

Morgan and Jonathan gave them both that new start, showed them what a real home and family are supposed to look like. They've loved them like family. And Felitia, she was in prison too, before she came here. Same story. Drug addictions. She's clean now and doing really well. If you let them, Morgan and Jonathan will help you start a new life. Think of it, Mom. They helped me start over when things were really bad."

Sheila brought her tear-filled eyes to Sadie's face. "You're different, baby. More confident. More mature. You sure didn't get that from me." She pulled Sadie into a hug.

Finally, she let her go, and her gaze strayed back to the window. "Go for a walk with me, Sadie. Show me this island paradise you've been writing me about."

Sadie couldn't think of anything she wanted to do more.

53

"Ben Jackson's mistress is a business owner somewhere on this island." Clara Montgomery wiped her oiled cloth over the antique dresser she had gotten at the Methodist church bazaar, and looked up at Blair. "You mark my word, she's someone we all know."

Blair had come by to pick Clara's brain about the mystery woman, since Clara was the biggest gossip in town. It seemed that everyone in town had heard the rumors, but no one had a name. "Come on, Clara. You know everything that goes on in this town. Don't you even have some idea?"

"It's a well-kept secret, that's all I know. I gleaned as much as I could from the hints I've gotten from people all over the island." She got finished wiping the wood and turned to an iron headboard propped against the wall. "Did you see this, Blair? It's lovely, isn't it? It would look so pretty in your bedroom. Especially if you were to

get married. That brass one you have right now is a little too feminine for a macho man like Cade, don't you think?"

Blair gasped. She didn't know whether to deny the rumor about a wedding with Cade or ask how the woman knew about her bedroom furnishings. "Clara, Cade and I are not engaged!"

"Just a matter of time, dear. Just a matter of time."

Blair decided to get out of there before Clara "gleaned" anything more. She said a hurried goodbye and rushed out to her car.

For a moment, she sat behind the wheel, letting Clara's words sink in. Was this confirmation that Carson's prediction was real? Could Blair really count on a wedding?

If so, why weren't things moving faster? Why wasn't there a commitment? Why hadn't Cade ever uttered a word about love or marriage?

Was she simply being an idiot to put any stock at all in Carson's or Clara's assumptions?

As she pulled out of the parking lot of the Trash to Treasures Antique Shop, she glanced across the street to Carson Graham's house, with its huge, faded Palm Reading sign. The dirt parking lot seemed

full of cars. She wondered if his visitors were media or people lined up waiting for readings.

Then she saw the front door open, and Carson stepped out with Vince Barr. What was he doing there? Digging up more dirt for his new television career? Manufacturing more lies?

She decided to ask him herself, so she pulled across the street. Carson went back in, and Vince crossed the parking lot to his car. Blair pulled in front of him and rolled her window down.

"Anything going on I should know about, Vince?"

He grinned. "Don't you wish?"

"Hey, I'm just trying to learn from the professionals. Don't tell me you were just getting your palm read."

He leaned into her window. "Carson's the man of the day. Everybody wants a piece of him. You'll have to stand in line."

"Oh, I'm not that interested in Carson. I'm more interested in Ben Jackson's alleged mistress."

"Have you got a name?" His question suggested he didn't.

She decided to play that game. "Maybe."

He grinned. "Did Sam Sullivan finally spill it?"

Blair shifted her car into park. Sam Sullivan? How did he figure into this? "I don't reveal my sources. You know that."

Vince straightened up and peered down at her. "I should have listened to him when he came to me three weeks ago, wanting me to do a story on the affair to blow Ben out of the campaign."

Blair almost caught her breath. So Sam Sullivan was behind the rumors. No wonder no one knew the woman's name. There probably *wasn't* a woman. He'd probably made the whole thing up just to ruin Ben's chances in the campaign.

"I told him I wasn't interested in local politics," Vince went on. "The *Observer* is a national publication. It didn't pique my interest until Lisa turned up missing. Come on, Blair. You got a name, tell me who it is."

"I don't have a name, Vince. I don't even know if I believe there was an affair. Her name would have come out by now if there really was someone."

"Then why are you wasting my time?"

She had expected as much. She watched him get into his car, and she turned hers around before he could pull out.

Cade needed to hear about this. If Sam Sullivan had anything to do with these ru-

mors, then maybe he wrote the letters — and if Sam wrote the letters, maybe he'd been involved in the murder.

She found Cade in a briefing session with McCormick and some of his men. He looked happy to see her when she came in, and he took her into his office.

"I found out some things that might be of interest to you," she said, taking the chair across from his desk. "It's about the alleged mistress. I've been digging around town, trying to find out who she is. No one knows, Cade. No one. Wouldn't you think *someone* would know something if Ben were having an affair?"

"What are you getting at?"

"I'm thinking that maybe it really is all a hoax. But who's behind it? Cade, do you know whose name kept coming up as I was questioning people about this rumor?"

"Who?"

"Sam Sullivan. He told Vince Barr about the affair even before Lisa went missing, hoping to derail Ben's chances in the campaign. Maybe he also sent the letters."

Cade sat back hard and stared at her for a moment. "So what I need to do is get a sample of Sam's handwriting and compare it to the letters."

"Just what I was thinking. Do you think

he just did this to make Ben look bad during the election? Or could he have had something to do with the murder?"

Cade leaned his head back on his chair and stared up at the ceiling.

"Just what you need, huh? Another suspect."

He ran his hands through his hair. "You don't know the half of it."

"Anything I can do?"

He leaned on his desk, rubbing his face until it was red. Looking at her over his fingertips, he said, "There might be."

"What?"

"Tell me about Jonathan and Morgan. Have they been seeing Dr. Sims?"

The shift in subject surprised her. "Yes, as a matter of fact."

"And what has he told them?"

Disappointed that he wasn't going to enlist more of her help in the investigation of Sam and the letters, she sighed. "Well, he's told Morgan that she has a problem producing eggs. They're considering their options."

"Has he suggested any big procedures?"

Blair didn't really know if she should be sharing this. "He suggested in vitro. I think Morgan's considering it."

"I thought so." Cade got up, went

around his desk, and closed the door. He bent over her chair, inches from her face. "Blair, I think Sims is a fraud. I need Morgan and Jonathan to help me prove it."

"A fraud? What do you mean?"

"I mean that I want her to get a second opinion. Have those tests done again."

"Why?"

He sat on the edge of his desk. "Blair, this is off the record. You can't repeat it to anyone, and you sure can't write about it."

Off the record. Again. She considered objecting, but figured silence was a small price to pay if this involved Morgan. "Okay, I won't. Cade, what is it?"

"Lisa's autopsy showed that she had what's called a bicornuate uterus. It's a condition she had since birth, and it kept her from being able to carry a child. Yet Sims never told her what her real problem was, and the IVF procedures wouldn't have helped. He lied to her for years, when surgery might have helped her, and he milked a lot of money out of them in the process."

Blair caught her breath and slowly got to her feet. "Do you think he's been lying to Morgan?"

"The procedures are expensive, Blair. He deals with desperate people who are

willing to do whatever it takes to have a baby."

She felt her scars burning, tears stinging her eyes. Had he given Morgan false hope? Had he preyed on her greatest fears?

"So . . . what? Do you think he's the killer?"

Cade drew in a deep breath. "I've got a medical fraud milking desperate people out of their money; I've got a mayoral candidate who may be stirring up scandals behind the scenes; and I've got a supposed psychic with inside information. Three con artists, and a husband with a weak alibi and a pair of dirty shoes. One of them could be the killer. But I don't know which one."

54

As Cade waited to hear back from the DA's office, he studied the phone records for the Jacksons' telephone number for the days prior to and since Lisa's disappearance. He'd hoped to see a pattern of calls to Ben's mystery mistress, but there didn't seem to be any. But there was one call the morning of her disappearance that caught his attention.

She'd gotten a call from a Dr. Ralph Anderson.

He looked up the practice on his database and saw that it was from another fertility clinic in Savannah. Had Lisa sought another opinion? If so, did Ben know about it? And if she had gone to another doctor, why was she keeping her appointments with Sims each day?

Cade went into the jail at the back of the small building and found Ben lying on his cot. He had been subdued ever since he'd locked him up, with no outbursts of rage

and no desperate pleas for freedom. Now and then Cade had come back here to check on him and had heard his deep, wet weeping. He told himself that the man's grief didn't necessarily proclaim his innocence. Guilty people could grieve, too.

But Ben wasn't crying now. He lay perfectly still, as if he slept with open eyes. He made no move at Cade's approach.

"How ya doing, Ben?" Cade asked him.

"How do you think?"

"Ben, I need to ask you something about Lisa."

That got his attention. Ben sat up and looked at him. "What?"

"It's about her infertility treatments. I need to know if Lisa ever sought a second opinion from another doctor."

Ben slumped over, set his elbows on his knees, and rubbed his stubbled jaw. "As it happens, she *had* decided to get a second opinion. She went the week before her disappearance to a doctor named Anderson in Savannah. He just gave her the runaround."

Dr. Anderson. The one the phone call had come from that morning. Cade pulled a chair close to the cell bars and sat down. "Could you tell me what prompted that?"

"Yeah," he said. "We were going to the

Resolve support group — a support group for infertile couples — and there was a woman in the group who convinced her to do it. She claimed she'd gotten a second opinion and that doctor had found what was wrong with her husband, something that Dr. Sims hadn't found. It was something minor that could be fixed in surgery, and now the woman was pregnant. Lisa thought it was worth a try, though she wasn't entirely sure she needed to give up on Dr. Sims. That's why we didn't cancel any of our appointments, and we were going ahead with the protocol."

"And how did he give her the run-around?"

"Well, he gave her a hysterogram and some other tests, but then she couldn't seem to get the results. Sims always gave them to her on the spot. But it was like an act of congress with Anderson. She'd just about given up on him."

"Are you aware that Dr. Anderson called your house the morning of Lisa's death?"

"No." Ben got up and came to the bars. "How do you know?"

"Phone records."

Ben stared at him for a moment as he processed the information. "He must have called after I left. Maybe he gave her the

results of her tests."

Cade wondered if he had finally told her about the problem with her uterus. Had his phone call prompted Lisa to confront Dr. Sims?

"Can you go see him, Cade? Find out what he told her? Maybe it had something to do with what happened to her."

Again, Cade's gut told him he had locked up the wrong man. He got up, put the chair back. "I will, Ben. That's first on my agenda today."

55

Cade found Dr. Anderson's office on the fourth floor of a building that housed dozens of medical practices. From the looks of the decor, every practice there was established and lucrative. He found the sign that said "Women's Diagnostic Health Clinic" and saw Anderson's name listed as one of three doctors in the practice.

He pushed open the heavy mahogany door and stepped into the big waiting room. It was full of couples of various ages — from their mid-twenties to mid-forties — talking quietly and flipping through magazines that probably didn't interest them.

Some of them looked up at him, and he wondered if he should have worn his uniform. He went to the reception desk and waited for the receptionist to slide open the glass panel. "I'm Chief Cade with the Cape Refuge Police Department —" he showed her his badge — "I need to see Dr.

Anderson as soon as possible."

The receptionist looked fascinated at his credentials, and a little frightened — the way one might look if Mike Wallace came into the office with the *60 Minutes* crew. "Of course. Come this way."

He followed her back into Dr. Anderson's office.

"Have a seat, Chief Cade. He's with a patient, but I'll tell him you're here. Unless it can't wait. I could go get him right now . . ."

"No, that's all right. He can finish with the patient."

She looked relieved, as if that meant that he wasn't in any kind of trouble. She closed the door, but Cade didn't sit down. Instead, he perused the framed degrees on the wall behind the doctor's desk, the pictures of his family. His wife looked about forty-five. They had two boys that looked college age. From the other framed snapshots around the room, he gleaned that they played baseball.

The door opened, and a small man with a bald head and a lab coat that looked too big for him came scurrying in. "Sorry to keep you waiting, Chief Cade." He closed the door behind him, then reached out to shake Cade's hand. "I've seen you on television."

Cade didn't know what to say to that. He'd never wanted to be a celebrity. He sat down, and Anderson took the seat behind his desk. It looked a little too high for him. "Then you know that I'm investigating the murder of Lisa Jackson. I understand she was a patient of yours."

"As a matter of fact, yes. She just came to see me the week before her death. I was shocked when I saw that she'd been murdered."

"I was wondering if you could tell me why she got a call from your office the morning of her disappearance."

"Oh, yes." Anderson reached into a stack on his desk and pulled out Lisa's file. "I had called her that morning with the results of her tests. Spoke to her myself."

Cade sat up straighter. "Is that right?"

"Yes. You see, she'd been through all these fertility treatments, very painful and difficult procedures, literally for years. But when I did her hysterogram I saw immediately why she'd never had a child."

"A bicornuate uterus," Cade said. "It showed up in the autopsy."

"That's right. I should have told her the day I did the test, but I decided to wait until I had all of her results. I was reluctant to accuse Alan Sims of lying to her. I tried

343

to fathom how he could have made a mistake like that. But it was impossible. He had done the same tests on her, so he knew what I knew."

"And you told her that morning?"

"Yes. It was a difficult thing to tell her. She could have had surgery years ago. The surgery has a high rate of success. But now, at her age, she had other factors against her. I told her we could still try, that there was much more hope with the surgery than there was with IVF."

"Doctor, if there was fraud involved, is it possible that he could have pulled it off without help from his nurses and technicians?"

"I suppose it's possible. I understand Sims does all his own lab work, instead of using outside labs like I do. If he falsified her results, it may be that no one knew."

Cade studied the man's face. "Dr. Anderson, why didn't you come forward with this before?"

The man leaned back in his chair, crossing his hands in front of him. "I decided to take a different approach."

"And what would that be?"

"I launched an inquiry with the American Medical Association. That's how we physicians normally do things, Chief Cade.

344

They have means for investigating these things, and if Sims is judged to be guilty of fraud, the appropriate authorities will be notified."

"I understand that, Doctor, but I would think that Lisa's murder might have made you rethink that approach."

He sighed. "Perhaps it should have. But I have a very busy practice, and I admit I didn't give it that much more thought. Once Lisa died, I figured her reproductive system wasn't an issue anymore. Surely you don't think that this had something to do with her murder."

"I don't know that, but right now everything is relevant."

Cade got a copy of her records and left the office, deep in thought as he drove back to Cape Refuge. On his way back he radioed McCormick at the station.

"Yeah, Chief, what you got?"

"I want you to go to get a list of every person scheduled to see our man on May 16." He hoped McCormick understood. The police scanner wasn't all that private, so he didn't want to spell it out.

There was a moment of silence, then McCormick came back. "Good idea, Cade. I'll get right on it."

56

Blair heard Cade's call on her police scanner. She recognized his attempt to keep his orders private from those like her who listened in. Dozens of private citizens had police scanners and kept up with the calls — retired or off-duty cops who still wanted to be a part of things, reporters like her looking for stories, and stringers hoping they could rush to crime scenes and get pictures to sell to her paper or others.

Who was *our man?* Was Cade telling McCormick to get the patient list from Dr. Sims' office for the day of May 16 or the list of clients Carson Graham had seen? Or did this have something to do with Ben or Sam Sullivan's business appointments?

It was unlikely he was talking about Ben or Sam, since they weren't in businesses that relied on frequent appointments. No, it had to be Graham or Sims, and since he'd just told her about suspecting Sims of fraud, she decided it was probably him.

Did he think that one of the patients had killed Lisa, or was he simply looking for a witness? Had he come to the conclusion that Sims was the culprit?

She went by the newspaper office to check her messages before deciding which story to cover next. There was one from the postmaster about the post office closing on Wednesday afternoons. "Would you put a notice in the paper that they'll have to do their mailing on Wednesday mornings instead, Blair? I don't want any angry residents banging on our doors."

Amy Matheson had left her weekly update about her daughter's latest accomplishments. "Blair, I'm sending you a picture and a paragraph about Courtney's soccer team's win last week. Also, I thought I'd stick in the list of the straight-A honor students from the high school. Courtney was among them, of course. Next week she's in the Chatham County Junior Miss Pageant. I know you'll want to cover that."

Blair sighed. Amy would love it if Blair devoted every page to her daughter. She needed an entire staff to keep up with these mundane stories. If she ever did expand into a daily, statewide paper, maybe she wouldn't need this kind of drivel to fill up the pages.

She waited for the next message. "Blair, it's me." It was Morgan's voice, flat and listless. "I wondered if you could come by and house-sit while I go to Dr. Sims this afternoon. I'm not comfortable leaving Sheila here alone with Caleb, and Jonathan's going with me. Sadie's here too, but I would feel a lot better if you were here. I have to be there at three."

Blair wondered why she was going to Dr. Sims. She hadn't had an appointment scheduled. Unless . . .

Blair's heart jolted. Had her sister decided to do something drastic? Was she going to tell him that she wanted in vitro?

She didn't bother to call her back. Instead, she called Cade's cell phone, hoping he was still in Savannah and could get the signal. When he picked up, she burst out of her chair.

"Cade, this is Blair. I hope I'm not interrupting anything."

"No, I'm just driving back. What's up?"

"It's Morgan. She's made an appointment to see Dr. Sims this afternoon. I'm afraid she's decided to go through with the in vitro. She needs to know what you told me."

He hesitated for a moment. "What time's her appointment?"

"Three o'clock."

"It's one now. Tell you what, I'll go straight to the house, and we'll tell her together. Maybe she can keep that appointment and help us out a little."

Blair grunted. "No, Cade. She's too fragile right now. She might not be able to handle it."

"Don't underestimate your sister, Blair. She's almost as tough as you are."

57

Morgan stared out through the glass window in the kitchen, across the sun porch to the backyard. She could see Caleb chattering while he played on his plastic playground. Sheila stood back, as if she didn't know how to involve herself in his play. Morgan hoped she wouldn't let him fall.

She started to turn away, but just as she did, she saw Sheila bring something to her mouth. Was that another cigarette?

Morgan opened the screen door and stepped out, letting it bounce shut behind her. Sheila jumped and dropped what she'd been holding, but a thin cloud of smoke lingered around her.

Morgan almost didn't say anything, but then she realized that Gus and Karen and Felitia had all been smokers too, when they'd come. They all quit as a requirement of living in the home. If she let Sheila get away with it, how would she face them?

She stepped down the steps into the

yard. "Sheila, you were smoking."

Sheila stepped on the butt, hiding the evidence. "No, I wasn't."

Morgan picked Caleb up. "He's never been around cigarette smoke, not since he's been with me. He doesn't need to be inhaling that stuff."

"Hey, I didn't do it, okay? I'm being falsely accused."

Morgan touched her arm and moved her aside. The butt lay on the ground like an indictment. "Then what is that?"

Sheila shoved her hair back from her face. "Look, there's no sin against smoking. I haven't done anything wrong."

Morgan tried not to react in her anger. She swallowed back her ire and took a deep breath. "Sheila, I really want this to work. Not just for Caleb and Sadie, but for you, too. We're not asking that much of you. We'll give you a nice place to live, food and clothing, and all the time in the world to be with your children. You don't even have to work until you get your bearings."

The screen door opened and Blair called out, "Hey, Sis."

Thank goodness Blair had come. Now she could leave without worrying. "I'll be in in a second," she called. Blair went back

in, and Morgan turned back to Sheila.

Caleb was fighting to get down. Morgan set him on his feet, and he bolted back to the playground.

Sheila sighed. "Look, I'm sorry. I won't smoke anymore. It's just stressful, this whole thing. I know I've been clean for a year, but I still have those cravings for . . . the drugs. And the cigarettes. I figure there's no harm in the cigarettes." She shoved her hair back from her face. "Oh, man. I can't believe I just told you that. You can't understand those cravings."

"No one's judging you, Sheila. Almost everybody who comes here has them, but I really believe the cigarettes make the cravings worse instead of better. Just the smell of matches starts the cravings in some people. In order to change your life, things have to be different. It's my job to help you with that. Don't you want to do better by your children? Don't you want to stop letting yourself down?"

Sheila's face softened, and she looked helpless as she stared back at her son. "Of course I do. I'll do better. I promise."

Morgan sighed as she went back into the house. She didn't want to talk to Blair or anyone else about all the negative feelings pulsing through her. She had only been at

this for a few months, since her mother had died. Before, she had just helped her parents deal with the problems the residents presented. She had watched and learned, but when they died, she had felt called to take over. But she wasn't a seasoned veteran, and she wasn't as wise as they were. She could only draw on the wisdom of the policies they'd set in place, and the strength she drew from her Bible study and prayer early each morning. Without that, she knew she would have closed the home months ago.

She stepped back into the kitchen and saw Blair waiting for her. She heard men's voices in the front room. "Is Jonathan home?"

"Yeah, he drove up when we did. He's talking to Cade. Morgan, we need to talk to you in private."

"What about?"

"It's about Lisa. Let's go into the parlor."

What now? Morgan followed Blair into the parlor and listened, horrified, as Cade told them about Lisa's uterus and the second opinion she'd gotten.

"Whoa, wait a minute," Jonathan said. "You're telling us that Sims is a liar? A fraud?"

"It looks that way," Cade said.

Morgan felt as if an eighteen-wheeler going ninety miles an hour had just broadsided her. She stared in front of her, searching her memory of every encounter with the doctor for some sign of guile. He'd seemed so sincere, so down-to-earth, so compassionate. He'd acted as if he really wanted them to have a child. For Lisa . . .

"He manipulated Lisa, lied to her, kept her from getting the help she needed that would have helped her get pregnant? How could anyone be that cruel?"

Blair spoke quietly, as if she feared setting Morgan off. "I told Cade that you had an appointment this afternoon. I wanted him to share this with you before you invested any more into this."

Tears came to Morgan's eyes. "We were going to have IVF. He convinced us that was the best thing."

"Can we trust him with the results of the tests?" Jonathan asked. "Any of them?"

"I wouldn't," Cade said.

New hope blossomed inside Morgan. Maybe he was wrong about her hormones. Maybe it wasn't as bad as he'd made it sound. Maybe she *could* have a family.

Jonathan got up and went across the room. He turned back, rubbing his tanned

neck. "Wow. This is unbelievable. What do you want us to do, Cade?"

"I want you to keep that appointment today. Tell him you've decided to do the in vitro. I'll put a wire on you, Jonathan, so we can record whatever he says. I want you to ask specific questions. Get him to tell you Morgan's condition again. Ask who does the ultrasounds, who fertilizes the egg after its harvested, which labs they work with, and how long before you get the results."

"I'll go along with this," Jonathan said, "as long as he doesn't touch my wife again. I don't want him doing anymore tests or injecting anything into her or drawing blood —"

"That's fine. I just want him to indict himself with his words."

"I can't promise I won't reach across that desk and throttle him."

Morgan knew her husband wasn't exaggerating. "Jonathan, we can't do this if you act angry."

"She's right, man," Cade said. "I need you to stay calm. Act like you would have before. He thinks he's getting away with it."

Jonathan's jaw popped. "Do you think he killed Lisa?"

Cade rubbed his face. "I don't know. We may be talking about two different cases that have nothing to do with each other. But it's real coincidental that Lisa found out on the same day she disappeared."

Morgan sat down. "I'm going to be sick."

Jonathan looked down at her. "Honey, are you sure you're up to this?"

"You *bet* I am —" She bit the words out. "If he killed my friend, or even just lied to her — or to us — he needs to be stopped."

Cade got up. "I'm going to get you an appointment with Dr. Anderson, Lisa's other doctor. He's going to do some preliminary testing of you and Jonathan and see if he can confirm what Sims has already told you. Will you do that, Morgan?"

"Of course. Just tell me when to show up."

58

Morgan's heart hammered out a triple-time cadence as she followed Jonathan into Dr. Sims' waiting room. As always, the room was full. How many people in here were clinging to false hope, and how many had been lied to about their conditions? She fought the urge to scream out that they needed to flee from this office and get second opinions immediately. She hoped they would know to do so when Cade got through with Sims.

Jonathan guided her to two of the last available seats. Morgan's palms were wet. She hoped the doctor didn't try to shake her hand. She glanced at Jonathan. He wore a dress shirt and jacket, not his usual attire, but it helped hide the wire that Cade had put on him. It wasn't visible at all. There would be no reason for the doctor to suspect anything.

She glanced around for something to read — anything to keep her hands and eyes busy while they waited — and found a

copy of the latest *Cape Refuge Journal*. She picked it up and saw the picture of Lisa Jackson on the front page.

"That's so sad about Lisa Jackson." The woman next to her pointed to the picture. "She was a friend of mine."

"Really? How did you know her?"

"From here. I used to see her here from time to time. We had a lot in common."

Morgan didn't want to get into her own relationship with Lisa. Her throat was too tight, and her heart still sprinted. She hoped her nerves didn't show on her face.

"Life is so short," the woman said. "You just never know what's going to happen. Here she was, struggling so hard to have a baby, and if she had gotten pregnant, she wouldn't have even lived to see it be born."

The irony had not escaped Morgan, either. "Maybe all those babies she miscarried were waiting for her in heaven."

The woman got tears in her eyes. "That's a nice thought."

"Yes, it is." Morgan smiled and patted her hand.

"I saw her the morning she disappeared."

Jonathan put his hand over Morgan's and leaned forward to see the woman. "You saw her that day? Are you sure?"

"Oh, yes. I'll never forget that."

"Where did you see her?" Morgan asked.

"Right here. In this very office."

Morgan couldn't speak, so Jonathan did. "But I read that the appointment she missed was for that afternoon."

"Oh, she wasn't here for an appointment. In fact, the doctor wasn't in until after noon. I just came in to get some blood work done. Lisa came storming in. She looked like she was fuming."

Morgan turned and looked at Jonathan. This was new information. Even Cade didn't know about this.

The woman lowered her voice. "She didn't even speak to me. She walked right past me to the receptionist's desk and told them that she needed to see the doctor immediately. They told her he wasn't in, that he was off that morning, so she hurried back out. That was the last time I ever saw her. The next day, when I heard she was missing, I was stunned."

"Did you hear her say where she was going?"

"No, nothing."

"Was she alone?" Morgan asked.

"Yes, as far as I could tell. I didn't see her drive away, though." She sighed. "I've

thought about it a million times. Maybe if I'd stopped her, asked her what was wrong, invited her for a cup of coffee . . . maybe she wouldn't have gotten murdered."

The nurse came to the door and called out, "Laura Gulley."

The woman next to Morgan sprang up, whispered goodbye, and headed back to see the doctor.

Morgan stared at Jonathan. Whispering, she said, "The question is, did she find the doctor after she left here?"

"I hope Cade is getting this," Jonathan said in a low voice.

59

"So you've decided to try IVF!" Dr. Sims looked almost jubilant at the decision. He sat down at his desk and folded his hands in front of him. "Tell me what prompted this decision."

Morgan swallowed and looked at Jonathan. He took her hand. She was trembling. "Well, it was a very hard decision, but you convinced us it was the right thing. I'll be thirty soon, and I want so much to have children. Not just one, but three or four. Maybe even more. I'm ready to get started."

"And how do you feel about that, Jonathan?"

Jonathan was calmer than she was. She could feel the heat of his anger in his hand. "I wasn't so sure. For one thing, we'll have to mortgage our house to do this. We just barely make ends meet as it is. I'm not sure it's the right thing to do. Are you sure it's not too soon to try this?"

Sims took off his reading glasses and leaned forward on his desk. He looked like a pastor, counseling them on their covenant. His eyes held no guile. He seemed compassionate, caring. Could he really be a liar? A killer?

"It has to be your call," he said. "I can't really say what's right for you. All I know is that Morgan's FSH is too high. Her ovaries are not producing mature eggs on their own. They need help. Even if you did manage to conceive, more miscarriages could happen. If we harvest mature eggs and fertilize them outside her body, there's a greater chance that she could carry the baby to term." He turned his hands palms up. "But you do have the option to wait. We can do it a year from now. Two years."

"But even if it works," Jonathan said, "won't we have to do it with every child we have?"

"Maybe she would have multiple births," he said with a grin. "One of my patients had triplets just last night. She sold her car and cashed in her 401(k) to pay for it, but she has no regrets. None at all. She was almost forty, though. If it had happened ten years ago, it would have been much better for her. She waited until it was the absolute last resort. I'm glad she finally went

through with it."

"And then there's Lisa." Morgan hadn't expected the words to come out of her mouth. "She'd had two procedures and none of them worked."

"I had every hope that the third one would. We were so close. We had gotten her FSH levels low enough and were ready to harvest the egg. And then this."

Morgan fought the urge to ask him if Lisa had found him that morning, if she'd confronted him about her misshapen uterus and the false hope he'd given her, and all the money he had taken from her. She bit her lip until it almost drew blood.

He went on about what she could expect from the drugs he would give her and when he estimated the procedure could actually take place. Morgan sat like a statue, her hands folded in her lap. As he went on, she prayed that Cade would get enough from this conversation to lock the man up for life.

Jonathan interrogated him like a pro, probing him with pointed questions, making the man talk long enough to hang himself. "Do you use a lab, Doctor, or do you do everything yourself?"

"We do it here, in the office. Most doctors do have outside labs, but I've hired

some of the best technicians in the area, and we do all our own work. I'm very hands-on. I see the results immediately, and I oversee all of it. I do a lot of the actual lab work myself. Morgan, you've come to the best possible place to make your dreams come true. Do you believe that?"

She hesitated for a moment. "I want to," she whispered.

"Good. You're going to have to trust me. But I won't let you down."

60

Riley Holmes, Chatham County's DA, was new to his office, and while he was tough in the courtroom, he was more cautious than most of the cops in his jurisdiction would have liked.

"I do think you're onto something here, Cade," he said, looking down at the report Cade and McCormick had brought him. "But I don't think we'll have probable cause to arrest Sims for medical fraud until we get confirmation that he lied to not one, but many patients. Any lawyer could make a case for a doctor making a mistake. Interview some of his patients, get them to go for second opinions, subpoena his records, his lab reports —"

"We'll do that," Cade said. "But before we give him a heads-up on the fraud thing, I want to question him about whether Lisa found him that morning or not, and I want to get his alibi."

Holmes nodded. "Yes. We don't have

enough on the fraud case, and we have even less on the murder. I need something concrete, guys. I can't even get a grand jury indictment with any of what you've brought me. You're close, and I know you're headed in the right direction — but you still have a lot of work to do."

Cade had known that would be the answer. He looked at McCormick, whose expression was irritated but not surprised.

"Meanwhile," McCormick said, "he's going to keep seeing patients."

"All the more incentive for you to get your work done quickly."

Cade almost laughed as they left the office — as if they hadn't been working night and day with every resource they had already.

"The man's got a point," Cade said as they strode back to their car. "We don't want to make an arrest only to have some slick lawyer get it thrown out of court."

McCormick only grunted as they got into the car.

61

The Saturday debate for the mayoral race brought out hundreds of Cape Refuge citizens. Morgan supposed that was a good thing for Jonathan since he hadn't had the advertising budget that Sam Sullivan had. Hopefully, some minds would be swayed today.

It was a nice day. The temperature was low, hovering around seventy-five to eighty degrees, rather than the usual ninety-five. Even though the weather forecast had predicted rain, there wasn't a cloud in sight.

Annabelle Cotton's Dance Club was on the stage, the ladies decked out in their frilly square-dancing skirts and their Mary Jane shoes, and their partners wearing short-sleeved white shirts with sweat rings under the arms. They danced with gusto to Otis Peabody's calls. Some of the audience danced along, missing the calls and laughing with glee.

Jonathan was too busy mingling to dance, so Morgan just stood near their

campaign tent and clapped to the music, trying to keep her mind off the events of the last few days and on the task at hand. As she did, she kept her eyes on Sheila and Caleb. Sheila had taken the toddler down to the water and held his hand as he romped in the waves licking at his feet. They were, indeed, bonding. Morgan had to give Sheila credit for being attentive to the baby. She hoped Sheila didn't take her eyes off him today. So much could go wrong in a crowd at the beach.

She looked for Sadie through the crowd and saw her with her camera hanging from her neck. Blair was paying her to photograph the event for the paper. She seemed deep in conversation with Matt, the guy who helped out at the florist shop while he attended college in Savannah. He was a nice kid, a Christian, and Morgan hoped that something might come of it. Sadie needed a young man to find her attractive, one who wasn't controlled by his hormones, but she hoped the girl wouldn't get too busy with him or her pictures to forget about Caleb and her mother. Morgan wanted her to jump in if Sheila turned away for a second.

Ben Jackson's absence was conspicuous. The stage looked different than it had two

weeks ago for the original debate. Instead of three microphones and three chairs, there were only two. Instead of an organized debate moderated by an objective party, it looked as if Sarah Williford was going to moderate, which meant it would probably turn into more of a back-and-forth between the two candidates themselves. Morgan hoped Jonathan was prepared, but with all the other distractions, she feared he wasn't.

"It's all set up, Morgan."

She turned and saw that Gus had set up the table under Jonathan's tent and was unpacking stacks of campaign flyers and cards. Karen sat in one of the folding chairs behind the table, holding Emory.

"Thank you, Gus."

"I'm going to get my bride-to-be something to drink. You want something, too?"

Morgan smiled and winked at Karen. "No, thanks. I'm fine."

She turned back to the square dancing, wishing she felt more festive. She needed to be mingling, talking up Jonathan's ideas, and sticking close to his side. But she couldn't seem to drag herself out of her depression.

Blair stepped into the shade of the tent. "So where's Cade?"

Morgan looked around at the people. "I haven't seen him."

"Guess he decided not to come since he's one of the issues they'll be debating." Blair's disappointment was clear. "He should have shown up to defend himself, though."

"Don't worry, Jonathan will defend him. He probably did the right thing, staying away. Besides, he's really busy, isn't he?"

"Yeah. The DA's got him jumping through hoops." Blair paused and gave Morgan a long look. "Are you okay, Sis?"

"Yeah. Just a lot on my mind." Her eyes strayed back to the water. Caleb had plopped down in the wet, packed sand, and Sheila was helping him make a little mountain. Morgan hoped he didn't try to eat any of it.

"Stop watching them. He'll be all right."

Morgan forced her eyes away. "I know he will."

Blair stroked her back as if wishing she could offer something to lift Morgan's spirits. She needed to look happier, Morgan thought. The candidate's wife shouldn't look so melancholy.

The music ended and the square dancers curtsied and bowed. The crowd whistled and applauded.

Then Councilwoman Sarah Williford — decked out in a hot-pink sundress and a big straw hat — took the stage, clapping as the dancers exited. "Thank you, dancers. Annabelle, you work wonders with this group. I went to the high school prom with ol' Jake Pryne, and doggone if my toes weren't black and blue. You've turned him into a Fred Astaire."

The man laughed and gave another mock bow.

"Welcome to the Cape Refuge mayoral debate," she said over the PA system. "Will the candidates please come to the stage?"

She saw Jonathan shaking hands with the people he'd been talking to, and quickly he ran up to the stage. Sam Sullivan took his place as well. Sam had worn a big Hawaiian shirt and a gold chain around his neck. He had an even tan and little round white circles over his eyelids. It was a tanning bed tan, Morgan thought, carefully planned for the purpose of looking like one of the islanders. But Morgan knew he rarely spent time outdoors. He was a white-collar, at-his-desk kind of businessman.

Jonathan's tan was real, from all the hours he spent out at sea on his fishing tours. He wore a white short-sleeved dress

shirt, which probably had been a mistake since sweat rings were already visible under his arms. She hoped he looked more like a citizen who wanted to serve than a politician who wanted to take over.

"In case you guys are hungry," Sarah said into the microphone, "we have hot dogs over here to the right, only a dollar apiece, courtesy of Mac's Hot Dog Stand, and the Colonel from Cricket's has graciously offered to sell us drinks over here to the left. And Nemo from the concession stand down the beach has offered us cotton candy and popcorn."

"Give me a break," Blair said under her breath. "This is a forty-five-minute debate, for heaven's sake. What, are we gonna starve to death?"

"It's a town event, Blair," Morgan said. "Food makes it more festive."

Morgan glanced over at Sheila again. Caleb was on his feet, sand sticking to the back of his diaper. He walked toward the water, and Sheila did nothing to stop him.

Morgan caught her breath and started toward them, but suddenly Sheila got up and grabbed him before he could get slapped by a wave. His mother was doing fine — so why didn't that make her happier than it did?

"All right, ladies and gentlemen," Sarah Williford said. "I hope you all realize the importance of this debate. Since we're without a mayor right now — due to his run-ins with the law — the newly elected mayor will be sworn in just a few days after the election and will begin serving immediately. The direction of our town hangs on your decision."

"Would you get on with it, Sarah?" somebody yelled from the audience. "It's getting hot out here."

Sarah lifted her chin and kept talking. "As moderator of this debate, I'm going to start off by asking the candidates to comment on several issues. The first issue concerns the police department. We've heard Sam Sullivan saying that he would like to revamp it, that he's not satisfied with how it's running. Jonathan Cleary seems to be happy with the status quo. Sam, would you go first and please comment on your stand on this issue?"

Sam moved his heavy frame up to the microphone. "As most of you know, I'm for getting Chief Matthew Cade out of our police force and bringing in some new blood with more experience. Cade was fine when all he had to take care of was an occasional car theft and disturbing the peace

violations, but in the last year we've had five murders here, including Lisa's — God rest her soul — and as far as I can see, they're not letting up."

"Oh, brother," Blair bit out. "Somebody needs to throw a tomato at that guy."

Morgan touched her arm to calm her. "Don't say anything, Blair. Let Jonathan refute that."

The scars on Blair's face burned crimson.

Sam raised his hand dramatically. "And to make matters worse, he's running this city into some serious debt by hiring outside people to help with this investigation, even though he's already arrested the killer, my former opponent. Every day that goes by is costing this city thousands and thousands of dollars. I say it's time we got somebody who knows what they're doing in here and get the police department back on track, where it can protect our citizens and our money."

Sullivan stepped back from the microphone. Jonathan came forward, and slid his hands into his pockets. Morgan knew that he was nervous.

"As most of you know, I have great faith in our police department. Three of those murders that Sam just referred to were very

personal to me. As most of you know, my mother- and father-in-law were the first two victims, and one of our residents at Hanover House was the third. Chief Cade and his police force worked as professionally and as quickly as any police force I've ever seen to bring those cases to a resolution, just as he's done on the other two cases."

"Way to go, Jonathan," Blair muttered.

"As for the money he's spending, if I'm elected mayor, this town will get behind our police force and stop balking about giving them the resources they need to fight crime. The department is still housed in a laundromat, for Pete's sake, and their cars are all over ten years old. There is all sorts of technology available to them, but their computers are outdated. We need to hire more officers and send them to schools where they can get more training and certifications. I say we need to keep Cade in office and support him whole-heartedly."

"How you gonna pay for all that, Jonathan?" Sam mopped his forehead with a handkerchief and stuffed it back into his pocket. "You plan to raise property taxes?"

The crowd muttered disapproval, and Morgan saw the tension on Jonathan's face. "No, I'm not. The town can mark my

word. We get enough taxes from our citizens, but under my leadership, the City Council will stop wasting it."

Applause and whistles and yells roared up from the crowd, and Morgan found her spirits lifting. Jonathan could hold his own with Sam. The voters were seeing what he was made of.

Sam Sullivan's smug smile seemed to say he would shoot down Jonathan's little victory as soon as he got the microphone back.

Sarah Williford went on to ask them about parking on the island, about tourism and their approach to it, about real-estate development, and the kinds of businesses they should attract to the island. Sullivan got his licks in regarding the cell phone company he had already wooed to the island, taking absolute credit for the fact that the tower would be completed and Cape Refuge would have cellular service within a matter of days.

Morgan glanced around to see where Caleb was. She saw that Sadie had him now. She was standing back from the crowd with a concerned look on her face. As Morgan watched Sadie's eyes scan the crowd, she realized the girl was looking for her mother.

Morgan looked around, searching the crowd for Sheila's face. "Blair, do you see Sheila?"

"No, and frankly, I need Sadie to be taking pictures, not watching her brother."

"I'll get him." Morgan cut through the people and got to Sadie. "Honey, where's your mother?"

Sadie looked close to tears. "I'm not sure. She gave Caleb to me and said she'd be right back. Maybe she went to the bathroom or something."

Morgan took Caleb from her arms and kissed him on the cheek. He was getting hot. He needed to be in the shade before he got sunburned. Had Sheila done as she'd reminded her and put sunscreen on the boy?

"Morgan, I know she didn't run off. I'm not sure where she went, but she'll be right back. I know she will."

"Why don't I take Caleb and go stand under our tent? He needs something to drink."

"Okay, and I'll go look for Mom. I'm sure she's around here somewhere." Sadie took off her camera and handed it to Morgan. "Will you give this to Blair, in case she needs to get something? Tell her I'll be back in a minute."

62

The moment the debate was over, Blair saw Vince Barr, complete with a cameraman, conducting interviews among the people. Since he was a print journalist — and she used that term loosely — he'd have no reason to film unless he planned to sell the video footage to the news channels. He was probably drilling townspeople on their opinions about the murder and why Ben may have done it, whether there were others involved, or whether the police even had the right person. Anything he could find to keep the story going.

She hoped no one said anything stupid. Heading to her car to change the film in Sadie's camera, she cut through the line of cars in the parking lot and heard giggling from Carson Graham's Palm Reading van parked under a tree. As she hurried by, she glanced over.

Sheila sat in the doorway with a bottle of beer and a cigarette in one hand. Carson

held her other one and seemed to be studying her palm.

"So there you are, Sheila!" she called as if she'd been looking for her.

The woman dropped her cigarette as if it had stung her. She pulled her hand from Carson's and set the bottle down behind her in the van.

Blair stepped between the two. "My sister's been looking all over for you."

Sheila didn't get up. "I told Sadie I'd be right back."

Blair reached into the van and pulled out the beer. She held it up to Carson. "So, what are you doing, Carson? Contributing to the delinquency of one of the Hanover House residents?"

"Hey, I didn't know she lived at Hanover House."

Blair gave a sarcastic grunt. "You didn't see it in her palm?"

He smiled. "Let's just say hers wasn't as clear as yours was."

Sudden shame swept through her.

"So you had a reading too, huh?" Sheila seemed amused.

"No, I did not. I went there to interview him."

Graham's smug grin told her he enjoyed her discomfort. "I gave her one on the house."

"You did not read my palm," Blair bit out. "And any prediction you made about my life was unsolicited."

Sheila was laughing now. "Don't be so defensive, Blair. I believe in it, too."

Blair felt the fight deflating out of her. "I *don't* believe in it! And you're changing the subject."

Sheila got up. "Okay, so I saw his 'Palm Reading' sign on his van, and I asked him to give me a reading. He had an ice chest with beer, so I took one. It's not the end of the world. You don't have to tell Morgan."

Blair couldn't believe the gall of the woman. Sheila turned back to Carson. "Look, I'll see you later, okay? Feel free to call anytime. I could use the diversion."

Carson chuckled. "Maybe I will. We can finish your reading."

Blair's chin shot up at the man. "Where's your *wife*, Carson?"

He stiffened slightly. "She's here, over with the crowd. I haven't done anything wrong, Blair. By the way, I saw you and Cade at my show the other night. Hope you enjoyed it."

Sheila breathed a laugh then, as if he'd just knocked Blair down, and started to walk away. Blair launched out after her and stopped her before she reached the sand.

"What is wrong with you?"

Sheila swung around. "What do you mean?"

"I mean you have a lot of nerve doing this after Morgan has been taking care of your children for the last year. You're throwing her kindness back in her face. You had no place else to go and you know it. If you had gone back to Atlanta, you would have gone right into the arms of some other man who would get you back hooked on drugs and abuse you in every possible way. And if history repeats itself, he might also abuse your children. But instead, you get to come here to a place that's practically paradise on earth and live in a house that you would never have even *dreamed* of living in before, where your child is getting an education and your baby has been cared for and loved. All you have to do is abide by certain rules of their program, which are designed for your good. But you can't even do that!"

"I have a life, okay? I'm not some Hanover House robot. I get to think of myself sometimes."

"Isn't that what got you put in jail? Isn't that what almost got your daughter killed? Maybe it's time you started thinking of your children for a change and doing

what's right for them."

"How is my drinking an occasional beer and smoking a cigarette wrong for my children? It has nothing to do with them."

"It has *everything* to do with them," Blair said, "because if Morgan and Jonathan throw you out of the home, it's not just you who's going to lose out. It's your children."

Sheila gritted her teeth. "If I leave Hanover House, my children are going with me."

Blair threw up her hands. "*That's* what I'm talking about. There's no way on earth you could think that was best for them, not by any stretch of the imagination. They're going to lose, and you're going to lose, too. Why can't you be grateful for all Morgan and Jonathan have done for you and just abide by a few little easy rules?"

Sheila took a step closer, her face inches from Blair's. "I don't have to take this stuff from you. I'm not your inferior. You're not better than me just because you came from that family."

"I know I'm not better than you. Just a couple of months ago I was a lot like you — a sham who considered myself wise. I was stupid enough to believe the world's lies. I didn't want to be accountable to God, but you know what? I was anyway.

And so are you. If you could stop being stupid, you might actually make something of your life!"

Sheila just stared at her as if Blair had struck her in the face. Blair tried to take a deep breath. It wasn't exactly the way Morgan would have shared her faith, but it was the best Blair could do.

"You know —" she tried to calm her voice — "by all rights, you should have been in jail for four more years. The fact that you got out early was a gift from God. Look at your life, Sheila!"

"Mom!"

Blair turned and saw Sadie coming toward them. Sheila's expression changed and she started toward her daughter. "Hey, I was just on my way back."

Sadie was clearly upset. "Where were you?"

"I was looking for a bathroom."

"There's one on the Pier. All you had to do was ask me."

"Next time I'll know."

Sheila shot Blair a look that told her to keep her mouth shut, and started walking back to the crowd. Sadie exchanged looks with Blair. She clearly knew something unpleasant had occurred, but she just followed her mother back to the group.

Blair stood there a moment, wondering why she felt like a faithless hypocrite. Here she was, holding up Sheila's shortcomings like a mirror, forcing her to look into it. But she didn't want to look at her own.

The shame that someone like Carson Graham had seduced her with his uninvited reading and caused her to dwell on it, hope for it, even plan for it, sickened her. Wasn't she stronger in her faith than Sheila? Didn't she, indeed, know better?

She saw Jonathan greeting people at his table. Blair swallowed and followed Sadie and Sheila to his tent. When Sheila marched in and took Caleb out of Morgan's arms, Jonathan excused himself. She started away, but he grabbed her arm. "Sheila, have you been drinking?" he asked quietly.

"Of course not. Where would I get alcohol?"

"I don't know, but you smell like beer and cigarettes."

"What is wrong with you people?" Sheila said. "Even if I did, I'm not going to hell just because I smoke a cigarette and drink a beer!"

"Of course not," Jonathan said. "Beer and cigarettes are not what keep you out of heaven, but they are things that will keep

you out of Hanover House."

"Fine," Sheila spouted back. "Just let me know when you want me to leave, and I'll pack my bags."

She stormed off, Caleb on her hip.

Morgan looked helplessly at Jonathan.

"Is she a piece of work or what?" Blair muttered.

"Did you see where she was?" Morgan asked.

"Oh, yeah. She was in Carson Graham's van, sipping on one of his beers."

"That's it." Jonathan's voice brooked no debate. "She's out."

A look of stark-raving fear came over Morgan's face. "No, Jonathan! We *can't* throw her out."

"Either she abides by the rules or she doesn't. Look at Karen and Felitia and Gus. They're following the rules. What if they see Sheila breaking them and getting away with it?"

She had told herself the same thing, but when it came right down to it, she couldn't risk losing Caleb. "Sheila's different," she whispered harshly. "She's Caleb and Sadie's mother."

Jonathan just stared down at her. "Morgan, you can't possibly think that we should back down."

"We didn't throw Sadie out when she broke the rules."

"That was different. Sadie was our foster daughter. She was just a kid trying to grow up. Sheila is *not* a kid. She supposedly wants to change her life, but if I don't see any commitment from her, I am not willing to give her a free ride."

He went back to his constituents, forcing himself to look cordial.

Morgan turned away and looked at Blair. "What am I going to do?"

"I don't know, but I had a little talk with her. Maybe some of what I said will penetrate."

"What did you say to her?"

Blair looked back at Sheila and saw that she was whispering through her teeth to Sadie. There was anger on her face, and she knew that her words hadn't made a difference. Why should they, when she was no better than Sheila?

"Well, I sort of witnessed to her. In my own way."

"You did?" Morgan asked hopefully. "Good, Blair. Maybe coming from you, she'll listen."

"Yeah, well, my methods leave a little to be desired, I think, and I haven't exactly painted myself as the shining role model."

"What do you mean?"

"Nothing. Never mind." Blair hoped it hadn't done further damage.

Karen approached Morgan from the crowd. "Morgan, Gus is gonna take me and Emory home. It's getting too hot out here, and it's time for Emory to go down for his nap."

Morgan nodded. "Would you see if Sheila wants to go with you and take Caleb? He's looking a little peaked himself. You can take our car and we'll get a ride."

"Sure."

They watched Karen approach Sheila. Sheila looked their way, squinting in the sun. She nodded as if she was anxious to get away from this place.

"Are you okay, Morgan?" Blair asked.

Morgan sighed. "I've got to be. Jonathan needs me."

63

Blair found Sadie sitting at the end of the Pier, staring down into the water. She sat down next to her. "Want to talk about it?"

Sadie had been crying, but she tried to hide it. "I don't know why she's being like this. I'm afraid she's going to leave — or get thrown out."

Blair thought about Jonathan's decision to throw Sheila out but decided not to mention it. Maybe Morgan would talk him out of it. "She's just adjusting."

"She needs Jesus," Sadie whispered. "He's all that's really going to change her life."

Blair looked out across the ocean. Three sailboats drifted on the horizon, and toward the west she saw a schooner and a speedboat crossing paths. "It can happen," Blair said. "I'm a living example. I found myself at my lowest point of desperation, panic-stricken, with nowhere to turn, feeling like my life was totally out of my

control. That was when I looked to Christ. That was when he saved me."

Sadie nodded. "Me too. My mother's been like that for a long time. Her life has been out of her control and she's been at her lowest point. She says she's a Christian, but I don't really think she gets it. I saw her at that psychic's van. She'd rather get her palm read than pray."

Blair's throat was dry. She swallowed hard. There it was again — that shame. She didn't know why. Sadie knew she'd gone to interview Carson Graham — but she didn't know that she'd paid him any heed. She would be so disappointed if she knew.

Blair was disappointed with herself.

The warm wind blew through Sadie's hair as she studied Blair for a moment. "What was it that worked for you, Blair?"

"People were praying for me," Blair said. "Lots of people who loved me were praying hard. Those prayers were heard, Sadie. If you pray for your mom, God's going to hear."

"But will he answer?" Sadie asked.

Blair picked up a piece of hot dog bun someone had dropped next to her on the Pier and tossed it into the ocean. "I don't know the Bible as well as my sister and my

parents did, but I was raised on it just like Morgan was. I didn't always heed it, but I did hear it. I always heard that the Lord answers prayers that glorify him and are according to his will. If you pray for your mother to know Christ, God's going to answer that prayer. It's not his will for any to perish. So why wouldn't he answer that?"

"I hope that's true," Sadie said. "What a family we could have if Mom believed and lived for Jesus. I wouldn't have to worry about her so much, and I wouldn't have to worry about Caleb. She would always want to do the right thing for him, even if it meant staying at Hanover House with Morgan and Jonathan."

A strong gust of wind blew the hair back from their faces. Blair saw a dark cloud moving in from the horizon.

"Looks like it's going to storm, after all," Sadie whispered.

Blair gave the girl a hug. "We've survived storms before, haven't we?"

Sadie got up and looked back toward the crowd. Tears still ran down her face. "Can you do without me, Blair? I really need to get back home to keep an eye on Caleb and my mom."

"Sure, go ahead. I can take it from here."

She watched Sadie head back up the

Pier. The girl was clueless about who she had asked for spiritual advice.

Blair turned back to the water and thought of the way Carson's predictions had gripped and manipulated her mind, the greed and ambition and discontent they had fostered in her. Suddenly it was clear to her — none of that had been from God. They were sinful pipe dreams that, if pursued, might destroy all the blessings she had.

Her flesh was still so weak. She loved Jesus and had given her life to him, but avoiding sin was still harder than she thought.

She started to cry as the sky grew grayer and the wind whipped harder against her face.

"You okay, Sis?"

Blair hadn't heard her sister coming. Quickly, she wiped her face and looked back. "Yeah. You?"

"Not really." Morgan had been crying too, and her nose was red. She set one foot on the bottom rail and leaned on the top one.

Blair sighed, put her arms around Morgan's neck, and laid her head on her shoulder.

"We're some pair," Morgan whispered.

"You're not crying over the Sheila thing too, are you?"

Blair let her go. "No, that's not it. But it's going to be all right. You'll talk Jonathan out of throwing her out."

"How, when I know perfectly well that she *should* be thrown out?"

"Maybe this was a wake-up call for her. Maybe it's just what she needed to straighten up."

Morgan didn't answer. The wind kicked up her long brown curls, and she pushed them back from her face. "So if you weren't crying about Sheila, then what's wrong?"

Blair pulled herself up and sat on the rail, her back to the ocean. "I'm crying because I don't understand why I'm such a weak Christian."

"What? You're not weak."

"Oh, yes, I am. I'm horribly weak." She looked toward the crowd still milling around on the beach. Anabelle's clogging class had taken the stage in their red and white checkered dresses. "Morgan, the other day when I went to interview Carson Graham, he made some predictions."

"What kind of predictions?"

"About my business and my relationship with Cade. He told me that I was going to

expand my business to a statewide paper, and that Cade and I would get married soon. Ever since, I've been thinking of increasing my staff — not just by two or three people — but by dozens. Buying property, new equipment, going from twice a week to every day . . ."

Morgan looked at her like she was crazy. "Blair, you know you're not ready for that. Buying the paper in the first place was a huge step, and it's only been a few weeks."

"I know, you're absolutely right. But I've been thinking about it anyway . . . wanting it. Trying to figure a way to make it work. My ambitions have become greedy and unrealistic, just because of him. When I was a librarian, I never had these kinds of ambitions. I just loved my work. If they hadn't practically fired me, I'd still be perfectly content stacking books and doing research."

"They didn't fire you. You quit."

"Only because they were unhappy with my work." She slid down from the rail and turned around, looking out at the water. "But that's beside the point. What is wrong with me, listening to that guy? He also told me that Cade and I would get married, and now I've been picturing myself walking down the aisle, impatient about

our relationship . . . I keep thinking about when he's going to propose, like it's some kind of destiny and he's just not getting with the program. For all I know, he may not feel that way about me. We haven't made any commitments or even talked about our feelings."

"Blair, you've only been dating for a little over a month. It's not time. There are steps you have to go through. You can't just jump straight to the wedding. This kind of thing can't be short-circuited — not unless you're both ready."

"Exactly," Blair said. "And rushing things is not Cade's style, and it's not mine, either. Instead of shopping for wedding gowns I need to just enjoy the way things are developing now. But these ambitions — these crazy hopes and dreams — are making me crazy. If it weren't for Carson, I never would have been thinking this way — and that's why I'm so upset. How is it that he affected me that way?"

"Well, it probably has something to do with your listening to him in the first place. The Bible says somewhere that the pagans listen to those who practice witchcraft and to diviners, but you — meaning believers — are not allowed to."

"It's Deuteronomy 18," Blair said. "I

read it. Didn't sink in, though, apparently. And the really sick thing is that I caught Sheila getting a reading, and I acted all shocked and judgmental, and then Carson made it sound like he had read my palm too. Boy, did that make her smug."

"Oh, no."

"Yeah. Only, for the record, he did not read my palm. I didn't ask for his predictions and didn't want them. But she thinks I went to him for that. And as much as he affected me, I might as well have." Tears sprang to her eyes again. "I'm no better than her, and she knows it. Morgan, I'm so sorry."

Morgan shook her head and pushed Blair's hair out of her eyes. "Sheila has a lot of problems. You're not the cause of them, Blair."

"It's just that I hate myself for falling for it." She swallowed back the tears in her throat, and looked at her sister. "Morgan, do you remember when we were little, and Mama would wake us up and walk us through 'putting on' our helmet of salvation, our belt of truth . . ."

Morgan nodded. "Our breastplate of righteousness, and our shoes of peace."

Blair smiled. "When we headed out the door to school, she would hand us our

shields of faith and our swords of the spirit, like she expected us to run into some angry fallen angels on the way to the bus."

Morgan laughed. "And you would use that imaginary sword to stab me and throw your invisible shield like a Frisbee."

"I'd forgotten that." She laughed softly, but then her amusement faded. "Guess I never took it all that seriously, but it never made sense to me. I might as well have been putting on an imaginary crown and fairy wings. But now I see that I need that armor. Our struggle is not against flesh and blood. It's against the rulers and principalities. Apparently even against the psychics."

"That's right," Morgan said. "Mama knew what she was talking about."

"But I still don't understand how you get it. The only armor I have lying around is the imaginary kind. No pretend armor is going to stop the enemy's arrows. It certainly didn't help me against Carson."

Morgan looked surprised that she would ask such a thing. "Sis, you do have the armor. But maybe it's just weak. Look at it piece by piece. The helmet of salvation — you got that the minute you gave your life to Christ. You don't have to pretend to put some imaginary steel cap on your head in

the mornings. It's already there."

Blair thought about that for a moment. "Okay, I'll buy that, but what about the rest? The belt of truth, for instance. I sure didn't know truth when Carson was telling me what I wanted to hear."

"The truth is in God's Word. You get it from studying it, learning it, knowing what it says. Not whipping it out of some pretend closet."

"I guess that's the problem. I don't know the Bible that well, and even since I became a Christian, I haven't spent that much time reading it."

"That's easy to change. As for your breastplate, you do have that protection, because you exchanged your sin for Christ's righteousness . . . and your shoes of the gospel of peace —"

"They don't fit very well," Blair cut in. "Because my peace quotient is low. All I've had lately is anxiety and discontent. How can I take peace to anyone else when I'm in such a mess?"

"Again, you study God's Word, make it a part of you. But the shoes are about spreading the Word, telling others about the peace you've found. You have something they need."

"So what about the shield of faith? How

do I strengthen mine?"

"You have to feed it the things that make it grow stronger. Again, you have to study God's Word as if it were your very lifeline. Because it is."

Blair looked out across the water and saw that the clouds were starting to break up, revealing a fissure of bright blue sky. Morgan was so wise. Blair knew she was right, that the armor was there for her taking, if only she spent time learning God's Word and getting to know him better.

"Okay, so I'm protected if I do that. But what about the sword? It's the only offensive weapon, but I don't feel like I'm any threat at all to the enemy."

"As you get to know the Word of God, front to back, layer upon layer — hunger for it, breathe it — that sword will get sharper and more effective. If you don't arm yourself with God's Word, it's about as effective as that imaginary one you used to poke me with."

Blair felt hope seeping back into her heart. Maybe all wasn't lost. "But then why did Mama wake us with that every morning? Like it was something we could do that day?"

"She wanted to remind us what we had,

and maybe she assumed that we were more spiritually mature than we were, that our weapons and armor were ready. But the truth is, you have to build up those weapons before you need them, so you'll be ready when you're face-to-face with someone like Carson Graham."

"You're right. I was unarmed with him. Completely unequipped." She looked down at the waves crashing past the posts. "I guess occasional curiosity about something in the Bible doesn't cut it, huh? And neither does regurgitating what someone else told me. Not even if I hear it from you or Jonathan, or even Cade."

"You're getting it, Sis. It's a hands-on project, and you're responsible to keep your armor in good condition. You're a member of God's army, and that's what a good soldier does."

She deserved a court-martial, a dishonorable discharge, or maybe even a firing squad. "That does it. I'm not going to be found unarmed again. The next time the Devil tries to attack me, he's gonna have a real fight on his hands." She considered her sister for a long moment. "Maybe I need to be in the Hanover House program. Your graduates come out more grounded in their faith than I am."

"God's growing you, Blair, and you're letting him. You're not kicking against the goads, like Sheila."

Blair realized she'd been mouthing off about her own problems when her sister was hurting. She settled her eyes on Morgan. "What are you going to do?"

Morgan's tears filled her eyes again. "I don't know. I honestly don't. But please pray for me — and for Caleb and Sadie. God's worked miracles in our lives before. We could use another one, right about now."

64

Alan Sims was in much better shape than he'd been in the last time Cade had interviewed him. Cade and McCormick found him at home. Though it still looked cluttered, it was cleaner than it had been just after Lisa's death.

"No, I didn't see Lisa the day she disappeared. I told you she canceled that appointment."

"One of your patients told us that she saw Lisa come into your office that morning."

Sims looked startled. "That morning? No, it couldn't be. I wasn't working that morning."

"That's what she said," Cade went on. "They told her you were off, and she left. She said Lisa looked angry and upset and that she was intent on speaking to you. You sure she didn't come to find you?"

Sims huffed and poked his chin in the air. "*Quite* sure. As I said, I would have

told you something like that."

"Dr. Sims, what were you doing the morning Lisa Jackson disappeared?"

"I was here, puttering around in my yard. My wife went to Europe for a month, and I've been building her a fountain in the backyard to surprise her. Would you like to see it?"

Cade looked at McCormick, and the detective got up. "I would. I've thought of building one of those myself."

Cade knew his detective wanted a look at more of the house, the back door, the yard, anything that might offer him a clue.

Sims led them out and showed them the finished fountain. There was no way to tell when it was built, though it did appear new.

"Was anyone with you that morning?"

"No. My maid, Kylie, had already taken the day off. Up and quit after that. I was here alone and kind of enjoying it."

"Did anyone see you at any time that morning? Did you talk to anyone on the phone?"

"Yes, my office called a couple of times, but I didn't leave the house until about noon."

"When your office called, did they tell

you that Lisa had come in looking for you?"

"Of course not." He led them back in. "I get angry patients in all the time. They go ballistic when they start their menstrual cycles after they hoped they were pregnant. Talk about PMS. You haven't seen the half of it until you've worked with angry, hormonal, infertile women."

Cade knew the doctor expected him to laugh, but he couldn't bring himself to do it. He wished he could nail him with questions about Lisa's second opinion, about the results that suggested he was a fraud. But he couldn't. Not yet. He couldn't risk having him go back to the office and start destroying evidence.

"They certainly don't notify me of every one of them. Besides, they knew I was seeing her that afternoon. Whatever she came to see me about could have waited."

"Don't you find it odd that she would have come in that morning when she could have waited until her appointment?" McCormick asked. "Sort of sounds urgent, doesn't it?"

He rubbed his jaw and nodded his head. "Yes, it does. I wish I'd had the chance to find out what it was about. But I didn't, officers. I didn't."

★ ★ ★

Later, Cade and McCormick sat at their desks and conducted phone interviews with patients who'd been to Sims' office the day of Lisa's death. So far, only the woman Morgan met in the office claimed to have seen her that morning. The receptionist and all of the nurses had denied seeing her. Either Sims had warned them to lie, or it hadn't really happened.

After he'd talked to a dozen or so women, he hung up and studied his notes. McCormick stuck his head in Cade's office. "Have you gotten anything yet, Chief?"

"Nothing to work with. You?"

McCormick looked down at his own list. "Afraid not, and everybody I'm talking to thinks this doctor hung the moon. You wouldn't believe the loyalty."

"Well, who can blame them? A lot of these women have invested a number of their biological years in this man. To admit that he may have cheated them would be admitting they had wasted a lot of time and money."

"You don't think this guy's *responsible* for their infertility, do you?"

Cade shook his head. "Who knows? Maybe he's just in the business of giving

false hope. Or maybe he doesn't lie to all of them. Maybe it's just a select few."

"What a sleazeball."

Cade picked up his phone again. "The DA is considering subpoenaing his office for his patient files. He's reluctant to do it until we can come up with a little more evidence. Before he shuts the guy down, he wants a smoking gun."

"Let's hope we can find one before he uses it again."

65

Sheila took advantage of Caleb's nap time to make some phone calls. Since Jonathan and Morgan were still at the Pier, and Karen was lying down while Emory napped, she knew she wouldn't get caught if she slipped into that master bedroom that no one used and called her friends in Atlanta.

She closed the door quietly behind her. Sadie had told her this was the bedroom of Morgan's parents who had been murdered less than a year ago. The family had left it like a shrine, with all their belongings still in place. It was downright creepy, but it had a telephone.

Sheila sat down on the bed and dialed her best friend in Atlanta.

"Hello?"

"Marlene!" She kept her voice low. "You'll never guess who this is."

Marlene paused for a moment. "Sheila, is that you?"

"Yes, it's me. I'm out of jail. Can you be-

lieve it? They let me out early. Some law by the legislature. Whoever thought those people were good for anything?"

Marlene gave a hoarse victory yell. "Well, when are you coming home, kid?"

"That's just it. I'm not. I had to come to Cape Refuge to be with Sadie and Caleb. I'm staying in a home that's almost like a prison itself. I really miss you guys. What's going on there?"

"I've got a new guy," Marlene said. "His name's Harley, and he moved in with me last week. I'm glad you're not here. You'd probably steal him from me."

"Well, why don't you bring him east and let me check him out? I could use some company, and you could probably use a little beach time."

"We might do that," Marlene said, "only I'm working weekends now and most nights. Harley had a good job, but he got laid off a couple of weeks ago. I'm trying to keep us both above water."

It sounded like a typical scenario. The men in Marlene's life — Sheila's too, for that matter — had always had trouble holding jobs. "Man, I'd give anything to come home."

"Hey, if you do, you can stay with me. I can clean out the back room. It'll be

just like old times."

"What about Sadie and Caleb? I can't leave without them."

"Hey, we can work it out. I love babies." She'd had three of her own, but two had been removed from her home and the other one lived with his no-account father.

The door opened, and Sheila jumped. Morgan stepped into the room, staring at her as if she'd caught her stealing from her purse.

"What are you doing in here?"

Sheila dropped the phone. "I just wanted to see what was in here." She fumbled for the phone, then quickly hung it up. "It's a nice room. Why doesn't anybody ever use it?"

Pain flashed across Morgan's eyes. "It's off limits, that's why. I don't want anybody in here."

"Okay, okay." Sheila got up and started to the door.

"You were on the telephone."

Here it came. Sheila stopped in the doorway. "Yeah? So?"

"Sheila, you're allowed to make local calls, and we have phones all over the house. Why did you come in here to make a call?"

"Because I wanted my privacy."

Morgan picked up the phone, pressed redial, and read the readout. "Privacy to make a long distance call to Atlanta?" She hung the phone back in its cradle.

"I just wanted to talk to my friend."

Morgan struggled with tears in her eyes. Sheila couldn't imagine why. Was this just a battle of wills? Morgan hated losing that much?

"This was my parents' room." Her voice rasped as she got the words out. "I don't like for anybody to come in here except family."

Sheila didn't know why that stung her. Sadie had talked so much about Hanover House being a family, but she had known it couldn't be true. People didn't treat strangers like family. Especially not people like her.

"I've had a hard time with their deaths," Morgan whispered. "I want . . . I need . . . to leave things in here exactly as they left them. It gives me comfort."

Sheila didn't want to see Morgan's grief. It was better if she kept her distance. She started toward the door.

"Sheila, the home is supported by donations and the money that Jonathan makes on his fishing tours. We barely make ends meet as it is. We can't afford long distance

bills for the residents."

"Then add it to my list of broken rules and throw me out. My friend says I can come and live with her. She has a room for me, and Sadie and Caleb will be happy there. The more I think about it, the more I think it's a really good idea."

Morgan just stared at her. "Sheila, why are you so hostile?"

"Hostile? *Me?* You're the one riding me about everything."

Morgan sat down on the bed and started to cry. "I'm begging you, please don't do this to Caleb and Sadie."

"I'm not doing anything to them except clearing their heads! You've brainwashed them both. If I get them out of here, it might be the best thing that ever happened to them."

"What are you doing, Mom?"

Sheila swung around and saw Sadie standing in the doorway. How much had she heard?

"I was just having a few words with Morgan." She left the room and headed for her bedroom. Grabbing the bag she'd brought from jail, she pulled open her dresser drawers and started packing. There wasn't much, since even the clothes on her back were borrowed. Sadie came in behind

her. "I've decided I'm leaving here. I've had enough. Marlene says we can move in with her. All I have to do is call her and tell her to clean out the back room. Pack your stuff."

She looked over her shoulder at Sadie, and saw that she was crying now too. She softened. "Honey, it'll be fun. You remember Marlene, all the times we used to have."

"I won't go with you, Mom. I'm staying here."

Sheila stopped packing and turned back to her. "How can you say that? After all this time that I've been in jail, not able to see you . . . ? Are you trying to break my heart?"

"No. I'm trying to change it."

"Well, you can't change me! There's nothing wrong with me. I know what you're afraid of. You think I'm going to go back to drugs, but I'm not, Sadie. I'm stronger now. I've been sober all this time, and I know I can do it."

"You knew you could do it last time too, Mom, only you didn't. Jack came along and he ruined you, and you wound up in jail." She smeared the tears across her face. "You can go, if you have to, Mom, but you'll go alone. I won't let you take Caleb."

Sheila stood stiffer now, facing off with her. "You can't stop me, Sadie. He's my son."

"That's right!" Sadie cried. "He's your *son*. Be a mother to him! I'm asking you to put his welfare first. It's not good for him to move in with Marlene and her boy-friend-of-the-week and her drugs, and you know it. If you cared about him, you wouldn't even *think* of it."

Sheila felt as she had in jail when someone had waltzed into her cell and stolen her hard-earned commissary items. "You have no right to talk to me that way. After all I've been through, the sacrifices I've made."

"The only sacrifices you've made have been forced on you," Sadie cried. "They've been because you were backed into a corner and you had no choices. You *have* choices now, Mom. You can do the right thing for Caleb. I'm old enough to make my own decisions, and I don't have to go with you. But so help me, if you take Caleb out of here and disrupt his life, you'll never see me again."

Sheila gaped at her. "You would turn your back on your mother and your little brother?"

"I wouldn't want to, Mom, but you've

got to think about what you're doing. He's just a baby. He's seen some hard times, but he doesn't even remember them because the last few months have been so good. He doesn't need to go to some place where the people can't be trusted and he can't have any peace. He loves Morgan and Jonathan, and he loves me, and he doesn't even know you anymore!"

The words stung like the bite of a viper. "Sadie . . ."

Her daughter could hardly speak through her sobs. "I know it hurts to hear that, Mom, but it's true. You can't say you love him if you're going to take him out of this home. It would be a lie. I'm asking you to do the right thing. The hard thing. I want you to stay, but if you can't do that, leave him here. If you don't, you can quit calling me your daughter, because I don't want to have anything to do with you!"

The words slammed hard into Sheila's heart, almost knocking her back. She watched her daughter turn and run back down the stairs. The front door slammed. She looked out her window and saw Sadie running across the street to the beach, sobbing her heart out.

It only made her angry.

"You really gonna leave?"

413

She swung around and saw Karen standing in her doorway, her arms crossed.

Sheila wiped her face. "What's it to you?"

Karen came in, looked at the bag she'd been packing. "I'll tell you what it is to me. When I got out of jail I wanted to do the same thing. I had the choice of coming here or going back to the old neighborhood. I decided to go back. Wound up moving back in with my boyfriend, and every night he got high and slapped me around."

Sheila had been there. She hadn't forgotten what that was like.

"And then I went and got pregnant." Karen sat down on her bed. "And I kept telling myself that he was gonna change, because I was having his baby and he was gonna care. Only he had a few other women, and some of them had babies, too. One of them had her baby before me. She had to go back to work two weeks after the baby was born because he wasn't about to support her."

"Why are you telling me this? I didn't ask you to come in here."

"She left her baby with him while she went to work, Sheila. The baby was two weeks old when he took him on a drug

414

deal with him, and somebody hurt him. That night he had a seizure, and his mama took him to the hospital. He had a cracked skull."

Sheila didn't want to hear this. It sounded too familiar. She thought of Sadie's broken ribs, her broken arm, the bruises on her face.

"That's when I knew my baby wasn't gonna make it if I stayed there. I had to make a choice, just like you have to make now. I decided to do what was best for my baby and get him out of that environment before he was even born. I showed up here nine months pregnant, begging them to take me in, and they did. The minute I gave my life back to God and started letting him call the shots, things turned around for me."

Sheila didn't want to keep crying in front of this woman she hardly knew. She turned back to the window and peered out. Sadie was long out of sight.

"It could happen to you, too. But if you choose to be stupid like I was stupid and go back to the place you came from — the same place that got your family torn apart and you thrown in jail — then you deserve to lose your daughter and your baby."

"How *dare* you?" Sheila bit out the

words. "You don't know me."

"Oh, I know you. I know you because you're just like me. You could take Caleb out of here and back to that neighborhood. But you better know he's gonna grow up just like you — shooting up, snorting, beating women . . . in and out of jail. You need to decide if it's worth it."

Sheila jerked up the bag and shoved the rest of her things into it.

Karen got up, touched her shoulder, and made Sheila look at her. "Sheila, you do the right thing for your kids, and you'll be doing the right thing for you, too. You need to look at your sins, girl. You need to repent and thank God that he's stepped in as much as he has to break that cycle for your babies."

Sheila just gritted her teeth. "Get out of my way." She threw the bag aside and bolted out of the room. Morgan stood at the top of the stairs, and Sheila knew she'd heard everything. Sheila pushed past her and went down the stairs and out the front door.

66

Fury propelled Sheila across the street and down the beach. Sadie was nowhere in sight, so she strode as fast as she could on the sand, cursing under her breath and replaying those conversations in her mind. Who did these people think they were? How did they know she couldn't do the right thing? How in the world could they anticipate the way she would bring up her child? They barely knew her.

The sun bore down on her, making her sweat. Summer was closing in. She wished she could move up north, where the summers were dry and cool. She could get a little house in the mountains and start over. All she had to do was work a while in Atlanta and she could make it happen.

She lifted her hair from her neck and slogged through the sand. The beach was four miles long, and she walked all the way down it, then up along the river. She was soaked and breathing hard as she went

past the Bull Bridge.

She wasn't going to find her daughter.

But maybe that was best.

After all, she was letting her down again. She knew it from the depths of her heart, but she felt powerless to change it. She couldn't stay here. It was out of the question.

She walked and walked, hating herself more with each step. It would have been better for everyone if she'd stayed in jail. Her daughter had been settled, well adjusted, until she'd come back. Caleb couldn't have been healthier or happier.

If she went back to Atlanta, would she do what Karen predicted? Would she fall back into the habit of using again, bringing men home, letting them ruin her life again? Was that her nature? She didn't want to believe it, yet she knew it was true.

Sadie was right. How had her daughter gotten her head screwed on so straight? She thought about that day that Sadie came to see her in jail, with her arm broken and her eye swollen shut. Jack had beaten her, and she'd barely escaped.

Sheila felt so helpless and so frightened for her baby, still in Jack's care. She'd told Sadie to run, to get as far from him as she could.

That's how Sadie wound up in Cape Refuge.

Sheila had moments of repentance in jail. She went to religious counseling and talked the talk. She had even meant it at times. From inside her cell, she'd had clarity of mind and had seen the provisions that had been made for her children. She'd even been thankful.

Why now did she feel so angry, so out of control, so *oppressed?* After all this time, why couldn't she get Atlanta out of her mind? Why couldn't she let herself start over?

It would be so simple just to follow the rules and be there for her children, but she didn't know if she had the character to be what they expected her to be.

She followed the river through the trees, hoping Sadie had not come back here. It was near the place where that Jackson woman had been found. Sadie had shown it to her yesterday. She came to the flowers placed at the sight where the woman's car had gone in.

She paused for a moment, noting the tire tracks in the grass and trying to picture where the car had plunged into the water. It didn't look like a place of death. She'd seen places that did — crack houses and

419

dirty hotel rooms and the alleys behind the strip clubs.

She'd kicked her crack habit once, when Sadie was a little girl, but when she'd started to gain weight, she'd changed her drug of choice to methamphetamine. That led her to Jack, a dealer with a lab, and she allowed him to come into her home and set up shop there.

What had she been thinking?

She stood at the edge of the water, staring down into it, and suddenly the reality of that horrible decision washed over her again — the shame that she felt when she was arrested in front of her daughter and taken off in handcuffs, the screams of her baby as she was driven away.

Her mother was an alcoholic, so Sheila always consoled herself with the idea that addiction was a family disease and she had no control over it. But the truth was that selfishness had more to do with her addiction than genes. She cared more about her drugs than she cared about her children.

That wasn't who she wanted to be.

She stared down the bank into the water. If she were to jump in right now, plummet straight to the bottom, Sadie would be the only one to mourn her passing.

She wanted to be a person people would

miss when she was gone, someone for whom they would bring flowers, someone who left a legacy of good things and not bad.

But that was never going to be who she was. Maybe throwing herself in the river would be the noblest act she'd ever done. Though they'd probably never say it out loud, they'd probably secretly thank God that she wasn't causing problems anymore.

She stared at the water as it rushed by to join the sea. She wondered what it felt like to jump in. It was probably warm enough, and the river rushed fast and hard enough to keep her from changing her mind and struggling back to the bank. No, if she did it, she needed to make sure it worked. Her cowardice could be no excuse for living.

She thought of the water closing over her head, fighting to catch her breath as the current swept her down river and then out to sea. Would a shark come along and end things quickly? Would they think she'd run away, until her body washed up several days later?

No, that was no better for Sadie than going to Atlanta.

She stepped back from the river's edge and wiped the tears from her face. What had Karen said, about her having a choice?

She'd said there was nothing noble about snatching Caleb and going back to Atlanta. She'd probably say there was nothing noble about making your daughter suffer through a suicide, especially after they'd exchanged harsh words, either. Sadie would blame herself. It would change the rest of her life. Nothing good could come of it.

What Karen was doing was noble — coming here and committing herself to starting a new life for the sake of her little baby. And now she was planning her wedding. Maybe the prison chaplain had been right. Maybe there were blessings in living right.

Breaking her daughter's heart for the hundredth time in her life was not noble. Staying here and submitting to Jonathan and Morgan's authority would be. The sacrifice would be theirs, not hers.

They'd offered her a life, a second chance, a new beginning. She'd thrown it back in their faces.

Her mind sorted through the possibilities. If she went back, begged their forgiveness, promised Sadie she would do better . . . would they let her stay? Or were they already making plans to throw her out?

She heard a screen door slam and looked up to the pier just around the bend of the river. There must be a house hidden in the trees there.

Then she saw him, coming through the trees, walking the path straight toward her.

Carson Graham.

He looked startled when he saw her standing there. She started to speak, but then she heard a woman's voice. "Carson! You forgot your wallet!"

He turned back, and Sheila saw a pretty blonde woman hurrying out to meet him. She handed him his wallet, then reached up to kiss him. Carson pulled back and nodded toward Sheila. The woman jumped away, then hurried back into the house. Carson followed her.

Was he fooling around? He'd told her that he lived in that Palm Reading house, and at the beach she could have sworn that his wife was a brunette.

It wasn't surprising that he'd have an affair. He'd certainly put out the signals with her, and she hadn't dissuaded him. In fact, she had told him to call her, even though she knew he wasn't single.

It didn't matter. Carson Graham's fidelity wasn't her concern. She had enough problems of her own.

She left the river to keep from walking through that yard, and followed the road back to Hanover House. Her feet hurt and she needed water. She hadn't meant to walk so far.

She'd been gone for over two hours by the time she made it back to Hanover House. She walked into the house and found everyone seated around the kitchen table. Sadie was home, but her eyes were swollen, and disappointment seemed etched into her young face.

It was an awful sight, that disappointment. That acceptance that her mother was a loser. Sheila wanted to erase that from her face.

They all looked up at her. They were angry, and she couldn't blame them for it anymore.

Caleb sat in his highchair between Morgan and Jonathan, feeding himself with a spoon. He was the only one who didn't look at her as if bracing himself. Instead, he ignored her, as if she had nothing to do with him.

Sheila drew a deep breath. "I used to think that all the bad things in my life were other people's fault, and I guess I blamed everybody but myself. But it's no one else's fault. It's just mine. I'm the one who's

failed myself. I'm the one who's failed my children."

It clearly wasn't what they'd expected her to say. She went around the table to Sadie. Her daughter looked up at her, tears streaming from her red eyes. Sheila's mouth trembled. "Honey, I'm so sorry that I've broken your heart so many times. You don't deserve it. If you'll give me another chance, I'll do better. I promise."

Sadie just looked at her as if she'd heard this before, and Sheila knew she would have to prove it. She turned to Morgan and Jonathan.

"Morgan and Jonathan . . ." She looked away, ashamed to meet their eyes. "I made up my mind in jail that when I got out I was gonna be somebody. I was gonna turn my life around and start taking care of my children. But the fact is, Morgan, you take a lot better care of my children than I do, and I've been having a hard time with that."

Morgan sighed and looked at Jonathan. "Sheila, I appreciate your saying that. I know it's not easy."

"No, it's not easy, but it should be. I mean, why is it so hard for me to admit things? I ought to be down on my knees, thanking you."

Jonathan got up and stepped toward her. "Sheila, why don't we start over? If you'll commit to our program and stop seeing us as the enemy, then we'd love for you to stay."

A sob caught in her throat, and she covered her mouth. "I promise. Thank you."

"All right then. Welcome back."

Morgan got up and hugged her, and she wept against her shoulder. How could Morgan stand to hold her after the way she'd spoken to her, the things she'd said?

But Morgan wasn't like anyone else she'd ever known.

Sheila went to Sadie, touched her shoulder. "Will you forgive me, honey?"

Sadie was crying so hard she could hardly speak. She got up too, and came to put her arms around her mother. Sheila clung longer than she needed to. She almost didn't dare let her go. Sadie felt so small in her arms, so vulnerable, so broken. She swore to herself — and to God — that she would never hurt her again.

67

"Curiouser and curiouser." McCormick came into Cade's office and sat down. "Another twist in this continuing saga."

Cade didn't need another twist. He'd been too busy trying to untwist the things they already knew. "All right. Let's hear it."

"We've got a match on the handwriting. Sam Sullivan wrote the letters to Lisa Jackson, all right, and his prints were all over them. He tried to disguise his handwriting, but the analyst says that it's definitely his."

Cade laced his fingers in front of his face. He couldn't say he was surprised. After all, he'd had enough suspicion to give Sam's sample to the analyst. Sam had been bonded for his work, so his prints had already been in the system.

"Okay, so we have Sam Sullivan, Jackson's opponent in the race, stirring up trouble for the front-runner. I guess the

question is, how far was he willing to go? There are miles between mail fraud and murder."

"You want to come with me to question him?"

Cade thought that over for a moment. "No, I'd rather you picked him up and brought him in for questioning. That'll be better than getting his whole office involved. Meanwhile, I'll get on the phone with the DA and see about getting an arrest warrant for mail fraud. Anything to hold him."

Half an hour later, they brought Sam in, still wearing the Hawaiian shirt he'd had on during the debate that morning. His neck and face were sunburned after a full day of campaigning door-to-door. He announced that he didn't know what this was about, but he wasn't saying a word until his lawyer joined him. Sam clearly knew that he'd been found out — but just how deep did his guilt run?

His lawyer, Richard Mason from Savannah, got there an hour later, and they all assembled in the interview room, as if they were sitting down to negotiate a deal.

"What's this all about, Cade?" Sullivan demanded.

Cade pulled out the letters that had been

sent to Lisa Jackson. "Sam, have you ever seen these?"

Sam glanced at his lawyer. A thin sheen of perspiration glistened on his lip. "No, I haven't. What are they?"

"They're letters that were sent to Lisa from someone who claimed to be Ben's lover."

Sam wiped his mouth. "So the rumors were true?"

Cade didn't answer. "Sam, your fingerprints are on these letters, and we have it on good authority that they're in your handwriting."

"No way!" Sam got to his feet and looked at his lawyer. "Why would I do a thing like that?"

Cade didn't move. "Sit down, Sam. Tell us where you were on the morning of May 16."

"Oh, you've got to be kidding me!"

His attorney touched his arm to silence him. "Chief, I'd rather my client didn't answer that until I've had the chance to confer with him."

Sam slapped his hand on the table. "No, I'll answer it. I have nothing to hide, Cade. I was in my office on the morning of May 16, and my secretary and a dozen others can vouch for it. In fact, that was the morning I had the cell phone people in." A

sweat drop ran from his hairline to his jaw. "You gotta believe me, Cade."

"We'll talk to them, and if it's true, we'll find out. But for now, I'd like to know how you explain those letters."

His lawyer tried to silence him again, but Sam shook him off. "If I don't talk, they're going to think I'm guilty of murder!" He rubbed the sweat off of his mouth and took a deep breath. "Okay, Cade. I'm gonna lay all my cards on the table, because I don't need a murder rap. I did something stupid, but not *murder*. I sent the letters, okay? I admit it."

Cade met McCormick's eyes. Now they were getting somewhere.

"It was a lousy thing to do, I admit. I was trying to get a leg up in the race. I thought if I stirred up a little trouble in paradise, that might knock Ben's legs out from under him. If I'd known that Lisa was gonna wind up dead, I never would have done it. It was unethical, but it wasn't criminal."

"Ever heard of mail fraud?" Cade asked. "How about harassment?"

McCormick agreed. "How about murder one? Lining up things to make it look like Ben had a motive for killing his wife."

"I wouldn't be that stupid!" Sam sat

back down and made an effort to calm himself. "I just wanted to start a rumor to sway opinion. I approached Vince Barr and tried to get him to write about it, but he wouldn't. Said he wasn't interested in local politics — and the *Savannah Morning News* wouldn't print it because they couldn't confirm it. I knew better than to approach Blair Owens with it. I never expected police involvement. If there hadn't been a murder, this would have been a harmless prank."

"A prank that might have broken up a marriage and ruined a man's life," Cade said.

McCormick chuckled. "And you didn't have much faith in the police department, did you, Sam? This Podunk outfit couldn't figure out anything that complicated."

"Oh, boy." Sam sat back hard in his chair. Despite his tanning-bed tan, he was beginning to pale. "Cade, I know you don't have good feelings toward me, after all I've said about you during the race, but so help me, if you try to pin this murder on me, I'll scream harassment so loud that they'll hear it all the way in Atlanta."

Cade leaned his elbows on the table and leveled his eyes on him. "That sounds like a threat, Sam."

Sam backed off. "That's not how I meant it, Cade. I'm just saying that people might *perceive* it wrong."

"They might perceive it right," McCormick said, "and then where would you be?"

When they'd finished questioning Sam, Cade realized holding him would invite accusations that Cade had worked things so Jonathan would win the election. If he let him go, they could keep an eye on him until they could corroborate his alibi. Cade watched Sam drive off with his attorney.

McCormick shook his head. "What a guy."

Cade looked around at the other cops in the squad room. They all watched him for a rundown of what they'd found out. "McCormick, I want you to check out Sullivan's alibi with every person he claims he saw that morning. Check his phone records, see who called him. Johnson, Caldwell, you interview everybody who talked to him, see if they spoke to him personally. I want this done before you go home tonight."

"So he did send the letters?" Caldwell asked him.

"Yeah, he sent them. He confessed to that much."

"You think he's the killer, Chief?" Johnson asked.

"He's got an alibi. We just have to see if it's real. At best, he's a scumbag who would lie and cheat to win an election. At worst, he's a murderer."

McCormick rubbed his hand over his bald head. "I say we leak it to the press. Let the voters know who they're dealing with before the election Tuesday."

"He's got a point, Chief," Johnson said.

Cade stared out the window. It was a temptation. A sure win for Jonathan. A way to ensure he kept his job. Didn't the voters have the right to know? Wasn't it critical information?

The room seemed to go quiet. The printers stopped printing, the radio ceased to crackle, the air-conditioner cycled off. Everyone waited for an answer.

"Hear me and hear me good, every one of you," Cade said. "Every bit of evidence we've uncovered is part of a criminal investigation. We don't do leaks, not in my department. If I hear of any, trust me, I'll find out who did it, and your career in law enforcement will be a thing of the past. Any questions?"

There weren't any.

"Good. Now get on it."

68

The Sunday morning crowd for the Church on the Dock had already assembled as Cade pulled into the small parking lot. He'd thought of missing church again today, since there was still so much pressing business in the investigation, but it was the Lord's Day and he needed to worship.

He got out of his truck and heard the sound of believers' voices lifting in song. His spirit quickened, and he felt instant relief and power . . . a filling up . . . a drawing in.

He went in and saw that the pews were full. Dock workers and transient sailors sat among the longtime members, offering their sacrifices of praise.

And Vince Barr, the illustrious tabloid reporter and recent television star, was there among them. Cade knew he wasn't there to worship or seek the Lord. He was, no doubt, looking for more trouble to stir up, more rumors, more yarns to spin on

his next television appearance, things that would keep the national media focused on him and his investigation.

Cade thought of leaving, but he wouldn't let that guy hinder his worship.

There was an empty seat beside Blair. Her eyes were closed as she sang to the Lord. He didn't want to disrupt her focus or distract her, so he waited at the back of the room until the song was finished. Then he slipped in beside her.

She smiled up at him, and his heart warmed.

Jonathan led them from the praise chorus into a hymn that filled Cade with comfort and reminded him of the joy of his salvation.

He was glad he had taken the time to come.

He'd half expected Jonathan to mention Tuesday's election, contend for the vote of the people in that room. But he never brought it up. He had to hand it to him. His friend would campaign outside of these walls, but this hour was only for the Lord.

When the service was over, Cade felt equipped to go back to the investigation.

Blair smiled. "Did you see our *Observer* friend?"

Cade shot him a look. He was already talking to some of the members in the corner. "Yeah, I saw him."

"At least he came to church."

"You think he learned anything?" Cade asked without hope.

"Nothing he could use to get on CNN." She looked back at Cade. "Want to get a bite to eat?"

He shook his head. "Better not. There's too much going on."

"Anything you want to share?" She grinned.

He matched it. "Can't think of anything."

"How about why Sam Sullivan was taken into the police station last night?"

His smile faded. "Blair, you know we've been interviewing everybody."

"Everybody didn't feel the need to get a lawyer."

Cade breathed a laugh. "This town. Nothing is sacred. Give it up, Blair. You know you're barking up the wrong tree."

"Just tell me if the handwriting matched his."

He leaned down, putting his face close to hers. "If I have something to say about this investigation, I'll call a press conference — and you'll get the first question."

Her grin crept back across her face. "All right, Cade. You win. Guess I'll go eat at Hanover House and figure it out for myself."

He watched her leave, then looked back toward the front of the chapel. Jonathan looked tired. Cade waited until Vince had followed some chatty resident out, and most of the congregation had left, then he approached his best friend. "How you doing, man?"

Jonathan sighed. "Okay. How about you?"

"Been kind of busy."

"Glad you were able to make it today."

"Me too. Your sermon was inspired, Jonathan. I don't know how you do it. So how's the campaigning going?"

Jonathan looked around. A few members still stood across the room, and Morgan was apparently introducing Sheila. "Let's talk outside."

"Sure." Cade followed him out to the boardwalk behind the warehouse, and Jonathan sat down on the bench that looked out over the river. He leaned his elbows on his knees, and his shoulders slumped, like they carried too much weight.

"What's up, buddy?"

"It's the election," Jonathan said. "Cade,

I owe you an apology."

"For what?"

"For losing."

Cade grunted. "Jonathan, it's not Tuesday yet."

"No, but I can see the writing on the wall." Jonathan leaned down and picked up a stick from the planks and threw it into the water. "Sam Sullivan's the favorite. Mr. Cell Phone hero himself. I let you down, man. I'm really sorry."

"What do you mean, you let me down? Why would you say that?"

"Because if Sullivan wins the election, you're probably going to lose your job. I hate that for you, Cade. It's flat-out wrong."

Cade sat down beside him and looked out over the water. "I haven't sent out resumés yet, Jonathan. Don't give up. Things could turn around."

"That's easy to say now, but what are you going to do if he wins?"

"Deal with it, I guess." Cade squinted in the sunlight. "He's not going to fire me until I solve this crime, but I guess in a way a vote for him is a vote against me. Maybe it is time I moved on, if that's what the people want."

"You've got it all wrong, Cade. A vote

for Sam is a vote for cell phones. It's as simple as that, I think."

"Hey, it's not like he's going to kill the deal for the phones if he loses the election. It's not one or the other."

"Yeah, well. I have two more days to get that word out."

Cade wished he could resolve this case in time for election day. It could only help. He thought about Sam's duplicity, his deceit, his cruel scheme to hijack the election. All he had to do was drop the secret to one person . . .

But that wasn't how he did business.

"I'll pray for you, buddy," he said, "if you keep praying for me. It's all in God's hands."

Jonathan couldn't argue with that.

69

Election day was grueling. Morgan and Jonathan had campaigned all day, standing in the hot sun with signs that made one last plea as voters drove down the road to the polling booths at the church gyms. Blair and Sadie had been manning both voting centers for the newspaper, polling people as they came out.

Blair conveyed to Morgan around mid-afternoon that the news might not be good. It was way too close and could go either way.

Still, Morgan had a party to throw that night. They'd invited dozens of people who had helped with the campaign to come and wait for the results. Melba Jefferson had done all the cooking, and hors d'oeuvres were passed around the house with abundance. Madelyn Short played piano in the corner, singing patriotic tunes, as if this were a national election. Several children raced through the house, balloons flying

behind them. Everyone was in a festive mood.

Everyone except Jonathan.

The polls closed at seven, but the counting wouldn't be finished for several hours yet. The town's voting equipment was antiquated, so they had to be hand counted, hanging chads and all. Morgan hoped Jonathan had the chance to replace the equipment before they had to vote again.

She went into the kitchen to check on the food, and saw that Melba and several of the ladies from the church had things under control. She wondered where Sheila had gone with Caleb, so she started up the stairs to look for them.

She saw that the door to Caleb's room was closed. She leaned against it, listening, but heard nothing. Finally, she turned the knob and pushed it open.

Sheila sat in the rocker, singing softly as she held her sleeping son in her arms.

"Hey," Sheila whispered. "He was getting sleepy so I brought him up where it's quiet."

Morgan gave her a weak smile. "That's good. He's had a long day."

She watched as Sheila got up, laid him carefully in his bed without waking him,

and then gently stroked his hair. "He's so beautiful, isn't he?"

Morgan got tears in her eyes and nodded. "Yes, he is." She swallowed hard. "He looks just like you."

Sheila's glistening eyes showed her gratitude.

"Well, I'll go back down."

Sheila smiled. "I'll be down in a minute."

Morgan stepped out into the hall, closing the door behind her, and leaned back against the wall, the reality of the moment washing over her. This was as it should be — Sheila mothering her child.

It was the best thing for Caleb.

She breathed a silent prayer that God would give her the strength to accept that, and a strange peace fell over her.

In that moment, she vowed to stop thinking of herself. She would decrease so that Sheila could increase.

Wiping the tear that rolled down her face, she forced herself to rejoin the party.

She found Jonathan sitting on the back porch with Cade and Blair.

She tried to look upbeat. "What are you guys doing?"

"Commiserating," Jonathan said. "Wondering what we'll do if they fire Cade."

"They're not going to fire him, Jonathan," Morgan said. "Because you're going to win."

Jonathan clearly wasn't holding his breath.

Blair groaned. "It's insane. It would be absolutely ludicrous if they fired you, Cade. We can't let this happen."

"I don't see what we can do about it," Cade said. "I'm going to be at the mercy of the mayor, whoever it is."

They heard the phone ringing inside, and Jonathan started to get up.

Melba burst through the screen door. "It's the early part of the returns, Jonathan!" She handed the cordless phone to him. The piano stopped playing, the children stopped laughing, and all of the soft conversations ceased.

"Jonathan Cleary." His voice was tight, nervous.

Morgan said a silent prayer as she waited for the verdict. Suddenly a smile broke across Jonathan's face. "You're kidding me! Thanks, man. I appreciate it. Keep us updated."

He clicked off the phone and looked at the crowd who had suddenly come to bottleneck in the doorway to the porch.

"The votes at the high school have been

counted, and I'm a few dozen votes ahead."

Everybody sent up a cheer, and Morgan threw her arms around Jonathan's neck. He laughed and swung her around.

"Can you believe it? I thought it was impossible."

"Nothing is impossible with God," she said.

He let her go, then looked around at the others. "There's still several voting centers that haven't reported yet, so we need to be cautiously optimistic."

For the first time in over two weeks, a bubble of joy fluttered up inside Morgan, but it was a fragile joy. She prayed it would last.

The party atmosphere grew more tense as the night progressed. Each time Lance from the circuit clerk's office called with an update, that tension was turned up a notch. Sam Sullivan and Jonathan had been running neck and neck for the whole night. Sometimes Jonathan was a few votes ahead, causing a celebration at Hanover House. Then things would turn and Sam would be in the lead. No one could guess who might be the victor.

When Vince Barr showed up at nine-

thirty, Morgan graciously let him in. Blair cut across the room and took her aside. "What is wrong with you? Why would you let *him* in here?"

"I can't tell him to go away. Besides, when you're in politics, you have to be willing to talk to the media."

"But he's here to dig up dirt about the murder. He doesn't care about our mayoral election!"

Morgan's gaze drifted across the room to the man who was already engaged in conversation with some of her guests. "Then watch him for me. I'm really busy, Blair. We're going to hear the returns soon. Maybe he'll be able to write about a victory celebration."

Blair said a few words to Vince, then excused herself and went back to Cade, who stood talking to Sheila.

"Did you see who's here?" she whispered harshly.

Cade glanced across the room at the reporter who seemed to be making his way toward them. "Maybe it's time for me to leave."

"You can't leave before we know the results," Sheila said. "Maybe somebody needs to get in touch with that fortune-teller. Maybe he could tell us who the

winner's going to be."

Blair shot the woman a look. All night, she had flicked her hair as she'd followed Cade around like a groupie. Ever since Blair caught her sitting in Carson's van, she hadn't trusted her.

"Fortune-teller or not, that Vince guy's waiting for the returns just like we are," Blair bit out.

"But didn't Graham give you the information that helped you find that woman's body, Cade?"

The familiar way Sheila used Cade's name made Blair angry. She was being territorial, she knew, but Sheila was a flirt, and she was good at it. Sheila locked her blue eyes into Cade's with that sultry teasing look that sent Blair over the edge.

Cade was noncommittal. "I can't really comment on his involvement."

"Oh, of course you can't." Sheila touched his arm and leaned in. "Frankly, that guy's involvements seem to be all over the place. Some of them even extramarital, if you know what I mean."

Blair bristled. Was Sheila hinting she'd been involved with him? Would she admit that right here in front of Blair, knowing she would tell Jonathan and Morgan? "No. Why don't you tell us what you mean?"

Sheila crossed her arms and, with a coy grin, offered a shrug. "I'm just saying . . . I saw him with a cute little thing who was not his wife. Not unless she'd bleached her hair blonde since the debate that morning."

Blair looked at Cade. He was interested now, squinting as he stared at Sheila. "Where did you see him, Sheila?"

"I was walking around the island Saturday, trying to vent a little steam, and I was over there by the river. You know, where that woman's car was found? Sadie had shown it to me, and there were flowers marking the place. Just past that, there he came. The palm reader himself, bopping along the path, coming right toward me."

Blair felt Cade stiffening. "Where was he coming from?"

"From that house around the bend of the river."

Melanie Adams' house? Blair shot an alarmed look at Cade, then turned back to Sheila. "You say there was a blonde there?"

"Yes. He was walking toward me, and all of a sudden this Miss America–type calls to him and she comes running and says, 'You forgot your wallet.' She kisses him right on the mouth, and then he sees me and disappears back into her house."

"Melanie Adams." Cade looked at Blair, a million thoughts running through his eyes.

"You don't think . . ."

Sadie called Sheila from across the room, and Sheila hurried away.

Blair watched the dots connecting in Cade's mind.

"If Carson's having an affair with Melanie Adams, then we may have an answer about how he got his vision."

Blair lowered her voice to a whisper. "Do you think he just witnessed the murder, or was he actually the one who committed it?"

"I don't know, but I'm sure going to find out." He pulled his keys out of his pocket. "I've got to go, Blair."

She started walking him to the door, when the telephone rang again.

A hush fell over the room again, and Cade froze, waiting to see what the news was.

Jonathan picked it up. "Jonathan Cleary. Yeah, Lance?"

There was a long pause.

Jonathan swallowed. "So that's it? The final result?"

Blair's heart plunged. She knew he'd lost.

He hung up the phone and looked around at the crowd. She felt sorry for him. These things should be handled in private, not with fifty people staring you down.

He set his hands on his hips and drew in a deep breath. "It's over. Sam won by fifty-two votes."

Reactions flared up from everyone in the room. Morgan started to cry.

Jonathan put his arm around her. "It's okay, everybody. Really, I appreciate all the work that you all did and all the confidence you put in me. I especially appreciate those of you who convinced me to run. Maybe God just knew that I'd bitten off more than I could chew, what with running Hanover House, running a tour business, and trying to be the pastor of a growing church. I'm fine, really."

Cade crossed the room and pulled Jonathan into a hug. "I'm sorry, man."

"Me too. I tried."

Cade stepped back as others descended on Jonathan with soft words of encouragement and loving hugs. When he looked back at Blair, he saw that her scars had gone crimson.

"I can't believe it," she said under her breath. "I can't believe that jerk won. What

is wrong with the people of this town?"

Cade just shook his head. "The town needs a lot of prayer. And he'll take office within the week."

She threw her chin up in defiance. "It's not over, Cade. I'm going to fight Sam Sullivan tooth and nail. If he thinks he's going to replace you —"

Cade took her hand. "Leave it alone, Blair. I can fight my own battles."

"But he's going to fire you!"

"Until he does, I have a job to do, and I'm going to do it." He got his cane and headed for the door. "I'll call you later."

70

The rumor about Carson Graham's affair brought things into focus. Cade still couldn't see a motive, but Graham may well have lied about his whereabouts on the morning of May 16. They had never been able to confirm it. Either he witnessed the murder and saw Lisa's car going into the river from the vantage point of Melanie's property, or he'd been in place when Lisa came along, and had murdered her himself. And what was Melanie's part in the crime?

Carson Graham wasn't answering the door, even though his Palm Reading van was parked in his parking lot. Cade banged on the door. "Open up, Carson! We know you're there. We want to talk to you."

There was still no answer. He thought of having Caldwell kick the door in, but it was too visible from the busy street, and he didn't want to call attention to what they were doing. Besides, he didn't have an arrest warrant. Theoretically, Graham could

evade them all he wanted until he got one.

But Cade wasn't going to let him off that easily. "Let's try the side door."

He led McCormick and Caldwell around to the side of the house, where a warped door sat above concrete steps. The window was broken out, and the glass had fallen into the house. Someone from outside had smashed it in.

McCormick frowned at him. "What do you think?"

"I don't know. Maybe a burglary. Question is, is he in there?" Cade drew his weapon and radioed for backup. Then, pulling a handkerchief out of his pocket, he tested the knob. The door came open easily.

He led with his gun, checking all around him. Stepping over the glass, he moved into the kitchen. McCormick and Caldwell spread out, checking the laundry room, the pantry. Cade moved into the living room . . .

Carson Graham lay in the middle of the floor, a pool of blood under his head.

"In here!" He went to Carson's side and felt for a pulse.

But it was too late.

The palm reader was dead.

71

The phone rang just as Blair was getting ready for bed. Hoping it was Cade, she grabbed it up.

"Hello?"

"Blair, this is Clara Montgomery." The woman sounded excited. "I'm so sorry to bother you so late, honey, but I thought I'd give you a heads-up. There's something going on across the street at Carson Graham's. Police cars everywhere. Even an ambulance, but no one's been brought out."

Blair caught her breath. She couldn't imagine what could have happened. Had Cade's men gone to arrest him? Had he resisted arrest?

She thanked Clara, then grabbed her camera and rushed out to her car. She turned on her police scanner and listened to the chatter.

". . . homicide . . . gunshot wound to the head . . . notify his wife . . ."

Was Carson Graham dead?

She made it to his house on Ocean Boulevard in just a few minutes and saw the glut of squad cars, a fire truck, and a rescue unit blocking the road. She pulled her car over and saw that Vince Barr had already beaten her there. He stood talking to a neighbor who stood in the street.

Blair bolted up to the first cop she saw, standing at the edge of the crime scene tape. "Ed, what happened?"

He hesitated. "Blair, I can't talk to you. You'll have to wait until Cade makes a statement."

"I know it was a gunshot wound to the head. What caliber weapon was used? Have they got a suspect in custody?"

Ed looked agitated. "No comment, Blair."

"Were they making an arrest, Ed? Was there gunplay between Graham and the police?"

"No. Absolutely not. They found him dead." Ed turned away, ending her interview, so Blair started snapping pictures.

She heard the screeching of tires, a door slamming, feet running. Carson's wife had come home from working at the hospital. Amber tore aside the crime scene tape and cut across the grass. One of the officers

tried to stop her, but she wrestled away from him. "Carson!"

Blair just stood there, camera in hand, unable to photograph the woman in her terror. She watched as they escorted her into the house. Blair heard a loud, anguished scream and knew that Amber had seen her husband's body.

Suddenly, the spectacle turned from drama to reality. She knew how it felt to be notified by the police, led to the scene of the crime, and shocked by the sight of a loved one's lifeless body. She knew the grief that would follow.

She didn't know Amber very well, but she wished she could cross that tape and comfort her somehow.

"Where's Chief Cade?" a voice bellowed from behind her. She turned and saw Sam Sullivan stalking toward her. "I want to talk to him."

"He's kind of busy," Ed said.

"Go get him!"

"I'm sorry, but you'll have to wait until he comes out."

"Young fella, you must not know who I am," Sam bit out. "I am this town's newly elected mayor. You're my employee, and I told you to go in there and get Chief Cade, or I'll do it myself."

The young cop finally capitulated and went toward the house.

Blair stepped toward him. "Nice going, Sam. Way to flex those newly acquired muscles. You really know how to win friends and influence people."

"Hey, I influenced enough to win the election, Blair — and I do appreciate all the paper's support."

Blair bit her lip and walked away. She gave Sam ad space because he'd paid for it fair and square, but now she wondered at the merits of unbiased reporting. Maybe she should have given more of her opinion.

She knew better than that. She'd vowed when she bought the paper that she would be an old-fashioned reporter, the kind who was objective and factual. But sometimes it just didn't seem to pay.

She saw Ed coming back with Cade on his heels, so she slipped into the shadows behind some trees so her snooping around wouldn't set him off. Her heart surged with compassion for Cade. He looked as if he'd had about all he could take.

"What can I do for you, Sam?"

"I want to know what happened here."

"I'll be making a statement when I have something to say. You're welcome to wait here until I do."

"Do you know who did this?"

"Not yet, Sam."

"Does this have anything to do with the Lisa Jackson case?"

"We haven't ruled anything out. Everyone related to this case will be questioned — and since you're here, we can start with you."

She would have expected a calm response, an easy flowing of information that might help. Instead, Sam looked as if he'd been slapped. "I know you've checked out my alibi, Cade. You know by now that I was telling the truth about where I was May 16. I've had a hundred people around me all night tonight. I didn't leave my victory party once until now, and I got to tell you, if you keep harassing me, you're going to be in the unemployment lines even faster than you thought."

She could see Cade's jaw popping. "Wait here," he said. "I'm sending McCormick out to question you."

"Cade, I'm warning you!"

Shaking his head, Cade just turned and went back into the house.

Sam kicked the sawhorse holding up the yellow crime scene tape and knocked it over. Then he thought better of it and quickly picked it back up.

McCormick came out a moment later, and Blair stayed in her hiding place behind the tree. "Cade said you were here," he said. "Why don't you come sit in my car with me and answer a few questions?"

She saw Sam looking around to make sure no one heard. Blair stayed hidden, but strained to hear. "McCormick, Cade isn't trying to connect me with this, is he?"

McCormick just looked at him. "Why do you ask that, Sam?"

"Because he knew that if I got elected I was going to fire him. Tell me that he's not misinterpreting my little letter-writing hoax. I never would have written them if I'd known it was going to make me a murder suspect."

"Of course you wouldn't. You only did it because you thought you wouldn't get caught."

"Hey, I was forthright with you people. I admitted everything. That's got to count for something."

Blair let the words sink in. So Sam *had* written the letters. He'd hung a motive on Ben. He'd made him look guilty — and he'd confessed to the police.

Could the mayor-elect be the killer?

She didn't know, but her readers were about to find out what kind of man they'd

elected. It would be worth staying up all night to get out a special edition. Sam's first act as mayor would be picking up the pieces of his own character.

She looked around to make sure Vince hadn't heard the same thing. He stood in the next-door neighbor's yard, trying to take pictures of the palm reader's side door. He hadn't heard a word of the exchange.

She hurried back to her newspaper office. Normally, she would have confirmed this with at least two other sources, but she'd heard it from the horse's mouth. What could be greater confirmation than the man's own confession? As fast as she could type, she wrote the headline article about Carson's murder. She wrote furiously, trying to get everything down. At the bottom of the front page, she wrote about how Sam Sullivan had confessed to sending the letters to Lisa Jackson claiming her husband was having an affair. By morning, the residents of Cape Refuge would know what kind of man their new mayor was.

Half watching FOX News as she worked, she set about to paste in the articles that hadn't fit in yesterday's regular issue, including local club news and items about high school athletes and academic awards

— anything to fill up this issue so it wouldn't look so sparse.

Then she heard the News Alert.

"We have breaking news in the Lisa Jackson case. FOX News has just learned that Carson Graham, the psychic who led police to Lisa's body, was found dead tonight in his home. Joining us now from our FOX affiliate in Savannah is Vince Barr of the *Observer*. Welcome back, Vince."

She turned from her computer and gaped at the screen. How had he gotten to them so quickly? She turned up the set, and held her breath, praying that Vince wouldn't report what she'd just spent the last hours writing.

"Good to be here, John. First, let me backtrack a little to explain that the police force of Cape Refuge had gone to question Carson Graham. It's not clear what information led them to that. When Graham didn't answer the door, they looked around and found that the glass on one of his doors had been shattered from the outside. When they went in, they found the psychic dead on the floor."

"How was he killed?"

"A gunshot wound to the head."

"Do they have any leads on who may have killed him?"

"If they do, they're not saying, John. My question, as I'm sure yours is, is why no one heard the sound of the gunshot. But his house is in a business district, if you will, and his next-door neighbors include an exterminator's office and an insurance office. Both of these offices were closed, so no one would have heard. There's also a lot of traffic on that street, so anyone across the street may not have heard, either."

"Any theories on who might have killed him and why? And do we know for sure it has anything to do with the Lisa Jackson murder?"

"If it doesn't, it's quite a coincidence," Vince said on a chuckle.

Blair leaned back hard in her chair, relieved that he didn't seem to know about Sam's writing the letters to Lisa. He would surely have told it if he'd known.

She had scooped him, she thought with a smile. And maybe now she had a chance to save Cade's job.

72

Dawn had just broken when Cade reported to the police station. He'd been at Carson Graham's all night, working with the detectives to gather enough evidence to determine his killer, but they made little progress.

Billy Caldwell met him at the door with a newspaper in his hand. "Chief, you need to see something."

Cade glanced at the paper. It was the *Cape Refuge Journal*, hot off the press. The headline read, "Psychic Found Murdered."

"Where did you get this?"

"Paper guy just delivered it. Special edition."

Cade scanned the article, saw that it had no surprises. "She's good. She had the scoop before the *Savannah Morning News*, or even the *Observer*. Guess she couldn't wait to get it out."

Caldwell pointed at the article at the bottom of the page. "Check *this* out."

Cade glanced at the secondary headline. " 'Mayor-Elect Confesses to Fraud.' Aw, no!" He grabbed a chair and sank into it as his eyes ran over the article. "Tell me she didn't write that." Anger shot through him, stamping out his fatigue. "I want to know who leaked this."

"It wasn't me, Chief. I swear it."

Cade bolted into his office and grabbed the telephone. He dialed Blair's number, but she wasn't home, so he tried her at the office.

"*Cape Refuge Journal,*" she said in a tired voice. "Blair speaking."

"I want to know where you got this information," Cade bit out. "Give me a name, Blair."

She hesitated. "What are you talking about?"

"Who leaked the Sam Sullivan story to you?"

"Nobody, Cade. I heard it for myself. Sam was spouting off to Joe, saying that he hoped you didn't think his letter-writing scheme connected him to the murder."

"Blair, you should not have reported this. It was police business."

"I found it out fair and square, Cade, and the voters need to know what kind of

man they just elected. It's important news to this community."

"Blair, nothing good can come of this. He's going to think I leaked it in some feeble attempt to save my job. That's not how I operate."

"Cade, the article clearly says that I heard it myself. I'm sorry that you're not comfortable with it, but it's the truth — and it probably *will* save your job!"

"I told you to let me fight my own battles. Between you and Vince Barr, it's a wonder I still *have* a job."

That set her off. "Come on, Cade. This has all been a reporter's dream, but I'm not the one who's exploited it. I've been responsible with my reporting. You haven't seen me milking this into a national story, parading myself on the major news shows like that Vince jerk has done. I'm tired of taking the heat from you for the stuff he's doing. It's not fair, and you know it."

Maybe it *wasn't* fair . . . Maybe Vince *had* gotten famous over this, and maybe it was all making him look bad. Maybe he *was* taking it out on her.

But he was tired, and he didn't want to deal with these distractions anymore. He just wanted the case to be resolved.

"So where are we on Carson's murder?"

she asked. "I've been listening to the scanner all night, but nothing seems to be happening."

"You're not getting a thing out of me, Blair. I don't want you reporting an arrest before it's even made."

With that, he hung up the phone and tried to swallow his anger so he could do his job.

73

The facts about Carson Graham had filed in after his murder. His bank and phone records showed that he'd made a $30,000 deposit into his account on May 16 — the day of Lisa's murder.

"So either somebody paid him for killing Lisa," Cade told McCormick, "or he witnessed the murder and was blackmailing the killer."

Cade looked at the phone records scrolling across his computer screen. From May 16 on, there were several calls to newspapers across Georgia, placed after the body was found. It was his attempt to make himself a hero, and it had pretty much worked. Had he exploited something he'd only witnessed? If so, had Lisa's killer murdered him?

Cade had plenty of questions by the time he went with McCormick to visit Melanie Adams. When she answered the door, it was clear they had woken her up. She

clutched her robe shut and squinted out at them. "What's going on?"

"Melanie, we need to talk to you. Police business."

She opened the door further. "I'm not even dressed . . ." She stepped back to let them in.

Cade could see that the woman had been crying.

She turned on the light in her front room. Still clutching her robe, she sat down.

"Melanie, Carson Graham was murdered last night."

She swallowed hard and nodded. "I know. I saw it on the news." Her face twisted. "We were . . . friends. I couldn't believe it."

"Melanie, we know about your affair."

She just stared at them for a long moment, dread pulling at her expression. "My husband . . . he doesn't know. Is there any way to keep this quiet? He's out of town for a few more days. I really can't let him find out." Her lower lip began to quiver, and she started to cry. She covered her mouth, and her brow pleated as she stared at them.

"Do you think he knows already?"

She looked at them then, her eyes

rounding. "You think . . . No, it wasn't my husband! He's not a killer. He's been in Canada on business for the last three weeks. He has no idea. It's not him, Cade."

"Do you have any idea who might have wanted Carson dead?"

She got up, grabbed a tissue. "I told him. I told him to be careful, that he was playing with fire."

Cade glanced up at McCormick. His muscles were rigid with attention. He looked back at the woman. "Melanie, what did he tell you about Lisa Jackson's murder?"

She was sobbing now, clearly losing control. "He was a witness. He spent the night with me that night. My husband wasn't home, and Carson's wife was working a double shift at the hospital. He walked over so no one would see his van here. He was leaving my house around ten that morning, walking home, when he saw someone pushing Lisa's car into the river." She looked at Cade through her tears. "That person has to be the one who killed Carson!"

Cade wanted to be careful now. He didn't want to frighten her away from giving him a name. "I think he could have

been, Melanie. That's why your account is so important."

"I knew it." She got up again and walked across the room. "I told him! When Carson tried to get money out of him, I told him he was dealing with a killer. That he was putting his life in danger! He thought he had it all under control."

Cade's heart stopped. "So he was blackmailing the killer?"

"Yes! Only he wouldn't tell me who it was. I really don't know, Cade. You've got to believe me." She went to the front window as she spoke and peered out, as if she feared someone was watching her.

Cade shot McCormick a look. She knew who it was. She knew and wasn't telling, but her own fear spoke volumes.

"Melanie, I'm afraid we need to take you in to the station and take a statement from you."

She swung around. "You're arresting me?"

"Not yet. Not unless we think you're lying . . . or withholding important information about a homicide case."

She grunted and looked at him as if she couldn't believe he distrusted her. "I'm telling you, Cade, I don't know a thing."

"Then why are you looking out that

window like you know someone's going to come for you?"

"Because he might know about me. He might *think* Carson told me."

"Then you'll be safer at the police station anyway," McCormick said.

Her face changed as she saw the wisdom in his words. "All right. Let me get dressed, and I'll come with you."

74

By the time they got Melanie back to the police station, there was a message waiting for Cade. "Chief, this woman named Kylie Hyatt said she needs to talk to you," Alex Johnson said. "She says she knows who killed Lisa Jackson."

Cade grabbed the message and stared down at it. "Who is she?"

"I don't know. She wouldn't say."

Cade called the number, and a man answered in a gruff, phlegmy voice. "Yeah?"

"This is Chief Cade of the Cape Refuge Police Department. I'm calling for Kylie Hyatt."

"She wants to talk to you in person," the man said. He gave him an address in Savannah.

Cade frowned. "All right, but first tell me who she is and what she has to do with this case."

There was a long pause, then, "She's Dr. Alan Sims' maid — and that's all I'm going

to say until you get here."

The phone went dead in his hand, and he stared down at it. Sims' maid?

He rolled the tapes back through his mind, of his visit to Sims' house right after the murder. *"Excuse the mess. My maid is AWOL, and my wife has been in Europe for the past week. It doesn't usually look like this."* On his last visit, Sims had mentioned that his maid "up and quit."

Maybe there was a reason she was AWOL.

Maybe she'd witnessed a murder.

Cade hurried out of his office to the interview room where McCormick sat with Melanie. He motioned him out and closed the door.

"I just got a call from Sims' maid. She wants to talk to me. I think this might be our smoking gun. Let's leave Melanie here to stew in her juices while we go interview this woman."

75

Kylie Hyatt lived in a neighborhood of HUD houses and low-income rental units in Savannah. It was early in the evening, but even now, several men loitered out on the street, and women who looked as if they had long ago traded in their dignity for a drug fix stood on the corners. They all scattered at the sight of Cade's police vehicle, as if he'd come to make a sweep.

Cade had notified Savannah police that they'd be questioning Hyatt, and invited them to escort him and McCormick since it was their turf. They opted out, since it was Cade's case. McCormick followed him to the ramshackle door, and he knocked. Heavy footsteps shook the house, and then the door came open.

An obese man with a dingy white tank top and a cigarette in his mouth looked out at them. "You're here."

Cade showed him his badge. "I'm Chief Cade, and this is Detective McCormick."

473

"Come in." The door opened, and a small, plump woman peered past the man. "I'm Kylie," she said as they came into the dimly lit house.

The place reeked of tobacco and mold, and had decades of dirt ground into the vinyl tiles. The paint on the walls was peeling. But there was no clutter. Everything seemed in its place.

The woman had a nervous tick that kept twitching in her cheek. "I should have called you sooner, but I was scared. After I heard about that woman's murder, I didn't know what to do. Now that there's a second murder . . . well, I just couldn't stay quiet any longer."

She sat down, and Cade sat next to her on the dirty couch.

"Excuse the way the place looks. This is my brother's house." She looked up at the obese man. "Roy isn't as neat as I'd like for him to be. I've been trying to clean up since I've been here."

"Don't go apologizing for my place, Sis. It ain't none of their business how I keep house."

Cade didn't want to get sidetracked. "Miss Hyatt, you said you had something to tell us."

Kylie went to the window and peered

out as if she expected the killer to come walking up her porch steps. The nervous gesture was so similar to what Melanie had done this morning. "I was supposed to be off that day —"

"What day?" Cade asked.

"The day that lady was murdered."

"May 16," Cade said, and Kylie nodded.

"I hadn't left yet, though. Mrs. Sims went to Europe a couple of days before, and they'd given me a long weekend. Dr. Sims thought I was already gone, but Roy hadn't come to get me yet, and when that woman came banging on the door, I listened."

"What woman? Lisa Jackson?"

"Yes. He let her in, and she was hysterical. She called him a fraud and accused him of tricking her and deceiving her for money. Said he had robbed her of her childbearing years, that she was going to expose him. I felt like I was eavesdropping — and I didn't want Dr. Sims to get mad and fire me — so I went on outside and waited for Roy on the street."

"Did you see anything else?"

"No, that's all. Just an argument. She was very angry."

"Was she still there when Roy came?"

"Yes. I was so glad to get out of there."

Kylie burst into tears and covered her mouth with a trembling hand. "And then when I heard about her disappearance, and when she was found . . . I knew he killed her."

Cade's heart fell. "But you didn't see him do it."

She shook her head. "No, but she was so angry, and the things she was accusing him of were terrible. He must have snapped . . ."

He looked at McCormick. This was not the smoking gun they'd hoped for. Too bad she hadn't stuck around to see what else had happened, but the fact that Sims had lied about Lisa coming to see him didn't look good. If only they'd known all this earlier. "Miss Hyatt, why didn't you call the police before now?"

"I was scared. I didn't know what to do. I couldn't go back there, but I was afraid to come forward." She started to fall apart then, and her brother came over and put his arms around her.

"It's okay, Sis. You've done the right thing now." He looked up at them over her head. "You get him, officers. You lock him up so he can't hurt my sister."

Cade intended to do just that.

76

The waiting room in the fertility clinic was full of patients, both men and women, waiting for Sims to play God with their reproductive systems and give them hope — or take it away. They all looked up as Cade came in with two uniformed officers.

Armed with an arrest warrant, which the DA had finally granted him, he bypassed the receptionist's desk and pushed through the door into the back. A nurse was coming toward them, and she stepped back, startled.

"I need to see Dr. Sims," Cade said in a low voice. "Where is he?"

"He's with a patient right now."

"Which room?"

She pointed to the room, but stepped in front of him. "You can't go in there!"

"Knock on the door. Tell him to step out here."

She did as she was told, and after a moment, Sims stepped through the door. His

face drained of color as he saw his visitors. "Chief Cade, what are you doing — ?"

"Alan Sims, you are under arrest for the murder of Lisa Jackson. You have the right to remain silent . . ."

"You're out of your mind!"

One of the officers snapped a cuff over one of Sims' wrists, but he twisted away before he could click the other one into place. Cade's men descended on him, wrestling him to the ground.

"I didn't do it, you idiots! I didn't kill anybody!"

He fought to get away, but within seconds the other cuff snapped around his wrist, and Sims was jerked to his feet. His face was red and he breathed hard. "Elaine, call my lawyer! Tell him they're trying to frame me for Lisa Jackson's murder!" He swung back to Cade. "You're going to regret this, Cade! We're going to sue the socks off of you for this."

Cade grabbed his arm and led him back through the nurses. The doorway to Sims' waiting room came open, and the patients who'd put their faith in him watched, stunned, as their doctor was dragged away.

77

"Okay, she came to see me, but I didn't kill her."

Sims sat in the interview room at the police station, rubbing his sweating face with both hands. He'd finally confessed that he saw Lisa the morning of her death, but in the last hour of grilling, he hadn't confessed to anything else.

"Why did you lie to us when we asked you when you'd last seen her?" Cade demanded.

"Because I was scared. If you knew she came to see me that morning, you would have thought I did it. I'm not stupid. When I first heard she'd disappeared, I thought she'd gone off somewhere and killed herself."

"Why would she kill herself when Dr. Anderson had finally given her hope?"

"I didn't know. She was crazed with anger and rage, not thinking rationally. Then when she was found murdered . . ."

He rubbed his face again. "I was shocked. It was too much of a coincidence that it would happen on the same day."

"Coincidence, all right," McCormick said. "But I don't really believe in coincidences. You, Cade?"

"No, I don't. Not in murder cases."

"Come on," Sims said. "I know it looks terrible. It couldn't look worse, but I did not kill her."

"So she confronted you about lying to her."

"I made a mistake with her diagnosis."

Cade thought of the tape he'd heard of him trying to convince Morgan to mortgage her life to pay for IVF, the lies he'd probably told her about her fertility, and that same rage boiled up inside him. Slowly, he stood up and leaned over the table. "You didn't make a mistake with Lisa, Sims. You lied flat out. Falsified her test results. Exploited her fears to get money out of her. And you kept her from getting the help she needed so she could have a family."

Sims looked at the ceiling, shaking his head. "I'll fight this. I'll get the best lawyers money can buy."

"They won't help you, Sims. We have too much on you."

He considered that a moment, then his hand closed into a fist, and he gritted his teeth. "Even if everything you said was true, I did not kill her. She came to me rabidly angry, shouting threats and accusing me of . . . all those things. I never touched her. Then she left my house. I followed her out, trying to convince her it was a mistake, begging her not to go public with her accusations, but she got into her car and sped off. I never saw her again."

"Pretty convenient that she died before she could have you arrested."

"I didn't do it! But Ben probably did. She probably went home and had it out with him. I'm telling you, she was in a rage. Maybe he was defending himself, then didn't know what to do."

Cade believed she might have been killed in self-defense, but he was certain that Sims had been the one to do it. Nothing else made any sense.

A knock sounded on the door, and Cade looked up.

"Chief, can I see you for a minute?"

Cade got up and went out into the squad room. Caldwell nodded toward the television on in the corner. "Vince Barr is on again."

Cade moaned and limped over to the

set. "Man, he doesn't waste any time."

"The drama continues to unfold," Vince said to Shepherd Smith. "But if Dr. Sims is the man, then he very well could have killed both Lisa and Carson Graham. Kylie Hyatt, the woman who worked as Alan Sims' maid, told me just a few minutes ago that she reported to police that Lisa Jackson paid Sims a visit the morning of her disappearance. She had just gotten the results of a second opinion she'd obtained from another doctor, and learned that Sims had been lying to her about her fertility problem for the last thirteen years . . ."

Cade almost turned the set off. He turned back to the others in the squad room and saw that they all anticipated an explosion. "If one of you has been talking to this man, so help me . . ."

"Though Miss Hyatt left before it came to blows, she feels certain that her employer is the one who strangled Lisa Jackson with a telephone cord, and then disposed of her body, in order to keep her from exposing him as a fraud."

Cade swung back around and stared at the set. How had Barr known about the telephone cord? They found it on the floor of the car, bagged it as evidence, and kept

it quiet. Only McCormick and two of the detectives from the State Police knew about it. Cade hadn't even told his men.

It was something only the killer could know.

His heart started to pound, and sweat broke out on his face. He turned back to the interview room and looked at that door. Was it possible . . . could Sims and Jackson and Melanie Adams all be telling the truth? Could the killer be someone else entirely?

He turned back to the screen. Could it be someone who'd gotten famous from the story, who'd carefully orchestrated events so that it would garner national attention? Could it be the man who was reporting the story almost as fast as Cade was uncovering the facts?

"McCormick!" He limped to his office.

McCormick came out of the interview room. "What is it, Cade?"

"We've got more work to do. There's been a new development."

78

Vince Barr's background only added to Cade's suspicion. The man had a history of blowing mediocre stories into spectacular headlines, but he'd failed at getting much attention out of any of them. Cade did a search for Barr's name on the Internet, and amid the hundreds of articles Barr had written, Cade found a few about the writer, himself.

"Take a look at this." Cade turned his monitor so McCormick could see it. "Here's an AP report that came out an hour or so ago about the Lisa Jackson case and the media coverage of it. They're talking about how a local case turned into a national drama, and they quote Barr. He says, 'The timing was perfect for this case to break. No war news, no terrorist attacks, no hurricanes, no interesting politics filling the news. So when this attractive woman is killed and her husband is the immediate suspect, it can't help pique national interest. And as awful as this sounds, even

the murder of Carson Graham couldn't have come at a more perfect time. For those of us writing about it, it's like a dream come true.' "

McCormick rubbed his hand over his shaven head. "Okay, so let me get this straight. Didn't Sam Sullivan tell us that he went to Vince Barr with the rumor of Ben's affair?"

"Yes he did. Said Vince wasn't interested in local politics."

"But maybe that was the springboard Vince needed to set up the perfect story. One that he could help unfold, so he could give the national news shows a play-by-play."

Cade couldn't believe they'd been chasing down the wrong trails. "So you think he mulled this alleged affair over in his mind, then decided that it really would be a story if the candidate's wife turned up dead?"

"So he makes it happen — and he's on top of the story from Day One."

"What about Carson Graham?"

"I think he witnessed it, just like Melanie told us he did, and he seized the opportunity to blackmail the guy. Hence, the thirty thousand dollars that showed up in his account."

"Question is, did thirty thousand dollars leave Barr's account?"

"We'll soon see." He pulled up the man's bank records and studied them until he came to May 16. "Interesting. Looks like he had several accounts. A 401(k), a savings account, a couple of CDs. Pulled a little from each of them that day. And you'll never guess what it totals."

"Thirty K?"

"You got it."

McCormick drew in a deep, ragged breath. "Unbelievable."

Cade nodded. "So Graham agrees to keep quiet, and Barr agrees to use his own immediate fame to boost the reputation and notoriety of the psychic. They scratch each other's backs."

"Until we were about to bring Graham in for the murder. Then he was afraid Graham would cave. But how did he know we were going to do that? The timing was perfect. He got him before he could spill his guts to us."

Cade thought back over the night at Hanover House, the moment he'd realized that Carson Graham was having an affair with Melanie Adams. Sheila had been talking more loudly than she needed to . . .

"Vince Barr heard Sheila telling me

about Graham's affair. He was at Jonathan's party. He knew that information raised a red flag in my mind, and he probably saw the writing on the wall."

"So he beat us to Carson Graham's house."

"Looks like it."

McCormick handed Cade his cane. "I think we have one more arrest to make."

79

Through Vince Barr's office at the *Observer*, they were able to locate him at the local NBC affiliate. He was gearing up to do a satellite-linked segment on MSNBC.

Cade and McCormick hoped to take him peacefully, without making a huge media circus out of it.

But Vince *was* the circus, and he wasn't ready to give up the center ring. The moment he saw Cade and McCormick coming in, he headed toward them. "Chief Cade, I'd love to interview you during my segment. How about coming on with me?"

Cade thought of acquiescing, getting on national television, and asking the man where he was on the morning of Lisa's death and how he knew about the telephone cord. He imagined reading him his rights and cuffing him as the cameras rolled. Vince Barr wanted to be famous — well, this would be news for days.

"Vince, this isn't a social visit. We're

here to question you about where you were on the morning of May 16."

The smug look on Barr's face faded, and he frowned. "What do you mean where I was? The morning of . . . Lisa Jackson's murder?" Fear flashed across his face. "Oh, you've got to be kidding. No, you can't be serious."

"Where were you, Vince?"

Vince took another two steps back and almost tripped over a cord. "I was out doing a story. I don't remember which one."

Cade had expected as much. "Are you sure you weren't out *creating* a story?"

He laughed nervously. "I don't know what you're talking about. This is ludicrous."

"Vince, how did you know that Lisa was strangled with a telephone cord?"

His face turned white. The young blonde standing on the set looked fascinated, and one of the cameramen got interested, too.

"It was at the scene of the crime. In the car. I took pictures — didn't you see them?"

"There was no telephone cord in those pictures. No one had any way of knowing about that cord, except for the killer."

Cade wasn't sure, but he thought the cameraman had turned on his camera and was rolling now as Vince began to back further away.

"It was leaked to me. One of your own men told me about it."

"No one leaked it," Cade said. "You had inside information. Carson Graham knew, and that's why he's dead now. Where did you get the thirty thousand dollars to keep him quiet, Vince?"

He'd almost expected the man to break and run for it, but instead, he froze, staring at Cade, a stricken look on his face. A calm seemed to settle over him as he glanced back toward the set and realized the camera was rolling.

Vince was already miked up, so he turned to the camera. "As you can see, ladies and gentlemen, I'm here with Cape Refuge's finest, who've found a creative way of shutting up the press."

Cade glanced at the monitors on the wall, and realized that MSNBC had halted their normal reporting and was playing the unfolding scene. If Cade arrested Vince now, he would do it on national television.

Vince backed away and stepped onto the set and into the bright lights. "Well, you guys love drama. Here it is." He was

starting to sweat. "As you've probably already seen, they're accusing me of creating a story by murdering Lisa Jackson myself. As ludicrous as that sounds, I find I have to defend myself." He turned back to Cade. "Chief Cade, why don't we hash this out right now, on national television? Step up here with me and interrogate me publicly."

Another camera came on and swung around to Cade.

"I'm not here to interrogate you, Barr. I'm here to arrest you — and grandstanding on television isn't going to save you."

"Okay, look —" Vince chuckled — "I don't mind explaining myself right here and now. This is all because of the information I had about the telephone cord. As I told you, one of your own men leaked that to me, but I cannot reveal my sources. So arrest me if you must, but the viewers know you're coming after me because you can kill two birds with one stone. You need a scapegoat, and you can shut up the reporter."

Cade stood there, knowing the cameras were on him. He figured by now all of the news stations had live coverage of the scene. Vince was trying to make him look

stupid, figuring Cade would back off, not make the arrest.

But Vince had him all wrong.

Cade stepped up to the stage, into the lights, and went straight to the first camera. He pulled the plug that gave it power, and the red light died.

"Hey, you can't do that!"

"Watch." He walked to the other one and yanked it, too. The monitors went black, and then he saw the national anchors coming back on, commenting on what they'd just seen.

They were off the air.

"Arrest him," Cade said.

His men stepped onto the stage, fully armed, and surrounded the tabloid star. But Vince had no intention of going quietly. He bolted forward and knocked over the camera, leaped over it, and took off toward an exit door.

Cade had brought plenty of backup. "Freeze!" McCormick shouted, his gun aimed dead center.

Vince hesitated, then groped at the waistband of his pants just under his blazer.

"He's got a gun!" Cade yelled. "Drop it now, Barr!"

A camerawoman rushed in with a

camera on her shoulder, recording Vince's panic as he backed up with that gun. "You're making it worse," Cade shouted. "You're resisting arrest on live television."

The word *live* startled Vince, and he lowered his gun long enough to look back at the monitors. His own panicked, sweaty face stared back at him. The camerawoman moved closer . . . showing the world Vince Barr's pathetic attempt to save himself.

Suddenly he sprang forward, knocking the camera out of her hands and shoving the gun to her head.

"Get your men out of my way, or I'll blow her head off!"

80

The young woman Vince had taken hostage screamed out her horror as he dragged her across the floor. "Get back, all of you." He backed up with her, toward a door behind the lighted set. "I don't want to kill her."

"Vince, please," the woman cried. "Please, let me go."

"No! I'm taking you with me. If they make one wrong move, your blood will be on their hands."

"What do you think you're going to do?" Cade inched toward him. "You'll never get out of this building."

"Watch me."

Vince opened the door behind him and backed into the hallway. Cade followed him, his gun trained dead center. But the woman was in the way.

Barr kept backing up the hall, heading toward the exit door.

"Let me go, Vince!" the woman screamed. "I'm not your enemy!"

Cade came toward him. "Don't make it worse for yourself, Barr."

But the reporter had a look of crazed panic in his eyes. He wasn't going to surrender easily. "You're not going to make me tomorrow's headline!"

"You've already made yourself a part of this story," Cade said, "but if you let her go, if you cooperate with us . . ."

Barr got to the exit door and tried to open the door, but it was jammed. He looked around, his arm clamped across the woman's neck as he kept the gun on Cade.

Cade lowered his gun. "All right, let's slow down and take a deep breath," he said in a calming voice. "You don't have to do this, Barr. Maybe a judge will show you mercy if you stop resisting. Just let her go."

Vince tried shoving the exit door again. This time it fell open. He pulled the woman out into the daylight — and found himself staring at dozens of guns, pointed straight at him. Savannah police had arrived on the scene and had cordoned off the area.

"Hold your fire!" Cade shouted. "He's got a hostage."

Barr thought better of his decision to leave the building, and pulled the woman back inside. He looked around and saw a

staircase. Walking backward, he dragged the woman up the stairs, then backed into the stairwell, intent on escape.

Cade spoke softly into his radio. "Go up the other fire escape and cover every floor of the building."

He'd have no place to go except the roof. Where did he think he would go once he got there?

The woman screamed as her captor went further up, and McCormick and his men followed him, guns still drawn. Cade followed a few paces behind, his leg killing him as he made his way up four flights of stairs.

Barr got into daylight and dragged the fighting woman to the edge of the roof. McCormick stopped at the door, afraid to go further. "He's going to kill himself and take her with him."

"Oh, no, he's not." Cade pushed past him and went out on the roof. The woman's screams vibrated through his body. "Let her go, Vince! Come on, let her go. We don't need a third murder."

But Vince wasn't listening. He was teetering on the edge of the roof, looking down at what lay below him. Finally, he pulled his cell phone off of his belt and made a call.

"Send me the helicopter, now. I'm on the roof of Channel 3 — and hurry!"

Cade knew Barr had access to the *Observer*'s helicopter. But would they listen to him? Wouldn't they be keenly aware of what was going on?

Cade heard McCormick, still in the stairwell, making the radio call. "Get word to the *Observer* that any helicopter that touches down on this building will be fired upon."

"Vince, please let me go," the woman cried. "They'll come for you, and you'll be home free. Just let me go now."

"Shut up!"

He still stood dangerously close to the edge. Was he keeping open his option of jumping if the helicopter let him down?

Cade heard the sound of rudders overhead and saw the aircraft approaching. It had probably been en route even before Vince called, anxious to get the story as it moved outside the building.

Cade's hair blew wildly as the copter hovered overhead. McCormick and the others came out of the stairwell, some of their guns aimed high, and the others still trained on Barr.

"They're coming, Vince," the woman screamed. "Please, let me go now!"

Vince looked hopeful as the copter came closer, but it never got within gunshot range. Cade watched Vince's face as the man realized the *Observer* had not come to his rescue. Instead, they were filming his demise.

"No, you morons!" He raised his gun to fire on the helicopter.

Cade dove toward him, knocking the gun and the woman out of his hands and flinging him to the concrete. He screamed and struggled, but the other officers descended on him, fighting his arms behind him and grinding his chin into the roof.

Finally, Cade got off him and got up, jerking the man to his feet. Pulling his head back so that the helicopter's camera could get a good view, he said through his teeth, "Smile, Vince. Now you're really a star."

81

The calm after the storm left Cade feeling strangely empty and melancholy. If he'd thought the media circus was bad before Barr's arrest, it had been ridiculous since. They got footage of Cade's confrontation with Barr, then security tape that showed him dragging the woman through the building. Then from the helicopter they caught the drama on the roof. Every news station played the footage over and over, several times a day.

The story Vince Barr created had, indeed, made him famous.

Alan Sims was charged with medical fraud, then released on bond pending his trial. Meanwhile, the DA subpoenaed records from his office, and was building a rock-solid case that was sure to put Sims out of business and behind bars. Cade was finally able to let Ben go to finish grieving his wife's death.

And then there was Sam Sullivan.

Cade hadn't spoken to Blair since she'd written the piece about Sullivan in the paper, but the firestorm from that continued. The phone had rung off the hook since, mostly from local reporters who wanted Cade to confirm that Sullivan had confessed to fraud. He'd heard that Ben Jackson had filed a lawsuit against the mayor-elect. He hoped Sam got what he deserved.

He knew that the solving of the murder probably meant the end of his job. Any day now Sam would ask for Cade's resignation and put some yes-man in to replace him. He supposed it was inevitable. Though public opinion had shifted against the mayor-elect, he supposed he still had the power to take away Cade's position.

McCormick sat in his office now, helping him sort through all the papers on his desk. "Best I can figure, Chief, Barr killed Lisa in her own home. Must have been waiting for her there after she confronted Sims. Killed her right there with her own telephone cord. Piled her body into the car, grabbed a pair of Ben's shoes and his baseball cap, drove her to the river, not drawing anybody's attention, and pushed her car into the river. Must have put the shoes back in the house after the crime."

"We need to run the cap that was in the car through forensics. Maybe there's a hair or something —"

"Doubtful, Cade. It was underwater, remember."

"You never know. Doesn't matter, though. We've got enough to nail him. The DA says it's cut and dried. I guess the rumor Sam Sullivan started was what gave Barr the idea. The mayoral candidate who murders his wife for his mistress. Made a great story."

McCormick grinned. "We did it again, man. We're good."

Cade laughed for the first time in days.

"Hey, Chief, Art Russell from the City Council is on the phone." Cade looked up at Alex Johnson, leaning in his doorway. "Wants to talk to you."

"Well, here it comes." Cade grabbed a bottle of Tylenol out of his desk drawer. Pouring two pills into his hand, he shot McCormick a look.

"He said it was urgent."

"Yeah, I'll bet." Cade swallowed the pills and bottomed the glass of water on his desk. Finally, he picked up the phone. "Yeah, Art. What is it?"

"Cade, there's been a new development

at City Hall, and I wanted you to be the first to know."

Cade closed his eyes. "All right."

"Sam Sullivan resigned this morning."

"He *what?*"

"Came in and resigned. He really had no choice. The phone has been ringing off the hook ever since Blair's article came out about him. Everywhere he went, he faced attacks about what he'd done. There was no way he could be effective as mayor under the circumstances."

Cade put his hand over the phone and told McCormick. McCormick started to laugh. Cade held up a hand to quiet him, so McCormick rushed out to tell the others. "So what happens now?"

"We may have to call another election, but we've got Judge Evers looking at things, trying to decide what the proper course of action will be. We hope he'll rule sometime today."

Cade thanked him for the information, then hung up and stared at the phone. Maybe his job was going to be saved, after all.

The phone rang again, and McCormick stuck his head back in. "Chief, I know you don't want to be bothered again, but it's FOX News."

Cade groaned. He wasn't in the mood to make a statement, but he supposed they needed information about the murderer-reporter they had helped make a hero. He picked up the phone. "Chief Cade."

"Chief, this is Mike Lassiter from FOX News. We wondered if we could get you to come on this afternoon and talk about Vince Barr."

"I don't think so. I'll give you a statement on the phone, but that's it."

The reporter grunted. "What is it with you people? We tried to get Blair Owens earlier, but she refused, too. You know, it served Chief Moose of Virginia well to come on our network when he solved the sniper case. Now he has a huge book deal, and there are rumors of a movie."

Blair had turned them down? When she'd had the chance to go on FOX News and comment on the story, she'd declined?

He leaned forward, setting his elbows on his desk. Why hadn't she seized that opportunity to build up her subscriber base?

"Chief? Did you hear me?"

"Yeah, I heard you. I'm not looking for a book or movie deal, Lassiter. I just did my job."

"All right, then we'll have to make do with the phone interview. Chief Cade, tell

us how you learned that Vince Barr was the actual murderer in the Jackson case."

Cade told him about the interview their network had done with Vince, in which he'd mentioned the telephone cord. He explained how the media had played into the man's hands, aiding and abetting as he'd built himself into a media star, using the simple avenue of murder.

When he'd said all he was going to say and the man had stopped recording, he leaned back wearily in his chair. "So you say Blair refused to talk to you? Did she say why?"

Lassiter sounded amused. "She said she was too busy, but I'm guessing it was because of her scars. Who could blame her, really? She doesn't exactly have a face for television."

White-hot anger whipped through him at the remark, and he ground his teeth and thought of telling the man that he wouldn't know beauty if it bit his nose off, because if he had the slightest taste he'd realize that Blair Owens was the most beautiful woman in the entire state, and she didn't need some screaming news show to elevate her self-esteem.

Instead, he slammed down the phone. How dare he say that about her? Cade

hoped Lassiter hadn't said those things to her face. She didn't deserve that.

He thought of all the things he'd said to her himself, when he'd chewed her out about her special edition that had wound up saving the day.

And he realized that solving the murders and closing the case meant little to him, after all, if he didn't have Blair to share it with.

82

Morgan felt a little shaky when she came back to herself after the laparoscopy. She had been awake through the whole procedure, but couldn't remember a moment of it. The hypnotic drug they gave her in the place of anesthesia had an amnesiac effect.

Jonathan helped her get dressed, and they waited for the results.

Dr. Anderson looked sober as he came into the room. "How you feeling?"

"Fine." She clutched Jonathan's hand. "Did you find anything, Doctor?"

His smile was tentative. "As a matter of fact, I did. Morgan, the results of all of your tests — including your FSH — were normal. I'm afraid it was as we thought. Dr. Sims falsified the results he gave you."

Morgan caught her breath. "But if that's true, what caused my miscarriage? My infertility?"

Dr. Anderson's eyes had a pleasant twinkle as he regarded her. "It may be due

to the small fibroids I found in your uterus."

"Fibroids?" Jonathan asked. "Tumors, you mean?"

"Benign tumors."

Morgan got tears in her eyes. It was structural, then. Physical.

"I'd like to schedule you for a procedure called a hysteroscopy. We can do it next week, if you'd like. We'll go in and remove the fibroids with lasers. I can't promise that this will solve your fertility problem, but the chances are very good that it will. It's worked for quite a few of my patients."

Morgan stared at him for a moment, letting the hope sink in. "Really, Doctor?"

Jonathan wanted to make sure he understood. "Are you telling us that this could be resolved in one minor surgical procedure? That after that, we might be able to have a family without problems?"

"Again, I can't guarantee anything, but that's my hope."

Morgan started to laugh and threw her arms around Jonathan. And the bright light of joy began to shine on their lives again.

That afternoon, Morgan came home to an early dinner cooked by the residents of

Hanover House. Even Sheila had helped.

Sheila attended to Caleb over dinner. He had warmed up to her now, and sent her frequent smiles and giggles. The mother–son bond was renewing itself. It was a miracle of grace to Sheila, and as difficult as it was for Morgan, she found herself happy for Caleb.

When Blair burst in, everyone stopped what they were doing.

"I was just at the courthouse! The judge made his decision about the mayoral race!"

Jonathan groaned. "Don't tell me, let me guess. He's going to put us through another election."

"Wrong!" Blair crossed the room, took hold of his shoulders, and looked him squarely in the face. "Congratulations, Jonathan. You're the new mayor."

Morgan's mouth fell open, and she gaped at Jonathan. He stared at Blair as if he didn't believe. "But . . . how can that be? Sam was elected. I wasn't."

"The judge cited the city's bylaws, which say that if something happens to a candidate-elect to keep him from serving, a new election would be held, *unless* another candidate had gotten at least forty-five percent of the votes. In that case, that candidate

would win the race. Jonathan, you got forty-six percent!"

The residents sent up a loud cheer, whooping and hollering and congratulating the new mayor. Even Caleb joined in the celebration.

83

There was so much to celebrate, yet Blair found herself wanting to be alone later that evening. She left Hanover House as everyone fluttered into action preparing for Karen and Gus's wedding on Saturday. Church members filled the house to help decorate, insisting that Morgan not lift a finger after her procedure that morning. Karen seemed to walk on a cloud.

Blair wondered if that day would ever come for her.

The sun was dropping over the horizon, but it would still be light for a couple more hours. What was Cade doing? Was he floating in the aftermath of solving the murder? Had he heard that Jonathan was going to be his new boss?

Was he still nursing his anger toward her?

She went to the boathouse and fired up the boat. She hadn't used it in quite a while. They'd used it as a ski boat during

her teenage years, but mostly her father used it for fishing. Jonathan kept the motor well maintained, so it started right up. She guided it down river, out toward the sea, and headed through the waves to Breaker's Reef. It was one of her favorite places on earth — a cavern you had to dive underwater to get into. The payoff was inside, glorious in its beauty. Her father used to love anchoring his boat there and enjoying the quiet — and the occasional glimpse of a sea turtle — when he needed to think or pray. He used to bring her here sometimes to fish, and they would sit for hours in perfect stillness, listening to the whisper of the breeze stirring up frothy waves that hit the rocks of the cave. Sometimes he would forget she was there — or maybe he hadn't forgotten at all — and would talk aloud to Jesus, as if he sat in the boat with them. She hadn't recognized the value of that then, but now, as she looked out over the brilliant horizon, she knew it was true. Jesus had a thing for boats, after all.

Her boat rocked in the water as she looked up at the setting sun, its red-gold hues bursting across the water. It was glorious, like the grace God had bestowed on her ever since she had given her heart to

Christ. She had no right to ask for anything else.

Still, she did.

"I never expected to have somebody fall in love with me," she whispered. "A girl like me with her face all disfigured, is happy just to live a normal life without people gawking and staring wherever she goes. But then Cade came along . . . and I guess I got my hopes up."

Tears came to her eyes and she blinked them back.

It wasn't just Carson Graham who had buoyed her hopes. She had hoped it before Graham uttered his predictions. That's why she wanted to believe him.

"I thought maybe you were behind this. After all, it was a miracle that Cade would even look twice at me. An act of God. But maybe I jumped the gun just a little."

She drew in a deep breath and closed her eyes. The breeze blew her tears dry. "I'll try to be okay with him not being my long-lost love, the future father of my children, the one I grow old with, if you'll just let him be my friend. Everyone who knows Cade is blessed to be his friend."

The tears came harder then, and she realized that friendship wasn't going to be enough. Not for her. The pain that would

cause would be so deep that she didn't know if she could stay in town to endure it. Maybe she would have to leave, after all. Maybe she could sell the paper, start over somewhere else . . .

Then she heard a motor on the wind.

She turned, shaded her eyes, and saw another boat in the distance, coming toward her. As it moved closer, she realized it was Cade in the department's speedboat. Her heart burst.

He slowed and came to her boat, stopping beside her. "I figured you'd be here."

She hadn't seen him out of uniform since the night they'd gone to Carson's show. Now he wore a yellow tank top and a pair of navy shorts. He looked younger in the waning sunlight, more relaxed and at ease. But his face held a trace of tension.

"Jonathan said you were taking the boat out," he said. "Can I come on board?"

"Of course."

She watched him tie their boats together, and then he climbed over, careful not to bump his leg. The scar down his flesh was healing, but it would forever remind her of how close he'd come to death, not so long ago.

As he stepped into her boat, hope fired in her heart like a fourth of July display.

He stood there looking at her, the boat rocking beneath his feet. Her heart constricted her throat as she waited for him to speak. Instead, he reached out, slid his fingers through the roots of her hair and pulled her into a kiss.

She melted into it, realizing that God had answered a prayer she wasn't even confident enough to pray. The kiss said things they'd never uttered, made promises they'd never made. Could it be that it wasn't over?

He pulled back, breathless, and touched those flaming scars as if he didn't even see them. His eyes were misty as he gazed down at her. "I'm sorry I yelled at you," he whispered. "Can you forgive me?"

She tried to blink back the tears in her eyes. It was stupid to cry right here in front of him like this. He would think she was some sappy heartsick teenager. But the mist in his own eyes was glistening. Did he feel the same way?

"Of course I forgive you."

"I had no right to jump on you like that. You saved the day. Instead of fighting with you, I should have trusted you. We've always made a great team before."

"We have, haven't we?"

His eyes were soft as he gazed into hers.

"I'm tired of this surface dating game, Blair. I'm ready to put my cards on the table. The truth is, I think of you constantly. I want to be with you all the time, even when I'm mad at you. I want to assume that you're my girl, and that this is going somewhere."

She swallowed and breathed in a sob. "I want that, too."

"And the town, they'll know we're an item. They'll rib us, tease us, even try to marry us off before we're ready."

She grinned as a tear rolled down her cheek. "I'm tough, remember? I can take it."

He kissed her again, and she melted in his arms, thinking that if she fell over into the ocean and died right then, she would have had almost everything she'd ever wanted.

He broke the kiss and held her against his chest, his breath gentle against her ear. "I'm taking you to dinner tonight, and I'm going to hold your hand in public and let everyone know that I'm in love."

Her heart burst with the sheer grace of it. She started to cry so hard that she could hardly get the words out. "I love you, too."

She kept her head against his chest and watched as the sun melted into the water,

sending a twilight of gold that beckoned the night.

It was like a smile from God.

Afterword

At this writing I've been crafting novels for over twenty years. People often ask me where I get my ideas, and I always tell them that my gift consists of a fertile imagination and an ability to see and hear things around me that others may miss. Like most other writers, I get ideas when I least expect them, then I "what-if" my way to a complete plot.

But it doesn't stop with those ideas. Writing a novel is a lengthy, meticulous process that might never end if it weren't for deadlines that force me to turn the book in. Though I've written a number of books over my career, I can tell you that each one is harder than the one before. And the work never gets easier.

I write each book several times over, printing out copies and writing all over it like a bitter teacher who finds fault with every essay her student turns in. I'm brutal with my own work, and never satisfied, and I spend sleepless nights worrying over plot

twists and wondering if the story is too predictable or too boring. My mind wanders when I'm in places where it shouldn't as I work through problems and conversations and character interactions.

When I finally turn it in, I practically throw it into the mailbox and run away before I can change my mind. Once it's gone, I sweat until I hear from my publishers that they like it. But their praise is always tempered with criticism, and so — armed with their feedback — I tear into the book again, striving to take it to another level, to polish yet again, examining every plot device to see if it truly is the best I can do.

By the time it reaches publication, I practically have the work memorized. I know if one word has been changed in editorial, if one comma has been moved, if one apostrophe has been edited. And for all of my jealous protection of my work and my pursuit of excellence in my writing, I sometimes wind up with mistakes. I'm not the best writer around, nor am I the cleverest. I do the best I can, within the bounds of my own skill.

So why am I telling you this?

Because God is an author, too. He is the author of the most important, bestselling book of all time. And I believe that he is

even more careful with his work than I am with mine.

With the advent of cable television, the world is bombarded with documentaries regarding the authenticity of the Bible, whether it's fiction or fact, whether all of it is true or just some of it. People make a smorgasbord out of God's Word and choose which things to believe — a little here, a little there. They decide that some of it — the parts they like — are inspired by God, and that the rest is written by flawed men and compiled by corrupt committees with their own selfish agendas.

In making those claims, they are saying that God is not powerful, that he doesn't care enough about us to watch over his Word, that he doesn't care if we're confused or lied to or misled. That he didn't even strive for as much excellence as I strive for in my work. That it's okay with him if it isn't quite right, because the basic gist of what he was trying to say lies within those pages. That the musings of David and the instructions of Paul and the history of Moses are all just myth and entertainment.

Proverbs 14:12 says, "There is a way that seems right to man, that in the end leads to destruction."

I believe the Bible is true, every word of it — so far as it's translated accurately. I believe our Lord chose every word with great care and precision, and that each verse holds layer upon layer of meaning, truths so deep it would take us a lifetime to mine them — and still we wouldn't have seen it all.

I believe God gave us his Word because of his great love for us and his desire to help us know him better. And I think he also cares about our entertainment. He gave us minds that like to puzzle, uncover, discover things we haven't seen before. The Bible is available to every level of intellect — it can be as meaningful to the mathematical genius as it is to the little child. It is full of connections, threads that tie one thing to another, prophecies made and revisited (many, many of which have already come true), and signs all along the way that point to Jesus. From Creation itself, to the sacrificial system, to the Law and the covenants, the Cross, and the description of the final days of earth and our entrance into heaven, the Bible has a running theme of God's sovereignty, his love for those who break his heart, and his plan for our redemption even though we don't deserve it.

"All Scripture is God-breathed and is useful for teaching, rebuking, correcting and training in righteousness, so that the man of God may be thoroughly equipped for every good work" (2 Timothy 3:16–17).

We can choose to discount it if we want, pick and choose the parts we'll believe, or even ignore it entirely so that it doesn't interfere with our lives, but our denial doesn't make it less true. The consequence of being wrong is destruction.

My prayer for my books is that God will use them to whisper truth into your ear, and stir your soul to a longing for him and his Word. I pray that the next book you open will be the one he wrote for you.

Then you will be richly blessed, and I will have succeeded.

May the God of peace, who through the blood of the eternal covenant brought back from the dead our Lord Jesus, that great Shepherd of the sheep, equip you with every good thing for doing his will, and may he work in us what is pleasing to him, through Jesus Christ, to whom be glory for ever and ever. Amen.

Hebrews 13:20–21